Accession no

D1626141

M. Memet Özek · Giuseppe Cinalli · Wirginia J. Maixner

The Spina Bifida
Management and Outcome

Forewords by
C. Sainte-Rose
C. di Rocco

Preface by
M. Necmettin Pamir

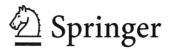
Springer

M. MEMET ÖZEK
Division of Paediatric Neurosurgery
Marmara University Medical Center and
Department of Neurosurgery
Acıbadem University
School of Medicine
Istanbul, Turkey

GIUSEPPE CINALLI
Department of Paediatric Neurosurgery
Santobono-Pausilipon Children's Hospital
Naples, Italy

WIRGINIA J. MAIXNER
Department of Paediatric Neurosurgery
Royal Children's Hospital
Parkville, Australia

Library of Congress Control Number: 2008926860

ISBN 978-88-470-0650-8 Springer Milan Berlin Heidelberg New York
e-ISBN 978-88-470-0651-5

Springer is a part of Springer Science+Business Media
springer.com
© Springer-Verlag Italia 2008

Cover design: Simona Colombo, Milan, Italy
Typesetting: C & G di Cerri e Galassi, Cremona, Italy
Printing and binding: Printer Trento S.r.l., Italy

Printed in Italy
Springer-Verlag Italia S.r.l., Via Decembrio 28, I-20137 Milan, Italy

Foreword

By C. Sainte-Rose

As we stand at the dawn of the 21st century, one may ponder the rationale of writing a book on spina bifida. Once commonplace in European countries prior to the era of ultrasonography, this disease became increasingly rare in developed countries as a result of improvements in antenatal diagnosis, to the point that we believed it to be disappearing. Knowledge of spina bifida and of its treatment, once so richly diffused only 30 years ago, began to fade. Young neurosurgeons who had never seen such a malformation at its initial presentation were hesitant, and did not understand the protean clinical signs of these patients presenting to the emergency department or outpatient clinics. This situation, however, did not last for long. As a consequence of the political and economic events of the final years of the 20th century, the advent of globalisation, and the significant desire for immigration, we realised that spina bifida had not disappeared at all in the rest of the world. Migration was, and is, bringing it back onto our doorstep, to our everyday clinical and surgical practice. It is important therefore, not to lose the knowledge gained by our masters, to try and assemble it in one place in order to understand the disease from its inception in utero through until adulthood and the reproductive age.

The chronology of the book, in reflection of this aim, is well organised, and ranges from history and embryology, to prenatal diagnosis and treatment, perinatal care, initial treatment and management, and middle- and long-term complications, and finally provides insights for the future. The authors, by not merely focusing on the neurosurgical issues but also on the urologic and orthopaedic consequences of this malformation, have allowed for a more global approach to these patients.

Through a greater understanding of the disease, through the improved quality of initial care, and through the dedication of the surgeons and physicians who manage these children from infancy into adulthood, children inflicted with spina bifida, whilst heavily burdened, may nevertheless lead happy and full lives.

Paris, May 2008

Christian Sainte-Rose
Department of Neurosurgery
Hospital Necker-Enfants Malades
Paris, France

Foreword

By C. di Rocco

Spina bifida refers to a cohort of pathological conditions that vary in severity from the dramatic and life-threatening myelomeningoceles to relatively mild defects such as dermal sinuses. This book aims to cover the whole spectrum although, as expected, most of its content is devoted to the management of myelomeningocele. With regard to this last type of malformation, the treatment of very few diseases in the history of medicine has been characterized by such an intimate relationship between scientific and technical problems and ethical and social considerations. Myelomeningocele is one of a very few congenital malformations that require the neurosurgeon and parents to face the fundamental dilemma of whether to promote survival, at a very high cost, or to deny treatment in the belief that it is better to prevent the newborn suffering unacceptable and lifelong physical and emotional suffering. It is unusual as it has been associated with such mutually exclusive therapeutic approaches – from treatment refusal to the use of sophisticated surgical and rehabilitative care. The management of the disease has been marked by oscillations between hope and dejection, despair and jubilation. These opposing emotions are also likely to affect the individual surgeon in his/her professional life, with cases of early success turning to late failures and, conversely, cases of satisfactory lives with rich social interaction following initially poor prognoses.

Before the 1960s, in common with other children with hydrocephalus, newborns with myelomeningocele had little hope of survival. Indeed, most of the affected subjects died from the uncontrolled progression of the associated ventricular dilation; death also resulted from sepsis, meningitis, and renal failure. The same secondary complications accounted for the extremely serious disabilities that blighted survivors' lives, in addition to the congenital neurological, orthopedic, and urologic deficits. It is not surprising, therefore, that at the beginning of the 1970s Lorber commented pessimistically on a series of patients followed in the previous decade. He considered that only 7% of the survivors had acceptable disabilities, while the majority of them "had a quality of life inconsistent with self-respect, learning capacity, happiness, and even marriage". A generation of pediatricians as well as the public opinion of the time was deeply influenced by the so-called "Lorber's selection criteria". Macrocrania, severe paraplegia, severe kyphosis or scoliosis, the presence of concomitant significant congenital anomalies, or the history of birth damage were all regarded as criteria for excluding any active treatment for myelodysplasic newborns. The echo of this negative attitude can also be found in more recent experiences, as demonstrated by the "Baby Jane Doe" case at the beginning of the 1980s, and by the "Baby Rianne" case in 1993. In this context, the protocol approved by the Dutch Association of Paediatrics in 2005, known as the Groningen protocol, on deliberate life termination for newborns with severe forms of spina bifida, is even more significant.

On the other hand, although these years were dominated by this negative attitude in most centres, some neurosurgical departments produced results that were much more optimistic. In a small number of neurosurgical centres, series of surgical unselected patients were managed with more advanced techniques and a multidisciplinary approach. The results unequivocally demonstrated that most of the children operated on could reach normal levels of intellectual ability, and that even individuals with severe myelomeningoceles could, after this treatment, lead meaningful lives.

These patients benefited from the surgical advances made in assuring a more effective closure of the back defect. They also had the advantage of improved control of the impaired cerebrospinal fluid (CSF) dynamics by means of more reliable CSF shunting apparatus, and, recently, endoscopy, early recognition and treatment of complications such as Chiari type II malformation or syringomyelia, and prevention and early treatment of spinal cord retethering. They gained further benefit from timely orthopedic correction for club feet, scoliosis, or kyphosis, as well as adequate prevention of damage to urological function. Furthermore, they also received strong support for reaching independence and social integration from the development of ad hoc rehabilitation and educational programs, which were additionally promoted by the establishment of myelomeningocele clinics; more generally, they also benefited from the combined efforts of multidisciplinary teams assisted by a more sympathetic public opinion.

The spirit that has inspired multidisciplinary myelomeningocele teams over the last two decades can be found in this multiauthored volume devoted to the management of spina bifida. The book conveys all the best information currently available in the field, and integrates the most specialized knowledge, from the basic sciences to the various surgical, medical, and psychosocial skills, in a unique well-organized source of information .

As a result of understanding the role of alpha-feto-protein in preventing spina bifida, and the introduction of routine prenatal ultrasound diagnosis, the number of children born with myelomeningocele is continuously decreasing in many western countries. This phenomenon is likely to result in a decreased interest in the management of spina bifida and there will almost certainly be fewer specialized scientific contributions. Consequently, the experience accrued over recent years faces the risk of not being sufficiently updated. Spina bifida, however, still continues to represent an important problem in several countries where preventive measures have not yet been adopted. In these countries, the need for specialized knowledge will persist for the foreseeable future. The present book then may cover an impending gap by helping to preserve the body of relevant scientific knowledge and expertise acquired over the last three decades in a society that may not have so much need of it in future years. By transmitting this skill and knowledge to countries that need it the book will help these countries to avoid retracing the false steps that in the past prevented many children with spina bifida from reaching the best possible outcomes.

Rome, May 2008

Concezio Di Rocco
Pediatric Neurosurgery
Catholic University Medical School
Rome, Italy

Preface

By M. Necmettin Pamir

This book presents the current understanding, diagnosis and treatment of spina bifida and related pathologies to the neurosurgical literature.

The book has two important qualities: first of all it provides a thorough analysis of the historical experience in the field, and secondly it presents to the reader the most up-to date conclusions, standards, and trends. Although this disease has been known to mankind since antiquity, the treatment is still not straightforward and experts still disagree on various fields. The discussion of modern diagnostic technologies, treatment modalities, and complications, presented in 39 chapters, will guide the reader to tailor an optimal treatment strategy to their patients. The book covers a wide range of topics in the field, starting from preventive measures and progressing to issues like the social adaptation of the patients. The extremely detailed nature of each chapter will be easily appreciated by the reader, whether this is the neurosurgeon, pediatrician, pediatric neurologist, pathologist, neuroradiologist, or any other professional who is involved in the diagnosis or treatment. Therefore, the reader will find answers to almost all his questions on spina bifida and related pathologies in this book. In this regard, it is a significant contribution to the medical literature.

I take great pleasure in congratulating the editors, Professor Özek, Professor Cinalli and Professor Maixner for the quality of the book and for their superb and unique work. It is an honor for me to introduce this excellent book to neurosurgical literature.

Istanbul, May 2008

M. Necmettin Pamir
Department of Neurosurgery
Acıbadem University
School of Medicine
Istanbul, Turkey

Preface

By the Editors

Spina bifida has been an issue of concern for thousands of years. The treatment for this malady begins at birth, or in some cases even before birth, and continues throughout the patients' lives. Over years of investigations and studies in our spina bifida outpatient clinics, we have come to realize the importance of understanding and preparing for the long-term difficulties awaiting our patients. As we are aware that the treatment is multidisciplinary, it is no surprise that the spark of an idea for a spina bifida book was generated during meetings between members of the subspecialties in our spina bifida team. With this inspiration, the decision was shaped further and finalized during the 2006 ESPN meeting in Martinique.

With the aim of promoting the academic success of our book, deciding on the authors for the specific chapters and depending on their expertise was of utmost importance. For this reason, we would like to acknowledge the invaluable contribution of all our authors. We express our heartfelt gratitude to Springer-Verlag Italy, and particularly Dr. Donatella Rizza and the whole editorial team for their skilfulness and tolerance. Lastly, we would like to sincerely thank our patients and their families from whose endurance we get all our clinical experience.

May 2008

M. Memet Özek
Giuseppe Cinalli
Wirginia J. Maixner

Table of Contents

List of Contributors

CARLOS G. ALMODIN
Department of Fetal Medicine
Federal University of São Paulo
São Paulo, Brazil

GIULIANA C. ANTOLOVICH
Department of Developmental Medicine
Royal Children's Hospital Melbourne
Parkville, Australia

STUART BAUER
Department of Urology
Boston Children's Hospital
Harvard Medical School
Boston, MA, USA

NIGAR BAYKAN
Division of Neuroanesthesiology
Acıbadem University
School of Medicine
Hospital for Neurological Sciences
Istanbul, Turkey

RICHARD BEAUCHAMP
Department of Orthopedics
University of British Columbia and
British Columbia's Children's Hospital
Vancouver, BC, Canada

MUHITTIN BELIRGEN
Division of Pediatric Neurosurgery
Marmara University Medical Center
Istanbul, Turkey

LIAT BEN SIRA
Department of Pediatric Neurosurgery
Dana Children's Hospital
Tel-Aviv Sourasky Medical Center
Tel-Aviv, Israel

LIANA BENI-ADANI
Department of Pediatric Neurosurgery
Dana Children's Hospital
Tel-Aviv Sourasky Medical Center
Tel-Aviv, Israel

ABDULLAH BEREKET
Division of Pediatric Endocrinology
Department of Pediatrics
Marmara University Medical Center
Istanbul, Turkey

ROBIN M. BOWMAN
Department of Neurosurgery
Children's Memorial Hospital
Northwestern University
Feinberg School of Medicine
Chicago, IL, USA

MARIA CONSIGLIO BUONOCORE
Department of Neuroradiology
Santobono-Pausilipon Children's Hospital
Naples, Italy

MASSIMO CALDARELLI
Department of Pediatric Neurosurgery
and Centre for Spina Bifida
Catholic University Medical School
Rome, Italy

BANU CANKAYA
Department of Psychiatry
University of Rochester Medical Center
Rochester, NY, USA

MARTIN CATALA
UMR Paris 6/CNRS Biologie du
Développement
Paris, France

SERGIO CAVALHEIRO
Department of Neurology and Neurosurgery
Federal University of São Paulo
São Paulo, Brazil

EMILIO CIANCIULLI
Department of Neuroradiology
Santobono-Pausilipon Children's Hospital
Naples, Italy

GIUSEPPE CINALLI
Department of Paediatric Neurosurgery
Santobono-Pausilipon Children's Hospital
Naples, Italy

DAVID D. COCHRANE
Division of Neurosurgery
Department of Surgery
University of British Columbia and
British Columbia's Children's Hospital
Vancouver, BC, Canada

SHLOMI CONSTANTINI
Department of Pediatric Neurosurgery
Dana Children's Hospital
Tel-Aviv Sourasky Medical Center
Tel-Aviv, Israel

ANN DE VYLDER
Department of Urology
Jeroen Bosch Hospital's
Hertogenbosch, The Netherlands

PATRICK DHELLEMMES
Department of Pediatric Neurosurgery
University Hospital
Lille, France

CONCEZIO DI ROCCO
Department of Pediatric Neurosurgery and
Centre for Spina Bifida
Catholic University Medical School
Rome, Italy

BÜLENT EROL
Department of Orthopaedics and
Traumatology
Marmara University Medical Center
Istanbul, Turkey

ANTONIO FERNANDES MORON
Department of Fetal Medicine
Federal University of São Paulo
São Paulo, Brazil

JAMES L. FRAZIER
Department of Neurosurgery
Johns Hopkins University
Baltimore, MD, USA

JAMES T. GOODRICH
Division of Pediatric Neurosurgery
Plastic Surgery and Pediatrics
Children's Hospital at Montefiore
Montefiore Medical Center
Albert Einstein College of Medicine
Bronx, NY, USA

WAGNER J. HISABA
Department of Fetal Medicine
Federal University of São Paulo
São Paulo, Brazil

UĞUR IŞIK
Section of Pediatric Epileptology and
Video-EEG Lab
Acıbadem University
School of Medicine
Hospital for Neurological Sciences
Istanbul, Turkey

GEORGE I. JALLO
Division of Pediatric Neurosurgery
Johns Hopkins Hospital
Baltimore, MD, USA

VIVEK JOSAN
Department of Paediatric Neurosurgery
Royal Children's Hospital
Parkville, Australia

JOON-KI KANG
Department of Neurosurgery
Catholic University Medical College
Kangnam St. Peter's Hospital
Seoul, Korea

CAROL KING
Spinal Cord Clinic
British Columbia's Children's Hospital
Vancouver, BC, Canada

MEHMET KEMAL KUŞCU
Department of Psychiatry Family and
Community Mental Health Unit
Marmara University Medical Center
Istanbul, Turkey

ANDREW MacNEILY
Department of Urology
University of British Columbia and
British Columbia's Children's Hospital
Vancouver, BC, Canada

WIRGINIA J. MAIXNER
Department of Paediatric Neurosurgery
Royal Children's Hospital
Parkville, Australia

DAVID G. McLONE
Department of Pediatric Neurosurgery
Spina Bifida Center
Children's Memorial Hospital
Department of Neurological Surgery
Northwestern University
Feinberg School of Medicine
Chicago, IL, USA

ELKA MILLER
Hospital for Sick Children and
University of Toronto
Ontario, Canada

ANDREW MOROKOFF
Department of Paediatric Neurosurgery
Children's Neuroscience Centre
Royal Children's Hospital
Parkville, Australia

TOBA NIAZI
Department of Neurological Surgery
University of Utah
Division of Pediatric Neurosurgery
Primary Children's Medical Center
Salt Lake City, UT, USA

EREN ÖZEK
Division of Neonatology
Marmara University Medical Center
Istanbul, Turkey

M. MEMET ÖZEK
Division of Pediatric Neurosurgery
Marmara University Medical Center and
Department of Neurosurgery
Acıbadem University
School of Medicine
Istanbul, Turkey

DARIO PALADINI
Fetal Medicine Unit
Department of Obstetrics and Gynecology
University Federico II
Naples, Italy

DAVID PHILLIPS
Orthotic Innovations
Surrey Hills, Australia

ALAIN PIERRE-KAHN
Department of Pediatric Neurosurgery
Hospital Necker-Enfants Malades
Paris, France

CHARLES RAYBAUD
Hospital for Sick Children and
University of Toronto
Ontario, Canada

HAROLD L. REKATE
Pediatric Neurosciences
Barrow Neurologic Institute
Phoenix, AZ, USA
Department of Surgery
Section of Neurosurgery
University of Arizona School
of Medicine
Tucson, AZ, USA

BENEDICT RILLIET
Service de Neurochirurgie Geneve and
Lausanne
Hôpital Cantonal Universitaire
Geneve, Switzerland

JONATHAN ROTH
Department of Pediatric Neurosurgery
Dana Children's Hospital
Tel-Aviv Sourasky Medical Center
Tel-Aviv, Israel

THOMAS ROUJEAU
Department of Pediatric Neurosurgery
Hospital Necker-Enfants Malades
Paris, France

HELIO RUBENS MACHADO
Division of Pediatric Neurosurgery
Department of Surgery and Anatomy
Ribeirão Preto School of Medicine
University of São Paulo
São Paulo, Brazil

CHRISTIAN SAINTE-ROSE
Department of Neurosurgery
Hospital Necker-Enfants Malades
Paris, France

RICARDO SANTOS DE OLIVEIRA
Division of Pediatric Neurosurgery
Department of Surgery and Anatomy
Ribeirão Preto School of Medicine
University of São Paulo
São Paulo, Brazil

AYDIN SAV
Department of Pathology and
Division of Neuropathology
Marmara University Medical Center
Istanbul, Turkey

LUCIANO SAVARESE
Department of Pediatric Neurosurgery
Santobono-Pausilipon Children's Hospital
Naples, Italy

SPYROS SGOUROS
Institute of Child Health and
Department of Neurosurgery
Birmingham Children's Hospital
Birmingham, UK
Department of Neurosurgery
University of Athens
Athens, Greece

ROGER F. SOLL
Division of Neonatal Perinatal Medicine
University of Vermont College of
Medicine
Burlington, VT, USA

PIETRO SPENNATO
Department of Pediatric Neurosurgery
Santobono-Pausilipon Children's Hospital
Naples, Italy

DAVID A. STAFFENBERG
Division of Plastic and
Reconstructive Surgery
Children's Hospital at Montefiore
Montefiore Medical Center
Department of Clinical Plastic Surgery
Neurosurgery and Pediatrics
Albert Einstein College of Medicine
Bronx, NY, USA

JUNICHI TAMAI
Department of Orthopaedic Surgery
Cincinnati Children's Hospital Medical
Center
Cincinnati, OH, USA

TUFAN TARCAN
Department of Urology
Marmara University Medical Center
Istanbul, Turkey

MATTHIEU VINCHON
Department of Pediatric Neurosurgery
University Hospital
Lille, France

SHARON VLADUSIC
Department of Orthopaedics
Royal Children's Hospital
Melbourne, Australia

MARION L. WALKER
Department of Neurological Surgery
University of Utah
Division of Pediatric Neurosurgery
Primary Children's Medical Center
Salt Lake City, UT, USA

BENJAMIN WARF
Department of Neurosurgery
A.I. Dupont Hospital for Children
Wilmington, DE, USA

ALISON C. WRAY
Children's Neuroscience Centre
Royal Children's Hospital Melbourne
Parkville, Australia

BO XIAO
Department of Pediatric Neurosurgery
Dana Children's Hospital
Tel-Aviv Sourasky Medical Center
Tel-Aviv, Israel

MICHEL ZERAH
Department of Neurosurgery
Hospital Necker-Enfants Malades
Paris, France

Section I
GENERAL CONSIDERATIONS

CHAPTER 1
A Historical Review of the Surgical Treatment of Spina Bifida

James T. Goodrich

Spina Bifida in Antiquity

Spina bifida or spinal dysraphisms have been present as long as man has walked the planet. A number of anthropological excavations have uncovered spines with stigmata typically seen in infants born with myelomeningoceles. As these children were born in an era where little or no treatment was available we can only assume that most did not survive. Having said that, there are a large number of surviving anthropological figures sculpted in stone, terracotta and other materials from early civilizations. These sculptures provide evidence of individuals who

survived with what would be a normally devastating disease. Over the years the author has collected a number of terracotta figures from the Americas that show clear evidence of surviving children with stigmata of spinal dysraphism. These figures are seated in the typical position of a paraplegic child or adult with the typical lumbar kyphosis. Some of the figures have been incorrectly described as patients with tuberculosis or Pott's disease. A careful examination of these figures clearly shows the physical characteristics of individuals with chronic myelomeningocele. We have included several examples that come from Meso-American cultures where figures of this type are not at all uncommon (Figs. 1.1-1.5).

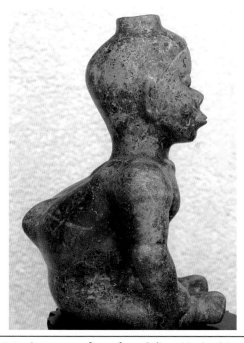

Fig. 1.1. A terracotta figure from Colima, Mexico (circa 200 A.D.), revealing findings classic for a child or adult with a spinal dysraphism. The forward posture with hands resting on the knees and the severe kyphosis of the lumbar spine are classic findings. From the author's personal collection

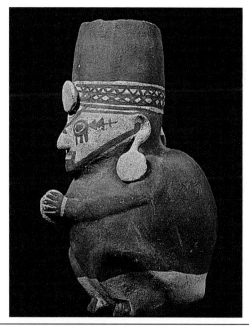

Fig. 1.2. A terracotta figure from Chancay, Peru (circa 1000 A.D.), showing an individual with classic findings of spina bifida, including the typical forward posture with hands resting on the knees as a result of paraplegia. The thoraco-lumbar kyphotic spine can be seen in the profile. From the author's personal collection

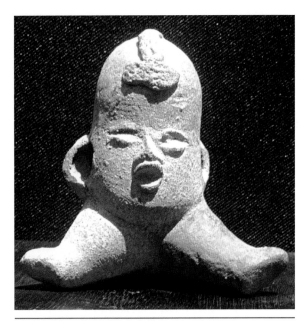

Fig. 1.3. An Olmec child with spina bifida in the typical seating position with severe lumbosacral kyphosis. The child also appears to have hydrocephalus. From the Olmec culture (circa 1500 B.C., Meso-America). From the author's personal collection

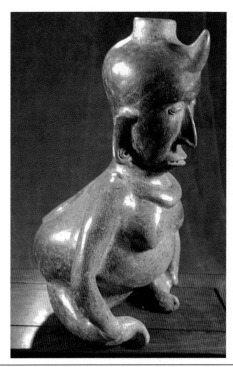

Fig. 1.5. An example of a "shaman" represented by the horn on the forehead, a large hydrocephalic head and the typical characteristics of a spina bifida. On the backside, where the myelomeningocele is located, is a large medallion-like character that lies over the severe lumbosacral kyphosis. The patient is sitting in the classic forward pitched position as a result of weak abdominal muscles, with hands resting on the legs – a typical sitting position for a child with a severe myelomeningocele. From the author's personal collection

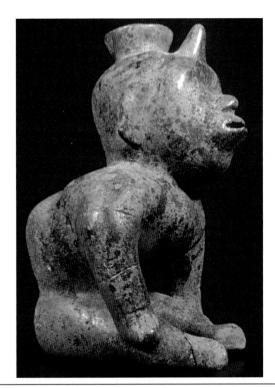

Fig. 1.4. A terracotta pottery piece from Colima, Mexico (circa 200 A.D.), showing a "shaman" figure with the typical horn on the forehead. The seating position with plegic legs and the lumbosacral kyphosis are indicative of an individual with a spinal dysraphism. From the author's personal collection

"Alius morbus oritur ex defluxione capitis per venas in spinalem medullam. Inde autem in sacrum os impetum facit, quo medulla ipsa fluxionem perdit". – Hippocrates [1] (Another disease springs out as an outflow from the head through the veins into the spinal cord. From there moreover it attacks the sacral bone, where the spinal cord itself contains the flow).

Descriptions of what appear to be spinal dysraphisms are found in the early writings of Hippocrates (see quotation above), Galen and others. Review of these early writings indicates that these authors clearly lacked any formal comprehension of the disorder. Surgical treatment for the condition appears to have been virtually nonexistent in the early Greco-Roman era. The earliest definitive description of spina bifida that we have located is that of the Dutch clinician Peter van Forest (1522-1597). In a posthumous work published in 1610, van Forest gave an account of a 2-year-old child with a neck malformation that appears to have been a form of spina bifida. Van Forest surgically ligated the mass at the base but the child went on to die [2].

The first illustrated example of spinal dysraphism appeared in a textbook entitled *Observationes Medicae*, first published in 1641, which went through many editions [3]. The author of this book was Nicholaas Tulp (1593-1674). Tulp (real name, Claes Piereszoon) is best remembered as the main figure in Rembrandt's painting of "The Anatomy Lesson of Dr. Tulp", from 1632, Tulp's second year in practice as an anatomical lecturer. To Tulp we also owe the introduction of the term "spina bifida" [3]. In his textbook, Tulp described six cases, one of which was that of a child with a large lumbar myelomeningocele arising from a narrow pedicle (Fig. 1.6). Tulp described this lesion as "*nervorum propagines tam varie per tumorem dispersas*" (the prolongations of the nerves scattered in different directions through the tumor). For its treatment he described dissecting the myelomeningocele sac and ligating the pedicle; the patient soon died of infection. As a result of this experience, Tulp recommended approaching such lesions with caution as consequences could be dire. Tulp's illustration shows the sac and dissected nerves at autopsy. In reviewing the legend to this plate we find the first printed use of the descriptive term "spina bifida" [3, 4].

To Marco Aurelio Severino (1580-1656), we owe the first textbook on surgical pathology, originally published in 1632 [5]. This work underwent many editions because of its widespread popularity, which is believed to reflect the high quality of the illustrations and the elegant discussions of the case presentations. This remarkable work contains one of the earliest published illustrations of a child with a cervical myelomeningocele (Fig. 1.7). Severino was a widely known and respected teacher in Naples, Italy. He was also an early and important supporter of

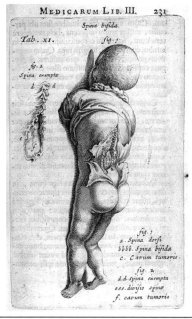

Fig. 1.6. One of the earliest known printed examples of spina bifida, from Tulp's *Observationes Medicae* [3]. In the legend (*bottom right of image*) of this image is the first use of the term "spina bifida". This diagram was based on a patient in whom, after Tulp attempted to repair the myelomeningocele, sepsis prevailed shortly after surgery. The child also appears to have hydrocephalus, a commonly associated pathological condition

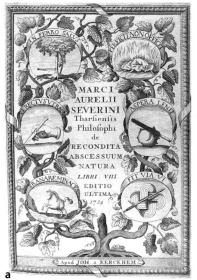
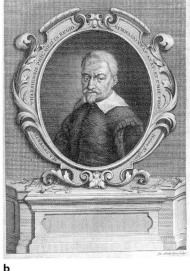
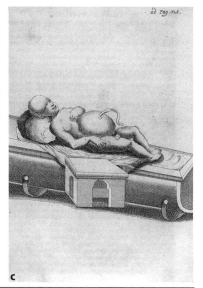

Fig. 1.7 a-c. The first textbook on surgical pathology. **a** Titlepage. **b** Frontispiece portrait of Severino. **c** A classic illustration of a child with a cervical myelomeningocele

William Harvey and his ideas on the circulation of the blood. In this book on the "obscure nature of tumors", we find some of the most remarkable and early depictions of pathological lesions and tumors, often called "swellings". In addition, he often added the history of the patient and, if surgery was indicated, the techniques he used. Reflecting a then-prevailing view of spina bifida, however, he rarely considered it as a surgical entity. Even so, his illustration of this disorder is one of the earliest printed examples [5, 6].

Another prominent Dutch surgeon and anatomist, Frederik Ruysch (1638-1731), published the first extensive spina bifida series, ten cases, in 1691 [7]. While Ruysch clearly described the condition, he offered nothing in the way of treatment, as he considered it untreatable. He did, however, associate the pathology of the paralytic limbs with the "want of the spinal medulla". Ruysch was professor of anatomy at Leiden and Amsterdam and is best remembered for his technique of injecting anatomical structures to outline the anatomy. Among his great accomplishments was discovering the concept of fetal nutrition via the umbilical cord. Ruysch gave the following description of spina bifida [8]:

"A tumor frequently arises in the loins of a foetus, while it is yet an inhabitant of the uterus… If we rightly examine this tumor, it will appear as plain as the Noon Sun to be a dropsy, in part of the spinal medulla and is almost the same disorder, allowing for the difference of situation with that which in the head of the foetus is commonly called an hydrocephalus. Whereas, it is surprising that I should often find the spinal medulla well conditioned below the tumor; whence some children retain the motion of their lower limbs, whereas I have found others with their lower limbs paralytic for want of the spinal medulla. With respect to the cure of this disorder, little or nothing can be done toward it".

During this period, a number of midwifery manuals were issued, the most popular of which was a work by Jacques Guillemeau (1550-1613), namely, *"Child-Birth, Or, The Happy Delivery of Women Wherein is set downe the Government of Women in the time of their breeding Childe: of their Travaile, both Natural and contrary to Nature: and of their lying in Together with the diseases"*, published in London in 1635 (Fig. 1.8) [9]. Guillemeau was a prominent Paris surgeon, successor to Ambroise Paré as surgeon to King Charles IX. A review of the text yields only one case discussion of a child with hydrocephalus; no cases of spina bifida were identified, leading one to ask whether this author considered this a "hopeless" disease and hence not treatable.

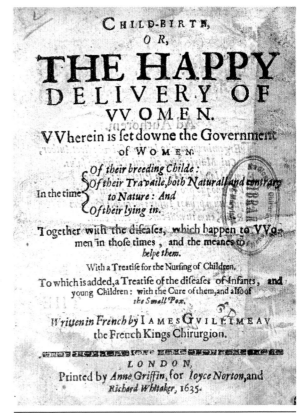

Fig. 1.8. Midwifery manual by Jacques Guillemeau:"Child-Birth; or, The Happy Delivery of Women Wherein is set downe the Government of Women in the time of their breeding Childe: of their Travaile, both Natural and contrary to Nature: and of their lying in Together with the diseases", London, 1635 [9]

To Giovanni Baptiste Morgagni (1682-1771), a teacher of anatomy at Padua, we owe the first solid clinical description of the association of hydrocephalus and spina bifida. In his book on the *Seats and Causes of Diseases*, he gave a clear and vivid description of a child in the post-mortem state who had been born with spina bifida and hydrocephalus [10, 11]. In a section entitled *"Sermo de Hydrocephalus et de Aqueis Spinae Tumoribus"*, he discussed several cases of associated hydrocephalus and spina bifida. However, he did not recognize cerebrospinal fluid (CSF) as a physiological entity; rather, he described this fluid collection in the brain and spine as *"hydrops cerebri et medullaris"*, or an excessive collection of fluid. As an anatomist he described only the clinical findings and offered no advice as to how to treat this disorder (Fig. 1.9).

One of the finest and earliest illustrated examples of spina bifida, with hand-colored drawings, was prepared by Jean Cruveilhier (1791-1874), the son of a military surgeon. These important and elegant rep-

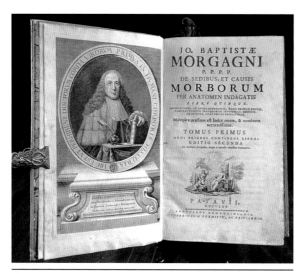

Fig. 1.9. The second edition of Morgagni's masterpiece "On the Seats and Causes of Disease" with a nice frontispiece engraving of Morgagni – *De sedibus, et causis morboum per anatomen indagatis libri quinque.* Patavii: Sumptibus Remondiananis, 1765 [11]

resentations were published in a series of fascicles published over 14 years, 1829-1842 [12, 13]. Detailed case presentations and clinical findings were included, along with case summaries. Cruveilhier added his own comments on the disease process and observations about treatment. As a result of his considerable clinical acumen Cruveilheir was appointed the first professor of descriptive anatomy (i.e., pathology) at the University of Paris. In addition he worked at the Charité and Salpetrière. In his remarkable two-volume folio work he described a number of significant early pathological conditions. The only criticism of this work could be lack of organization, as a number of unrelated cases were put together in a fascicle. However, it is the only fault that can be found with this remarkable treatise. Among his contributions were a series of illustrations showing dramatic presentations of spina bifida and hydrocephalus. He devoted four sections to these subjects. Two cases of myelomeningocele are discussed along with the clinical course (see Livraison 6, plate 3). One child was seen at three days of age and followed for two weeks when the child died of meningitis. At autopsy Cruveilhier found massive hydrocephalus with flattened gyri and sulci. In addition, there was purulent material in the ventricles that he felt had spread through the subarachnoid space from the spina bifida to the ventricles. He noted that the infection probably coursed through the foramen of Magendie – interestingly, this foramen had only just been recently described.

A second case description of spina bifida is most interesting as Cruveilhier clearly describes what we now call the Chiari Type II malformation nearly 55 years before Arnold and Chiari provide the definitive anatomical description (to be discussed below). The case involved a child with a myelomeningocele who died of sepsis. At autopsy he described the bony anomalies of spina bifida and associated diastematomyelia. The further description of the posterior fossa and cerebellum are typical of what we now call a Chiari Type II malformation. His description: "… the upper part of the cervical region, considerably enlarged, contained both the medulla oblongata and the corresponding parts of the cerebellum which was elongated and covered the fourth ventricle which itself became longer and wider". Cruveilhier described two other cases in which his findings were similar: "… this type of descent of the elongated medulla and cerebellum into the upper part of the spinal canal". Cruveilhier believed that spina bifida occurred secondary to an abnormality of development, in retrospect, a remarkably early insight.

An important further clinical observation by Cruveilhier was that the child with myelomeningocele who did best was the one with a closed non-leaking sac. Once the sac opened, the course was disastrous, with infection, sepsis, paraplegia, seizures and death. He commented on the celebrated case of Sir Astley Cooper, who claimed to have cured a child of this problem by repeated punctures of the sac – his observation was that this was a singular fortunate event and not the rule (see Livraison 16 plate 4) (Fig. 1.10).

A surgeon, M. Baxter, likely unaware of the earlier findings of Morgagni in 1761 and of Cruveilhier, published a note in 1882 in which he described the association of hydrocephalus with meningocele [14]. Another anomaly not uncommonly associated with spina bifida was first described by Lebedeff in a case of spina bifida with anencephaly [15].

In more recent times, anatomical studies have further elucidated spina bifida. Such studies include the classic studies by Kermauner [16], Keiller [17] and Bohnstedt [18]. In an effort to enlarge the concept of spina bifida, Fuchs introduced the term "myelodysplasia" in 1910 to denote spina bifida, enuresis, and associated deformities of the feet [19]. This clinical syndrome was further refined in the classic paper by de Vries in 1928 [20]. Lichtenstein used the term "spinal dysraphism" to describe a pleomorphic group of disorders of cutaneous, mesodermal or neural origin [21]. Lichtenstein was among the first to discuss the neuroanatomic effects of spina bifida on distant parts of the central nervous system [22].

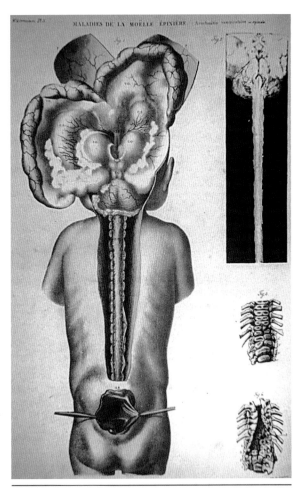

Fig. 1.10. An important illustration of a child with a myelomeningocele and hydrocephalus. In the smaller drawings to the right are examples of spina bifida of the spine. Not well appreciated is the tonsillar herniation of the cerebellum at the cervico-medullary junction – the first description of what we now call a Chiari Type II malformation [12]

Review of the surgical treatment of spina bifida over the years indicates that the most common treatment has involved nothing more than ligation or amputation of the sac. The outcome has almost always been fatal, either because of CSF leakage and infection, or the secondary progressive untreated hydrocephalus. Looking back at the literature, we find a typical eighteenth century case of surgical treatment of spina bifida as described by a prominent London surgeon, Benjamin Bell (1749-1806). Bell's treatment was to place a tight snare ligature around the base of the sac and then allow it to slough off. Interestingly, Bell commented that hydrocephalus was not uncommonly associated with myelomeningoceles. The outcome was fatal in all the cases Bell described, leading him to comment: "This is perhaps the most

fatal disease to which infancy is liable; for as yet no remedy has been discovered for it... Experience shows, however, that every attempt of this kind should be avoided for hitherto the practice has uniformly proved unsuccessful. The patient has either died suddenly, or in the course of a few hours after the operation" [23].

Sir Astley Paston Cooper (1768-1841), a London Guy's Hospital surgeon well known for his surgical prowess, presented a paper to the Royal College of Surgeons in 1811 on spina bifida [24]. Despite being a skilled surgeon who trained under John Hunter, he summarized a number of prevalent views, all of which culminated in the conclusion that this was an untreatable disease that was best left alone. Cooper had only one successful surgical treatment, a child in whom he performed multiple punctures of the sac. The child's survival represented an amazing feat considering this was in the pre-Listerian era of no antisepsis. In Cooper's view this disorder was only to be treated with measures that are "palliative, by pressure, or curative, by puncture". In his paper he provided a lithograph of the disorder (Fig. 1.11).

Samuel Cooper (1780-1848), a prominent English surgeon and former president of the Royal College of Surgeons, provided an excellent nineteenth century clinical view of spina bifida. In the following statement [25], he clearly summed up the clinical problems related to spina bifida and the contemporary lack of successful surgical treatment: "The generality of children, affected with spina bifida, are deficient in strength, and subject to frequent diarrhoae. Incontinence of urine and the feces, emaciation, weakness, and even complete paralysis, are sometimes the concomitants of this serious complaint. However, some of the patients are, in every respect, except the tumor, perfectly healthy, and well formed". In discussing surgery, Cooper remarked [26]: "Experience has fully proved, that puncturing the tumor with a lancet, and thus discharging the fluid, either at once, or gradually, cannot be done without putting the patient in the greatest danger, the consequences being for the most part fatal in a very short space of time". Surgeons continued to be inventive, offering other techniques for treating spina bifida that included injecting the sac with sclerosing solutions (typically iodine, potassium iodide). Although the reported mortality was less in such cases, nonetheless the frequency of neurological deficits was reported as significantly increased [27].

Following up on earlier injection techniques, Palasciano proposed a "new" method to treat spina bifida cystica and encephalocele in the 1850s [28]. He first emptied the dysraphic sac of CSF, and then

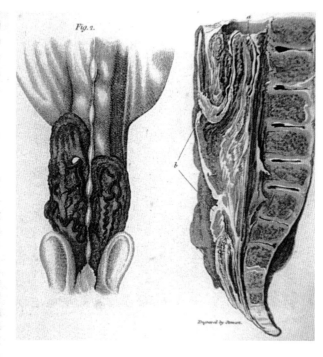

ON

SPINA BIFIDA.

By ASTLEY COOPER, Esq. F.R.S.

SURGEON TO GUY'S HOSPITAL.

Read *May* 21, 1811.

I PROBABLY should not have read to the Society the following remarks on Spina Bifida at the present time, had not I been urged to it by those on whose judgment and friendship I have been accustomed to rely. The cases which form the basis of this paper having been shewn to Drs. Marcet, Yelloly, and Farre; to Mr. George Young, and to Mr. Barlow of Blackburn; they were of opinion that they not only deserved publication, but strongly urged that they ought not in justice to remain concealed, as there were,

Fig. 1.11. Title page and illustration of spina bifida from Astley Cooper's monograph on spina bifida [24]

concentrically compressed the sac to bring together either the cranial or the vertebral margins of the defect. He then injected iodine into the sac to induce sclerosis. A surgical technique for myelomeningocele was further refined by Francesco Rizzoli (1809-1880) in 1869 [29]. He abandoned the technique of using sclerosing iodine as he felt it was too damaging to the nervous elements. As an alternative method he designed and applied a "Rizzoli enterotome" to the dysraphic sac and slowly closed it, allowing the sac to necrose and slough off (Fig. 1.12).

In the nineteenth century a number of atlases were produced that dealt with "human monsters" and a number of these illustrated various cases of myelomeningoceles. One of the most popular atlases was by Friedrich Ahlfeld, entitled *Atlas zu die Miss-bildungen des Menschen*, published in Leipzig in 1880-1882 [30]. The work was on a number of human malformations with some elegant lithographic plates. Some examples of spina bifida from this volume are included (Figs. 1.13-1.15). Ahlfeld felt this disorder was due to an excess collection of fluid, not recognizing the physiology of CSF: "*Man muss für die Mehrzahl der Fälle die primäre Ursache im spinalen Hydrops suchen*". There is no discussion of surgical management in this work. It was not until the work of Lebedeff (1881-1882) that the concept

was put forward that spina bifida resulted from a failure of neural tube closure in early fetal development [15]. Lebedeff commented on this disorder as "*Entstehung der Hemicephalie und Spina Bifida zurück auf Anomalie Krümmungen des Medullar-rohrs in der frühesten fötalen Period*" [31].

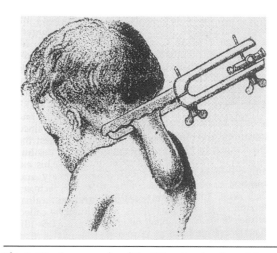

Fig. 1.12. An example of the "Rizzoli enterotome" for removing a myelomeningocele. The instrument was applied and then "slowly" closed, causing the sac to necrose and eventually fall off

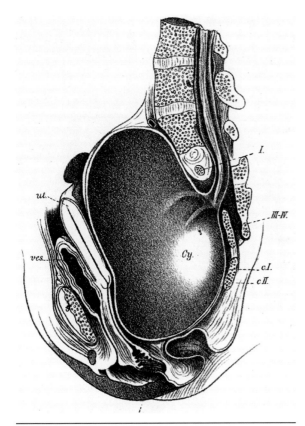

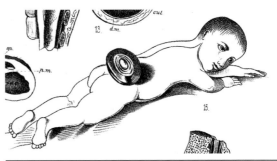

Fig. 1.14. From Ahlfeld's *Atlas zu die Missbildungen...* (1880-1882) illustrating a newborn child with a large untreated myelomeningocele

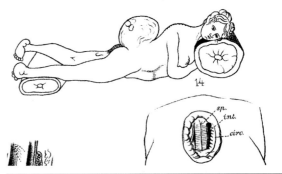

Fig. 1.13. From Ahlfeld's *Atlas zu die Missbildungen...* (1880-1882) showing a nice example of a rare anterior myelomeningocele

Fig. 1.15. From Ahlfeld's *Atlas zu die Missbildungen...* (1880-1882) showing a nice example of an adult female with a large untreated myelomeningocele with clinical lower extremities weakness and deformation

One of the most important nineteenth monographs on spina bifida was published by Friedrich von Recklinghausen (1833-1910) [32]. Von Recklinghausen was a pupil of Rudolf Virchow (1821-1902) at the Pathological Institute in Berlin, Germany. Often forgotten is the fact that it was Virchow who coined the term "spina bifida occulta", now part of our standard nomenclature [33]. Von Recklinghausen eventually settled in Strasbourg, where he remained for the rest of his career, producing his monograph on spina bifida in 1886 [32]. He is probably better remembered for his work on neurofibromatosis, now called "von Recklinghausen disease". In his monograph he described a remarkable case of an adult with spina bifida occulta and hypertrichosis. The patient had a club foot that lacked sensation because of the spina bifida. An ulcer of the foot developed and became septic and the patient died from septicemia. At autopsy, von Recklinghausen found an occult spina bifida of L5 into the sacrum. The conus medullaris was tethered at S2 with a "fatty tumor", likely a lipomyelomeningocele. He made some interesting pathological postulates in that he felt the lipoma was due

to abnormal separation of the mesoderm during early embryological development. Von Recklinghausen made a number of other important points in that he appreciated that the fluid in spina bifida came from the subarachnoid space, i.e., it was CSF. He also observed that some patients with spina bifida survived into adulthood as functioning individuals. He noted that hydrocephalus was not always associated with spina bifida. Included in this work are some remarkable illustrations, including two folding plates that clearly outline both the internal and the external pathology of spina bifida. In the monograph von Recklinghausen presented a clear, detailed analysis of the formation of the neuroaxis in myelomeningoceles and spina bifida (Figs. 1.16, 1.17).

The concept of treating a myelomeningocele with a "sclerosis" injection was an old one, but was further embedded in the surgical literature by Morton in 1877 [34]. Morton felt that the surgical outcomes of ligation, amputation, and related procedures in relation to myelomeningoceles led to unacceptable outcomes. He therefore devised a solution that consisted of iodine in glycerine for injection into the "tu-

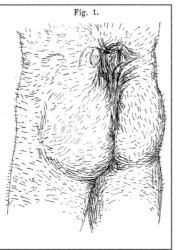

An den beiden Ober-
schenkeln namentlich an ihrer
hinteren Seite ist der Haar-
wuchs, ebenso wie an den
Genitalien stärker wie ge-
wöhnlich bei Erwachsenen,
ganz unverhältnissmässig aber
auf den Hinterbacken, in der
Gesässfalte und über dem
Kreuzbein bis hinauf zu den
Lenden. Während die Haare
an den Seitentheilen des
Steisses sehr fein, wenn auch
bis 2 cm lang, ausserdem nur
wenig gefärbt sind, werden
sie auf der Mitte des Kreuzes
dichter, dunkelbraun, bis zu
6 cm lang und biegen sich
an ihrem Ende um, so dass
sie mit einander Locken bil-
den. Der stärkste Haar-
busch liegt median über

Fig. 1.

Fig. 1.16. An illustration of the adult case that von Recklinghausen presented with a lipomyelomeningocele, spina bifida, and hypertrichosis [32]

mour". This technique became quite popular and was used throughout the United Kingdom and Europe.

A late nineteenth century advocate for surgical closure of myelomeningoceles was a Boston surgeon, Henry O. Marcy. In a paper published in *Annals of Surgery* in March of 1895, he came out strongly in favor of surgical repair, in order, so to speak, to cre-

ate in the closure what nature had failed to do [35]. He felt that failure to do so led to "sepsis *in loco*" and the death of the patient. His argument, and a legitimate one, was that "A priori reasoning would lead to the conclusion that art could supplement nature in her defective development". The case report he presented was that of an 18-year-old female born with a "soft swelling under the skin in the lumbar region". Because the swelling's steady growth had recently become more rapid, resulting in thinning of the sac with the danger of rupture, he decided on surgical intervention. Clinically she had only club feet and was otherwise normal. She "has consulted many surgeons, who have invariably advised against surgical interference". At surgery, the sac contained "one gallon of perfectly clear colorless fluid, which was drawn off by means of a trocar". It is interesting to note that he did the operation on October 16, 1895 and wrote his report and published it on November 9, 1895! He noted that the patient was still in bed with her only complaint that of burning in the feet. Marcy then comprehensively reviewed the nineteenth century surgical literature. He became a clear advocate of surgical closure, as pressure, sclerosis, taps and the like all led to mostly bad outcomes.

In England, a surgeon by the name of J. Cooper Forster presented a case of a child with lumbo-sacral myelomeningocele [36]. Included in his book was an

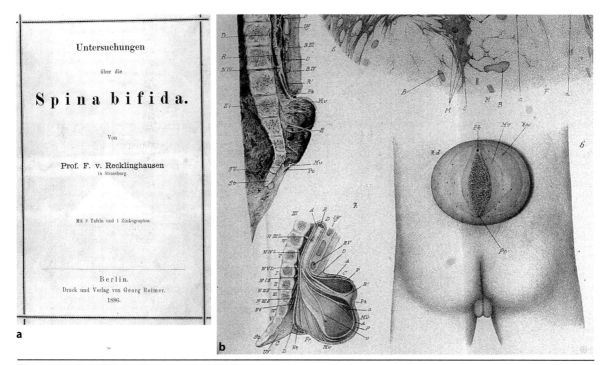

Fig. 1.17 a, b. a Title leaf from von Recklinghausen monograph [32] on spina bifida (from the author's personal collection). **b** Illustrated examples of spina bifida from von Recklinghausen

elegant hand-colored engraving of the lesion. The treatment he advocated was compression of the sac with gentle tapping off of the spinal fluid (Fig. 1.18).

Review of a prominent textbook of surgery from 1887, by John Wyeth of New York, reveals that the author was intrigued to see how little was offered in surgical treatment of myelomeningocele [37]. In most cases treatment was only palliative, with compression of the sac. In the large sac, tapping off of fluid was feasible, but required care and avoidance of the midline because of the nearby neural elements. Wyeth cautioned that the needle should always enter the sac from the side. The smallest needle should be used and only small quantities of fluid taken at any one time. In some cases, Wyeth suggested the injection of Morton's solution into the sac – a commonly recommended practice in the latter half of the nineteenth century. In discussing prognosis of patients with spina bifida, Wyeth commented, "The prognosis is, as a rule, very unfavorable".

Following a similar theme in treatment were the surgical thoughts of Roswell Park, whose volume on surgery was a popular text at the end of the nineteenth century [38]. In the chapter on spina bifida is a clear description of its various types, including illustrations of the anatomy and case presentations. In discussing treatment, one could be either "conservative or operative". Conservative treatment involved only tapping the sac, use of compression or injection of the ubiquitous Morton's solution. An additional thought in treatment was the addition of collodion and iodoform to the puncture site to help reduce further leakage and potential infection. Roswell Park's surgical technique involved freeing the neural elements and dropping them back into the canal. A wide-undermining of the skin flaps gave a primary closure over the defect. He also discussed the use of osteoplastic flaps to close the defective lamina. He felt this is a most difficult maneuver and did not recommend it. Park clearly stated that surgical intervention for spina bifida had only recently become possible with the introduction in the 1870s of aseptic techniques, since before this outcomes were almost always fatal because of septicemia (Fig. 1.19).

In his monograph on *Surgery of Childhood*, Sidney Wilcox, a New York homeopathic surgeon, summarized the surgical treatment of spina bifida at the turn of the century [39]. Wilcox felt this was a disorder that should be approached with some trepidation, as most authors had reported a dismal outcome when spina bifida was treated surgically. Techniques advocated at that time included injection into the sac of Morton's solution [34], which he described as a mixture of iodine, Kali iodide and glycerine. Other techniques included draining the sac and then "darning across the opening with silver wire". Wilcox described a successful case where "the tumour was removed, the laminae were united and the cord sutured end to end". But with some conservative insight he recommended that in those cases where surgery could not be done, to make a small wire cage and fit it over the myelomeningocele, which should be "… filled with cotton so as to make pressure and at the same time ward off blows, [and would thus] be of service" (Fig. 1.20).

The treatment and coverage of open myelomeningocele defects by rotating various skin and muscle flaps were first introduced in 1892, when a German surgeon, C. Bayer, reported on surgical repair of an open myelomeningocele using a series of rotating flap techniques [40]. This surgical technique introduced a new and important concept of placing the neural elements within the spinal canal and then covering the spinal elements with layers of surrounding tissues – a remarkable advance! (Fig. 1.21c).

Antoine Chipault (1866-1920) of Paris, France, prepared a number of important monographs on surgery. Of particular interest is his 1894-95 two-vol-

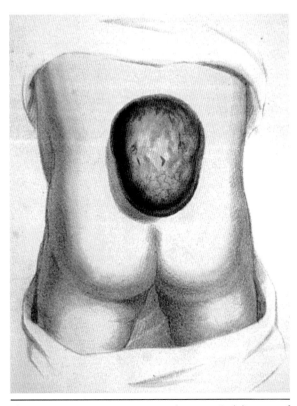

Fig. 1.18. From Forster monograph on surgical diseases of children [27]. A classic example of a lumbo-sacral myelomeningocele

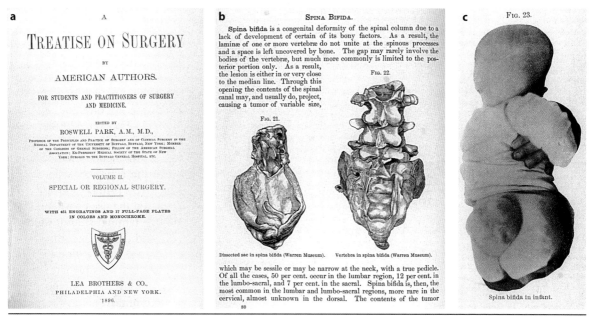

Fig. 1.19 a-c. Illustrations from Park's work on surgery. **a** Title page. **b** The anatomy of spina bifida. **c** A clinical example of a child with spina bifida [29]

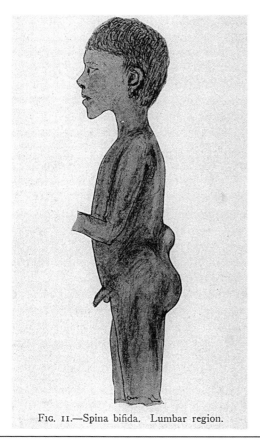

Fig. 11.—Spina bifida. Lumbar region.

Fig. 1.20. A child with an untreated myelomeningocele from Wilcox's *Surgery of Childhood*, 1909. In this case a "wire cage" would be placed over the lesion, filled with cotton to protect it from outside blows [30]

ume work entitled *Chirurgie Opératoire du Système Nerveux…* [41]. In this work he presented a number of examples of spina bifida along with a surgical treatment plan (Fig. 1.20). As was typical throughout the work, the anatomy and the surgical concepts were both impeccable and surgically insightful. Chipault became one of the first European surgeons to argue for a multi-layer closure of the myelomeningocele, adopting the techniques of Bayer [4]. Using aseptic techniques, just recently introduced, Chipault had reasonably good outcomes. Illustrations from his textbook showing the anatomy and techniques for a repair of a myelomeningocele are shown in Figure 1.21.

To Hans Chiari (1851-1916) we owe the development of the anatomical understanding of the "Chiari malformation", often seen in myelomeningoceles, among other disorders [42-46]. A skilled anatomist and pathologist, Chiari is credited with performing over 30,000 autopsies using the systematic autopsy techniques of Karl von Rokitansky (1804-1878) under whom he trained. Often forgotten is the fact that Chiari published the first case of traumatic pneumoencephaly, a publication that later influenced Walter Dandy's development of the pneumoencephalogram [47]. However, it is Chiari's studies on congenital brainstem anomalies associated with hydrocephalus that remain classic [42, 43]. On the basis of his work at the Kaiser Franz Joseph Children's Hospital in Prague he described three different malformations found in 63 patients with hydrocephalus.

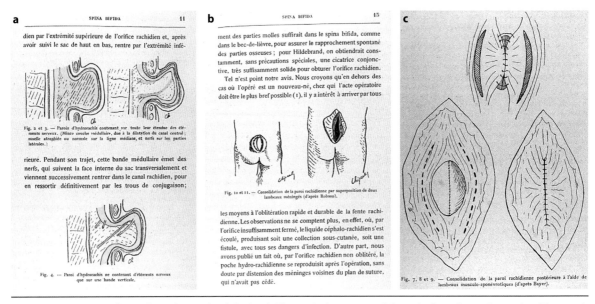

Fig. 1.21 a–c. Images from Chipault's textbook [41]. **a**, **b** The typical anatomy of the spinal myelomeningocele. **c** The repair of a myelomeningocele in a multi-layer closure is shown. Chipault adopted this technique from Bayer [40]

Currently we divide these hindbrain anomalies into four types, but the one germane to this paper is the type 2 malformation. Chiari described 14 cases of the type I malformation in patients aged 3 months to 68 years. Interestingly, all of the patients were adults and had hydrocephalus and only one had a myelomeningocele. He called this a deformity of the brain stem that resulted in hydrocephalus: *"Über Veränderungen des Kleinhirns infolge von Hydrocephalie des Grosshirns"*. Chiari's type II malformation was described in seven cases in patients ranging from the ages of birth to 6 months. The combination of hydrocephalus and spina bifida was seen in all seven cases. The anatomical findings were a prolongation of the cerebellar vermis and the tonsils (as seen in type I). Associated with this was an inferior prolongation of the fourth ventricle into the cervical spinal canal. Often seen was a kinking of the inferiorly displaced medulla oblongata. In type III there was inferior displacement of the brainstem with herniation of the cerebellum and myelomeningocele. The fourth ventricle was dilated. Type IV was described as cerebellar hypoplasia. Interestingly, Chiari had only one case of type III and described no cases of type IV. Type IV per se was not described until a later monograph in 1896 [43].

For the record, priority in the description of the Chiari type II malformation does not go to Chiari. Rather, this description was first published by John Cleland in 1883, some eight years before Chiari [48]. Chiari gave credit to Cleland's earlier description in

his first monograph [42]. Cleland was a Scottish surgeon and anatomist teaching at the University of Glasgow and based his findings on autopsies of nine infants. One of the cases was a child with spina bifida and hydrocephalus and findings that we would now call a Chiari type II.

Julius Arnold (1835–1915), whose name is often associated with this anomaly, published his findings on brain stem anomalies in an infant with multiple congenital anomalies including a large thoraco-lumbar spina bifida in 1894 [49]. Interestingly, the child described did not have hydocephalus. He attributed this anomaly to a primary disturbance in the organization, or disorganization, of the germ cells – a concept he called "monogerminal teratomatous malformation". Two pupils of Arnold, E. Schwalbe and M. Gredig, published a paper in 1907 discussing the association of the hindbrain anomalies with spina bifida and coined the term *"Arnold'sche und Chiari'sche Missbildung"*, which led to the "Arnold-Chiari malformation" [50]. Most modern writers have given priority for these descriptions to Chiari and hence the current use of "Chiari" when describing these various malformations [44–46].

By the early part of the twentieth century surgeons were developing better surgical concepts of the repair of myelomeningoceles, i.e., multilayer closures using dura, fascia, muscles and skin. A good example of these newer concepts appears in a classic textbook on the spine by Charles H. Frazier (1870–1936) [51]. Frazier was professor of surgery in Philadelphia and one of the early pioneers in American neurosurgery. A classic autodidact of the time, he continued his medical and surgical education in Europe working under giants such as Ernst von Bergmann, Rudolf Virchow and others. While at the University of Pennsylvania, he came under the influence of Charles Mills and William G. Spiller, two locally prominent neurologists. Although Frazier's interest remained mostly in adult neurosurgery, he did make some interesting contributions to pediatric neurosurgery, in particular, surgery of the myelomeningocele. Frazier first pointed out certain contraindications to operating on children with myelomeningoceles: presence of hydrocephalus,

sphincter paralysis, irreparable deformities and any form of ulcerative process in the region of the myelomeningocele [51]. For closure of the myelomeningocele he devised several different methods: small sacs were excised followed by a primary closure of the neck after overlying the spinal erector muscles. In the instance of larger, more complex defects, he mobilized the aponeurosis and paraspinal muscles to overlie the defect. In some cases Frazier would fracture the laminar arches of the vertebrae and sew them at the midline (Fig. 1.22). These techniques would become the primary types of repair used by surgeons in the first half of the twentieth century. With

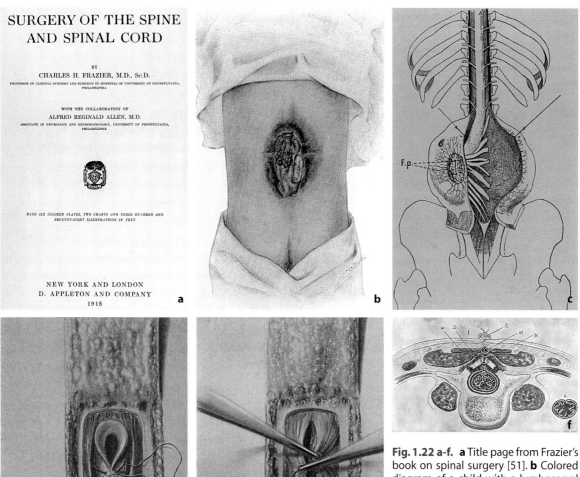

Fig. 1.22 a-f. **a** Title page from Frazier's book on spinal surgery [51]. **b** Colored diagram of a child with a lumbosacral myelomeningocele. **c** Frazier illustrates the anatomy of the various elements in an open myelomeningocele. **d** Frazier's technique of a multilayer closure starting here with the dural closure. **e** Frazier's technique of a multilayer closure showing here the fascia and muscle closure. **f** Frazier's technique of a multilayer closure showing here the fracture of the spinal lateral elements

the now classic paper of Ingraham and Hamlin in 1943 [52], the present technique of a multi-layer closure was introduced and standardized as further discussed in their monograph.

In the modern period (i.e., post World War II), concepts of the timing of surgery for spina bifida have changed a number of times. In 1943 Ingraham and Hamlin initially argued that surgical correction of a myelomeningocele should be delayed until 18 months of age, to allow adequate assessment of the patient's eventual neurological outcome [52]. If the neurological impairment was not too severe and the IQ was normal, surgical closure was recommended. In the 1960s earlier surgery, i.e., in the peri-natal period, was advocated by Lorber, Matson, Sharrard, and others; surgery was to be done within the first week of life in order to avoid complications. As a result, such timing has now become routine in most countries [53]. In many parts of the world these lesions are still repaired by pediatric surgeons rather than neurosurgeons. However, as a result of a better understanding of the complexity of these newborn disorders and their long-term follow-up, these lesions have now come more into the domain of the pediatric neurosurgeon.

It is interesting to review the surgical history of this disorder and the long period of time over which little was offered in the way of treatment. The medical treatment was typically cathartics or purging, and in some cases even bleeding, barbaric treatments in retrospect, but all that could be offered by a population of physicians who were clearly ignorant of the problem. Early treatment by surgeons mostly meant ignoring the disease as surgeons quickly found out that operative intervention often lead to death. To our twentieth century colleagues we really owe a debt of gratitude for being both adventurous and insightful in the management of this devastating disorder. As a result, now many of these children go on to live independent and productive lives. With the recent introduction of folic acid into the diet of expecting mothers and early diagnostic ultrasonograms, the incidence of this disorder has dropped dramatically in developed countries.

References

1. Hippocrates. In: Kühn CG (1825) Medicorum graecorum opera quae exstant. Leipzig, C, Cnoblochius, Volume 21, p 500
2. van Forestus P (1610) Observationum et curationum chirurgicarum Libri Quinque Lugduni Batavorum (i.e., Leyden), Ex. Officiana Plantiniana Raphelengii
3. Tulpius N (1641) Observationes medicae. Amsterdam Elzevirium, see Libri III, pp 231 for illustration and plate
4. Furukawa T (1987) First description of spina bifida by Nicolaas Tulp. Neurol 37:1816-1828. See also Rickham PP (1963) Nicolaas Tulp and spina bifida. Clin Peds 2:40-42
5. Severinus, Marcus Aurelius (1632) De Recondita abscessum natura. Neapoli, Beltranum
6. Severinus, Marcus Aurelius (1724) De Abscessuum Recondita Natura: Libri VIII, Editio novissima, Lugduni Batavorum, apud Joannem a Kerckhem
7. Ruysch F (1691) Observationum anatomico-chirurgicarum centuria. Amsterdam, Apud Hnricum & viduam Theodori Boom
8. Ruysch F (1751) The celebrated Dr. Frederic Ruysch's practical observations in surgery and midwifery. T. Osborne, London. See Walker, AE (ed) (1951) A History of Neurological Surgery. Baltimore, Williams and Wilkins, pp 352-353 for quote
9. Guillemeau, Jacques (1635) Child-Birth; or, The Happy Delivery of Women Wherein is set downe the Government of Women in the time of their breeding Childe: of their Travaile, both Natural and contrary to Nature: and of their lying in Together with the diseases. London, Anne Griffin for Joyce Norton and Richard Whitaker
10. Morgagni JB (1761) De sedibus, et causis morborum per anatomen indagatis libri quinque. Venice Ex. Typographia Remondiniana
11. Morgagni JB (1765) De sedibus, et causis morboum per anatomen indagatis libri quinque. Patavii: Sumptibus Remondiananis
12. Cruveilhier J (1829-1842) Anatomie pathologique du corps humain. JB Baillière, Paris
13. Flamm ES (1973) The neurology of Jean Cruveilhier. Medical History 17:343-355
14. Baxter M (1882) Chronic hydrocephalus with meningocele. Med Times Gaz I:239-249
15. Lebedeff A (1881) Über die Entstehung der Anencephalie und Spina bifida bei Vögeln und Menschen. Virchows Arch 86:263-273
16. Kermauner F (1909) In: Schwalbes: die Morphologie der Missbildungen des Menschen und der Tiere, III, Teil 3:86-94, Jena, Gustav Fischer
17. Keiller VH (1922) A contribution to the anatomy of spina bifida. Brain 45:31-41
18. Bohnstedt, G (1895) Beitrag zur Kasuistik der spina bifida occulta. Arch f Path Anat 140:47-57
19. Fuchs A (1910) Über Beziehungen der Enuresis nocturna zu Rudimentärformen der Spina bifida occulta (Myelodysplasie). Wien med Wochnschr 60:1569-1573
20. de Vries E (1928) Spina bifida occulta and myelodysplasia with unilateral clubfoot beginning in adult life. Am J M Sc 175:365-371
21. Lichtenstein BW (1940) Spinal dysraphism: Spina bifida and myelodysplasia. Arch Neurol Psychiatry 44:792-809

22. Lichtenstein BW (1942) Distant neuroanatomic complications of spina bifida (spinal dysraphism): Hydrocephalus, Arnold-Chiari deformity, stenosis of Aqueduct of Sylvius, etc. Pathogenesis and pathology. Arch Neurol Psychiatry 47:195-214

23. Bell B (1787) A system of surgery. Edinburgh: C. Elliott. See volume 1, pp 245-249 for operative technique on spina bifida. See p 246 for quote

24. Cooper A (1811) Some observations on spina bifida. Medico-Chirurgical Transactions 2:443-447

25. Cooper S (1830) The first lines of the practice of surgery; ... with notes by Alexander H. Stevens. Third American, from the fifth London edition. Philadelphia, John Grigg. See vol 2, pp 346-347

26. Cooper S (1830) The first lines of the practice of surgery; ... with notes by Alexander H. Stevens. Third American, from the fifth London edition. Philadelphia, John Grigg. See vol 2, pp 347

27. Morton J (1872) Case of spina bifida cured by injection. Brit MJ 1:632-633

28. Palasciano F (1897) Memorie ed osservazioni del Prof. Ferdinando Palasciano. Postmortem ed. Napoli: trani

29. Rizzoli F (1872) Memoires de chirurgie et d'obstétrique. Paris: Delahaye. For a further discussion on Rizzoli see also Guidetti B, Giuffrè B, Valente V (1983) Italian contribution to the origin of neurosurgery. Surg Neurol 20:335-336

30. Ahlfeld F (1880-1882) Atlas zu die Missbildungen des Menschen. Leipzig, Fr Wilh Grunow

31. Lebedeff A (1882) Lehrbuch des allgemeinen pathologische Anatomie. Berlin, Druck und Verlag von Georg Reimer, p 297

32. von Recklinghausen F (1886) Untersuchungen über die Spina Bifida. Berlin, Druck und Verlag von Georg Reimer. See also von Recklinghausen F (1886) Recherches sur le spina bifida. Arch f Path Anat und Physiol 105:31-41

33. Virchow R (1875) Ein fall von hypertrichosis circumscripta mediana, kombiniert mit spina bifida occulta. Ztschr f Ethnol 7:280-290

34. Morton J (1877) Treatment of spina bifida by a new method. Glasgow, J. Maclehose

35. Marcy HO (1895) The surgical treatment of spina bifida. Annals of Surgery 20:70-76

36. Forster JC (1860) The surgical diseases of children. Parker, London

37. Wyeth JA (1887) Text-book on surgery, general, operative, and mechanical. Appleton, New York, p 712

38. Park R (ed) (1896) A treatise on surgery by American authors. Lea Brothers & Co, Philadelphia, 2:80-84

39. Wilcox SF (1909) Surgery of childhood. Boericke and Runyon, New York

40. Bayer C (1892) Zur technik der operation der spina bifida und encephalocele. Prag med Wchnschr 17:317, 332, 345

41. Chipault A (1894-95) Chirurgie opératoire du système nerveux. Avec une preface de M. Le Professeur Terrier. Paris:Rueff et c. Editeurs

42. Chiari H (1891) Über Veränderungen des Kleinhirns in Folge won Hydrocephalie des Grosshirns. Dtsch med Wschr 17:1172-75. An English translation of this paper was published in 1987. Chiari H (1987) Concerning alterations in the cerebellum resulting from cerebral hydrocephalus. 1891. Pediatr Neurosci 13:3-8

43. Chiari H (1896) Über Veränderungen des Kleinhirns, des Pons und Medulla oblongata infolge von kongenitaler Hydrocephalie des Grosshirns. Denkschriften der Kais Akad Wiss math-naturw Wien 63:71-116

44. Carmel PW, Markesbery WR (1972) Early description of the Arnold-Chiari Malformation. J Neurosurgery 37:543-547

45. Burke JR, Massey EW (1990) Hans Chiari. In: Ashwal S (ed) The founders of child neurology. Norman Publishing, San Francisco, pp 190-195

46. Brockhurst G (1976) Spina bifida for the clinician. Clinics in developmental medicine No. 57. William Heineman Medical Books, London, pp 7-11

47. Chiari H (1884) Ueber einen Fall von Luftansammlung in den Ventrikeln des menschlichen Gehirns. Ztschr F Heilk 5:383-390

48. Cleland J (1883) Contributions to the study of spina bifida, encephalocele, and anencephalus. J Anat Physiol 17:257-292. For a historical review see a paper by Koehler PJ (1991) Chiari's description of cerebellar ectopy (1819) with a summary of Cleland's and Arnold's contribution and some early observations on neural-tube defects. J Neurosurg 75:823-826

49. Arnold J (1894) Myelocyste, transposition von Gewebskeimen und Sympodie. Beitr path Anat allg Path 16:1-8

50. Schwalbe E, Gredig M (1907) Über Entwicklungsstörungen des Kleinhirns, Hirnstamms und Halsmarks bei Spina bifida. (Arnold'sche und Chiari'sche Missbildung) J Beitrage sur pathologischen Anatomie. 40:132-144

51. Frazier CH (1918) Surgery of the spine and spinal cord. D Appleton & Co, New York

52. Ingraham FD, Hamlin H (1943) Spina bifida and cranium bifidum; surgical treatment. N Engl J Med 228:631-641

53. Sharrard WJ, Zachary RB, Lorber J (1967) The long-term evaluation of a trial of immediate and delayed closure of spina bifida cystica. Clin Ortho Res 50:197-207

Chapter 2
Embryology Applied to Neural Tube Defects (NTDs)

Martin Catala

Spina bifida is a frequent congenital malformation involving the spinal cord. It was first described by Nicolas Tulp in 1651 (Figs. 2.1 and 2.2). Nicolas Tulp is also famous for the portrait Rembrandt painted of him during his anatomical lessons. The term spina bifida was suggested by Tulp and proposed solely to describe the vertebral anomaly that was considered a duplication of the spinous process of the vertebra. In fact, we will see that this interpretation is incorrect. However, the term spina bifida is still in use. Nowadays, spina bifida belongs to a super-family of malformations called neural tube defects (NTDs), which include anencephaly, exencephaly, encephaloceles and meningoceles.

Modern developmental biology deals with the mechanisms that are responsible for cell differentiation and migration, formation of organs, and con-

NICOLAI TVLPII
AMSTELREDAMENSIS
OBSERVATIONVM
MEDICARVM.
LIBRI TRES.
Cum Æneis figuris.
AMSTELREDAMI,
Apud LVDOVICVM ELZEVIRIVM,
CIↃ IↃ CXLI.

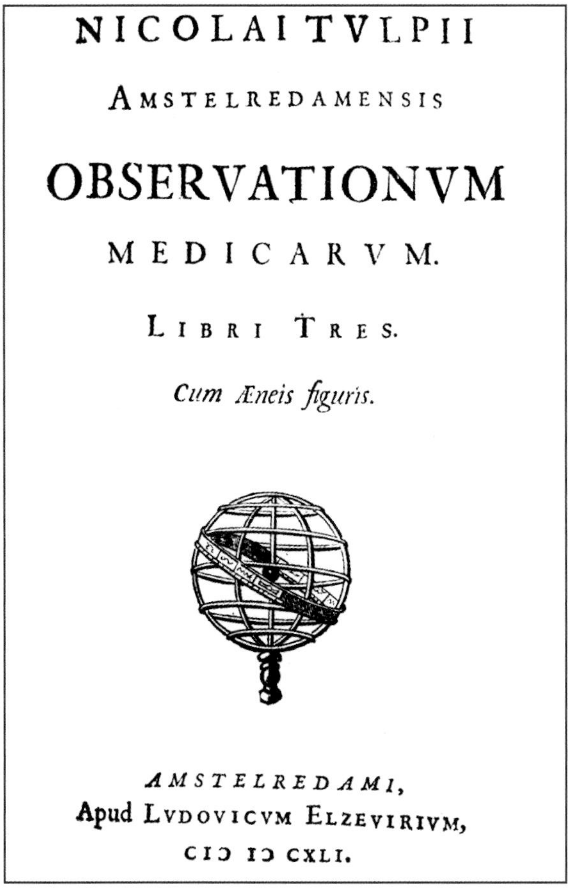

Fig. 2.1. *Observationum medicarum* (third book) published by Nicolas Tulp in 1651 (Ludovicum Elzevririum editor, Amsterdam)

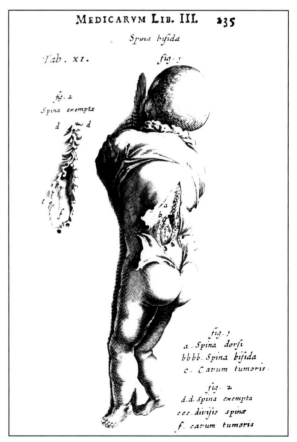

Fig. 2.2. The first description of a case of spina bifida. Nicolas Tulp proposed the term spina bifida. To describe the vertebral anomaly considered as a duplication of the spinous process of the vertebra

trol of growth. Defects affecting these elementary mechanisms are likely to account for congenital malformations. One of the complex concepts that should be kept in mind when trying to understand the cause of a malformation is that embryonic structures interact. Thus, the spine (derived from the paraxial mesoderm) and spinal cord (derived from the neural tube) interplay. This can explain why an abnormal development of one structure is usually associated with the maldevelopment of the other.

How Cells Differentiate during Embryonic Life

It is obviously beyond the scope of this chapter to present an overview of this highly complex and fascinating question. Differentiation can be summarized as follows:

1. From one cell (the fertilized egg), more than 250 different cell types should arise
2. The first cell is not differentiated
3. The unique cellular event that affects the egg is mitosis
4. Mitosis allows the duplication of one cell into two daughter-cells that are identical in terms of genetic material

The first cells of the embryo are identical and totipotent (each cell can generate a complete embryo). The first phase of differentiation takes place when the pre-implantation embryo is composed of eight to 16 cells. This differentiation is due to a mitosis that generates two different daughter-cells. This is achieved by an asymmetrical repartition of the cytoplasmic components between the two daughter-cells. This type of cell division is termed an asymmetric mitosis and may be explained by the polarization of the mother cell (namely, a cytoplasmic gradient exists which allows the asymmetric inheritance of the cytoplasmic components).

After the generation of a first diversity between cells, a second series of interactions can take place. One population of cells can modify the fate of a second population by producing secreted factors. This type of interaction is known as tissue induction. Neural tissue arises after an induction during the third week of gestation in humans. At the end of the second week of gestation, the human embryo presents as a disk with two cell layers: the superficial layer (or epiblast faces the amniotic cavity), the deep layer (or visceral endoderm faces the yolk sac). The definitive embryo derives exclusively from the epiblast.

Neural Induction during Gastrulation

Hans Spemann and Hilde Mangold put forward the concept of neural induction in the 1920s. They developed an experimental technique in amphibians consisting of grafting a region from a pigmented species into a non pigmented host [1]. They grafted the dorsal lip of the blastopore to the ventral region of a host and they found that the dorsal lip differentiated into notochord, medial somites and floor plate of the neural tube (Figs. 2.3 and 2.4). Further-

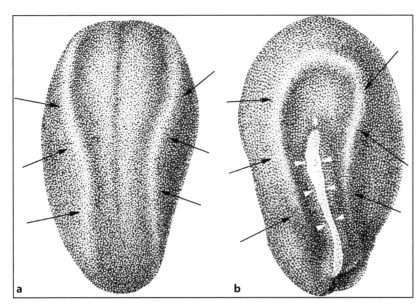

Fig. 2.3 a, b. The graft of an unpigmented dorsal lip of the blastopore into a pigmented host leads to the formation of a double axis. **a** The endogeneous axis derives exclusively from the host (*black arrows*); **b** the induced axis (*black arrows*) is from both origins. The midline derives from the graft (*white arrowheads*), whereas the rest of the neural plate arises from the host. Modified from [1]

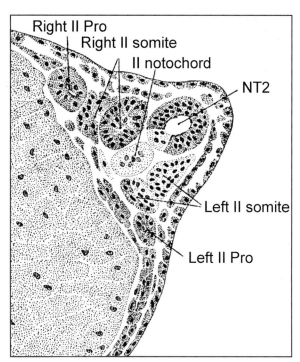

Fig. 2.4. Histological section of the secondary axis induced by the graft of an unpigmented blastoporal lip into a pigmented host. The graft gives rise to the floor plate of the neural tube (NT2), the notochord (*II notochord*) and a part of the somites (*Right II somite* and *left II somite*). Secondary pronephros (*Right II Pro* and *Left II Pro*). Modified from [1]

more, the graft forced the host ectoderm into neurectoderm. Spemann and Mangold defined the dorsal lip of the blastopore as an organizing region that is able to induce neural tissue.

A few years later, Conrad H. Waddington demonstrated that the most anterior part of the primitive streak (namely Hensen's node) is able to induce neural tissues in birds [2] and in mammals [3].

The general conclusions of these experiments are:
1. An organizer is necessary to form neural tissues in the embryo
2. This organizer is represented by the dorsal lip of the blastopore in amphibians and by Hensen's node in birds and mammals
3. The development of amniotes and anamniotes is very similar in terms of cell interactions.

Molecular Biology of Neural Induction

After describing this cell behaviour, the subsequent goal of the laboratories devoted to neural induction is to determine the molecule responsible for such an induction. This molecule has to fulfil different criteria:

1. To be produced by the organizer at the correct place and correct time
2. To be able to reproduce neural induction when ectopically expressed
3. To prevent neural induction if it is knocked down (whichever technique one uses)

In spite of multiple candidates discovered during the late 80s and the early 90s, no molecule fulfils all of these criteria.

Some puzzling results force us to reconsider neural induction. If you culture ectodermal cells after dissociation, these cells will adopt a neuronal type. Anne-Marie Duprat called this process autoneuralization [4]. This result leads to the construction of the so-called neural default model.

Bone morphogenic proteins (BMPs) are secreted by the lateral ectoderm and they promote the formation of epidermis [5, 6]. The organizer secretes anti-BMPs such as chordin, noggin and follistatin that prevent epidermalization of the future neural plate [7, 8]. This model is called the default model and is summarized as follows: "Vertebrate embryonic cells will become nerve cells unless told otherwise" [9].

This "default model" was challenged by the group of Claudio Stern. Indeed, it was observed that fibroblast growth factor (FGF) is mandatory for neural induction before gastrulation [10-12]. Furthermore, Wnt signalling has to be inhibited to permit the action of FGF on neural induction [13].

Whatever the model, the consequence of neural induction is to divide the primitive ectoderm into two derivatives: the neurectoderm (forming the neural plate), which is the primordium of the central nervous system; and the surface ectoderm (which represents the future epidermis).

About neural induction (NI):
- NI takes place very early during embryonic development
- NI precedes the ingression of axial mesoderm
- The notochord cannot be considered as responsible for the induction of the overlying ectoderm to form the neural plate.

Cell Fate during Gastrulation

Gastrulation consists of the formation of the three germinal layers from the epiblast (namely the most surperficial or dorsal tissue of the embryo at that stage). This process has pivotal importance for subsequent development. Indeed, if gastrulation is perturbed, the embryo will die.

The three germinal layers are the ectoderm (for the most dorsal tissue), the mesoderm (for the intermediate tissue) and the endoderm (for the most ventral one). The intermediate layer, i.e., the mesoderm, arises from an induction that takes place at the future caudal pole of the embryo.

The Primitive Streak Forms from Caudal to Rostral

Gastrulation in amniotes begins with the formation of the so-called primitive streak, a condensation of cells that marks the future antero-posterior axis. The primitive streak is also the future zone of mesodermal ingression (a morphogenetic movement that allows mesodermal cells to leave the superficial layer and to form the definitive mesoderm).

The cellular and molecular events that are responsible for the formation of the primitive streak have been particularly well studied in birds. The avian embryo before gastrulation forms a disk located at the upper side of the yolk. The embryonic disk is called the area pellucida, whereas the extra-embryonic region forms the area opaca (Fig. 2.5). The marginal zone is located between the areas opaca and pelluci-

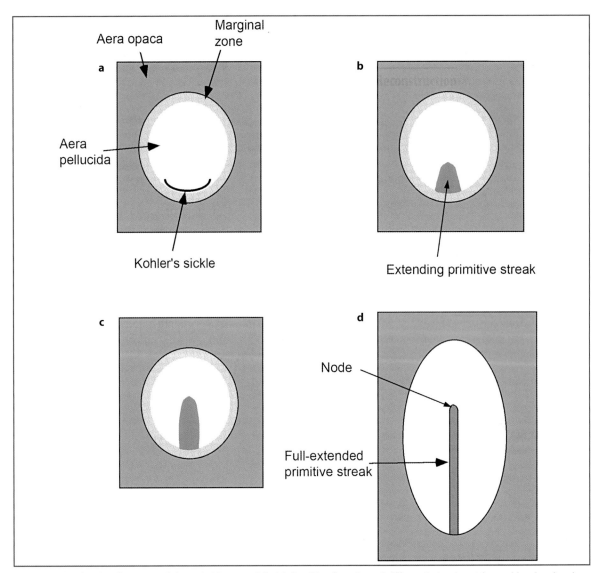

Fig. 2.5 a-d. The development of the primitive streak in birds. **a** The first sign of differentiation is evidenced by the development of the so-called Kohler's sickle located at the future caudal pole of the embryo. At that stage, the embryonic region is composed of the central area pellucida whereas the extra-embryonic region forms the area opaca. In between, one can observe the so-called marginal zone. **b, c** From the region of Kohler's sickle a dense mass of cells develops that migrates from caudal to rostral and forms the primordium of the primitive streak. **d** The streak is now fully elongated. Its extreme rostral region is the avian organizer, namely the node or Hensen's node. Modified from [13a], with permission from Elsevier, Masson, Paris

da. The posterior marginal zone can induce the formation of the primitive streak and does not participate in the formation of embryonic derivatives [14].

Such a result has prime importance in the search for homologies with amphibians in which mesodermal induction has been first described. In amphibians, the vegetative blastomeres (i.e., the more ventral cells of the embryo) induce mesoderm formation in the marginal zone (the region located between the vegetative blastomeres and the animal cap). The dorsal vegetative blastomeres induce the organizer (namely the dorsal lip of the blastopore) without participating in this structure. The dorsal vegetative blastomeres have been called Nieuwkoop's center in memory of the Dutch biologist who described the structure.

Claudio Stern and his group proposed that the posterior marginal zone in birds is homologous to Nieuwkoop's center. The avian marginal zone expresses two genes that code for secreted factors: *Vg1* and *Wnt8C* (limited at the most caudal region of this structure). Forcing the expression of these two genes leads to induction of *Nodal* (a gene that encodes a transforming growth factor beta [TGF-beta]-related protein) (Fig. 2.6) [15]. The cells that expressed *Nodal* will migrate from the caudal region of the embryonic disk to its center. These cells are fated to form the node, the amniotic homologous counterpart of the amphibian organizer. During their migration, these cells generate convergent movements to the midline allowing formation of the primitive streak (Fig. 2.7).

It is likely that these molecular systems are also involved in the control of the primitive streak formation in mammals. Indeed, *Wnt3* is mandatory for the expression of *T*, a key gene responsible for the development of mesodermal progenitors [16].

Formation of the Endoderm and the So-Called Neurenteric Canal

Formation of the Endoderm

At the very beginning of gastrulation, the mammalian embryo is composed of two layers: the superficially-located epiblast and the deeply-located visceral endoderm (Fig. 2.8).

The visceral endoderm does not participate in the formation of the definitive endoderm (or the embryonic endoderm) except for a few cells that pop-

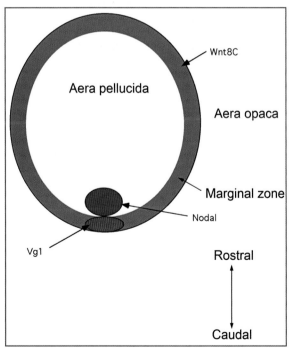

Fig. 2.6. The embryonic disk is in close contact with the marginal zone (an extra-embryonic region that expresses *Wnt8C*). Furthermore, the posterior marginal zone expresses also *Vg1*. The co-expression of these two genes (in *red*) leads to the up-regulation of *Nodal* in the overlying epiblast (in *blue*)

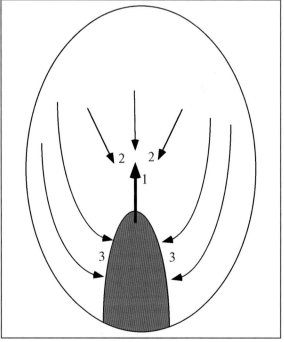

Fig. 2.7. Cell movements during the formation of the primitive streak. The primordium of the streak (*red*) moves from caudal to rostral (*1*). Along the way, cells converge at its rostral tip (*2*) contributing to the formation of the organizer. Furthermore, lateral cells converge to the midline (*3*) aggregating to participate in the formation of the streak

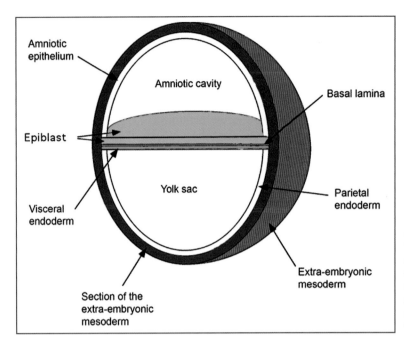

Fig. 2.8. The human embryo just before gastrulation. The embryonic region is represented as a disk composed of two layers: the epiblast that will give rise to the whole embryo and the visceral endoderm (or hypoblast), an extra-embryonic region fated to act as a potent inducer on the overlying epiblast

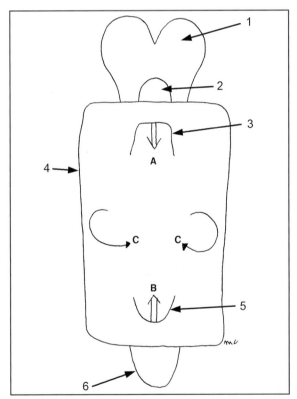

Fig. 2.9. Mouse embryo during the formation of the gut tube (ventral view). Anterior neural plate (*1*); developing foregut (*2*), anterior intestinal pocket (*3*); section of the yolk sac (*4*); posterior intestinal pocket (*5*); developing embryonic tail (*6*). Caudal movements of prospective ventral midline cells that will be eventually located rostral to the yolk sac (*A*). Rostral movements of prospective ventral midline cells that will eventually be located caudal to the yolk sac (*b*). Closure of the lateral endodermal cells (*C*). Redrawn from [20]

ulate both the fore and hindgut [17]. In both chicken and mouse embryos, definitive endodermal cells arise from the node and the most anterior part of the primitive streak [17-19].

The formation of the gut is established according to four major morphogenetic events [20]:

1. The most anterior cells of the definitive endoderm move ventrally and then caudally to give rise to ventral midline cells of the gut situated rostrally to the yolk sac (Fig. 2.9)
2. Endodermal cells that are located at the level of the node give rise to dorsal midline cells of the endoderm [21]
3. Midline cells of the posterior intestinal pocket move rostrally to form the endoderm ventral midline located caudally to the yolk sac
4. Lateral cells converge to the ventral midline and fuse with cells produced by the intestinal pockets.

There is growing evidence that cells in the anterior primitive streak (including the node) can give rise to both mesoderm (axial and paraxial) and endoderm. These cells are named mesendodermal cells [20].

The So-called Neurenteric Canal

The neurenteric canal was first described by Alexander Onoufrievich Kovalevski (1840-1901) in 1877 through observation of *Amphioxus lanceolatus* embryos [22]. This canal is also observed in amphibians and reptiles. The neurenteric canal represents a direct communication between neurectoderm and endoderm located at the caudal end of the notochord (Fig. 2.10) [23].

Such a direct communication has never been found in mammals. For example, the caudal section of a murine embryo does not display any neurenteric canal (Fig. 2.11) [23].

About endoderm formation:
– The so-called di-dermic stage is formed by a superficial epiblast and a deep visceral endoderm
– The epiblast gives rise to the three embryonic layers
– The visceral endoderm does not participate in the formation of the embryo (except for a few endodermic cells)

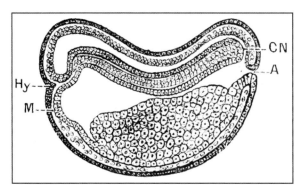

Fig. 2.10. Sagittal view of an embryo from *Bombinator igneus* according to Goette (quoted by Brachet [23]). The neurenteric canal (*CN*) allows a direct communication between the lumen of the neural tube (namely the neurocele) and the lumen of the gut. Anus (*A*); pituitary gland (*Hy*); pharyngeal membrane (*M*)

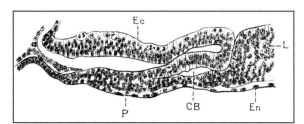

Fig. 2.11. Sagittal section of the caudal moiety of a murine embryo, according to Ed. Van Beneden (quoted by [23]). Blastoporal or chordal canal (*CB*), ectoderm (*Ec*), endoderm (*En*), primitive streak (*L*), axial mesoderm (*P*)

– A true neurenteric canal is never observed in mammals
– The communication between the amniotic cavity and the yolk sac is in fact a notochordal or chordal canal.

One of the salient conclusions of this analysis is that the neurenteric canal cannot account for the emergence of the so-called neurenteric cysts in humans. The genuine mechanism remains to be established.

Mesoderm Induction

In the mouse embryo, the epiblast that will form all the embryonic tissues is in close contact with the so-called extra-embryonic ectoderm. In humans, this region is represented by the amniotic epithelium that connects the epiblast (Fig. 2.8). The extra-embryonic region that is in contact with the epiblast secretes BMP4. Furthermore, the posterior visceral endoderm secretes BMP2, whereas the anterior visceral endoderm secretes anti-BMPs. Consequently, BMPs produced by both the extra-embryonic tissues and the posterior visceral endoderm act by promoting mesoderm formation. In contrast, the anterior is prevented from mesoderm induction by the production of anti-BMPs by the anterior visceral endoderm. This will explain why posterior tissues are converted into mesoderm whereas anterior tissues remain ectodermic.

Gastrulation Movements

The cells of the node and in the primitive streak will give rise to mesodermal derivatives. Cells from the node invaginate rostrally to form the axial mesoderm that is covered by the neural plate (Fig. 2.12) [24]. This mode of formation of the notochord accounts for the development of axial organs from the telencephalon to the hindbrain [24]. After this period, the morphogenetic movements that give rise to the notochord act in a reverse direction, i.e., from rostral to caudal (Fig. 2.13) [21]. An impairment of these axial elongating movements could explain the occurrence of the so-called caudal agenesis syndromes [25].

Lateral mesodermal cells invaginate through the primitive streak, diverge laterally and add to the already formed mesoderm (Figs. 2.12 and 2.13). This mode of growth is responsible for the development of the paraxial, intermediate and lateral domains of the mesoderm. It is interesting to note that the rostrocaudal organization of the primitive streak foreshadows the future medio-lateral mesodermal patterning: the more rostral a cell in the primitive streak, the more medial their derivatives will be (Figs. 2.12 and 2.13).

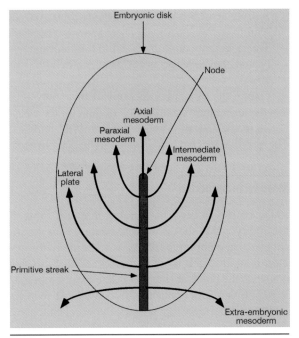

Fig. 2.12. Mesodermal movements at the beginning of gastrulation. The axial mesoderm originates from the node and grows from caudal to rostral. The rest of the mesoderm ingresses and diverges laterally to form the different domains of the mesoderm

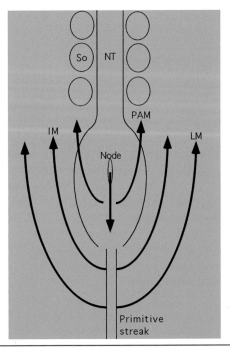

Fig. 2.13. Mesodermal movements from 6-somite stage onwards. The axial mesoderm derives from the node and moves from rostral to caudal. The other mesodermal domains set up as previously described. Neural tube (*NT*), somite (*So*), paraxial mesoderm (*PAM*), intermediate mesoderm (*IM*), lateral mesoderm (*LM*)

About mesoderm formation:

–   Mesoderm forms during gastrulation
–   The primitive streak is induced at the future posterior pole of the embryo
–   Gastrulation is associated with complex cell movements that allow deformation of the embryonic region

The Two Modes of Neurulation

Neurulation is the embryonic stage that allows the transformation of the flat neural plate into the neural tube. This is due to a series of morphogenetic movements. In fact, neurulation is far from being a simple process since different mechanisms act at different antero-posterior levels of the neural primordium. Two main types of neurulations have been described: primary and secondary.

Primary Neurulation

Gary Schoenwolf and his group have proposed the classic description of the morphogenetic movements affecting the neural plate during primary neurulation in the chick embryo [26-28]. Neural induction leads to the formation of the neurectoderm that appears as a flat sheet of cells forming an oval structure located anteriorly to Hensen's node. Two phases of morphogenetic movements allow the neural plate to produce the neural tube, namely shaping and bending.

Shaping of the Neural Plate

Shaping consists of the morphogenetic movements that are responsible for the conversion of the oval neural plate into the narrow spinal plate and the wide brain plate [29]. To illustrate such movements, it is possible to mark the neural plate with fluorescent dyes and study its subsequent deformation (Fig. 2.14) [30].

The result of this experiment shows that lateral cells converge to the midline and that medial tissue elongates according to the antero-posterior axis. Three events account for this deformation: apicobasal thickening, transverse narrowing and longitudinal lengthening [26, 28, 31-33].

Apicobasal Thickening

The thickening is mainly due to a change of the shape of the cells. Neural plate cells will transform from cubic to prismatic [34]. This transformation leads to

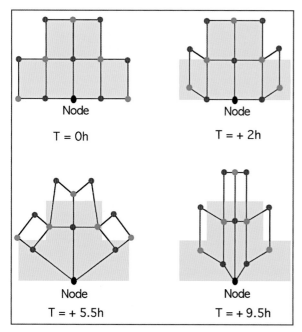

Fig. 2.14. The deformation of the avian neural plate during shaping showing both transverse narrowing and longitudinal lengthening. Modified from [30]

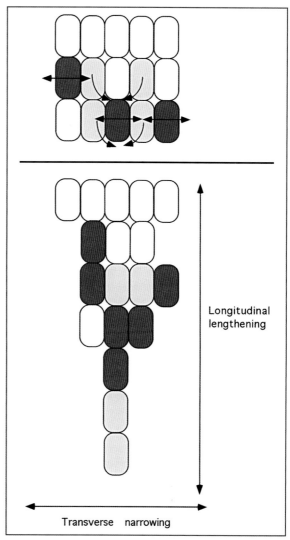

Fig. 2.15. Intercalation of cells accounting for both longitudinal lengthening and mediolateral narrowing. The respective movements of the cells are illustrated by *arrows*

an increase in the height of the neural cells. Such a feature is also observed in both amphibians, birds and mammals [34]. Treatments that depolarize microtubules prevent cell apicobasal thickening [35].

Transverse Narrowing

Apicobasal thickening leads to transverse narrowing as illustrated in Fig. 2.14. Furthermore, cell rearrangement (intercalation) also participates in this morphogenetic movement. During rearrangement, cells converge on the midline and intercalate with cells already present in this region (Fig. 2.15).

This cell event produces both transverse narrowing and longitudinal extension. Such coordinated movements are a general feature observed during vertebrate development. These are described as convergence-extension movements. They account for the major force that drives gastrulation and neurulation in amphibians. It is interesting to note that mutations of genes involved in the control of convergent-extension movements have been associated with neural tube defects in vertebrates [36, 37].

Longitudinal Lengthening

As already mentioned, intercalation accounts for longitudinal lengthening. Furthermore, cell mitoses are not randomly orientated, as the mitotic spindle is oriented according to the antero-posterior axis. Consequently, the two daughter cells are arranged along this axis allowing axial elongation [31].

When one separates the neural primordium from neighbouring tissues, the primordium underlies correct shaping [29, 31, 33, 38, 39]. This result demonstrates that shaping is due to intrinsic forces generated within the neural anlage.

Bending of the Neural Plate

Bending takes place after shaping and involves morphogenetic movements that allow the transformation of neural primoridum into the neural groove and then of the neural tube. Two events account for bending: furrowing and folding.

Furrowing

A medial furrow develops in the midline of the neural plate. This is due to a modification of the shape of midline cells that transform from prismatic to wedged-shape. The flat neural plate is deformed to adopt a V-shape, this structure is called the neural groove. The medial region of the neural plate is called the medial hinge point (Fig. 2.16) [39, 40].

This modification of the shape of the medial cells is accompanied by an increase in the duration of the cell cycle, whereas the cell cycle is not modified for the lateral cells of the neural plate [40]. Furrowing has been inhibited by the ablation of the node [41]. Although it is known that the node gives rise to both floor plate and notochord at the spinal level [21], it is possible to propose an alternative explanation. Removing the node will prevent the formation of both the floor plate and the notochord. It is thus impossible to be sure that the notochord is responsible for the wedging of midline neural plate cells. It is interesting to note that the group of Schoenwolf described furrowing as an intrinsic process of the neural primordium in subsequent papers [27, 31]. The role of microfilaments in the control of furrowing was also assessed by Schoenwolf's group [32]. Treating avian embryos with cytochalasin D does not prevent furrowing. Thus, the wedging of medial cells is largely independent of microfilaments.

Folding

Folding is characterized by the morphogenetic movement of upfolding of the lateral borders of the neural plate. This is due to the formation of the medial hinge point (Fig. 2.16) and to the successive lateral hinge points (Fig. 2.17). These lateral hinge points are very similar to the medial one in terms of cell shape. These movements allow the lateral borders of the neural plate (i.e., the neural folds) to converge on the dorsal midline and to fuse together (Fig. 2.17). It is interesting to note that these morphogenetic movements are driven by extrinsic forces mainly provided by the surface ectoderm [39].

The Mechanisms of Neurulation Differ According to the Position of the Neural Plate in the Antero-Posterior Axis

At the spinal level the mouse neural tube does not follow a uniform mode of neural tube formation [42]. A unique medial hinge point is formed at the rostral cervical levels. There are no lateral hinge points in this region. The classic model we describe applies to intermediate levels. Bending affects all the cells of the caudal neural tube leading to a region of the neural tube where the lumen is circular. This diversity in the mechanism of formation of the neural tube may explain the occurrence of neural tube defects at different levels of the spine without involvement of either rostral or caudal levels. For example, anencephaly is generally limited to the cephalic zone (Fig. 2.18) except for craniorachischisis (Fig. 2.19). In some cases, the malformative process is segmental, affecting the thoracic and upper lumbar regions but preserving the cervical and the lumbo-sacral ones (Fig. 2.20).

Consequently, it is of prime importance to note that the genes involved in the control of neurulation at the different antero-posterior levels are different [43]. For example, in the mouse, *AP-2*, *Cart1*, *Hes1* and *Twist* are involved in cranial neural tube defects whereas *Axd* and *vl* are linked with spinal defects.

The So-Called Multi-Site Closure Theory

To account for the emergence of segmented NTDs, some authors propose that fusion of the neural tube proceeds at different sites. This concept was first put forward in the mouse [44, 45]. However, the situation is far from being simple: the respective location of the different sites varies among mouse strains [45] and according to the species [46, 47]. In humans, some authors do not describe multiple sites of closure [48], whereas others do [49].

About primary neurulation:
– Shaping involves apicobasal thickening, transverse narrowing, and longitudinal lengthening

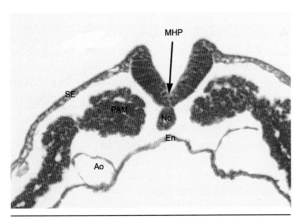

Fig. 2.16. Transverse section of a chick embryo. Aorta (*Ao*), endoderm (*En*), medial hinge point (*MHP*), notochord (*No*), paraxial mesoderm (*PAM*), superficial ectoderm (*SE*)

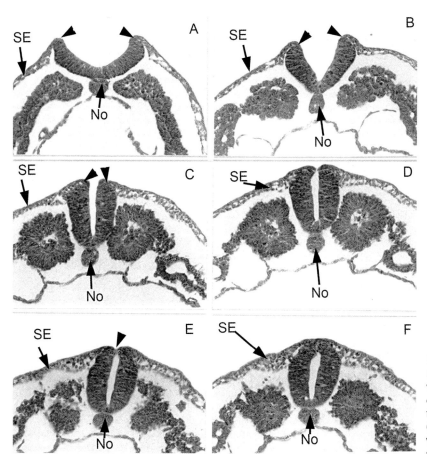

Fig. 2.17. A summary of primary neurulation on successive transverse sections of an 8-somite stage chick embryo. Notochord (*No*), surface ectoderm (*SE*), neural folds (*arrowhead*). Modified from [49a], with permission from Elsevier, Masson, Paris

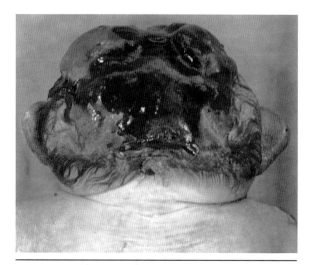

Fig. 2.18. Dorsal view of a fetus aged of 32 gestation weeks suffering anencephaly. Note that the neck is normal

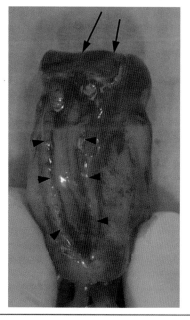

Fig. 2.19. Dorsal view of a fetus aged of 10 weeks of gestation suffering craniorachischisis. Cephalic area (*arrows*); spinal cord (*arrowheads*)

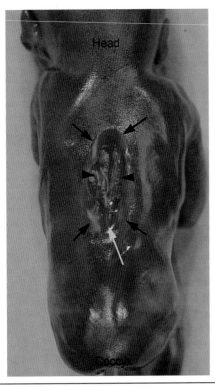

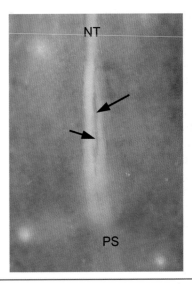

Fig. 2.21. Dorsal view of the caudal region of a chick embryo (15-somite stage). The neural tube (*NT*) is still open at its caudal end (*arrows*). Primitive streak (*PS*)

Fig. 2.20. Dorsal view of a fetus aged 16 weeks of gestation presenting a segmented spinal bifida. Neural plate (*arrowheads*); skin malformation (*black arrows*); and the caudal neural tube (*gray arrow*)

– Bending involves both furrowing and folding
– The mechanisms that account for neurulation are not the same along the antero-posterior axis
– The multi-site closure theory should be applied carefully for deciphering NTDs

Secondary Neurulation

Descriptive Embryology

Primary neurulation proceeds according to a cephalo-caudal gradient which is a general feature of amniote development. It is important to note that neurulation develops more rapidly than elongation of the embryonic axis. Consequently, the neural tube will close before axis extension is completed. The posterior neuropore corresponds to the last part of the primary neural plate that closes (Fig. 2.21).

After closure of the posterior neuropore, the caudal tissues, which are the remnants of Hensen's node and primitive streak, form the so-called tail bud or caudal eminence (Fig. 2.22) [50].

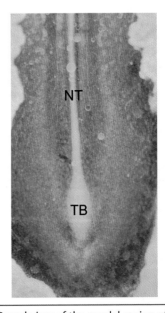

Fig. 2.22. Dorsal view of the caudal region of a chick embryo (20-somite stage). The neural tube (*NT*) is closed. The tail bud (*TB*) lies caudally to the NT

The stage of closure of the posterior neuropore depends on the species. In the chick, the neural tube closes at the 16-22 somite-stage [51]. In the mouse, it closes at the 27-29 somite-stage [52]. In the hamster, it closes at the 21 somite-stage [53] and lastly, in humans, at the 21-29 somite-stage (corresponding to 26 postovulatory days) [54].

The caudal part of the spinal cord derives from the development of the tail bud. In this region, neurulation proceeds according to a different morphological process called secondary neurulation [55]. Secondary neurulation was first described in the chick embryo in 1911 [56]. The cells from the tail bud (Figs. 2.22 and 2.23e) [57] aggregate in the midline (Fig. 2.23d) and participate in the formation of a cord (namely, the medullary cord). This cord undergoes cavitation with multiple lumens (Fig 2.23b) that communicate with the lumen formed by primary neurulation (Fig. 2.24). All the lumens then coalesce to form a neural tube with a single lumen (Figs. 2.23a and 2.24). This mode of formation explains why secondary neurulation is sometimes referred to as neurulation by cavitation.

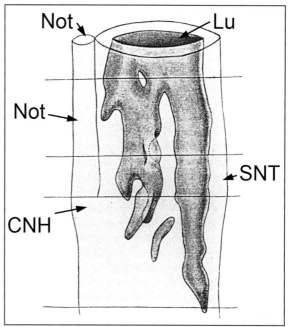

Fig. 2.24. Three-dimensional reconstruction of the lumens (*Lu*) produced by cavitation in the secondary neural tube (*SNT*) of a chick embryo. Chordo-neural hinge (*CNH*), notochord (*Not*). Modified from [57]

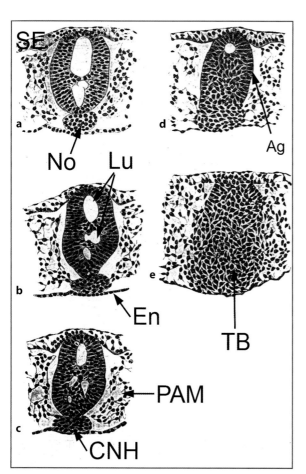

Fig. 2.23 a-e. Successive transverse sections of a chick embryo (**a** is the most rostral one and **e** is most caudal). Midline aggregation (*Ag*); chordo-neural hinge (*CNH*); endoderm (*En*); lumens (*Lu*); notocochord (*No*); paraxial mesoderm (*PAM*); surface ectoderm (*SE*); tail bud (*TB*). Modified from [57]

The Two Classic Conceptions of the Tail Bud

Until recently, there was controversy about the mode of formation of the caudal spinal cord from the tail bud.

The Tail Bud Functions as a Blastema

David Holmdahl [58] considered the cells of the tail bud as multipotent precursors that can give rise to the notochord, neural tube, endoderm and mesoderm. The tail bud is thus a blastema responsible for the growth of the caudal part of the body. Furthermore, the caudal region is built without forming the classical germinal layers. This constitutes an important exception to the general feature of gastrulation.

The Tail Bud is a Mosaic of Territories

The tail bud, according to Jean Pasteels [59], results from the morphogenetic movements taking place earlier during development. The uniformity of the structure is only due to the poorly-differentiated cells at this stage but Pasteels considered that the tail bud is in fact a mosaic of territories that are already engaged in a specific way in development. For him, gastrulation is still active in this region.

Constructing a Fate Map of the Tail Bud

To try to solve the discrepancy between these two theories, we used the quail-chick chimera technique (Fig. 2.25) in order to follow the fate of precise groups of cells (Fig. 2.26) [55] The salient features of this fate map are:

1. Both notochord and floor plate derive from the chordo-neural hinge (Figs. 2.23, 2.24, 2.27, 2.28), which represents Hensen's node remnants.
2. The rostral part of the tail bud (region 2 in Fig. 2.26) gives rise to the lateral walls and the roof of the neural tube. Furthermore, it also participates in the formation of the somites.
3. The caudal tail bud (region 3 in Fig. 2.26) is not able to generate neural structures and only participates in the formation of the somites.

These results are highly supportive of Pasteels' conception of the tail bud.

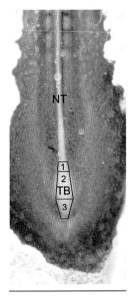

Fig. 2.26. The different grafted territories shown in Figure 2.22. Region *1* is rostral and involves the chordo-neural hinge, region *2* is intermediate, region *3* is caudal. Neural tube (*NT*); tail tube (*TB*)

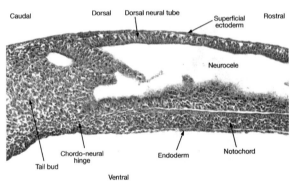

Fig. 2.27. Sagittal section of the caudal part of a chick embryo (25-somite stage) showing the location of the chordo-neural hinge and the tail bud

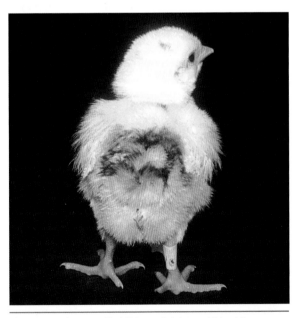

Fig. 2.25. The so-called "Pâques" chimera. This chimera was obtained after grafting a quail tail bud from a 25-somite stage quail into a chick host at the same stage. The pigmentation pattern shows that the graft contributes to the caudal part of the body

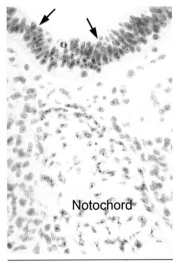

Fig. 2.28. A quail-chick chimera produced by grafting region 1 (see Fig. 2.26). The chordo-neural hinge gives rise to both notochord and floor plate (Feulgen-Rossenbeck staining)

Continuous Processes Act during both Primary and Secondary Neurulations

Fate mapping of the neural primordium at the 6-somite stage (Fig. 2.29) [21] shows that (1) Hensen's node differentiates into the notochord and floor plate of both the primary and the secondary neural tubes, (2) the primordium of the secondary neural tube lies initially at the caudal border of the neural plate and (3) that the cells located in the primitive streak generate all the mesodermal derivatives. So the primary organization of neural precursors does not differ even if they are fated to form a primary or a secondary neural tube. Furthermore, the node gives rise to a chordo-neural hinge indicating a high level of similarities between the two modes of neurulation.

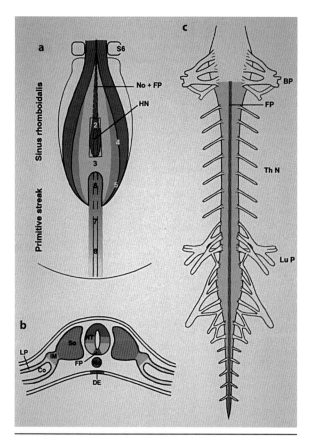

Fig. 2.29 a-c. a Dorsal view of a 6-somite stage chick embryo. Derivatives of the different regions grafted at 6-somite stage are evidenced on **b** transverse section of the embryo and **c** on a ventral view of the spinal cord. Brachial plexus (*BP*); coelome (*Co*); dorsal endoderm (*DE*); floor plate (*FP*); Hensen's node (*HN*); intermediate mesoderm (*IM*); lateral plate (*LP*); lumbar plexus (*LuP*); notochord (*No*); neural tube (*NT*); sixth somite (*S6*); somite (*So*); thoracic nerves (*ThN*). Reproduced from [21], with permission

About secondary neurulation:

– The secondary neural tube forms by cavitation
– The primordium of this tube is located at the caudal border of the neural plate
– There is growing evidence that primary and secondary neurulation proceed as continuous morphogenetic processes

Embryonic Interpretation of Open NTDs

It is now widely accepted that open NTDs are caused by an impairment of the morphogenetic movements taking place during neurulation (Fig. 2.30). The consequence of such a malformation is that the neural tissue is in contact with the amniotic fluid. Prolonged contact with this fluid is deleterious and leads to destruction of the neural tissue. Some groups, consequently, propose to cover the malformation in utero in order to limit the risks of secondary destruction.

Other malformations can be associated with myelomeningocele, namely Chiari II [60]: a portion of the cerebellum is located in an enlarged cervical vertebral canal. Furthermore, the fourth ventricle lies in the cervical canal. The posterior fossa is small with a low situated cerebellar tentorium (Fig. 3.31) [61]. Such a malformation is never observed in embryos but begins to appear during fetal life, indicating that this is not a primary abnormality but a secondary event [62].

Several explanations have been proposed to account for the emergence of Chiari II malformation in spina bifida: Penfield and Coburn [63] reported

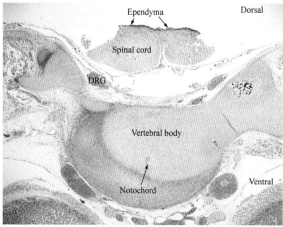

Fig. 2.30. Transverse section of a fetus (28 weeks of gestation) presenting a myelomeningocele. The ependyma is in contact with the amniotic fluid. The neural plate is destroyed as is the rule in this type of malformation. Dorsal root ganglion (*DRG*)

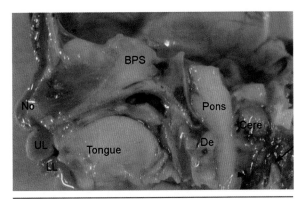

Fig. 2.31. Sagittal section of the head of a fetus interrupted at 20 weeks of gestation for a myelomeningocele. Posterior arch of C1 (*arrow*); most caudal tissue of the cerebellum (*arrowheads*) (*Cere*); basi-presphenoide (*BPS*); dens (*De*); lower lip (*LL*); nose (*No*); upper lip (*UL*)

the case of a 29 year old woman who had a thoracic (T4) spina bifida operated at the age of 3. The patient died and the autopsy showed a classic Chiari II malformation with hydrocephalus (Fig. 2.32). Furthermore, the authors reported that the direction of the cervical roots and nerves was abnormal, growing upwards instead of horizontally (Fig. 2.33). They proposed that the thoracic spina bifida led to a downward traction responsible for the descent of the cerebellum. However, this feature is far from constant in myelomeningocele, shedding doubt on this explanation. The most widely accepted theory was put forward by McLone and Knepper [64]. The open malformation leads to a leakage of cerebrospinal fluid (CSF), lowering pressure in the fourth ventricle. This prevents the correct expansion of the posterior fossa, which remains small with the tentorium in a low position. When the cerebellar primordium grows, the little posterior fossa cannot support this growth, leading to herniation in the cervical canal.

It is quite common to observe subependymal nodules at the level of the lateral ventricles [65]. In our fetal material, these nodules are preferentially located at the level of the occipital lobe (Fig. 2.34). Their position is subependymal (Fig. 2.35) and they are constituted of undifferentiated cells with various cells expressing glial fibrillary acidic protein (GFAP) (Fig. 2.36).

Hydrocephalus is a frequent complication of spina bifida. While it is never observed during embryonic life, it appears in fetuses [62]. Such is also the case for hydromyelia.

Craniolacunae can be observed in myelomeningocele (Fig. 2.37) [65]. The mechanism of their formation is largely unknown and they are not associated with hydrocephalus.

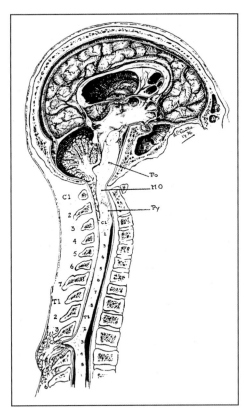

Fig. 2.32. Schematic drawing of the malformation. Reproduced from [63], with permission

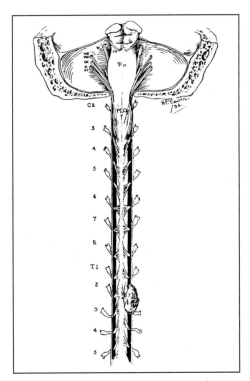

Fig. 2.33. The vertical trajectory of the cervical roots rostral to the malformation. Reproduced from [63], with permission

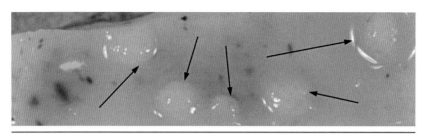

Fig. 2.34. A ventrionic view of the occipital horn in a fetus (33 weeks of gestation) suffering a lumbosacral myelomeningocele. *Arrows* point to periventricular heterotopias

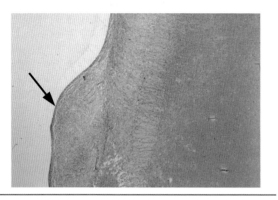

Fig. 2.35. Histological aspect of the previous case. The nodule (*arrow*) lies under the ependyma (H&E staining)

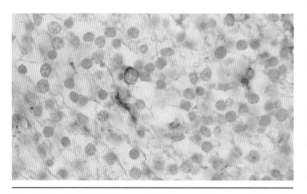

Fig. 2.36. Histological aspect of the previous case. The cells are undifferentiated. A few cells express GFAP (immunohistochemistry against GFAP)

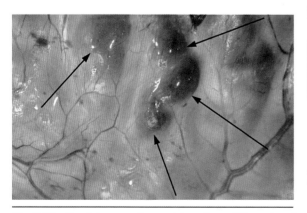

Fig. 2.37. Craniolacunae (*arrows*) in a fetus (35 weeks of gestation) presenting a lumbosacral myelomeningocele

The Neural Tube is Polarized According to the Ventro-dorsal Axis

After its formation by neurulation, the neural tube is composed of the roof (the most dorsal region), the alar plate, the basal plate and the floor (Fig. 2.38).

In fact, this polarization begins before neurulation. The notochord lies underneath the medial neural plate and acts by secreting ventralizing factors. The lateral regions of the neural plate undergo the dorsalizing action of the surface ectoderm that lies at the border of the neural plate. The genes that are expressed by the cells of the neural tube differ according to their position along the ventro-dorsal axis.

It is Possible to Induce an Extra Floor-Plate by Grafting either a Notochord or a Floor-Plate

Grafting a quail notochord close to the lateral wall of a neural tube in a chick embryo leads to the formation of an additional floor plate developed by the chick and facing the grafted quail notochord (Fig. 2.39) [40, 66-68]. Such a result can be mimicked by grafting a floor-plate instead of a notochord [68].

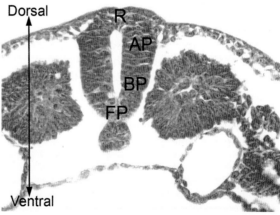

Fig. 2.38. Transverse section of a 10-somite stage chick embryo showing the ventrodorsal polarization of the neural tube. Alar plate (*AP*), basal plate (*BP*), floor plate (*FP*), roof (*R*) (violet cresyl staining)

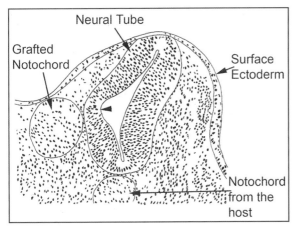

Fig. 2.39. Transverse section of a chick embryo in which a notochord was inserted in contact with the wall of the neural plate. After re-incubation, one sees the development of an extra floor-plate deriving from the host and in contact with the graft

Removing the Notochord Prevents the Formation of the Floor Plate

In the chick embryo, it is possible to microdissect the notochord and to remove it [40, 68-70]. These authors conclude that the floor-plate does form after removing the notochord. This confirms the concept of a mandatory induction of the floor-plate by the underlying notochord.

However, the correct interpretation of the extirpation experiments requires that only the notochord be removed, leaving the floor-plate primordium in the embryo. Furthermore, at the caudal pole of the body, the notochord is firmly attached to the floor-plate (see our Fig. 2.27). This prompted Teillet et al. [71] to reproduce the former experiments and to analyse the tissues that have been really removed. They found that it is technically impossible to selectively remove the notochord without removing the floor-plate.

About the relationships between the notochord and the floor-plate:
– A notochord is able to induce a floor-plate
– A floor-plate is able to induce a floor-plate
– The precise temporal pattern of this induction remains to be established during embryonic development

Sonic Hedgehog and the Floor-Plate

Sonic hedgehog (SHH) is a morphogene that is homologous to Drosophila's *hedgehog*. The protein needs post-translational modifications that are mandatory for its function [72]. It is cleaved into a C-terminal domain that stays in the cytoplasm and an N-terminal domain that is secreted and acts on a membranous receptor, namely Patched [73]. Patched acts with a co-receptor called Smoothened. The cytoplasmic effectors of the SHH pathways are mediated by GLI1, 2 or 3.

Some groups reported an induction of an ectopic floor-plate by adding SHH laterally to the neural tube [74, 75]. Furthermore, the mouse mutant *Gli2* -/- develops a notochord but no floor-plate [76]. Consequently, the SHH pathway plays a crucial role in controlling the interactions between notochord and floor-plate.

Sonic Hedgehog and the Ventral Development of the Neural Tube

The role of *SHH* is far from limited to the induction of a floor-plate. Indeed, if the SHH signal is impaired, Patched directly induces cell death in the ventral neural tube [77]. This shows the complexity of this molecular system (acting by an action produced by Patched and another action produced by the GLIs according to the absence or the presence of the ligand). In the case of deprivation of SHH, apoptosis removes all the ventral primordium. The remnants are thus the dorsal moiety of the neural tube and cannot be interpreted as a problem of dorsalization.

SHH plays a very important role in controlling the development of the so-called ventral subdomains [72]. SHH is able to activate the transcription of genes and to repress the transcription of others. Furthermore, there are pairs of genes that are mutually exclusively expressed (if one gene is activated the other is repressed and vice-versa). This leads to the definition of subdomains that are characterized by a unique molecular address. For example, the subdomain that is fated to form motoneurons expresses *Nkx6.1*, *Olig2* and *Pax6* [72]. Since the notochord is active before the movements of neurulation, it is thus possible to show differentiated motoneurons in the malformative spinal cord (Fig. 2.40).

Dorsalization of the Neural Tube Involved the TGF-β Family of Secreted Molecules

A very similar mechanism takes place at the dorsal part of the neural tube. Different members of the TGF-β family participate in the dorsalization of the neural tube [72, 78, 79] and are able to dorsalize the cells of the neural tube.

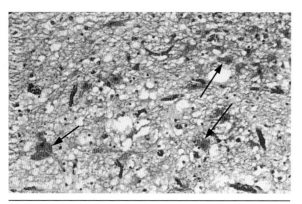

Fig. 2.40. Histological section of a myelomeningocele showing differentiated motoneurons (*arrows*). Hemateineosin staining

Since axial organs may produce anti-BMPs, the ventral region of the neural tube acts also to control the development of its dorsal moiety [80].

As for the basal plate of the neural tube, the BMP pathway leads to the development of different subdomains (dP1 to dP6) that represent the progenitors of dorsal interneurons in the spinal cord [72, 81].

The Peripheral Nervous System Develops from the Neural Crest

From the roof of the spinal neural tube, a population of cells is segregated and emerges to give rise to neural crest cells (Fig. 2.41) This population is able to extensively migrate to differentiate in situ into melanocytes, neurons of the dorsal root ganglia, neu-

rons of the vegetative ganglia and Schwann cells and into adrenal cells of the medulla gland. The situation is much more complex in the head and is obviously beyond the scope of this chapter.

The unique elements of the peripheral nervous system that is yielded by the neural tube are the axons arising from the motoneurons. Interested readers can find an extensive analysis of neural crest cells in Le Douarin and Kalcheim [82].

Migration of Neural Crest Cells

The Three Streams of Migration of the Trunk Neural Crest

Primordial cells located in the neural tube loose their epithelial characteristics. They are then isolated and migrate along the extra-cellular matrix. It is easy to recognize three streams of migration from the neural tube. The dorsal stream is located between the dermatome and the surface ectoderm. This stream will eventually give rise to melanocytes. The ventro-lateral stream invades the rostral moiety of the somite (the caudal moiety of this structure is not permeable to neural crest cells and does not allow the growth of motoneuronal axons). The cells that migrate in this location will differentiate into dorsal root ganglia. The last stream lies between the neural tube and the medial border of the somite. These cells will contribute to the formation of the vegetative elements of the peripheral nervous system.

The Molecular Control of Neural Crest Migration (see [83] for a review)

Extracellular Matrix and Migration

The components of the extracellular matrix are different in the rostral part of the somite compared to its caudal part [84-87]. Furthermore, the receptors expressed by the cells are different [88]. This explains why the rostral moiety of the somite is permeable whereas its caudal one is not.

The Formation of the Roots and the Plexus

Nerve Roots and Dorsal Root Ganglia are Patterned by the Intrinsic Properties of the Somites

Due to their specific molecular expression and by the molecules accumulated in the matrix, neural

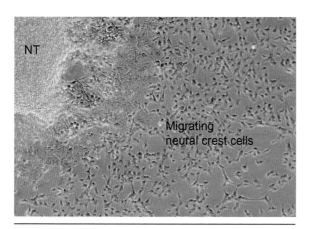

Fig. 2.41. A quail neural tube (*NT*) was dissected from the surrounding tissues and put in culture. After 3 days, migrating cells can be seen; they represent neural crest cells

crest cells can only migrate into the rostral half of the somite. The consequence of this is that the continuous flow of neural crest cells arising from the roof of the neural tube is separated into discrete foci. Each focus will give rise to a dorsal root ganglion, explaining why these peripheral nervous structures are segmented contrarily to neural crest cells. It is possible, experimentally, to disrupt this arrangement by grafting only rostral somites. This leads to the formation of a huge unsegmented ganglion [89].

What About the Most Caudal Part of the Spinal Cord?

The most caudal part of the spinal cord in mammals is characterized by the presence of the so-called filum terminale. This region derives from the caudal neural tube but is devoid of both motor and sensory nerves. Our group uses the chick caudal neural tube as a homolog of this region in order to try to understand why these anatomical features develop. One of the salient features of this region is that neural crest cells cannot generate any neurons (explaining the absence of dorsal root ganglia) [90]. Furthermore, this region cannot generate motoneurons. We are currently dissecting the molecular pathways that account for this fact.

The Spine Develops from the Somite

Early Somites Mature to Form Three Derivatives

The origin of pre-somitic cells before gastrulation is the rostral region of the primitive streak [19]. These undergo an epithelio-mesenchymatous transition allowing them to form the intermediate primordial layer (i.e., the medoserm). They then migrate laterally and adopt a paraxial phenotype. The fate of these cells differs according to the antero-posterior axis. The most anterior cells will eventually form the cephalic mesoderm that participates in the formation of the head region. However, this important developmental problem will not be discussed in this chapter.

First, the paraxial trunk mesoderm is unsegmented and as development proceeds, epithelial spheres, called somites, are formed in a cephalo-caudal gradient. An epithelial somite is constituted of an epithelial wall and a mesenchymatous core. These two regions are not true compartments since cells are intensively mixing and migrating from one part of the somite to the other and vice-versa. The epithelial somite matures during development and this maturation proceeds according to a cephalo-caudal gradient. This maturation leads to dissociation of the epithelial somite that forms the dermatome (dorsal), the myotome (intermediate) and the sclerotome (ventral). The dermatome is located underneath the surface ectoderm. It will give rise to dermal cells for the dorsal moiety of the body (the ventral dermal cells originate from the somatopleure). The myotome gives rise to all the striated muscle fibres of the body. The sclerotomal cells differentiate into cartilaginous cells of the vertebrae, cells of the intervertebral discs and ligaments, and cells of the spinal meninges. Furthermore, the somite gives rise to endothelial cells. It is important to note that the sclerotome is first located ventrally and then it spreads to enwrap the entire neural tube forming at its dorsal face the so-called dorsal mesoderm. This dorsal mesoderm is a late appearing structure because the neural tube and the surface ectoderm are tightly apposed just after neurulation, the interepithelial space being permeable late after the achievement of neurulation [91].

The Somite is not Polarized According to the Ventro-Dorsal Axis

The ventral part of the somite differentiates into the sclerotome, whereas its dorsal part will give rise to the dermatome and myotome. This difference between the fates of the hemi-somite is not fixed when the somite segments. Indeed, if one rotates the somite according to the ventro-dorsal axis, the new ventral hemi-somite (which was initially dorsal) gives rise to the sclerotome. The new dorsal hemi-somite (formerly ventral) differentiates into the dermatome and myotome. This shows that the fate of the hemi-somites is not fixed and can be changed by the environment.

The ventralization of the somite is promoted by notochord and floor plate [92] as is the case for neural tube ventralization. The dorsalization of the somite is promoted by the surface ectoderm and the dorsal neural tube [93, 94].

Which Molecules are Responsible for the Ventro-dorsal Polarity of the Somites?

The sclerotome formation is elicited by the secretion of Sonic hedgehog by the notochord and floor plate [94, 95]. If you perform a knock-out of the *Shh* gene in the mouse, no vertebral structures develop since their sclerotomes fail to form. The dorsal moiety of the somite (i.e., the dermatome and the myotome) are induced by BMPs [96]. SHH (which is secreted by both the floor plate and the notochord) induces the expression of *Gli1* whereas *Gli2* and *Gli3* are induced by the dorsal region mediated by the Wnts [97].

The Neural Tube and the Notochord Induce the Formation of the Vertebral Cartilage

It is well known from classic studies of tissue recombination that the neural tube and the notochord can induce (together or in isolation) the formation of cartilaginous cells from the somite [98, 99]. It is important to note that notochord and neural tube behave differently according to cartilage induction. The induced cartilage is contiguous with the notochord,

whereas it is always at some distance from the neural tissue [99]. It can be postulated that the neural tube induces meningeal tissue in close contact and cartilage at a distance.

One striking result about vertebra formation is that three domains can be recognized within the vertebrae [76, 100]. The ventral domain is responsible for the formation of the vertebral body and is controlled by *Gli2* [76, 101]. The neural arch of the vertebra forms the second domain and is under the control of *Gli3* [101]. At last, the dorsal domain (which derives from the so-called dorsal mesoderm) differentiates into the spinous process. This dorsal domain depends on the dorsal neural tube, on surface ectoderm and on BMP4 [100]. These different sub-domains in the development of the vertebrae may explain some human spine malformations selectively affecting the dorsal domain and sparing the ventrolateral one, as in the case of spina bifida with lipoma [102].

References

1. Spemann H, Mangold H (1924) Über Induktion von Embryonalanlagen durch Implantation artfremder Organisatoren. Wilhelm Roux Arch Entw Mech Org 100:599-638
2. Waddington CH (1933) Induction by the primitive streak and its derivatives in the chick. J Exp Biol 10:38-48
3. Waddington CH (1936) Organizers in mammalian development. Nature 138:125
4. Duprat AM, Kan P, Gualandris L et al (1985) Neural induction: embryonic determination elicits full expression of specific neuronal traits. J Embryol Exp Morpho 89; Supplement:167-183
5. Wilson PA, Hemmati-Brivanlou A (1995) Induction of epidermis and inhibition of neural fate by BMP-4. Nature 376:331-333
6. Suzuki A, Kaneko E, Ueno N, Hemmati-Brivanlou A (1997) Regulation of epidermal induction by BMP2 and BMP7 signaling. Dev Biol 189:112-122
7. Piccolo S, Sasai Y, Lu B, De Robertis EM (1996) Dorsoventral patterning in Xenopus: inhibition of ventral signals by direct binding of chordin to BMP-4. Cell 86:589-598
8. Zimerman LB, De Jesus-Escobar JM, Harland RM (1996) The Spemann organizer signal noggin binds and inactivates bone morphogenetic protein 4. Cell 86:599-606
9. Hemmati-Brivanlou A, Melton DA (1997) Vertebrate embryonic cells will become nerve cells unless told otherwise. Cell 88:13-17
10. Streit A, Berliner AJ, Papanayotou C et al (2000) Initiation of neural induction by FGF signalling before gastrulation. Nature 406:74-78
11. Mitchell TS, Sheets MD (2001) The FGFR pathway is required for the trunk-inducing functions of Spemann's organizer. Dev Biol 237:295-305

12. Stern CD (2006) Neural induction: 10 years on since the "default model". Curr Opin Cell Biol 18:692-697
13. Wilson SI, Rydström A, Trimborn T et al (2001) The status of Wnt signalling regulates neural and epidermal fates in the chick embryo. Nature 411:325-330
13a. Catala M (2006) Embryologie, développement précoce chez l'humain. 3th edn. Masson, Paris
14. Bachvarova RF, Skromme I, Stern CD (1998) Induction of primitive streak and Hensen's node by the posterior marginal zone in the early chick embryo. Development 125:3521-3534
15. Skromme I, Stern CD (2002) A hierarchy of gene expression accompanying induction of the primitive streak by Vg1 in the chick embryo. Mech Dev 114:115-118
16. Stappert J, Bauer A, Kispert A et al (2000) Brachyury is a target gene of the Wnt/beta-catenin signalling pathway. Mech Dev 91:249-258
17. Tam PP, Beddington RS (1992) Establishment and regionalization of germ layers in the gastrulating mouse embryo. Ciba Found Symp 165:27-41
18. Lawson KA, Meneses JJ, Pedersen RA (1991) Clonal analysis of epiblast fate during germ layers formation in the mouse embryo. Development 113:891-911
19. Psychoyos D, Stern CD (1996) Fates and migratory routes of primitive streak cells in the chick embryo. Development 122:1523-1534
20. Lewis SL, Tam PPL (2006) Definitive endoderm of the mouse embryo: formation, cells fates, and morphogenetic function. Dev Dyn 235:2315-2329
21. Catala M, Teillet M-A, De Robertis EM, Le Douarin NM (1996) A spinal cord fate map in the avian embryo: while regressing, Hensen's node lays down the notochord and floor plate thus joining the spinal cord lateral walls. Development 122:2599-2610

22. Neuhauser EBD, Kaufmann HJ (1961) A.O. Kovalevski and the neurenteric canal: a note on some historical inaccurancies. Proc R Soc Med 54:927-929

23. Brachet A (1935) Traité d'embryologie des vertébrés. Masson, Paris

24. Patten I, Kulesa P, Shen MM et al (2003) Distinct modes of floor plate induction in the chick embryo. Development 130:4809-4821

25. Catala M (2002) Genetic control of caudal development. Clin Genet 61:89-96

26. Schoenwolf GC, Smith JL (1990) Mechanisms of neurulation: traditional viewpoint and recent advances. Development 109:243-270

27. Schoenwolf GC (1991) Cell movements in the epiblast during gastrulation and neurulation in avian embryos. In: Keller R (ed) Gastrulation. Plenum Press, New York, pp 1-28

28. Colas J-F, Schoenwolf GC (2003) Towards a cellular and molecular understanding of neurulation. Dev Dynamics 221:117-145

29. Moury JD, Schoenwolf GC (1995) Cooperative model of epithelial shaping and bending during avian neurulation: autonomous movements of the neural plate, autonomous movements of the epidermis, and interactions in the neural plate/epidermis transition zone. Dev Dynamics 204:323-337

30. Schoenwolf GC, Sheard P (1989) Shaping and bending of the avian neural plate as analysed with a fluorescent-histochemical marker. Development 105:17-25

31. Schoenwolf GC, Alvarez IS (1989) Roles of the neuroepithelial cell rearrangement and division in shaping of the avian neural plate. Development 106:427-439

32. Schoenwolf GC, Alvarez IS (1992) Role of cell rearrangement in axial morphogenesis. Curr Top Dev Biol 27:129-173

33. Schoenwolf GC (1991) Cell movements during neurulation in avian embryos. Development Supplement 2:157-168

34. Schoenwolf GC (1985) Shaping and bending of the avian neuroepithelium: morphometric analyses. Dev Biol 109:127-139

35. Schoenwolf GC, Powers ML (1987) Shaping of the chick neuroepithelium during primary and sencondary neurulation: role of cell elongation. Anat Rec 218:182-195

36. Takeuchi M, Nakabayashi J, Sakaguchi T et al (2003) The prickle-related gene in vertebrates is essential for gastrulation cell movements. Curr Biol 13:674-679

37. Kibar Z, Capra V, Gros P (2007) Toward understanding the genetic basis of neural tube defects. Clin Genet 71:295-310

38. Schoenwolf GC (1988) Microsurgical analyses of avian neurulation: separation of medial and lateral tissues. J Comp Neurol 276:498-507

39. Alvarez IS, Schoenwolf GC (1992) Expansion of the surface epithelium provides the major extrinsic force for bending of the neural plate. J Exp Zool 261:340-348

40. Smith JL, Schoenwolf GC (1987) Cell cycle and neuroepithelial cell shape during bending of the chick neural plate. Anat Rec 218:196-206

41. Smith JL, Schoenwolf GC (1989) Notochordal induction of cell wedging in the chick neural plate and its role in neural tube formation. J Exp Zool 250:49-62

42. Shum AS, Copp AJ (1996) Regional differences in morphogenesis of the neuroepithelium suggests multiple mechanisms of spinal neurulation in the mouse. Anat Embryol 194:65-73

43. Ybot-Gonzalez P, Copp AJ (1999) Bending of the neural plate during mouse spinal neurulation is independent of actin microfilaments. Dev Dynamics 215:273-283

44. Sakai Y (1989) Neurulation in the mouse: manner and timing of neural tube closure. Anat Rec 223:194-203

45. Juriloff DM, Harris MJ, Tom C, Mc Donald KB (1991) Normal mouse strains differ in the site of initiation of closure of the cranial neural tube. Teratology 44:225-233

46. van Straaten HW, Peeters MC, Hekking JW, van der Lende T (2000) Neurulation in the pig embryo. Anat Embryol 202:75-84

47. Peeters MC, Viebahn C, Hekking JW, van Straaten HW (1998) Neurulation in the rabbit embryo. Anat Embryol 197:167-175

48. O'Rahilly R, Müller F (2002) The two sites of fusion, of the neural folds and the two neuropores in the human embryo. Teratology 64:162-170

49. Nakatsu T, Uwabe C, Shiota K (2000) Neural tube closure in humans initiates at multiple sites: evidence from human embryos and implication for the pathogenesis of neural tube defects. Anat Embryol 201 455-466

49a. Catala M (1995) Neurochirurgie, 41 (S1). Masson, Paris

50. Hughes AF, Freeman RB (1974) Comparative remarks on the development of the tail cord among higher vertebrates. J Embryol Exp Morph 32:355-363

51. Schoenwolf GC (1979) Observations on closure of the neuropores in the chick embryo. Am J Anat 155:445-466

52. Schoenwolf GC (1984) Histological and ultrastructural studies of secondary neurulation in mouse embryos. Am J Anat 169:361-376

53. Shedden PM, Wiley MJ (1987) Early stages of development in the caudal neural tube of the Golden Syrian Hamster (*Mesocricetus auratus*). Anat Rec 219:180-185

54. Müller F, O'Rahilly R (2004) The primitive streak, the caudal eminence and related structures in staged human embryos. Cell Tissues Organs 177:2-20

55. Catala M, Teillet M-A, Le Douarin NM (1995) Organization and development of the tail bud analysed with the quail-chick chimaera system. Mech Dev 51:51-65

56. Kelsey H (1911) Subdivision of the spinal canal in the lumbar region of chick embryos. Proc Royal Soc Victoria 24:152-155

57. Schumacher S (1927) Über die sogenannte Vervielfachung des Medullarrohres (bzw. Des Canalis centralis) bei Embryonen. Zeitschrift für mikroskopisch-anatomische Forschung 10:83-109

58. Holmdahl DE (1925) Experimentelle Untersuchungen über die lage der Grenze zwischen primärer und

sekundärer Körperentwicklung beim Huhn. Anatomischer Anzeiger 59:393-396

59. Pasteels J (1937) Études sur la gastrulation des vertébrés méroblastiques. III. Oiseaux. IV. Conclusions générales. Arch Biol 48:381-488

60. Chiari H (1891) Ueber Veränderungen des Kleinhirns infolge von Hydrocephalie des Grosshirns. Deustche Medicinische Wochenschrift 17:1172-1175

61. Daniel PM, Strich SJ (1958) Some observations on the congenital deformity of the central nervous system known as the Arnold-Chiari malformation. J Neuropath Exp Neurol 17:255-266

62. Osaka K, Tanimura T, Hirayama A, Matsumoto S (1978) Myelomeningocele before birth. J Neurosurg 49:711-724

63. Penfield W, Coburn DF (1938) Arnold-Chiari malformation and its operative treatment. Arch Neurol Psychiatry 40:328-336

64. McLone DG, Knepper PA (1989) The cause of Chiari II malformation: a unified theory. Pediatr Neurosurg 15:1-12

65. Cameron AH (1957) The Arnold-Chiari and other neuro-anatomical malformations associated with spina bifida. J Path Bact 73:195-211

66. van Straaten HWM, Thors F, Wiertz-Hoessels L et al (1985) Effect of a notochordal implant on the early morphogenesis of the neural tube and neuroblasts: histometrical and histological results. Dev Biol 110:247-254

67. Placzek M, Tessier-Lavigne M, Yamada T et al (1990) Mesodermal control of neural cell identity: floor plate induction by the notochord. Science 250:985-988

68. Yamada Y, Placzek M, Tanaka H et al (1991) Control of cell pattern in the developing nervous system: polarizing activity of the floor plate and notochord. Cell 64:635-647

69. van Straaten HW, Hekking JW (1991) Development of floor plate, neurons and axonal outgrowth pattern in the early spinal cord of the notochord-deficient chick embryo. Anat Embryol 184:55-63

70. Hirano S, Fuse S, Sohal GS (1991) The effect of the floor plate on pattern and polarity in the developing central nervous system. Science 251:310-313

71. Teillet M-A, Lapointe F, Le Douarin NM (1998) The relationships between notochord and floor plate in vertebrate development revisited. Proc Natl Acad Sci USA 95:11733-11738

72. Afonso ND (2003) Le contrôle moléculaire de la polarisation ventro-dorsale du tube neural spinal chez les vertébrés. Morphologie 87:47-56

73. Platt KA, Michaud J, Joyner AL (1997) Expression of the mouse *Gli* and *Ptc* genes is adjacent to embryonic sources of hedgehog suggesting a conservation of pathways between flies and mice. Mech Dev 62:121-135

74. Echelard Y, Epstein DJ, St-Jacques B et al (1993) Sonic hedgehog, a member of a family of putative signaling molecules, is implicated in the regulation of CNS polarity. Cell 75:1417-1430

75. Roelink H, Augsburger A, Heemskerk J et al (1994) Floor plate and motor neuron induction by *vhh-1*, a vertebrate homolog of *hedgehog* expressed by the notochord. Cell 76:761-775

76. Ding Q, Motoyama J, Gasca S et al (1998) Diminished Sonic hedgehog signalling and lack of floor plate differentiation in Gli2 mutant mice. Development 125:2533-2543

77. Thibert C, Teillet M-A, Lapointe F et al (2003) Inhibition of neuroepithelial Patched-induced apoptosis by Sonic hedgehog. Science 301:843-846

78. Basler K, Edlund T, Jessell TM, Yamada T (1993) Control of cell pattern in the neural tube: regulation of cell differentiation by *dorsalin-1*, a novel TGFβ family member. Cell 73:687-702

79. Liem KF, Tremmi G, Roelink H, Jessell TM (1995) Dorsal differentiation of neural plate cells induced by BMP-mediated signals from epidermal ectoderm. Cell 82:969-979

80. Liem KF, Jessell TM, Briscoe J (2000) Regulation of the neural patterning activity of sonic hedgehog by secreted BMP inhibitors expressed by notochord and somites. Development 127:4855-4866

81. Helms AW, Johnson JE (2003) Specification of dorsal spinal cord interneurons. Curr Opin Neurobiol 13:42-49

82. Le Douarin NM, Kalcheim C (1999) The neural crest, 2nd edn. Cambridge University Press, Cambridge

83. Krull CE (2001) Segmental organization of neural crest migration. Mech Dev 105:37-45

84. Debby-Brafman A, Burstyn-Cohen T, Klar A, Kalcheim C (1999) F-spondin, expressed in somite regions avoided by neural crest cells, mediates inhibition of distinct somite domains to neural crest migration. Neuron 22:475-488

85. Ring C, Hassell H, Hafter W (1996) Expression pattern of collagen IX and potential role in segmentation of the peripheral nervous system. Dev Biol 180:41-53

86. Tucker RP, Hagios C, Chiquet-Ehrismann R et al (1999) Thrombospondin-1 and neural crest cell migration. Dev Dynamics 214:312-322

87. Ranscht B, Bronner-Fraser M (1991) T-cadherin expression alternates with migrating neural crest cells in the trunk of the avian embryo. Development 111:15-22

88. Krull CE, Collazo A, Fraser SE, Bronner-Fraser M (1997) Interactions of Eph-related receptors and ligands confer rostrocaudal pattern to trunk neural crest migration. Curr Biol 7:571-580

89. Kalcheim C, Teillet M-A (1989) Consequences of somite manipulation on the pattern of dorsal root ganglion development. Development 106:85-93

90. Catala M, Ziller C, Lapointe F, Le Douarin NM (2000) The developmental potentials of the caudalmost part of the neural crest are restricted to melanocytes and glia. Mech Dev 95:77-87

91. Martins-Green M (1988) Origin of the dorsal surface of the neural tube by progressive delamination of epidermal ectoderm and neuroepithelium: implications for neurulation and neural tube defects. Development 103:687-706

92. Pourquié O, Coltey M, Teillet M-A et al (1993) Control of dorsoventral patterning of somatic derivatives by notochord and floor plate. Proc Natl Acad Sci USA 90:5242-5246

93. Fan C-M, Tessier-Lavigne M (1994) Patterning of mammalian somites by surface ectoderm and notochord: evidence for sclerotome induction by a hedgehog homolog. Cell 79:1175-1186

94. Spence MS, Yip J, Erickson CA (1996) The dorsal neural tube organizes the dermamyotome and induces axial myocytes in the avian embryo. Development 122:231-241

95. Johnson RL, Laufer E, Riddle RD, Tabin C (1994) Ectopic expression of *Sonic hedgehog* alters dorsal–ventral patterning of somites. Cell 79:1165-1173

96. Ikeya M, Takada S (1998) Wnt signaling from the dorsal neural tube is required for the formation of the medial dermomyotome. Development 125:4969-4976

97. Borycki A-G, Brown AMC, Emerson CP (2000) Shh and Wnt signalling pathways converge to control *Gli* gene activation in avian somites. Development 127:2075-2087

98. Holtzer H, Detwiler SR (1953) An experimental analysis of the development of the spinal column. III. Induction of skeletogenous cells. J Exp Zool 123:335-369

99. Lash J, Holtzer S, Holtzer H (1957) An experimental analysis of the development of the spinal column. VI. Aspects of cartilage induction. Exp Cell Res 13:292-303

100. Watanabe Y, Duprez D, Monsoro-Burq A-H et al (1998) Two domains in vertebral development: antagonistic regulation by SHH and BMP4 proteins. Development 125:2631-2639

101. Mo R, Freer AM, Zinyk DL et al (1997) Specific and redundant functions of *Gli2* and *Gli3* zinc finger genes in skeletal patterning and development. Development 124:113-123

102. Catala M (1997) Embryogenesis. Why do we need a new explanation for the emergence of spina bifida with lipoma? Childs Nerv Syst 13:336-340

CHAPTER 3

Pathological Anatomy of Spina Bifida

Aydın Sav

Definition

Spina bifida occulta results from incomplete closure of the neural tube around the twentieth day of embryonic development [1]. Spina bifida was described in the medieval literature and was recognized even earlier. Indeed, the association of foot deformities with sacral hypertrichosis may be the origin of the mythological figure of the satyr [2]. The term spina bifida encompasses the entire central nervous system, ranging from merely an absent spinous process through to myelomeningocele (MMC), Chiari malformation and hydrocephalus to cortical cytoarchitectural changes [2].

For the purpose of management, spina bifida had been classified into (1) spina bifida cystica, which refers to either MMC or meningocele, (2) spina bifida aperta, which involves lesions communicating with the environment, and (3) spina bifida occulta, which manifests as a concealed form of spinal dysraphism with few cutaneous stigmata of the underlying spinal anomaly, e.g., split cord malformation (SCM) [3]. Spina bifida aperta or cystica and spina bifida occulta were used to refer to open spinal dysraphism (OSD) and closed spinal dysraphism (CSD), respectively [4], but these terms are now obsolete.

A recent classification of spinal dysraphism was proposed by Tortori-Donati et al. [5]. In this classification, not only the clinico-neuroadiological correlations but also the importance of almost every lesion has been linked with the embryological aspects. Essentially, dysraphic anomalies are divided as open spinal dysraphism and closed spinal dysraphism as the main categories and with the latter subdivided into two further subcategories: with or without a subcutaneous mass.

MMC, the commonest anomaly of spinal dysraphism, has drawn a large amount of attention from pediatric neurosurgeons in recent decades and is well described in the literature. The coexistence of SCM and MMC is most probably suggestive of some developmental error in the third to fourth week (postovulation stages 8-12) of embryogenesis [6, 7].

Incidence and Prevalence

Statistics on the frequency of CSD vary from 2 to 24% of the population. This variation is to some extent age-related. CSD of the first sacral vertebra was found in 51.6% of the 7- to 8-year old group and in 26.4% of adults. CSD of the fifth lumbar vertebra occurred in 16.1% of the 7- to 8-year old group and in only 2.2% of adults [8]. Routine radiological examination of 1,172 consecutive autopsies, mostly adults, showed a 5% incidence of CSD [9]. The frequency of CSD averages between 1 and 2.5 per 1000 live births [10]. There are substantial racial and geographic variations. The disease is approximately 2.5 times more frequent in Caucasians than in Negroes and is particularly common (above 4.0) in Belfast, Liverpool and Dublin, and uncommon (0.2) in Japan. There were also reports of local epidemic increases of 2-6 times of normal in certain parts of the world [11, 12].

Sex Distribution

CSD in adults shows nearly equal distribution between sexes [8]. Timson collected 3,521 cases from nine studies and found an average female predilection of 65.5% [13]. This was statistically significant when compared with the general population or with their siblings. The predilection for females is greater the more severe the lesion. A greater number of affected females were found in stillbirths than in live births [14]. Female excess occurred among myelomeningoceles but was absent for meningoceles [15].

Main Lesions Forming the Basis of Classification

The lesions of spinal dysraphism are formed by combined malformations of the vertebral column and the spinal cord. The mesodermal and neuroectodermal malformations are usually comparable, but the cor-

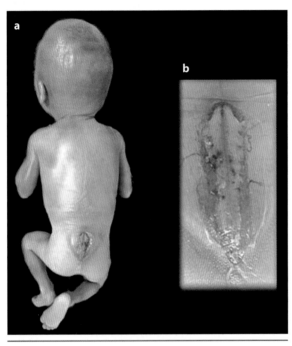

Fig. 3.1 a, b. a OSD, dorsal view. **b** Close-up of OSD, L1-L5 levels

relation is not precise. Either component may predominate or may even be presented as the one and only feature. The disease may be classified in terms of the deformity of the spine or that of the cord. It is widely accepted to use the spinal defect or dysraphism for classification:

1. Open spinal dysraphism (OSD) comprises myelomeningocele, myelocele, hemimyelomeningocele and hemimyelocele. Meningoceles are without spinal cord tissue but myelomeningoceles are the group in which the spinal cord is a component of the cyst wall. Rachischisis is the most severe defect. There is a widely patent dorsal opening of the spine with or without residual cord tissue (Fig. 3.1). Rachischisis is usually associated with anencephaly (Fig. 3.2) [16].

2. Closed spinal dysraphism (CSD) consists of unenclosed vertebral arches without an externally visible cystic lesion in the back. These lesions differ from spina bifida cystica, in which a vertebral defect combines with a cystic lesion on the back. CSD manifests with or without mass depending on clinical, radiological and pathological findings.

The deformities of the neuraxis may be termed as amyelia, nonfusion of the dorsal half of the cord, diastematomyelia, hydromyelia, tethering of cord, overgrowth of cord or nonspecific dysplasia. Any type of classification may lead to misconceptions if the mesodermal or the neuroectodermal lesions are emphasized to the point that their mutual relationship is no longer considered [16].

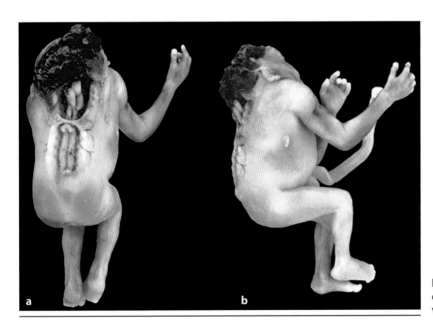

Fig. 3.2 a, b. a Rachischisis associated with anencephaly, dorsal view. **b** Lateral view

Classification

Numerous classifications have been proposed in the literature in order to capture all the associations of spinal dysraphism, considering the clinical, radiological and pathological aspects. Some of these mainly relate to abnormalities of specific structures in the embryological development of the human fetus and embryo. In fact, patients' daily demands shape more practical and realistic classifications that will expedite further clinical applications in the management of the patient. An easily understood scheme was offered by Tortori-Donati, simplifying not only the diagnosis but also the underlying pathological conditions of this burden (Table 3.1) [5].

The ratio of OSD/CSD is about 9:1 [5]. The key features of OSD patients are listed in Table 3.1 (note the lumbosacral prevalence). Additionally the Chiari II malformation was seen in all cases of OSD [17, 18]. On the other hand, CSD is manifested by a wide variety of complex lesions either represented as congenital malformations or as ensuing lesions with the development of complications in subsequent years.

The presence of a subcutaneous mass is the critical clue in the differential diagnosis of a group of lesions, including lipomyeloschisis, lipomyelomeningocele, meningocele and terminal myelocystocele. Although lipomyeloschisis and lipomyelomeningocele are rarely seen pathologies, they are accompanied by a lipoma, which in the former penetrates into the spinal canal through a bony defect and in the latter remains exterior in relation to the spinal canal [5]. CSD lesions unaccompanied by a subcutaneous mass include either simple or complex dysraphic conditions forming a list of until now unexplained pathogenetic considerations.

Open Spinal Dysraphism

Myelomeningocele

The first modern description, according to modern criteria, was provided by Von Recklinghausen (1886), who gave a detailed account of 32 patients with spina bifida cystica and its variants. Since then, consecutive series have been published in the literature [19]. Myelomeningocele refers to a bony defect in the vertebral column through which the meningeal membranes that cover the spinal cord and part of the spinal cord protrude. Almost all parts of the spine can be involved, but most involve the lumbosacral region (Figs. 3.3a-d). Surprisingly, not all the lesions are associated with bony malformations. The vertebral column is, for the most part, deranged at the sacral level [20]. Almost 1% of the cases show multisegmental involvement [21].

Most myelomeningoceles show a predilection for the sacral or lumbosacral regions. On the other hand, rare examples can occur at lumbar, thoracolumbar and thoracic levels (Fig. 3.3e) [5].

On naked eye examination, the degree of skin covering the outpouching is relative to its size. The myelomeningocele sac is normally unilocular but the presence of numerous septa is not unusual. Histologically the sac wall is lined by skin, dura proper and arachnoidal cells. In most of the cases spinal neural tissue does not protrude into this outpouching. Even though dilatation of the ependymal-lined central canal (hydromyelia) and bony spur (diastematomyelia) are rare, they may be accompanying lesions [16].

The surface of the myelomeningocele shows a characteristic central area devoid of epithelial lining,

Table 3.1. Cliniconeuroradiological and pathological classification of spinal dysraphism. Reprinted from [5]

Open spinal dysraphism (95%)
  Myelomeningocele
  Myelocele
  Hemimyelomeningocele, Hemimyelocele

Closed spinal dysraphism (5%)
  With a subcutaneous mass
    Lumbosacral
    Lipoma with dural defect
      Lipomyelomeningocele
      Lipomyeloschisis
    Terminal myelocystocele
    Meningocele
    Cervical
      Cervical myelocystocele
      Cervical myelomeningocele
      Meningocele
  Without a subcutaneous mass
    Simple dysraphic states
      Posterior spina bifida
      Intradural and intramedullary lipoma
      Filum terminale lipoma
      Tight filum terminale
      The abnormally long spinal cord
      Persistent terminal ventricle
    Complex dysraphic states
      Dorsal enteric fistula
      Neurenteric cysts
      Split cord malformations (diastematomyelia and diplomyelia)
      Dermal sinus
      Caudal regression syndrome
      Segmental spinal dysgenesis

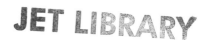

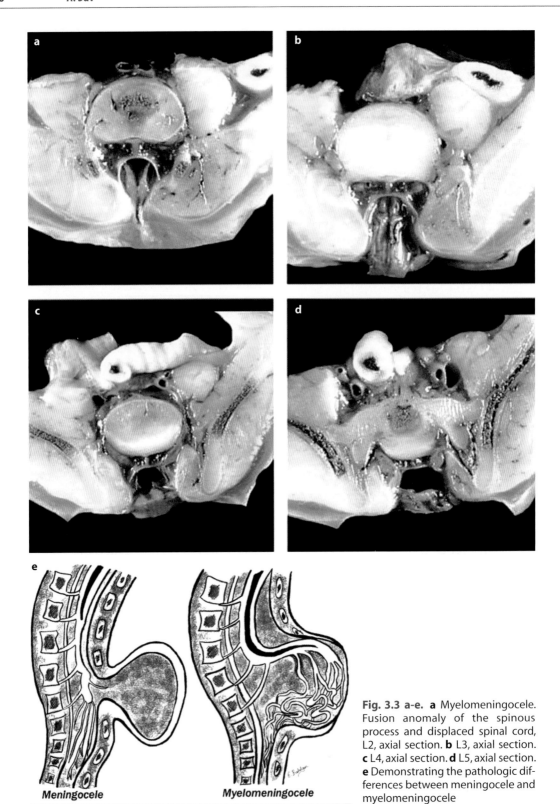

Fig. 3.3 a-e. a Myelomeningocele. Fusion anomaly of the spinous process and displaced spinal cord, L2, axial section. **b** L3, axial section. **c** L4, axial section. **d** L5, axial section. **e** Demonstrating the pathologic differences between meningocele and myelomeningocele

exposing vascular tissue, from which cerebrospinal fluid (CSF) or tissue transudate may ooze. An overt vascular proliferation of not only the dural but also the neural tissue is observed (Fig. 3.4). The specif-ic hypervascularity of the tissues, including the densely vascularized meninges, is called medullo-vasculosa, and mimics cerebrovasculosa of enen-cephalitic brains [16].

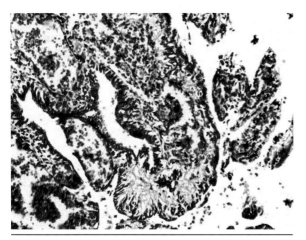

Fig. 3.4. Medullovasculosa. Overt vascular proliferation accompanied by neural tissue (HE, ×200 original magnification)

Myelocele

Although very rare in this malformation, in a myelocele the ventral region of the subarachnoid space is not expanded. Therefore the placode is not expanded so that the placode faces with the cutaneous surface [22]. Embryologically the same principles apply as for myelomeningoceles. Actually the myelocele is equivalent to the myelomeningocele, the only difference being the absence of expansion of the underlying subarachnoid space. Myelocele forms 1.2% of OSD in a series [5].

Hemimyelomeningocele

Both myelomeningoceles and myelocele are associated with SCM in 8-45% of cases [23, 24] (see Chapter 14).

Chiari II malformation

Almost all OSD are associated with a Chiari II malformation, which is typified by a group of abnormalities including a shallow posterior fossa accompanied by downward displacement of the cerebellar vermis, brain stem and fourth ventricle (Fig. 3.5). Some authors consider the Chiari II malformation as part of the OSD (Fig. 3.6) [18]. The hindbrain malformation may be inconsistent, with the size of the posterior fossa being almost within normal limits [17, 18]. It has to be emphasized therefore, that the Chiari II malformation is a constant feature of OSD, albeit in a minimal degree [5].

The bony and dural anomalies are distinctive and crucial for the radiological diagnosis. In addition to craniolacunia, irregular patches of thinning or complete erosion of the cranial vault, the falx is short and fenestrated [23]. The tentorial hiatus is widened but the tentorial insertion is low, near the rim of an enlarged foramen magnum. The posterior fossa is shallow; the torcula is low lying and the clivus concave and thinned. The herniated cerebellar tissue varies from a short peg to a long tail and involves the nodulus, pyramis and uvula, respectively [24]. It may extend down as far as

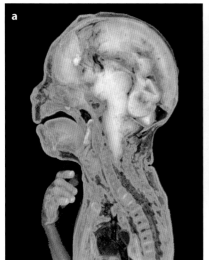
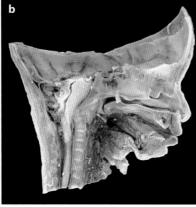

Fig. 3.5 a, b. a Chiari type II malformation. A constellation of lesions including shallow posterior fossa accompanied by downward displacement of the cerebellar vermis, brain stem and fourth ventricle. Sagittal section. **b** Close-up of Chiari type II malformation

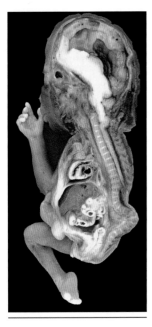

Fig. 3.6. OSD located at L2-L5 associated with Chiari type II malformation. Sagittal section

the upper thoracic vertebral segments. Rarely is there any cerebellar displacement, and the herniated tissue includes the tonsils as well as the vermis. The elongated tongue of flattened whitish cerebellar vermis, often associated with choroid plexus, lies on the dorsal surface of the lower medulla and cord, firmly bound to them by fibrous meningeal adhesions. Its upper end is often grooved by the edge of the foramen magnum. The cerebellar tail may cover the roof of the ventricle or may be intraventricular. In 50% of cases, just caudal to the ventricle, the lower medulla below the gracile and cuneate nuclei forms an S-shaped curve or kink over the cervical cord. The brainstem, particularly the medulla, fourth ventricle and its choroid plexus, is elongated and displaced caudally.

Histologically, the presence of focal cortical dysplasia and grey heterotopias in the hemispheric white matter is well recognized, as is distortion of brainstem tracts and nuclei. Purkinje and granule cell depletion with shrinkage and gliosis of the folia and absence of myelin are eye-catching features in the herniated cerebellar tissue. Hypoplasia or agenesis of cranial nerve nuclei and pontine nuclei in young infants may also be present in this setting.

The cerebellar hemispheres are often asymmetrical and flattened dorsally; the vermis may be buried between the hemispheres, which might extend around the brainstem over its ventral surface, sometimes meeting in the midline [24]. The pontomedullary junction is distracted with an elongated rod-shaped pons. Moreover, there may be a beaklike deformity of the corpora quadrigemina that is

directed backwards and downwards to a point formed by the fusion of inferior colliculi [25].

Although the upper cervical roots are normally placed, the fourth to sixth cervical spinal roots are angled upwards towards their intervertebral foramina. Other frequently described anomalies are subependymal nodular grey heterotopias in the lateral ventricles and thickening of the massa intermedia. Spina bifida almost invariably is present, although there are some extremely rare exceptions [26]. Myelomeningocele is more common than meningocele and typically occurs at a lumbar or lumbosacral level. Additional spinal anomalies like hydromyelia at C8 [27], syringomyelia just below the cervicomedullary junction, diastematomyelia and diplomyelia may be present [28, 29].

Hydrocephalus is usually present and might be explained in terms of obstruction of the aqueduct of Sylvius. The most common related changes are aqueduct atresia, forking and gliosis [23]. The dilated hemispheres often show an abnormal convolutional pattern consisting of an excessive number of small gyri and shallow sulci, most appropriately termed polygyria, since usually normal cytoarchitecture is preserved unlike the laminar abnormalities present in polymicrogyria.

Closed Spinal Dysraphism

As previously mentioned, the accompaniment of a subcutaneous mass is the criterion for classifying closed spinal malformations. Therefore in this section, malformations with and without a mass will be discussed.

Malformations with Subcutaneous Mass

The most remarkable mass lesions are located in two different sites: lumbosacral and cervical. In the former the most frequent malformations are either lipomyeloschisis or lipomyelomeningoceles, whereas a mass in the latter is most likely due to a myelomeningocele, myelocystocele or meningocele [30]. Mass lesions comprise almost 20% of all CSD [5]. On the other hand cervical lesions are relatively rare entities among this group [31].

Lipomas Accompanied by Dural Defect: Lipomyeloschisis and Lipomyelomeningocele

Lipomyeloschisis and lipomyelomeningocele are the most common malformations, although the incidence of the former is double that of the latter. The

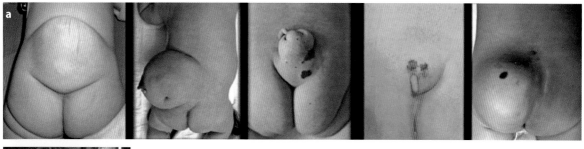

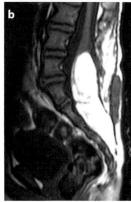

Fig. 3.7 a, b. a Lipomas in different locations and appearance. Courtesy of Prof. M.M. Özek.
b Lengthened and revolved segmental placode adjacent to lipoma and tethered spinal cord

common denominator of these lesions is the lipoma formed by proliferation of adipose tissue (Fig. 3.7) [5]. In principle, a midline subcutaneous mass asymmetrically extends into the buttock [32]. Almost 25% of subcutaneous masses are formed by mature adipose tissue. By and large, the remainder of the lesion is formed by the coexistence of germ cell layers in various ratios [33]. Lipomyeloschisis contains a subcutaneous mass formed by adipose tissue extending into the spinal canal through a bony defect and adhering to the spinal cord [5].

In lipomyelomeningocele the coexistence of a lengthened and rotated segmental placode adjacent to the lipoma and a tethered spinal cord are the main characteristic features [22]. The caudal part of the spinal cord above the malformation is not only normal in appearance but also in its position within spinal canal (Fig. 3.7b).

Other tissue elements, i.e., fibrocartilagenous, fibrosseous, neuromuscular, and vascular elements, may be accompanying features. Adipose tissue enveloping the spinal cord beneath the dural sac is called lipomatous dura mater [5].

Meningocele

This common malformation is located either posterior or anterior to the spinal canal. A posterior menin-

gocele is characteristically a sac made up of dura filled with CSF protruding through a posterior of spina bifida. The most common sites are lumbar and sacral. Although rare, other sites such as thoracic and cervical may be involved [5]. Although both nerve roots and, more rarely, a hypertrophic filum terminale may course within the meningocele; by definition, no part of the spinal cord is within the sac, and the spinal cord itself is completely normal structurally, although it is usually tethered to the neck of a sacral meningocele [34].

Conversely, anterior meningoceles that predominate in the presacral region are consistently found in the caudal regression syndrome [35]. Neither anterior meningocele nor intrasacral meningocele are associated with subcutaneous masses [36, 37].

Terminal Myelocystocele

The histological features of this extremely rare malformation consist of a subcutaneous mass located in the sacrococcygeal region comprising an ependyma-lined cyst representing dilatation of the terminal ventricle. It is also called a syringocele [38, 39]. This malformation is almost always associated with distention of the arachnoidal lining giving rise to herniation of the meninges and finally producing a meningocele [5]. Cross sectional view of a syringocele sac shows an outer layer comprised of pia and arachnoid, with the inner surface lined by ependyma. Fibrofatty tissue and skin attach directly to the ependyma. In almost all cases the syringocele occurs caudal to a meningocele [5].

Cervical Myelocystocele

Unlike terminal myelocystoceles, cervical myelocystoceles differ in that only part of the dorsal wall of the hydromyelic cavity protrudes into the meningocele. Nonetheless, this rare malformation bears an epithelial lining [22].

Cervical Myelomeningocele

The relative frequency of cervical myelomeningoceles is 3.7% in OSD [31]. They are strikingly different from the more frequent lumbosacral myelomeningoceles. The most common features of cervical myelomeningoceles are a fibroneurovascular stalk containing neurons, glia and peripheral nerves, emanating from a limited dorsal myeloschisis and penetrating through a narrow dorsal dural opening to fan out into the lining of a meningeal sac and frequently an underlying split cord malformation (Fig. 3.8). Moreover, a Chiari II malformation might accompany the condition. Some authors have speculated that the limited extent of the myeloschisis makes it unlikely that enough CSF leakage occurs to start the cascade of events leading to a Chiari II malformation[31].

So far, there is no consensus as to whether cervical myelomeningoceles are sufficiently different as to be considered a separate entity. Some authors found them to differ from the typical lumbosacral myelomeningocele in that the neural tissue was not exposed [40, 41] and concluded that these malformations actually represent limited dorsal myelocystoceles because of the limited spinal cord within the spinal canal. In addition, when compared with the proposal forwarded by Pang and Dias [31], a true "meningocele" would be unlikely, as meningoceles often contain some elements of neural tissue, such as aberrant nerve roots.

Malformations without Subcutaneous Mass

Simple Dysraphic States

This group contains seven major subgroups, all of which show different characteristics with heterogeneous embryological origins. Furthermore, as a group, they represent the most common abnormalities in children without significant lower back cutaneous stigmata, who presented with symptoms and signs of cord tethering [42-44].

Posterior Spina Bifida

This malformation forms almost 20% of CSD and is represented as a simple bony defect of fusion of the posterior arches of vertebra. It is mostly sited at the L5 or S1 level without associated clinical signs or symptoms [5].

Intradural and Intramedullary Lipoma

In general pathology a lipoma is a benign tumor of adipocytes forming an encapsulated mass with a blood vessel rich stroma. Most commonly, lipomas of the spinal cord lie at the lumbosacral level with the remainder located at any level within the canal. Rarely, some lie completely within the spinal cord or may invade as a diffuse proliferation known as diffuse medullary lipomatosis. The relative frequency of intradural lipomas is about 25% of all spinal lipomas (Fig. 3.9) [5].

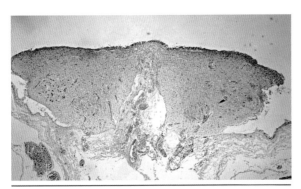

Fig. 3.8. Dorsal myeloschisis. Fibroneurovascular stalk containing neurons, glia and peripheral nerves (HE, x40 original magnification)

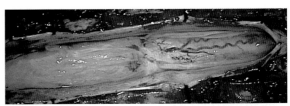

Fig. 3.9. Intradural lipoma. Courtesy of Prof. M.M. Özek

Filum Terminale Lipoma

This simple malformation is characterized by fibrolipomatous thickening of the filum terminale. It can be interpreted as an anatomical variant of a tethered cord syndrome. Some authors believe that this malformation is most likely due to residual totipotential cells of the caudal cell mass giving rise to mature adipose tissue, namely lipoma (Fig. 3.10) [45].

Tight Filum Terminale

This malformation is characterized by a short, hypertrophic filum terminale producing tethering and impaired ascent of the conus medullaris. In most cases, therefore, the conus lies below its expected level. Additionally, posterior spina bifida, scoliosis and kyphoscoliosis occur in the majority of cases [5].

The Abnormally Long Spinal Cord

This abnormality is characterized by the absence of a normally tapered conus medullaris. Surprisingly, the caliber of the spinal cord does not show any significant changes down to the sacrum where it ultimately unites with the lower end of the thecal sac.

Persistent Terminal Ventricle

The term "fifth ventricle" first described by Kernohan, encompasses an ependymal-lined small cavity in the conus medullaris, which is always identifiable on postmortem examination [46]. Theoretically, it represents incomplete regression of the terminal ventricle with preservation of its continuity with the central canal of the rostral spinal cord. It is not clear whether the "terminal ventricle cyst" is due to maldevelopment or as the end result of a pathological obstruction of the terminal ventricle [47]. Its differential diagnosis from hydromyelia is based on its site, which is immediately above the filum terminale.

Complex Dysraphic States

The development of the notochord takes place during weeks 2-3 of development. Inevitably spinal dysraphism originating in this period shows a complex picture comprising not only the spinal cord but also other organs deriving from or induced by the notochord. As a result, disorders of gastrulation are occasionally called complex dysraphic states [48]. Other than hemimyelocele and hemimyelomeningocele, most cases are covered by skin and no significant subcutaneous mass is present. In theory, various possible failures of midline notochordal integration may be responsible. These may give rise to longitudinal splitting or failures of notochordal formation resulting in the absence of a given notochordal segment [5].

Disorders of Midline Notochordal Integration

Embryologically the two paired notochordal anlagen fuse in the midline, giving rise to a single notochordal process. Unfortunately, if these notochordal precursors fail to integrate, they remain separate without developing a variable segment. With time, the intervening space will be filled by totipotential primitive streak cells [48]. The predisposing causes of notochordal splitting are a matter of debate. Several possible explanations have been put forward, such as endo-ectodermal adhesion within the primitive streak [49], initial teratogenic or spontaneous mutation of the developing notochord [50] and persistence or only partial obliteration of the neurenteric canal [29]. Recently, Dias and Walker [48] demonstrated that separation of Hensen's node into two independent halves during gastrulation resulted in a duplicated notochord and neuraxis. Regardless of the underlying cause, the type of malformation depends on the level and extent of the defect and on the success of subsequent reparative efforts [48, 49]. The split notochord syndrome includes several apparently quite different entities, such as the dorsal enteric fistula, neurenteric cysts, diastematomyelia, dermal sinuses and even intestinal duplication. The differences between these entities result from the different developmental fate of the intervening primitive-streak tissue towards endo-, meso- or ectoderm; however, they all share some degree of vertebral abnormality (block vertebrae, butterfly vertebrae, hemivertebrae), pointing to the original notochordal abnormality [5].

Dorsal Enteric Fistula

Although an exceedingly rare condition, dorsal enteric fistula is the most severe of the complex dysraphic states. Among the eye-catching features are a cleft con-

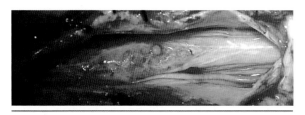

Fig. 3.10. Filum terminale lipoma. Courtesy of Prof. M.M. Özek

necting the bowel with the dorsal skin surface through the prevertebral soft tissues, vertebral bodies, spinal canal and its contents, neural arch and subcutaneous tissues. The involved segment of both the vertebral column and spinal cord is split to form two columns surrounding the cleft. Bifurcation of the spine and spinal cord at the lumbar level with bilateral continuation to the conus medullaris is reported [51].

Neurenteric Cysts

Neurenteric cysts may be due to endodermal differentiation of primitive streak remnants, possibly related to incomplete regression of the neurenteric canal, and representing an intraspinal counterpart of gut duplications. In fact, neurenteric cysts resemble the gastrointestinal tract more closely than the spinal cord, with the only reliable criterion used for differentiating neurenteric cysts from gut duplication being their location [52].

Histologically, neurenteric cysts are found within the spinal canal and are lined by mucin-secreting, cuboidal or columnar epithelium resembling the gastrointestinal tract (Fig. 3.11) [48, 53]. Some are lined

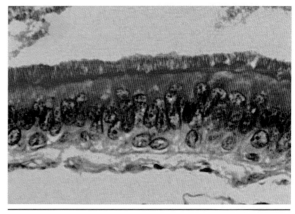

Fig. 3.12. Neurenteric cyst. Respiratory type epithelium with ciliated surface (HE, ×400 original magnification)

by respiratory type of epithelium (Fig. 3.12). Their contents are variable, and their chemical composition may be similar to CSF. The characteristic site is the intradural thoracic spine, anterior to the spinal cord [54, 55]. It might also be found in the cervical or lumbar spine. Vertebral abnormalities are commonly present [5].

Split Cord Malformations (SCM)

Diastematomyelia literally means spinal cord splitting, while diplomyelia represents cord duplication. Until now there has been no widespread consensus on the use of these terms in medical terminology. The relative frequency of SCM is about 4% of all CSD [5].

In 1992, Pang et al. [29] suggested that terms such as diastematomyelia and diplomyelia be abandoned, to make way for a new classification of SCM into two types, based on the state of the dural tube and the nature of the median septum.

Type I SCM (Diastematomyelia with Septum)

This malformation presents with scoliosis and the tethered cord syndrome. Cutaneous stigmata, including hemangioma, skin discolorations and hypertrichosis, are characteristic features. Vertebral abnormalities including butterfly vertebra, hemivertebrae, and posterior spina bifida are also prominent findings [29, 42]. An osseous or osteocartilagineous midline septum splits the spinal cord into two tubes each containing a hemicord. The spur may divide the spinal canal asymmetrically giving rise to two irregular hemicords (Fig. 3.13). The level of the split occurs in either the thoracic or lumbar regions. Beyond the bony spur the two hemicords adhere to each other and return to a normal anatomic position. Hydromyelia is a common finding, and may involve the

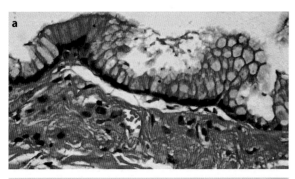

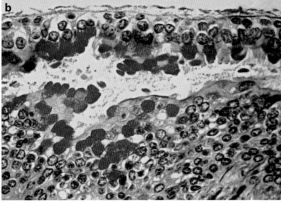

Fig. 3.11 a, b. **a** Neurenteric cyst. Columnar epithelium resting on a fibrous stroma containing telangiectatic capillaries (HE, ×400 original magnification). **b** Neurenteric cyst. Columnar cell cytoplasm filled with glycoprotein rich material (PAS, ×400 original magnification)

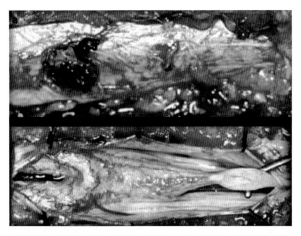

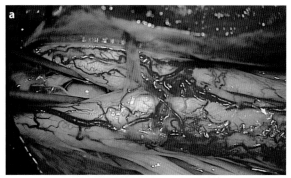

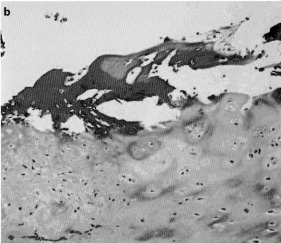

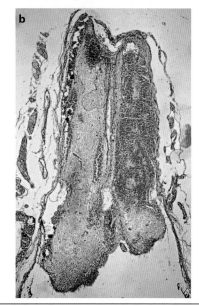

Fig. 3.13 a, b. **a** SCM Type I associated with filum terminale lipoma (courtesy of Prof. M.M. Özek). **b** SCM Type I (diastometamyelia). Bony spur formed by mature cartilage and ossified foci (HE, ×100 original magnification)

Fig. 3.14 a, b. **a** SCM Type II (diplomyelia). Hemicords within a single dural sheet (courtesy of Prof. M.M. Özek) **b** SCM Type II. Asymmetrical split hemicords are wrapped by a common arachnoidal membrane (HE, ×40 original magnification)

normal cord both above and below the split as well as one or both the hemicords [56].

Type II SCM (Diastematomyelia without Septum)

No osteocartilagineous spur is found in this malformation. Some cases display signs of tethered cord. Rarely, thin fibrous septae may form. Occasionally the cleft is partial and the split incomplete (Fig. 3.14); these are the mildest forms of diastematomyelia [57]. Hydromyelia may be present. Posterior spina bifida is often present [5].

To summarize this section, it is proposed that diastematomyelia and diplomyelia are two ends of a spectrum of split-cord malformations with a common embryonic mechanism. The common denominator of these entities is "incomplete duplications" of two hemicords. In each malformation, the existence of surface skin covering and presence of an ependyma-

lined central canal within the hemicords support the abovementioned observation [5, 58].

Dermal Sinus

This common malformation is mostly found in the lumbosacral region. By definition, the dermal sinus is a squamous epithelium-lined fistula extending inwards from the skin to the spinal cord and its coverings (Fig. 3.15) [59]. A midline dimple accompanied by a hairy nevus, capillary hemangioma, or skin discolorations are observed on the skin surface (Fig. 3.16). Dermal sinuses may open into the subarachnoid space leading to CSF leakage. In some instances sinuses may adhere to a fibrolipomatous filum terminale or a low conus medullaris. The portal of entry can be a harbinger of ascending meningitis. Nevertheless, progressive accumulation of exfoliated

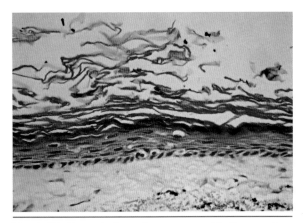

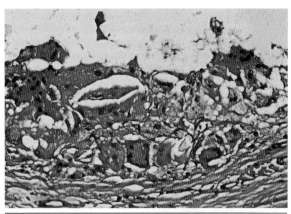

Fig. 3.15. Dermal sinus. Squamous epithelium surface with exfoliating anucleated squames (HE, ×200 original magnification)

Fig. 3.17. Dermal sinus. Ruptured sinus wall evoked inflammatory reaction containing histiocytes and foreign body giant cells (HE, ×200 original magnification)

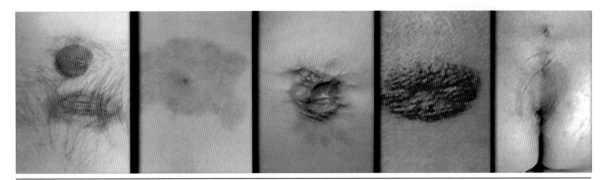

Fig. 3.16. Dermal sinus cases of different appearances. Courtesy of Prof. M.M. Özek

squames can rupture (Fig. 3.17). Unfortunately, abscess formation and rupture into the subarachnoid space with subsequent chemical meningitis may complicate the clinical picture [60].

Disorders of Notochord Formation

During early embryogenesis (week 2-3), cells that are incorrectly situated in terms of their rostrocaudal position are eliminated. This leads to a smaller group of cells left to form the notochord, and most likely as an end result a segmental notochordal pathology will ensue. If the prospective notochord or caudal cell mass is depopulated, a wide range of segmental vertebral malformations, including segmentation defects, i.e., hemivertebrae or isolated butterfly vertebrae, indeterminate or block vertebrae, or even absence of several vertebrae, will result [61].

Caudal Regression Syndrome (CRS)

By and large, this group is a heterogeneous collection of caudal malformations consisting of a wide variety of lesions, i.e., total or partial agenesis of the spinal column, anal imperforation, genital abnormalities, bilateral renal dysplasia or aplasia and pulmonary hypoplasia [61]. The lower extremities are usually dysplastic with distal atrophy and a short intergluteal cleft; fusion or agenesis results in the most severe cases (sirenomelia) [62]. Agenesis of the sacrococcygeal spine may be part of syndromic complexes such as OEIS (omphalocele, exstrophy, imperforate anus, spinal defects) [62], VACTERL (vertebral abnormality, anal imperforation, tracheoesophageal fistula, renal abnormalities, and limb deformities) [63] and the Currarino triad (partial sacral agenesis, anorectal malformation and sacrococcygeal teratoma) (Figs. 3.18)

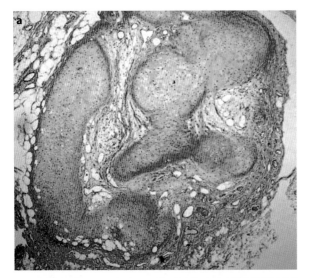

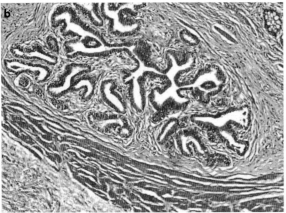

Fig. 3.18 a, b. Teratoma. **a** Irregular shaped mature cartilage tissue (HE, ×40 original magnification). **b** Malformed tumor tissue resembling colonic mucosa with papillary foldings and adjacent smooth muscle fibers forming bowel wall (HE, ×200 original magnification)

genesis of the bony structures, but also its proximity. In severe cases the spinal cord may be dissected into half [61]. Segmental dysgenetic conditions can be accompanied by partial sacrococcygeal agenesis, and renal abnormalities [5]. It has been postulated that SSD and CRS most likely represent two consecutive parts of a variety of segmental malformations of the spine and spinal cord (Fig. 3.19) [5].

Conclusion

After reviewing a wide variety of malformations occurring in spinal dysraphism, it is evident that the common denominator is the sequential disruption of neuroectodermal and mesodermal structures giving rise to developmental anomalies. Although different entities seem to share similar pathogenetic mechanisms, so far there is no satisfactory encompassing theory to explain the whole picture. Interestingly, the neural tube and related mesenchyme all appear to be vulnerable to in-situ impairment between the 22nd and 26th days. It appears that minor variations in time sequences and in extent of regional severity could account for the wide spectrum of dysraphic malformations. The abovementioned basic algorithmic approach to a child with spinal dysraphism is believed to be useful for daily clinical practice. Further definition of the pathological aspects of dysraphic anomalies from a molecular and neuroradiological viewpoint is needed. Future advancements including the use of cybernetics and the collaboration of interdisciplinary members of the scientific team focusing on spinal dysraphism will potentiate both the understanding and the solution of this particular problem.

[64-66]. Lipomyelomeningocele and terminal myelocystocele are present in 20% of cases [31].

Segmental Spinal Dysgenesis (SSD)

By definition, segmental spinal dysgenesis (SSD) is a group of abnormalities including segmental agenesis or dysgenesis of the lumbar or thoracolumbar spine, segmental abnormality of the underlying spinal cord and nerve roots, congenital paraplegia or paraparesis, and congenital lower limb deformities [61]. This group may involve the thoracolumbar, lumbar, or lumbosacral spine. Inevitably the adjacent spinal cord may be hypoplastic or completely absent at the level of the abnormality. The severity of the spinal cord lesions is dependent not only on the extent of the segmental dys-

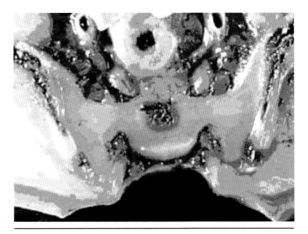

Fig. 3.19. Close-up view of segmental lumbar dysgenesis with total spinal cord agenesis

References

1. Banta JV, Lin R, Peterson M et al (1990) The team approach in the care of the child with myelomeningocele. JPO 2:263-73
2. von Recklinghausen (1886) In: Friede RL (ed) Developmental neuropathology. 2nd and revised edition. Springer-Verlag, Berlin Heidelberg New York, pp 248-262
3. Kumar R, Bansal KK, Chhabra DK (2002) Occurrence of split cord malformation in meningomyelocele: Complex spina bifida. Pediatr Neurosurg 36:119-127
4. Sattar MT, Bannister CM, Turnbull IW (1996) Occult spinal dysraphism-The common combination of lesions and the clinical manifestations in 50 patients. Eur J Pediatr Surg 6 Suppl 11:10-14
5. Tortori-Donati P, Rossi A, Cama A (2000) Spinal dysraphism: a review of neuroradiological features with embryological correlations and proposal for a new classification. Neuroradiol 42:471-491
6. Reigel DH, Rotenstien D (1994) Spina bifida. In: Section of pediatric neurosurgery of the American Association of Neurological Surgeons (ed) Pediatric neurosurgery, 3rd edn. Saunders, Philadelphia, pp 51-76
7. Iskandar BJ, McLaughlin C, Oakes WJ (2000). Split cord malformations in myelomeningocele patients. Br J Neurosurg 14:200-203
8. Sutow WW, Pryde AW (1956) Incidence of spina bifida occulta in relation to age. Am J Dis Child 91:211-217
9. James CC, Lassman LP (1972) Spinal dysraphism. Spina bifida occulta. Butterworth, London
10. Alter M (1962) Anencephalus, hydrocephalus, and spina bifida. Epidemiology, with special reference to a survey in Charleston. Arch Neurol 7:411-422
11. Boris M, Blumbcig R, Feldman DB, Sellers TF Jr (1963) Increased incidence of meningomyeloceles. JAMA 184:768
12. Lucey JF, Mann RW, Simmons GM, Friedman E (1964) An increased incidence of spina bifida in Vermont in 1962. Pediatrics 33:981-984
13. Timson J (1969) The sex ratio in spina bifida. Genetics 40:427-433
14. Record RG, McKeown T (1949) Congenital malformations of the central nervous system I. A survey of 930 cases. Br I Soc Med 3:183-219
15. Doran PA, Guthkelch AN (1961) Studies in spina bifida cystica. General survey and reassessment of the problem. J Neurol Neurosurg Psychiatry 24:331-345
16. Friede RL (1989) Developmental neuropathology. 2nd and revised edition. Springer-Verlag, Berlin Heidelberg New York
17. Cama A, Tortori-Donati P, Piatelli GL et al (1995) Chiari complex in children. Neuroradiological diagnosis, neurosurgical treatment and proposal of a new classification (312 cases). Eur J Pediatr Surg 5(Suppl 1):35-38
18. Tortori-Donati P, Cama A, Fondelli MP et al (1996) Le malformazioni di Chiari. In: Tortori-Donati P, Tacone A, Longo M (eds) Malformazioni cranio-encefaliche. Neuroradiologia. Minerva Medica, Turin, pp 209-236
19. Keiller VH (1922) A contribution to the anatomy of spina bifida. Brain 45:31-103
20. Barson AJ (1970) Spina bifida: the significance of the level and extent of the defect to the morphogenesis. Dev Med Child Neurol 12:129-144
21. Fisher RG, Uihlein A, Keith HM (1952) Spina bifida and cranium bifidum: study of 530 cases. Proc Staff Meet Mayo Clin 27:33-38
22. Naidich TP, Zimmerman RA, McLone DG et al (1996) Congenital anomalies of the spine and spinal cord. In: Atlas SW (ed) Magnetic resonance imaging of the brain and spine, 2nd edn. Lippincott-Raven, Philadelphia, pp 1265-1337
23. Cameron AH (1957) Arnold-Chiari and neuro-anatomical malformations associated with Spina bifida. J Pathol Bacteriol 73:195-211
24. Daniel PM, Strich SJ (1958) Some observations on the congenital deformity of the central nervous system known as the Arnold-Chiari malformation. J Neuropathol Exp Neurol 17:255-266
25. Cleland J (1883) Contribution to the study of spina bifida, encephalocele and anencaphalus. J Anat Physiol 17:257-292
26. Peach B (1965) Arnold-Chiari malformation: morphogenesis. Arch Neurol 12:527-35
27. MacKenzie NG, Emery JL (1971) Deformities of central nervous cord in children with neurospinal dysraphism. Dev Med Child Neurol 13(Suppl 25):58-61
28. Gibert JN, Jones KC, Rorke LB et al (1986) Central nervous system anomalies associated with meningomyelocele, hydrocephalus, and the Arnold-Chiari malformations: reappraisal of thesis regarding the pathogenesis of posterior neural tube closure defects. Neurosurgery 18:559-563
29. Pang D, Dias MS, Ahab-Barmada M (1992) Split cord malformation. I. A unified theory of embryogenesis for double spinal cord malformations. Neurosurgery 31:451-480
30. Breningstall GN, Marker SM, Tubman DE (1992) Hydrosyringomyelia and diastematomyelia detected by MRI in myelomeningocele. Pediatr Neurol 8:267-271
31. Pang D, Dias MS (1993) Cervical myelomeningoceles. Neurosurgery 33:363-373
32. Naidich TP, McLonc DG, Mutluer S (1983) A new understanding of dorsal dysraphism with lipoma (lipomyeloschisis): radiological evaluation and surgical correlation. AJNR 4:103-116
33. Pierre-Kahn A, Zerah M, Renier D et al (1997) Congenital lumbosacral lipomas. Childs Nerv Syst 13:298-334
34. Raimondi AJ (1989) Hamartomas and the dysraphic state. In: Raimondi AJ, Choux M, Di Rocco C (eds) The pediatric spine 1. Development and the dysraphic state. Springer, Berlin, pp 179-199

35. Lee KS, Gower DJ, McWhorter JM et al (1988) The role of MR imaging in the diagnosis and treatment of anterior sacral meningocele. Report of 2 cases. J Neurosurg 69:628-631
36. Castillo M, Mukherji SK (1996) Imaging of the pediatric head, neck, and spine. Lippincott-Raven, Philadelphia, pp 638-640
37. Okada T, Imae S, Igarashi S et al (1996) Occult intrasacral meningocele associated with spina bifida: a case report. Surg Neurol 46:147-149
38. Byrd SE, Harvey C, Darling CF (1995) MR of terminal myelocystoceles. Eur J Radiol 20:215-220
39. Peacock WJ, Murovic JA (1989) Magnetic resonance imaging in myelocystoceles. Report of two cases. J Neurosurg 70:804-807
40. McComb JG (1993) Comment on: Pang D, Dias MS. Cervical myelomeningoceles. Neurosurgery 33:373
41. Parent AD (1993) Comment on: Pang D, Dias MS. Cervical myelomeningoceles. Neurosurgery 33:372-373
42. Tortori-Donati P, Cama A, Rosa ML et al (1990) Occult spinal dysraphism: neuroradiological study. Neuroradiology 31:512-522
43. Raghavan N, Barkovich AJ, Edwards M, Norman D (1989) MR imaging in the tethered spinal cord syndrome. AJNR 10:27-36
44. Altman NR, Altman DH (1987) MR imaging of spinal dysraphism. AJNR 8:533-538
45. Uchino A, Mori T, Ohno M (1991) Thickened fatty filum terminale: MR imaging. Neuroradiology 33:331-333
46. Kernohan JW (1924) The ventriculus terminalis: its growth and development. J Comp Neurol 38:10-125
47. Coleman IT, Zimmerman RA, Rorke LB (1995) Ventriculus terminalis of the conus medullaris: MR findings in children. AJNR 16:1421-1426
48. Dias MS, Walker ML (1992) The embryogenesis of complex dysraphic malformations: a disorder of gastrulation? Pediatr Neurosurg 18:229-253
49. Prop N, Frensdorf EL (1967) A postvertebral endodermal cyst associated with axial deformities: a case showing the "endodermal-ectodermal adhesion syndrome". Pediatrics 39:555-562
50. Faris JC, Crowe JE (1975) The split notochord syndrome. J Pediatr Surg 10:467-472
51. Hoffman CH, Dietrich RB, Pais MJ et al (1993) The split notochord syndrome with dorsal enteric fistula. AJNR 14:622-627
52. Kincaid PK, Stanley P, Kovanlikaya A et al (1999) Coexistent neurenteric cyst and enterogenous cyst. Further support for a common embryologic error. Pediatr Radiol 29:539-541
53. Burger PC, Scheithauer BW, Vogel FS (2002) Surgical pathology of the nervous system and its coverings. Churchill Livingstone, New York
54. Brooks BS, Duvall ER, El Gammal T et al (1993) Neuroimaging features of neurenteric cysts: analysis of nine cases and review of the literature. AJNR 14:735-746
55. Ciao P, Osborn AG, Smirniotopoulos JG et al (1995) Neurenteric cysts. Pathology, imaging spectrum, and differential diagnosis. Int J Neuroradiol 1:17-27
56. Schlesinger AE, Naidich TP, Quencer RM (1986) Concurrent hydromyelia and diastematomyelia. AJNR 7:473-477
57. Tortori-Donati P, Fondelli MP, Rossi A (1998) Anomalie congenite del midollo spinale. In: Simonetti G, Del Maschio A, Bartolozzi C, Passariello R (eds) Trattato italiano di risonanza magnetica. Idelson Gnocchi, Naples, pp 517-553
58. Ersahin Y, Mutluer S, Kocaman S et al (1998) Split spinal cord malformations in children. J Neurosurg 88:57-65
59. Barkovich AJ, Edwards MSB, Cogen PH (1991) MR evaluation of spinal dermal sinus tracts in children. AJNR 12:123-129
60. Duhamel B (1961) From the mermaid to anal imperforation: the syndrome of caudal regression. Arch Dis Child 36:152-155
61. Tortori-Donati V, Fondelli MP, Rossi A et al (1999) Segmental spinal dysgenesis. Neuroradiologic findings with clinical and embryologic correlation. AJNR 20:445-456
62. Valenzano M, Paoletti R, Rossi A et al (1999) Sirenomelia. Pathological features, antenatal ultrasonographic clues, and a review of current embryogenic theories. Hum Reprod Update 5:82-86
63. Raffel C, Litofsky S, McComb JG (1991) Central nervous system malformations and the VATER association. Pediatr Neurosurg 16:174-173
64. Currarino G, Coln D, Votteler T (1981) Triad of anorectal, sacral, and presacral anomalies. AIR 137:395-398
65. Dias MS, Azizkhan RG (1998) A novel embryogenetic mechanism for Currarino's triad: inadequate dorsoventral separation of the caudal eminence from hindgut endoderm. Pediatr Neurosurg 28:223-229
66. Gudinchet F, Maeder I, Laurent T et al (1997) Magnetic resonance detection of myelodysplasia in children with Currarino triad. Pediatr Radiol 27:903-907

CHAPTER 4
Epidemiology and Aetiological Factors

Vivek Josan, Andrew Morokoff, Wirginia J. Maixner

Introduction

Spina bifida refers to a wide range of neural tube defects (NTDs) affecting the spine and spinal cord. These defects result from the maldevelopment of the neuropore and the adjacent mesodermal and ectodermal structures during embryogenesis. Spina bifida can be classified as either open or closed type according to the presence or absence of exposed neural tissue. These are called spina bifida aperta and spina bifida occulta, respectively. Spina bifida aperta is caused by the failure of primary neurulation resulting in exposed neural tissue or meninges with or without cerebrospinal fluid leakage. It includes two main types: myelomeningocele and meningocele. Myelomeningocele is the severest form in which the spinal cord and the meninges protrude from an opening in the spine. Meningocele is a less severe form in which only the meninges and non-functional nerves protrude into a sac.

Spina bifida occulta is caused by defects in secondary neurulation and includes various closed spinal defects such as diastematomyelia, diplomyelia, dorsal dermal sinus, spinal lipoma and a pure bone fusion defect of the dorsal spinal column. In these defects the neural tissue or meninges are not exposed and the defect is fully epithelialised, although the skin covering the defect may be dysplastic. Spina bifida occulta is much more prevalent than the open forms. In its simplest form with a pure bony dysraphism it occurs in about 17-30% of the population and is seen more commonly in males [1, 2].

Epidemiology

Spina bifida is a congenital malformation that occurs early during embryogenesis, resulting in a certain number of affected foetuses being spontaneously aborted. In addition, prenatal diagnosis has resulted in an increase in the number of therapeutic abortions [3, 4]. Establishing its true incidence, therefore, becomes very difficult. To assess the incidence accurately data collection should include all occurrences of NTDs within the population of live births, stillbirths, miscarriages and elective abortions. Prevalence at birth is a more practical estimate of the frequency of spina bifida in a population. This will include information on both live births and still births, though it will omit spontaneous and therapeutic abortions.

Epidemiological studies have revealed a wide variation in the prevalence of spina bifida based on ethnicity, race, geography and temporal trends. The incidence of spina bifida has a marked geographic variation. In Europe the highest rates are found in the British Isles, with an overall incidence of 2.4-3.8 cases of NTDs per 1000 live births [5]. Within the British Isles, higher rates are reported in the North West, particularly in Ireland, where the rate approaches 5 per 1000 live births. These higher rates are not observed with other congenital malformations. Within continental Europe, a lower incidence of 0.1-0.6 per 1000 live births is reported [6]. A higher incidence of spinal dysraphism has been reported in Eastern Canada compared to Western Canada. The incidence of spina bifida in the United States has been estimated at 0.3-0.4 per 1000 live births, with the East Coast reporting a higher incidence than the West Coast. In China the incidence rates north of the Yangtze River are six times those in the southern provinces. Pockets of higher incidence have also been seen in India, but these do not fit any broad geographic patterns [7].

Ethnicity also has an effect on the rates of spina bifida, with certain populations having a significantly increased incidence compared to others. In the United States the Hispanic population is at the highest risk, with African Americans and Asians at the lowest risk among all ethnic groups. An increased risk for neural tube defects remains among Hispanics even after controlling for other factors such as diabetes and obesity [8]. In the British Isles, populations of Irish, Scottish and Welsh descent have a higher risk of spinal dysraphism, which may explain the increased incidence seen in regions densely populated with these ethnic groups. When ethnic groups with low prevalence, such as Africans or Asians, migrate to a region of high incidence they tend to maintain their low rates. Dietary practices, the availability of health promotion programs and antenatal screening, as well as cultural views regarding termination, all play a part in determining variations in incidence, particularly in regions such as Europe.

Over the last three to four decades there has been an overall decline in the incidence of spina bifida in most industrialised countries. In the UK, Ireland [9] and the USA [10] peaks of prevalence and incidence of NTDs were recorded in the earlier half of the twentieth century and since the 1970s the number of NTDs at birth has been declining. As the beginning of these declining trends predated the introduction of antenatal testing and widespread folate supplementation, they can be attributed only partly to elective abortions and dietary changes [11]. Other reasons for these declining trends are not currently known.

Aetiology

Genetic Influences

Spina bifida is recognised to have a complex aetiological basis, with both genetic and environmental factors at play. A known chromosomal, teratogenic, or Mendelian malformation syndrome can be identified in a small minority of individuals with meningomyeloceles. Spina bifida occurs more frequently in trisomy 13 and trisomy 18. An increased association is also seen with acrocallosal syndrome, CHILD syndrome, Fraser syndrome, Waardenburg syndrome and Meckel-Gruber syndrome, among others. As most epidemiological studies include only cases of live births and stillbirths and not spontaneous abortions, it is difficult to estimate the true impact of chromosomal malformations on the prevalence of NTDs.

The genetic influence on the occurrence of spinal dysraphism is evidenced by the presence of a recurrence pattern within families, ethnic groupings in the incidence of spina bifida and an increased risk with alteration in genes involved in folate metabolism and other cellular processes.

A family history of spina bifida or anencephaly is one of the strongest risk factors for these disorders. Several studies have shown a clear increase in the incidence of spina bifida within families. This increased risk is seen in spite of low vertical transmission due to lower reproduction in affected individuals and a higher rate of spontaneous and therapeutic abortions. The risk for spina bifida in the siblings of affected individuals is about 3-4% [12] and this risk nearly triples [13] with each subsequent affected pregnancy.

Folate and its metabolites are important in purine and pyrimidine synthesis, as well as for the transfer of methyl groups in the processing of some amino acids. Mutations or genetic variations in genes for the folate-homocysteine pathway enzymes, such as methyltetrahydrofolate reductase (MTHFR) or methionine synthase, have been implicated in neural tube defects [14]. It is postulated that these mutations may lead to a relative lack of function that may be overcome by therapeutic high levels of folate. The first genetic risk factor for NTDs to be discovered was a single nucleotide polymorphism (C677T) in the MTHFR gene, which led to a mildly dysfunctional enzyme, increased levels of homocysteine in plasma and an increased risk of NTDs in those affected [15]. This single nucleotide polymorphism (SNP) is present in 10% of the North American population but there is considerable ethnic and geographic variation. Many other folate pathway gene polymorphisms have also been implicated as NTD risk factors, albeit inconclusively [16].

Variants of other genes that are involved in neural tube formation or genes involved in the metabolism of compounds needed for embryonic development are also candidate risk factors for spina bifida, but at this point in time no specific associations have been established. For instance, the genes encoding the Pax family gene products have been implicated in NTDs. Mice with homozygous *Pax-3* disruptions have neural tube defects and in humans, the *Pax-3* homolog gene has been weakly associated with Waardenburg syndrome and myelomeningocoele [17]. Mutation of the *Pax-1* gene has also been found in one patient with spina bifida [18]. However, large family linkage studies have failed to show any role for PAX genes [19].

The curly tail (ct) mouse represents a well-studied model of NTDs in which other genes besides the ct gene product, as well as environmental factors, influence NTD occurrence. Interestingly, NTDs in these mice are folic acid resistant, as is thought to be the case in 30% of human cases [20]. There are now over 190 mutants and strains of mice associated with NTDs, some of which respond to specific supplementation with folic acid, inositol, methionine or other dietary factors [21]. These suggest that the genetic and environmental causes of NTDs in humans are likely to be multifactorial as well.

Folate Deficiency

The vast majority of cases of spina bifida are thought to be due to complex polygenic interactions with environmental factors. Only a few potential clinical variables have been established as risk factors for NTDs. Inadequate intake of folate before conception and during early pregnancy is now a well established risk factor [22]. Folate and folic acid are forms of the water soluble vitamin B9, which is required for DNA replication in cells but as discussed above, the exact mechanism for its role in preventing spina bifida is not known.

In 1931, after studying the nutrition of women in India, Dr. Lucy Wills found that brewer's yeast could reverse pernicious anaemia of pregnancy [23]; subsequently, the active ingredient in the yeast was shown to be folate. Folate was isolated from spinach leaves in 1941 and synthesised in 1945. In 1952, therapeutic abortions with the folate antagonist aminopterin were found to cause a number of cases of anencephaly [24, 25]. Observations in the mid-1970s in the UK that lower red cell folate levels in women of lower socioeconomic status were associated with a higher prevalence of NTDs implicated folate deficiency as an aetiological factor [26].

In the early 1980s, initial randomised control trials in the UK were strongly suggestive of a role for folate supplements in preventing NTDs [25, 27]. From 1988 to 1995, a number of case-control studies indicated a NTD risk reduction of between 30 to 75% in those who took folic acid supplements [28]. The definitive trial was The Medical Research Council Vitamin Study Research Group (UK) that reported in 1991 the results of a double-blind randomised-controlled trial in 33 centres across seven countries. This showed that periconceptional folic acid supplementation (4 mg/d in mothers with a previous history of NTD) was associated with a risk reduction of 72% [22]. In 1991, the US Centers for Disease Control (CDC) therefore recommended 4 mg/d folic acid supplementation to those mothers with a high risk by virtue of a previously affected pregnancy.

It is important to note that the above studies only addressed the risk of recurrent NTDs in mothers with a previous history of affected births. Studies with much larger power would have been required to investigate the risk pattern of first occurrences, although these represent the vast majority (~95%) of

cases of spina bifida and the larger public health issue. Only one randomised study, of 4,156 Hungarian women planning pregnancy, looked at first occurrence and found a statistically significant reduction in NTDs with folic acid supplementation of 800 μg/d [29]. This led to the further recommendation by the CDC in 1992 that all reproductive-aged women should take 400 μg folic acid daily in addition to a folate-rich diet [28].

Other Risk Factors

Other maternal conditions implicated as risk factors for neural tube defects are obesity [30] and diabetes with hyperinsulinaemia as the potential underlying metabolic factor. A body mass index of more than 29 is estimated to double the risk of conceiving a child with a NTD. Maternal febrile illness in the early pregnancy has also been shown to increase the risk of NTDs [31].

Maternal intake of anticonvulsants, especially sodium valproate and carbamazepine, during the periconceptional period is well recognised as a risk factor for NTDs. The prevalence of spina bifida is approximately 1-2% with valproate exposure and 0.5% with carbamazepine [19]. Data concerning the risk for congenital malformations associated with the newer anti-epileptics (gabapentin, felbamate, lamotrigine, levetiracetam, oxcarbazepine, tiagabine, topiramate, and zonisamide) are still limited. Seizure control must not be neglected in a pregnant woman with epilepsy since seizures are associated with harm to the foetus as well as the mother. Risk may be minimised by using a single drug at the lowest effective dosage.

The epidemiological and aetiological factors relating to spina bifida are complex and incompletely understood. While spina bifida is among the most devastating congenital malformations, it is also the only birth defect where effective prevention has been successfully employed.

Prevention of Neural Tube Defects

Folate

Since folic acid supplementation has been definitively shown to reduce the risk of NTDs, the mainstay of prevention is now aimed at increasing the intake of folic acid in the target population of women. It is now almost universally recommended by health authorities that all women planning or able to become pregnant should have an additional intake of 400 µg of folic acid per day. This needs to be taken at least from one month prior to conception and continued throughout the first 3 months of pregnancy. Those with a history of previously affected children are recommended to take an even higher dose of 4 mg per day.

This addition can potentially be achieved with three options: increasing folate-rich foods in the diet, folic acid supplementation and fortification of foods with folic acid.

Foods high in folate include green leafy vegetables such as broccoli, spinach and salad greens. However, because dietary folate is less stable and bioavailable than supplementary folic acid, it is difficult to get enough folate from natural sources alone to reduce the risk of NTDs and therefore recommendations to increase folate intake via food are not an adequate public health measure [32].

Since 1993, public health strategies in many countries have aimed to promote the taking of folic acid supplements by women of child-bearing age. However, these have generally not been successful in significantly increasing the intake of folic acid or reducing the numbers of affected births [33]. The likely reason for this is that up to 50% of all pregnancies are unplanned, and folate must be taken prior to conception in order to have an effect.

Food fortification policies have therefore been used by regulatory bodies to provide a more widespread and reliable increase in folic acid intake. Voluntary fortification policies have been implemented in the UK and Australia, as well as Mongolia. In Europe, there has been reluctance to introduce folic acid fortification programs. Australia implemented voluntary folate fortification in grain products and fruit and vegetable juices in 1995, a policy which led to an increase of 30-40% in the proportion of women taking periconceptional folic acid supplements [34]. Fortified foods could also be labelled with a 'health claim' regarding the benefits of folate supplementation; however, this has not been taken up consistently by fortified product manufacturers [35]. These policies have led to a drop in NTD cases, but have disproportionately benefited those of higher socioeconomic standing, whereas there has not been a substantial improvement in the Australian Aboriginal community.

Mandatory Fortification

In January 1998, the United States introduced mandatory folic acid fortification of flour as well as a number of other grain-based foods, including corn-

meal, rice, pasta and breakfast cereals. Fortification is now also mandatory in Canada, Indonesia and some South American, African and Middle Eastern countries. The level of fortification in the USA was set at 150 µg/100 g flour, which was projected to provide on average an additional 100 µg/d of folic acid to the population. This relatively modest increase was chosen to minimise the potential adverse effects of increasing folate levels across the general population, while still providing an important decrease in the incidence of NTDs. The American Academy of Pediatrics considers fortification to only provide one quarter of the officially recommended (400 µg/d) additional intake. On the other hand, there is some evidence that the official recommendation of an additional 400 µg/d only provides little extra benefit in terms of predicted NTD risk compared to 200 µg/d [32]. In any case, women of reproductive age should still be counselled to increase their folic acid intake by supplementation, since mandatory fortification programs do not currently supply enough additional folic acid on their own.

In the USA, the National Health and Nutrition Examination Surveys (NHANES), conducted before and after fortification was introduced, confirmed a significant increase in both serum and red cell folate levels in adults [36]. More importantly, recent data has confirmed that rates of NTDs dropped in the USA by 26% and in Canada by 46%, compared to pre-fortification rates, indicating that these policies are having a substantial desired effect [37-39]. In Canada, the risk reduction was highest in those geographic areas in which the baseline risk of NTDs was highest [37]. In Chile, where mandatory fortification was introduced in 2000, there has been a 40% drop in NTD rates [40].

Proposals for mandatory fortification are under debate currently in the UK, Ireland, Australia and New Zealand. Each year in Australia approximately 300-350 babies are affected by NTDs. Currently, mandatory fortification has been recommended by Food Standards Australia New Zealand (FSANZ) and is now before the Australia and New Zealand Food Regulation Ministerial Council. The plan proposes to fortify flour for bread-making at a level of 200-300 µg folic acid per 100 g of flour, with organic flour being exempt. This is projected to increase levels of daily folic acid intake in women by 100 µg in Australia and 140 µg in New Zealand, which could potentially lead to a decrease of up to 49 (14%) cases per year in Australia and 14 (20%) per year in New Zealand [41]. Some argue that the level of proposed fortification is not adequate in part because, according to some surveys, Australian women eat only 11 slices of bread per week. This has led to calls for folic acid to be added to products like milk and yoghurt as well.

Those in favor of mandatory fortification have also pointed out potential health benefits of folic acid for the general population, including a possible risk reduction in heart disease, stroke and cancer. An additional 200 µg/d of folic acid (rather than the projected 100 µg/d with the current fortification plan) would also lower plasma homocysteine with potential cardiovascular benefits [42]. People taking methotrexate for rheumatoid arthritis and other diseases may also benefit from folate supplementation. Some studies have indicated a possible cognitive beneficial effect of folate in those over the age of 50 as well as a synergistic effect of folate with medication in the treatment of depression [43, 44].

However, a number of concerns regarding mandatory fortification have been raised:

1. There will be significant increased costs to the flour milling industry and governments. These will eventually be passed on to the consumer with an estimated increase in the price of a loaf of bread of 0.5-1% [45].
2. There may be an exacerbation of the effects of B12 deficiency, or an increase in the incidence of B12 deficiency or a masking of the symptoms of B12 deficiency. However, the incidence of B12 deficiency in the USA has not changed since mandatory fortification was introduced in 1998 [46]. An Australian study from 2006 also showed that those elderly people with high levels of folate intake did not have a higher incidence of B12 deficiency [47].
3. There is a risk of exceeding recommended upper limits of folate intake, particularly in children. The maximum daily recommended dose is 1 mg per day. The FSANZ report estimates that 9% of children 2-3 years old and 4-8% of older children may exceed the stated upper limit. In adults the proportion over the limit is projected to be very small (< 1%). The possible sequelae of too much serum folate in children where pernicious anaemia from B12 deficiency is not an issue is not definitely known, but no adverse effects have been reported. Furthermore, the recommended upper limit of levels is subject to much uncertainty.
4. Folic acid can potentially interact with anticonvulsant medication to reduce drug levels and increase the risk of seizures. Some anticonvulsants are also known to lower folate levels leading to megaloblastic anaemia. However, these effects are rare and subject to much individual variation. Furthermore, they are generally associated with very high doses of folate supplementation (e.g., 5,000-10,000 µg/d). The Folic Acid Subcommittee of the United States Department of Health and Human Services has concluded that 1,000 µg/day oral folic acid supplementation is safe for individuals with controlled epilepsy (Expert Group on Vitamins and Minerals 2002).
5. A recent study suggested that low serum folate levels may be protective against colon cancer [48].
6. There are ethical concerns about restriction of the right to make individual choices regarding one's health and food intake.

Conclusion

Although the incidence of NTDs has been decreasing in many areas around the world, challenges still remain, particularly in terms of public health policy regarding folate acid supplementation and fortification of food. It is now a generally accepted recommendation that women of child-bearing age should take 400 µg/day of folic acid, in addition to a folate-rich diet. Fortification in the USA and Canada since 1998 has shown definite efficacy in lowering the incidence of NTDs in the population and other countries are currently evaluating whether to follow this lead. Of particular importance is the imperative to provide effective health education strategies and outcomes for those populations who are at higher risk and for socio-economic reasons may not have adequate access to primary health care, such as the Hispanic community in the USA and the Australian Aboriginal population. From a scientific point of view, NTDs appear to have a complex multifactorial aetiology, most likely due to a number of genetic variations, together with environmental factors. These will hopefully be elucidated more clearly in the future and will potentially suggest new preventative measures.

References

1. Fidas A, MacDonald HL, Elton RA et al (1987) Prevalence and patterns of spina bifida occulta in 2707 normal adults. Clin Radiol 38:537-542

2. Boone D, Parsons D, Lachmann SM et al (1985) Spina bifida occulta: lesion or anomaly? Clin Radiol 36:159-161

3. Nikkila A, Rydhstrom H, Kallen B (2006) The incidence of spina bifida in Sweden 1973-2003: the effect of prenatal diagnosis. Eur J Pub Health 16:660-662

4. Bower C, Raymond M, Lumley J et al (1993) Trends in neural tube defects 1980-1989. Med J Aus 158:152-154

5. Prevalence of neural tube defects in 20 regions of Europe and the impact of prenatal diagnosis, 1980-1986. EUROCAT Working Group (1991) J Epidemiol Comm Health 45:52-58

6. Prevalence of neural tube defects in 16 regions of Europe, 1980-1983. The EUROCAT Working Group (1987) Int J Epidemiol 16:246-251

7. Frey L, Hauser WA (2003) Epidemiology of neural tube defects. Epilepsia 44:4-13

8. Canfield MA, Annegers JF, Brender JD et al (1996) Hispanic origin and neural tube defects in Houston/Harris County, Texas. II. Risk factors. Am J Epidemiol 143:12-24

9. Elwood JH (1973) Epidemics of anencephalus and spina bifida in Ireland since 1900. Int J Epidemiol 2:171-175

10. Janerich DT (1973) Epidemic waves in the prevalence of anencephaly and spina bifida in New York State. Teratology 8:253-256

11. Rosano A, Smithells D, Cacciani L et al (1999) Time trends in neural tube defects prevalence in relation to preventive strategies: an international study. J Epidemiol Comm Health 53:630-635

12. Papp C, Adam Z, Toth-Pal E et al (1997) Risk of recurrence of craniospinal anomalies. J Matern Fetal Med 6:53-57

13. Elwood JM, Little J, Elwood JH (1992) Epidemiology and control of neural tube defects. Oxford University Press

14. Schwahn B, Rozen R (2001) Polymorphisms in the methylenetetrahydrofolate reductase gene: clinical consequences. Am J Pharmacogenomics 1:189-201

15. van der Put NM, Steegers-Theunissen RP, Frosst P et al (1995) Mutated methylenetetrahydrofolate reductase as a risk factor for spina bifida. Lancet 346:1070-1071

16. van der Linden IJ, Afman LA, Heil SG et al (2006) Genetic variation in genes of folate metabolism and neural-tube defect risk. Proc Nutr Soc 65:204-215

17. Chatkupt S, Chatkupt S, Johnson WG (1993) Waardenburg syndrome and myelomeningocele in a family. J Med Gen 30:83-84

18. Hol FA, Geurds MP, Chatkupt S et al (1996) PAX genes and human neural tube defects: an amino acid substitution in PAX1 in a patient with spina bifida. J Med Gen 33:655-660

19. Melvin EC, George TM, Worley G et al (2000) Genetic studies in neural tube defects. NTD Collaborative Group. Pediatr Neurosurg 32:1-9

20. van Straaten HW, Copp AJ (2001) Curly tail: a 50-year history of the mouse spina bifida model. Anat Embryol 203:225-237

21. Harris MJ, Juriloff DM (2007) Mouse mutants with neural tube closure defects and their role in understanding human neural tube defects. Birth Defects Res 79:187-210

22. Prevention of neural tube defects: results of the Medical Research Council Vitamin Study (1991) MRC Vitamin Study Research Group. Lancet 338:131-137

23. Roe DA (1978) Lucy Wills (1888-1964). A biographical sketch. J Nutr 108:1379-1383

24. Thiersch JB (1952) Therapeutic abortions with a folic acid antagonist, 4-aminopteroylglutamic acid (4-amino PGA) administered by the oral route. Am J Obstet Gynecol 63:1298-1304

25. Laurence KM, James N, Miller MH et al (1981) Double-blind randomised controlled trial of folate treatment before conception to prevent recurrence of neural-tube defects. Br Med J (Clin Res Ed) 282:1509-1511

26. Smithells RW, Sheppard S, Schorah CJ (1976) Vitamin deficiencies and neural tube defects. Arch Dis Child 51:944-950

27. Smithells RW, Nevin NC, Seller MJ et al (1983) Further experience of vitamin supplementation for prevention of neural tube defect recurrences. Lancet 1:1027-1031

28. Pitkin RM (2007) Folate and neural tube defects. Am J Clin Nutr 85:285S-288S

29. Czeizel AE, Dudas I, Fritz G et al (1992) The effect of periconceptional multivitamin-mineral supplementation on vertigo, nausea and vomiting in the first trimester of pregnancy. Arch Gynecol Obstet 251:181-185

30. Shaw GM, Velie EM, Schaffer D (1996) Risk of neural tube defect-affected pregnancies among obese women. JAMA 275:1093-1096

31. Chambers CD, Johnson KA, Dick LM et al (1998) Maternal fever and birth outcome: a prospective study. Teratology 58:251-257

32. McNulty H, Cuskelly GJ, Ward M (2000) Response of red blood cell folate to intervention: implications for folate recommendations for the prevention of neural tube defects. Am J Clin Nutr 71:1308S-1311S

33. Botto LD, Lisi A, Bower C et al (2006) Trends of selected malformations in relation to folic acid recommendations and fortification: an international assessment. Birth Defects Res 76:693-705

34. Bower C, Stanley FJ (2004) Case for mandatory fortification of food with folate in Australia, for the prevention of neural tube defects. Birth Defects Res 70:842-843

35. Lawrence M (2006) Evaluation of the implementation of the folate-neural tube defect health claim and its impact on the availability of folate-fortified food in Australia. Aust N Z J Public Health 30:363-368

36. Dietrich M, Brown CJ, Block G et al (2005) The effect of folate fortification of cereal-grain products on blood folate status, dietary folate intake, and dietary folate sources among adult non-supplement users in the United States. J Am Coll Nutr 24:266-274

37. De Wals P, Tairou F, Van Allen MI et al (2007) Reduction in neural-tube defects after folic acid fortification in Canada. N Engl J Med 357:135-142

38. Spina bifida and anencephaly before and after folic acid mandate--United States, 1995-1996 and 1999-2000 (2004) MMWR 53:362-365
39. Ray JG, Meier C, Vermeulen MJ et al (2002) Association of neural tube defects and folic acid food fortification in Canada. Lancet 360:2047-2048
40. Hertrampf E, Cortes F (2004) Folic acid fortification of wheat flour: Chile. Nutr Rev 62:S44-48; discussion S49
41. Bower C, de Klerk N, Hickling S et al (2006) Assessment of the potential effect of incremental increases in folic acid intake on neural tube defects in Australia and New Zealand. Aust N Z J Public Health 30:369-374
42. Ward M, McNulty H, Pentieva K et al (2000) Fluctuations in dietary methionine intake do not alter plasma homocysteine concentration in healthy men. J Nutr 130:2653-2657
43. Taylor MJ, Carney SM, Goodwin GM et al (2004) Folate for depressive disorders: systematic review and meta-analysis of randomized controlled trials. J Psychopharmacol (Oxford, England) 18:251-256
44. Durga J, van Boxtel MP, Schouten EG et al (2007) Effect of 3-year folic acid supplementation on cognitive function in older adults in the FACIT trial: a randomised, double blind, controlled trial. Lancet 369:208-216
45. FSANZ: Food Standards Australia and New Zealand Report 23 May 2007. http://www.foodstandards.gov.au/_srcfiles/P295%20Folate%20Fortification%20FFR%20+%20Attach%201%20FINAL.pdf.
46. Mills JL, Von Kohorn I, Conley MR et al (2003) Low vitamin B-12 concentrations in patients without anemia: the effect of folic acid fortification of grain. Am J Clin Nutr 77:1474-1477
47. Flood VM, Smith WT, Webb KL et al (2006) Prevalence of low serum folate and vitamin B12 in an older Australian population. Aust N Z J Public Health 30:38-41
48. Van Guelpen B, Hultdin J, Johansson I et al (2006) Low folate levels may protect against colorectal cancer. Gut 55:1461-1466

CHAPTER 5
Myelomeningocele and Medical Ethics

Toba Niazi, Marion L. Walker

Throughout history, the treatment of infants born with serious neurological and physical medical ailments has been debated: to treat or not to treat? In the early nineteenth century, little could be done for these infants who often either died during the perinatal period or succumbed to the natural progression of their disease. With improvements in medical diagnosis and treatment, a shift in attitude has led to more aggressive medical intervention in the treatment of affected newborns and an ability to treat certain conditions in the prenatal period [1-3]. Despite our success in treating younger and younger babies, some cases nevertheless result in children with a degree of physical or mental disability, many of whom could not have been treated as recently as 50 years ago [4]. Social and financial stresses are thus imposed on the families of these children as well as on society as a result of these "successful" treatments. Furthermore, a conflict remains between the benefits that the child gains from being sustained, albeit in a disabled state, and the quality of life the child experiences because of the treatments necessitated by his/her disease. Critical issues and arguments must be considered on all sides of the debate when considering medical intervention in severely ill infants.

Neural tube defects are an excellent representation of this type of major medical condition that affects newborns, and a consideration of the associated issues offers a framework for discussion of medical ethics and the right to treatment and the right to life. In fact, myelomeningocele or spina bifida ranks second only to cerebral palsy as a cause of locomotor instability in childhood [4, 5]. Furthermore, not only is myelomeningocele associated with physical impediment, but affected children may also have associated cognitive disabilities and behavioral issues. Myelomeningocele has a broad spectrum of manifestations ranging from a physically and mentally normal infant to one who may be severely debilitated both physically and mentally. Myelomeningocele is not a new disease, having been described in ancient times [4, 6], but the evolution in the treatment of this disease from the end of the nineteenth century to the present day has progressed rapidly, providing the opportunity to consider how ethical and moral obligations to these infants have been molded with medical technological advancements. In fact, we now have in our armamentarium the ability not only to treat this defect after birth but also to prevent it prenatally or begin treatment during gestational development [2, 3, 5, 7, 8].

Myelomeningocele affects approximately 2,500 to 6,000 newborns per year in the United States and a higher proportion of infants in the developing world [3, 5]. Infants with myelomeningoceles are the most severely affected neurologically, physically, and mentally of all of the children in the dysraphic spectrum. For this reason, infants with myelomeningocele seem to be at the cusp of the debate regarding the initial treatment of serious neurological and physical diseases [3, 6, 9-13].

In the earliest days in the life of an infant with myelomeningocele, infection is the most imminent danger, with the possibility of meningitis secondary to infection of the exposed neural placode. The degree to which infants with myelomeningocele are affected by physical handicap depends on the spinal level of the lesion. Most myelomeningoceles (85%) are located in the caudal thoracolumbar spine or sacrum [5]. This, in turn, leads to the possibility that affected infants may be ambulatory. Most importantly, if L3 function is preserved, the ability to stand erect is saved, and if L4 and L5 function are preserved, the ability to walk is maintained. Depending on the level of spinal cord involvement, most children with myelomeningocele lack urinary continence because of either a neurogenic bladder or lower motor neuron damage. This is not only a medical problem because of concern over possible kidney damage or failure, but there are also major social implications to urinary incontinence. To complicate matters further, approximately 80% of infants with myelomeningocele also have hydrocephalus [3, 5, 12], which requires them to undergo cerebrospinal fluid shunting procedures and life-long neurosurgical care. Finally, myelomeningocele may also be associated with deformities of the vertebral column such as scoliosis and kyphosis that may require orthopedic intervention [4]. As is apparent from the aforementioned list of associated conditions, these infants, if treated, require a multidisciplinary team of compassionate physicians in all subspecialties to assist with medical care and with maintenance of their complicated medical condition [3, 12, 14, 15].

Of paramount importance to this debate is the advancement in the understanding of the disease process, pathophysiology, prevention, and prenatal diagnosis of spina bifida. In the early nineteenth century little was known regarding this disease, therefore prevention could not be undertaken. Over the course of the last century, however, the cause of spina bifida has been determined to be multifactorial in nature. A major breakthrough in the mid-1980s demonstrated an association between neural tube defects and deficiencies of certain nutrients such as folic acid and zinc [5, 8, 16, 17]. Since then, a worldwide emphasis has been placed on the prevention of neural tube defects with supplementation of prenatal vitamins before and after conception. The recommendation is that women who are of childbearing years consume at least 0.4 mg of folic acid daily, women who are pregnant consume 0.6 mg per day, and women who have had a child already afflicted with a neural tube defect consume 4 mg per day [5, 8, 16, 17].

Certain conditions may naturally predispose a woman to having a fetus with a neural tube defect. One such condition is epilepsy treated with anticonvulsants. Carbamazepine and valproic acid are two of the anticonvulsants documented to increase the likelihood of neural tube defects. Pregnant women afflicted with type I diabetes mellitus have also been linked to an increased incidence of having children with neural tube defects. Prepregnancy obesity has also been associated with pregnancies complicated by spina bifida. In fact, the greater the body mass index of the mother, the higher the association with pregnancies complicated by neural tube defects [5, 8, 16-18].

Diagnostic testing has revolutionized the diagnosis of neural tube defects during pregnancy. The use of maternal serum markers for alpha-fetoprotein (AFP), amniocentesis, ultrasonography, and magnetic resonance imaging (MRI) has made early detection possible. Maternal serum AFP (MSAFP) is the gold-standard initial screening test for neural tube defects. This test is performed at 16-18 weeks of gestation. If the MSAFP is elevated, then a high-resolution fetal ultrasound is performed. This test has a sensitivity of 100% for prenatal screening of neural tube defects and is also excellent at visualizing other sequelae associated with neural tube defects such as hydrocephalus and Chiari II malformation [5, 7, 10, 14, 15]. Amniocentesis serves as a further confirmatory test if both the MSAFP and high-resolution ultrasound are suggestive of neural tube defects. This is a more invasive test that measures the amniotic acetylcholinesterase level. If all three diagnostic tests point toward the presence of a neural tube defect, then the likelihood that the pregnancy is complicated by a neural tube defect is high. Although MSAFP as a marker for the presence of spinal dysraphism seems to be the gold-standard initial screening test in the United States, physicians in most Asian and some European countries forego this initial screening test in favor of diagnostic imaging techniques. In countries such as Japan, Korea, and France, MRI is used in lieu of MSAFP testing, ultrasound, and amniocentesis [8, 15]. Although we have a good understanding of the risks of bearing a child with myelomeningocele and the diagnostic tests to confirm or deny such a diagnosis, there remains a 0.1-0.2% incidence of spinal dysraphism in the United States. The eradication of all birth defects, especially neural tube defects, may not be achievable in reality because of the multifactorial nature of the disease process.

Once a prenatal diagnosis of a spinal dysraphism has been made, the weight of ethical and moral decisions falls squarely onto the shoulders of the parents and physicians as they consider which course to follow. In some instances, the parents may choose to terminate the pregnancy. The period of legal termination in the United States is until no later than the 24th week of gestation, although individual states may impose different restrictions [8, 14, 15]. The termination of a fetus has always been at the center of the moral debate about the right to life and hinges on the status of the fetus. If the fetus is considered to be devoid of rights because it is not thought to be an independent viable entity able to subsist and survive without the shelter of the womb, then termination of pregnancy is considered legally appropriate in many countries. To many people, however, the fetus has rights as a living being, and abortion concerns not only the freedom of the woman bearing the fetus but also the rights of the fetus. To holders of this viewpoint, termination of the fetus is considered unethical because it constitutes the deliberate destruction of life. Regardless of how these views are interpreted, the fetus's "physical interconnection" with a woman whose personhood is indisputable must be remembered [1, 2, 16, 17, 19, 20]. Failure to recognize the vital bond between the woman bearing the fetus and the fetus itself leads to what many refer to as the "fallacy of abstraction": considering a concept as if it were separable from another with which, in fact, it is intimately related [20, 21].

Another option available to parents when a neural tube defect is identified prenatally is maternal-fetal surgery that is undertaken in an attempt to minimize the neurological deficits associated with spinal dysraphism. It is postulated that some of the neurological deterioration associated with spina bifida may be due to the persistent exposure of the neural elements to the amniotic fluid. To date, intrauterine repair has not been shown to be beneficial in minimizing the motor deficits associated with myelomeningocele, but in some series has demonstrated some potential to decrease the degree of the associated Chiari II malformation [1, 2, 5, 16-21]. Some authors have suggested that infants treated in utero are less likely to require shunting procedures for hydrocephalus in the first year of life [1, 2, 5, 16-21].

Intrauterine surgery is also controversial in that it deals with the aforementioned fallacy of abstraction and personhood status of the fetus. There are inherent risks to the mother with any surgical procedure and those who opt to undergo maternal-fetal surgery face not one but two surgical procedures: a mid-trimester hysterotomy and, later, a cesarean section. Women who undergo a mid-trimester hysterotomy are at increased risk of uterine rupture, one of the true obstetrical surgical emergencies [1, 2, 5, 16-21]. The risk is at its height during labor, and for this reason cesarean sections are preferred over standard vaginal deliveries. Intrauterine surgery may also affect future fertility if abnormal placental attachment in future pregnancies requires emergent hysterectomy at the time of delivery and renders the mother unable to bear more children [20].

In addition to the risks to the mother, there are also associated risks to the fetus, including the risk of preterm labor. Premature birth has its own set of comorbidities with significant effects on the newborn. Clearly, maternal-fetal surgery has profound implications for the mother as well as the fetus. Given the paucity of demonstrable improvement in neonatal cognitive, neurological, or motor function, the procedure remains experimental until there is more evidence that demonstrates that the benefits of maternal-fetal surgery outweigh the risks to both the mother and the fetus.

Because of the ethical and medical dilemmas posed by abortion and intrauterine surgery, many parents of children with prenatally diagnosed spina bifida choose to wait until the birth of their child to intervene with aggressive medical treatment, while still others choose not to treat the child even after birth. This opens the door to other ethical questions: If medically successful treatment is available, is non-treatment ever justified when dealing with a viable newborn? Would non-treatment in the era of medical advancement be considered negligence on the part of the parents or physician? Finally, and perhaps most importantly: What is the definition of medically successful treatment? Can this be shown to be of benefit to the infant and the quality of life? As alluded to before, aggressive medical intervention must start in the first few hours of the infant's life to prevent life-threatening infection but spans the course of the child's life and encompasses a broad range of medical and surgical specialties. In fact, 10-15% of children afflicted with a spinal dysraphism die before the age of six years despite aggressive medical intervention [3-5, 7, 22, 23].

Historically, two main considerations, mental capacity and physical-bodily integrity, are used to assess quality of life in an individual, and any minimization of either would be considered a detraction from that quality of life [3, 6, 9-13, 23]. In order to form human relationships, mental functioning is paramount regardless of physical impairment, given that even severely physically disabled individuals can sustain healthy relationships. Most children (75-80%) afflicted with myelomeningocele have a normal intelligence quotient (IQ) if their hydrocephalus is managed aggressively; however, a direct correlation between repeated central nervous system infections and decrease in IQ has been shown. Regardless of the IQ of the individual, however, the ability of the mentally impaired to experience and enjoy interpersonal relationships reaches well down the IQ scale [3, 5].

Children with spina bifida can have a wide range of physical-bodily impediments depending on the level involved, including paralysis below the level of the lesion, loss of sensation, fecal and urinary incontinence, and kyphosis/scoliosis of the spine. Most of these physical debilities can now be treated with the aid of medical and surgical integration and intensive physical and occupational therapy. We must also remember that children born with spina bifida are disabled from birth and their disabilities will, in turn, affect the development of all of their abilities. The process of habilitation will help to maximize these abilities. This is in contrast to rehabilitation where skills and abilities that were once learned must now be relearned. Children who are disabled from birth whose habilitation is accomplished effectively will not feel as if their lives are devoid of skills and abilities they have never had and can prosper as valuable members of society [4]. The onus lies on society to not only see the disability but also to recognize the individual as a person.

Beyond the evaluation of treatment on the basis of physical and mental abilities and quality of life, the emotional and financial burdens that are placed on the parents and society will also often be weighed in the consideration of treatment for children with myelomeningocele. Many parents gain fulfillment by dedicating their lives to the care of their disabled children, while a few parents opt to physically or emotionally abandon the disabled child at birth. Although consideration should first and foremost be given to the right to life of the infant regardless of what the burden to the families or society may be, to say that parental and societal resources have no effect on the future well-being of the infant would be naïve. With a lack of emotional and financial resources these children will not flourish, but we should not justify denying the right to life based on the absence of either [3, 4, 22, 23].

In the early 1970s, John Lorber was at the frontier of the debate regarding the management of infants with myelomeningocele. In Sheffield, England, he instituted a "selective treatment" policy limiting treatment for infants afflicted with myelomeningoceles based on certain criteria: a large thoracolumbar lesion, severe paraplegia with no innervation below the L3 segment, kyphosis or scoliosis clinically evident at birth, gross hydrocephalus, additional congenital defects, severe cerebral birth injury, or intraventricular hemorrhage [3, 6, 9-13]. The main goal of selection was not to avoid treating those infants who would die early despite treatment but rather to avoid treating those who would survive with severe handicaps. Infants in the non-treatment arm were treated humanely, kept comfortable, and fed sufficiently, but no extreme measures were taken to prolong their lives. If a child survived to six months of age despite non-treatment, necessary treatment was initiated. A decision not to treat was not necessarily a final one, as long as the therapy was to enhance good health rather than to interfere with failing health. Some likened this policy to that of passive euthanasia and deemed it ethically and morally inhumane. In fact, this policy was embraced and then abandoned and eventually deemed medically and ethically inappropriate by the global medical community. Nevertheless, we are torn by the fact that our treatment for this disease is not perfect and results in children whose lives are filled with multiple medical and surgical procedures and who may experience various limitations [3, 6, 9-13].

Thirty years after Lorber's experiment we still have ethical and moral issues surrounding management of patients with this disease, but as a society we are devoted to our children and have abandoned non-treatment as an unacceptable option. Most infants born with myelomeningocele can have their outcome maximized by early intervention and close follow-up as they grow and mature. Intrauterine surgery offers some promise, but the data collection and analysis are not complete. The value of intrauterine intervention has yet to be proven to be the best and safest alternative for treatment of myelomeningocele. Prevention is a better alternative that needs to be emphasized through education and will hopefully decrease the incidence of this medically and ethically challenging disease.

References

1. Bliton Mark J (2003) Ethics: "life before birth" and moral complexity in maternal-fetal surgery for spina bifida. Clin Perinatol 30:449-464
2. Bliton MJ (2005) Parental hope confronting scientific uncertainty: A test of ethics in maternal fetal surgery for spina bifida. Clin Obstet Gynecol 48:595-607
3. Johnson PR (1981) Selective nontreatment and spina bifida: a case study in ethical theory and application. Bioethics Q 3:91-111
4. Morrissy RT (1978) Spina bifida: a new rehabilitation problem. Orthop Clin North Am 9:379-389
5. Choen AR, Robinson S (2003) Myelomeningocele and myelocystocele. Youmans Neurological Surgery, vol 3. Philadephia, pp 3215-3227
6. Lorber J (1975) Ethical problems in the management of myelomeningocele and hydrocephalus. J R Coll Physicians 10:47-60
7. Gallo A (1984) Spina bifida: The state of the art of medical management. The Hastings Center Report, pp 10-14
8. Steward CR, Ward AM, Lorber J (1975) Amniotic fluid A1-fetoprotein in the diagnosis of neural tract malformation. Br J Obstet Gynecol 82:257-261
9. Lorber J (1976) Ethical problems in the management of myelomeningocele and hydrocephalus-1. Nurs Times 72:S5-8
10. Lorber J (1975) Some pediatric aspects of myelomeningocele. Acta Orthop Scand 46:350-355
11. Lorber J (1985) Spina bifida-a vanishing nightmare? Childs Nerv Syst 1:242

12. Lorber J (1978) Spina bifida: To treat or not to treat? Selection – the best policy available. Nurs Mirror 147:14-17

13. Lorber J (1986) Where have all the spina bifida gone? Midwife Health Visit Community Nurse 22:94-95

14. Karmarkar SJ (1997) Spina bifida clinic-organizational aspects. Ind J Pediatr 64:83-85

15. Oi S (2003) Current status of prenatal management of fetal spina bifida in the world: worldwide cooperative survey on the medico-ethical issue. Child Nerv Syst 19:596-599

16. Bliton MJ, Zaner RM (2001) Over the cutting edge: how ethics consultation illuminates the moral complexity of open-uterine fetal repair of spina bifida and patients' decision making. J Clin Ethics 12:346-360

17. Chervenak FA, McCullough LB (2002) A comprehensive ethical framework for fetal research and its application to fetal surgery for spina bifida. Am J Obstet Gynecol 187:10-14

18. Pringle KC (1986) In utero surgery. Adv Surg 19:101-138

19. Chervenak FA, McCullough LB, Birnbach DJ (2004) Ethical issues in fetal surgery research. Best Prac Res Clin Anesthesiol 18:221-230

20. Lyerly AD, Mahowald MB (2001) Maternal fetal surgery: the fallacy of abstraction and the problem of equipoise. Health Care Anal 9:151-165

21. Patricolo P, Noia G, Perilli L et al (2002) Fetal surgery for spina bifida aperta: to be or not to be? Eur J Pediatr Surg 12:S22-S24

22. Fernandez-Serrats AA, Guthkelch AN, Parker SA (1968) Ethical and social aspects of treatment of spina bifida. Lancet 2(7572):827

23. Wickes IG (1968) Ethical and social aspects of treatment of spina bifida. Lancet 2(7569):677

Section II
ANTENATAL DIAGNOSIS AND TREATMENT

CHAPTER 6
Diagnosis of Spina Bifida and Other Dysraphic States in the Fetus

Dario Paladini

Neural tube defects (NTD) include anencephaly, encephaloceles and spinal dysraphism. Although this volume deals primarily with spina bifida, for the interest of the reader we include a brief summary of the current role of ultrasound in the assessment of the normal and abnormal spine. Furthermore, an overview of other entities, anencephaly and encephaloceles, and, at the end of the chapter, a small review of the prenatal diagnosis of closed spinal dysraphism, have been included.

Current Potential of Prenatal Ultrasound in the Diagnosis of Cranial and Spinal Dysraphism

The Normal Head and Spine

During the last decade ultrasound imaging techniques have undergone dramatic advances. The resolutive power has significantly increased, allowing the assessment of normal and abnormal fetal anatomy in earlier gestational ages, unthinkable as recently as ten years ago. Currently, prenatal diagnosis of major neural tube defects such as anencephaly and large encephaloceles is routinely carried out as early as 12-14 weeks of gestation, or shortly thereafter. The mean gestational age at diagnosis of open spina bifida has thus shifted considerably, with nowadays the overwhelming majority of cases being diagnosed before 23 weeks of gestation.

The assessment of the normal calvarium and spine is the basis for the diagnosis of their abnormal counterparts. This evaluation relies on the achievement of well-established ultrasound planes in two-dimensional and, more recently, three-dimensional ultrasound. If the former provides the operator with all the tools needed for a thorough screening for anomalies, which is carried out in most countries at 18-22 weeks of gestation [1, 2], the latter enables the expert to derive extra diagnostic and prognostic information. This information can then be advantageously used during the prenatal multidisciplinary counselling session in which the panel of experts informs the couple of the type of the anomaly, its prognosis and possible outcome.

We briefly report hereafter the conventional approach to the screening and the diagnosis of neural tube defects in the fetus, by illustrating the ultrasonic aspects of the calvarium, posterior fossa and spine in the normal fetus. A thorough illustration of fetal brain anatomy is beyond the scope of this volume, and the interested reader is referred to existent literature dealing with this aspect [3, 4].

1. Fetal head: On two-dimensional ultrasound, the trans-ventricular and the trans-cerebellar views are of interest in the screening and diagnosis of spina bifida and other neural tube defects [1] (Fig. 6.1a, b). On the former, the secondary ventriculomegaly, often associated with spina bifida, and the frontal scalloping sign (lemon sign) are diagnosed (Fig. 6.1c); on the trans-cerebellar view, the Chiari II malformation (banana sign) can be recognised (Fig. 6.1d). On the contrary, it is only with three-dimensional ultrasound that the prenatal assessment of cranial bones, in the normal and abnormal fetus, has become reproducible and adequate. This image modality allows at the same time a detailed evaluation of the fetal brain [4] and a clear characterization of the cranial bones, sutures and fontanelles (Fig. 6.2). In this way, both delayed ossification or premature closure of the fontanelles and/or sutures (synostosis) has become readily recognisable in utero. This imaging modality can similarly be advantageously employed to characterize the bony deficit in encephaloceles (see corresponding heading, below).

2. Spine: The spine can also be assessed by two- and three-dimensional ultrasound. With the former, which represents the technique of choice for midtrimester screening of congenital anomalies [1], the spine and individual vertebrae can be studied in

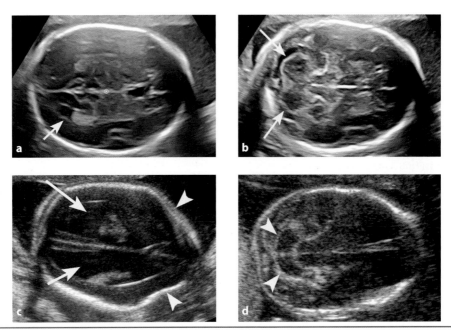

Fig. 6.1 a-d. Axial views of the fetal head used for mid-trimester ultrasound screening of central nervous system malformations in the fetus. **a** Normal fetus at 21 weeks of gestation. The axial trans-ventricular plane, cutting through the lateral ventricles (*arrow*), demonstrates absence of ventriculomegaly (atrial width less than 10 mm) and normal cerebral anatomy. **b** Normal fetus. The axial trans-cerebellar view demonstrates a normal posterior fossa, with an unremarkable cerebellum and a normal amount of fluid in the cisterna magna (*arrows*). **c** Fetus with open spina bifida at 20 weeks of gestation. The trans-ventricular plane demonstrates clear moderately-severe ventriculomegaly (*arrows*) and scalloping of the frontal bones (*arrowheads*), the so called lemon sign (from the shape of the fetal head). **d** Fetus with open spina bifida at 20 weeks of gestation. The trans-cerebellar plane demonstrates the Chiari II malformation, with obliteration of the cisterna magna, and the abnormal shape of the cerebellum (banana sign, from its shape - *arrowheads*)

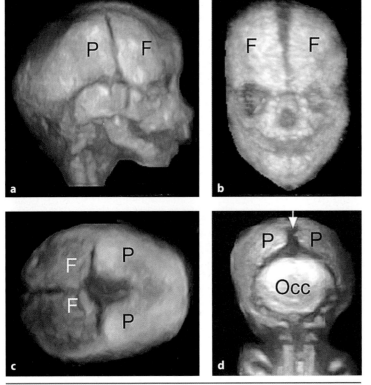

Fig. 6.2 a-d. Three-dimensional ultrasound enables clear visualization of the cranial bones, sutures and fontanelles. **a** Lateral view of the fetal head showing the coronal suture and the mastoid and temporal fontanelles. **b** Frontal view of the fetal head, demonstrating the frontal bones, the metopic sutures, and all the facial bones. **c** The fetal head seen from above, showing the anterior fontanelle. **d** Posterior view of the occipital region, showing the posterior fontanelle and the sagittal suture (*arrow*: posterior fontanelle; *F*: frontal bones; *Occ*: occipital bone; *P*: parietal bones)

detail in both the sagittal (Fig. 6.3) and axial planes. Three-dimensional imaging is able to provide the sonologist with even more self-evident images of the fetal spine and rib-cage (Figs. 6.4, 6.5). In most cases, a trans-abdominal approach suffices, but in obese women and in those in whom the fetus lies in a breech position (affording more direct access to the spine), trans-vaginal scanning is able to provide dramatic images of spinal anatomy, especially if three-dimensional ultrasound is used (Fig. 6.6). The main difference between two and three-dimensional ultrasound is that with the latter a volume dataset of the whole spine is acquired. After acquisition, the operator can choose to navigate through this volume dataset or, employing different post-processing (using his/her laptop) rendering modes, highlight the skin contour, the bony skeleton and reconstruct in the coronal plane, which is usually not accessible by two-dimensional

ultrasound (Figs. 6.4, 6.5). This, in turn, determines a higher degree of accuracy in reaching the final diagnosis and in its characterization both from a diagnostic and a prognostic standpoint.

ANENCEPHALY

- **Incidence:** Formerly 1 in 1,000, but rapidly decreasing due to prenatal diagnosis
- **Ultrasound diagnosis:** Absence of the cranial vault. Exencephaly: cerebral hemispheres visible in the amniotic fluid. Anencephaly: no cerebral cortex remaining. Frog appearance of the orbits in the second trimester (brain destroyed), Mickey mouse appearance in the first trimester (brain hemispheres still present)
- **Risk of chromosomal anomalies:** Low (2-11%)
- **Risk of non-chromosomal syndromes:** Low
- **Outcome:** Uniformly fatal

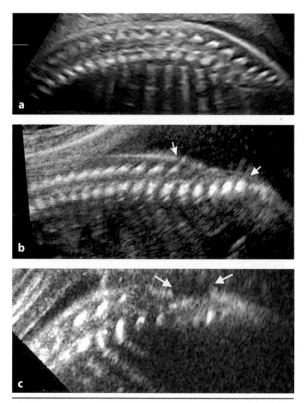

Fig. 6.3 a-c. Two-dimensional ultrasound of the fetal spine, employed during mid-trimester screening of spinal defects in the fetus (*sagittal view*) **a** Normal spine at 21 weeks of gestation: both the vertebral bodies and the posterior processes are clearly seen. **b** Fetus with open spinal defect: the *arrows* indicate the extent of the lesion, at the level of which the posterior processes are absent. **c** A small myelomeningocele (*arrows*), in which close contact with the uterine wall does not allow for clear visualization of the dorsal sac

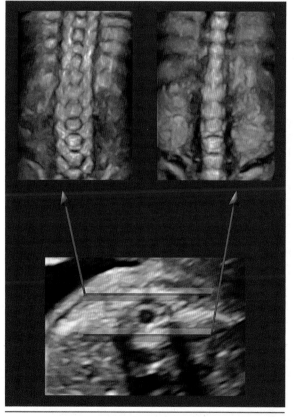

Fig. 6.4. Three-dimensional ultrasound of the normal fetal spine at 22 weeks of gestation. In the lower panel, a magnified axial view of a lower thoracic vertebra is shown. According to the depth of the three-dimensional reconstruction, either the lateral and posterior processes (*upper left*) or the vertebral bodies (*upper right*) can be displayed. Note the regular contour of all the vertebrae

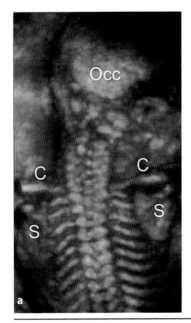
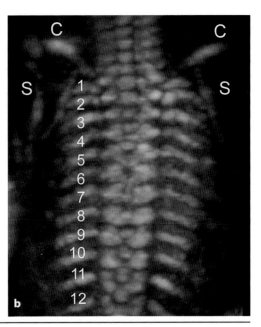

Fig. 6.5 a, b. Three-dimensional ultrasound of the normal fetal spine at 22 weeks of gestation. Maximum-mode reconstruction showing, with a posterior approach, the upper spine, ribcage and cranium **a** and the ribcage **b**. In this way abnormalities of rib number and shape, which can occur in a number of syndromic conditions, can be easily demonstrated (*C*: clavicles; *Occ*: occipital bone; *S*: scapulae; *1-12*: ribs)

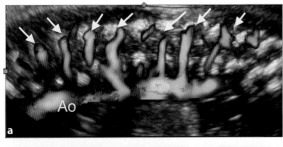

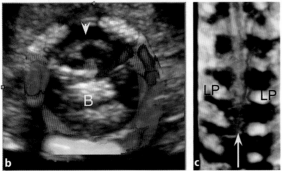

Fig. 6.6 a-c. Three-dimensional ultrasound of the normal spine at 18 weeks of gestation, transvaginal approach. **a** Longitudinal plane, showing vertebral feeding arteries (*arrows*) at the thoraco-lumbar level departing from the descending aorta (*Ao*).**b** Axial plane of a single vertebra, showing the blood supply to the vertebra (*B*) and the spinal cord (*arrowhead*).**c** Coronal view of the spinal canal, showing the spinal cord (*arrows*) between the lateral processes (*LP*)

Definition and Incidence

The term anencephaly generally refers to all the different stages of the sequence of destructive events which follow the failed development of the cranial vault, namely acrania. Exencephaly corresponds to the early stage, visible at the end of the first trimester (12-14 weeks of gestation), in which the brain hemispheres are virtually intact, though abnormally developed, and are visible above the fetal face, in direct contact with the amniotic fluid. Anencephaly is characterized by the complete destruction of the brain parenchyma, as visible from late second trimester onwards.

The incidence of anencephaly has been reported to be 1/1000 live births. This is dramatically decreasing due to an extremely high antenatal detection rate (at least in wealthy developed countries), which leads almost invariably to termination of pregnancy, in those countries in which this is allowed and if the couple does not opt for continuing the pregnancy on religious or moral grounds.

Etiology and Pathogenesis

The epidemiology and the etiology of anencephaly are those of NTDs, reported in a previous chapter. As for the pathogenesis of this condition, the most widely accepted theory is that acrania, exencephaly and anencephaly represent different stages of the same destructive sequence triggered by the failed development of the cranial vault bones. Owing to the absence of the cranial bones (acrania), the brain hemispheres, covered by meninges only, lie unprotected from chemical and traumatic insults in the amniotic fluid (exencephaly). This stage is visible at ultrasound until 13-14 weeks of gestation. From the eleventh week the fetal limbs are virtually complete and active flexion and extension movements begin. The result of these movements is that the fragile brain is crashed repeatedly onto the uterine walls, which leads to its rapid destruction. At the same time, the brain tissue is also exposed chemically to the amniotic fluid. The final result is that by 16-18 weeks anencephaly has developed, with virtually no cerebral tissue remaining.

Ultrasound Diagnosis

In the 80s, the diagnosis was usually made in the second trimester (19-22 weeks). On the trans-thalamic view, used for head biometry, the operator would not find the cranial outline, leading to referral and final diagnosis. The typical appearance was that of the so called frogs face sign, due to the association of absent cerebral tissue and cranial vault with concurrent macrophthalmos and proptosis (Fig. 6.7). Currently, the diagnosis is made in most cases at the end of the first trimester (12-14 weeks), at the acrania-exencephaly stage (Fig. 6.8), though it has been reported as early as the tenth week of pregnancy [5]. At this stage, the face appearance has been described as Mickey Mouse face, due to the fact that the almost intact cerebral hemispheres resemble, in the coronal plane, the large ears of Mickey Mouse (Fig. 6.8a) [6]. Three-dimensional imaging provides self-evident images useful for counselling, but does not add anything from diagnostic or prognostic standpoints (Figs. 6.7a, 6.8b).

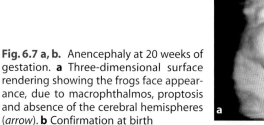

Fig. 6.7 a, b. Anencephaly at 20 weeks of gestation. **a** Three-dimensional surface rendering showing the frogs face appearance, due to macrophthalmos, proptosis and absence of the cerebral hemispheres (*arrow*). **b** Confirmation at birth

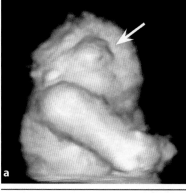 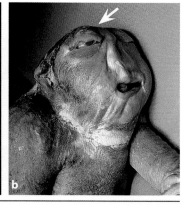

Fig. 6.8 a, b. Anencephaly. At 13 weeks of gestation, the lesion is still in the phase of exencephaly, with two hemispheres visible (*arrowheads*). **a** On the two-dimensional coronal image, the brain tissue floating in the amniotic fluid confers to the fetal face the classic Mickey Mouse aspect. **b** On three-dimensional rendering, with a lateral approach, the cerebral tissue is seen protruding above the fetal face (*arrow*)

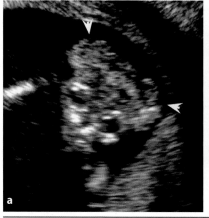 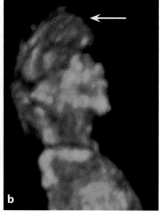

- Differential diagnosis: The diagnosis of anencephaly is usually straightforward. The only phase in which there is any diagnostic uncertainty is at the early exencephaly stage, when a large encephalocele may be mistaken for exencephaly. However, in the former the defect of the cranial vault is never complete and parts of the calvarial bones are always recognisable, which is not the case for anencephaly, where only the cranial base is present.
- Associated anomalies: Additional anomalies, mainly of the neural tube, may be associated in 25-50% of cases: spina bifida (27%) but also craniorachischisis, or iniencephaly [7]; cleft lip/palate, omphalocele, congenital heart disease, limb anomalies.

Risk of Chromosomal Anomalies

The risk of chromosomal anomalies is extremely low (2-3%), if the lesion is isolated, but reaches 11% if associated with other malformations [8, 9].

Risk of Non-Chromosomal Syndromes

The risk of non-chromosomal syndromes is relatively low. The most important condition not only associated but causative in some cases is an amniotic band syndrome. In this condition, the presence of amniotic bands in the uterine cavity may be responsible for anencephaly, limb amputation, and huge abdominal wall defects (body wall complex). The only real syndromic condition possibly associated with anencephaly is the Thoraco-abdominal syndrome, an extremely rare disorder in which anencephaly is associated with thoracic (e.g., diaphragmatic hernia, congenital heart disease), abdominal (e.g., omphalocele) and facial (cleftings) defects (Fig. 6.9).

Obstetric Management

Termination of pregnancy may be considered as an option, considering that this anomaly is incompatible with life. In fact, only few cases survive more than a week after birth.

ENCEPHALOCELE

- **Incidence:** 1/5,000-1/100,000 at birth, but decreasing due to prenatal diagnosis
- **Ultrasound diagnosis:** Cystic structure of variable dimensions protruding through a calvarial bone defect, most often in the occipital region
- **Risk of chromosomal anomalies:** Relatively high: 14-18%
- **Risk of non-chromosomal syndromes:** Relatively high
- **Outcome:** Postnatal mortality ranges 30-50% for encephalocele and 5-10% for meningocele

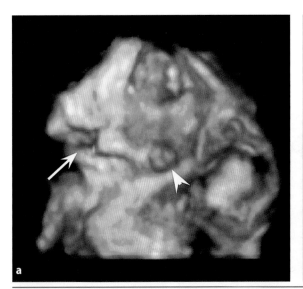 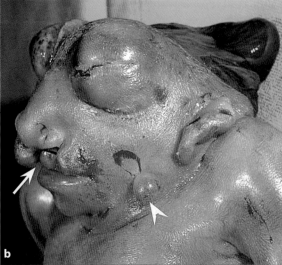

Fig. 6.9 a, b. Thoraco-abdominal syndrome at 22 weeks of gestation. **a** Three-dimensional rendering of the fetal face demonstrates the anencephaly, the cleft lip (*arrow*) and the pre-auricular tag (*arrowhead*). **b** Confirmation after termination of pregnancy (*arrow*: cleft lip; *arrowhead*: pre-auricular tag)

Definition and Incidence

Encephalocele is the protrusion of intracranial cerebral and/or meningeal (meningocele, encephalo-meningocele) structures through a cranial bone defect of variable size. Similar to anencephaly, the prevalence of encephalocele is decreasing due to the high antenatal detection rate leading to termination of pregnancy. Encephaloceles are more commonly occipital in location in Europe and USA, frontal in South-East Asia.

Etiology and Pathogenesis

Encephaloceles are thought to result from the failed neural tube fusion. Alternatively, according to some authors, this anomaly may occur due to abnormal mesenchymal induction in the post-neurulation phase. Encephaloceles may also be caused by amniotic bands, which secondarily disrupt the normal brain development; in this case the skull lesion is associated with other severe abnormalities, such as omphalocele and limb amputations. Encephaloceles are defined according to their anatomical location (frontal, parietal, occipital, fronto-ethmoidal, etc.).

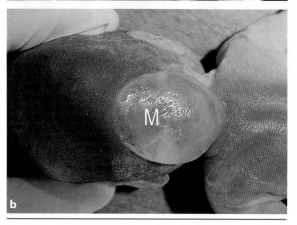

Fig. 6.10 a, b. Encephalocele. **a** Sagittal view of the fetal head at 18 weeks of gestation, showing a simple occipital meningocele (*M*). **b** Confirmation after termination of pregnancy

Ultrasound Diagnosis

At ultrasound, an encephalocele is diagnosed when a typically round mass is seen protruding from the fetal head, most commonly in the occipital region. The size of the encephalocele is extremely variable [10], and small lesions may escape prenatal diagnosis. The diagnosis can be made as early as week 12 of gestation. At diagnosis, the sonographic features of the herniated mass varies from completely anechoic (meningocele; Fig. 6.10) to mixed echoic structure (meningo-encephalocele; Fig. 6.11), depending on the herniated cerebral structures; it can also change sonographic appearance during gestation, with transition from a solid to a fluid pattern or showing transient disappearance [11]. The herniation of the cerebellum through the skull defect is often referred to as Chiari III malformation (Fig. 6.12). Occipital encephaloceles are usually revealed on a transthalamic view (Fig. 6.11), but the other planes are useful for a correct evaluation of the brain structures. In particular, the midsagittal view of the fetal head, if obtainable with a posterior approach, or a coronal one, may clearly demonstrate both the bony

defect and the myelomeningocele (Figs. 6.11d, 6.12). Three-dimensional ultrasound has enhanced the prenatal diagnosis of these defects. In particular, the use of multiplanar imaging allows a detailed assessment of the skull defect, whereas surface and maximum-mode renderings - which allow the highlighting of the outer surface or bony structures, respectively - can be used to further characterize the lesion (Fig. 6.12b, c). Anterior encephaloceles are rarely detected prenatally, due to their extremely low incidence, however there have been some case reports, particularly where the anterior encephaloceles occur in the context of syndromic conditions such as fronto-nasal dysplasia ([12], see below). Magnetic resonance imaging (MRI) is rarely needed prenatally to reach a final diagnosis of encephalocele; it may be used to assess its content and the overall development of the brain parenchyma and to rule out associated neuronal migration and proliferation abnormalities.

• Differential diagnosis: Prenatally, the most important lesions to differentiate occipital meningo-

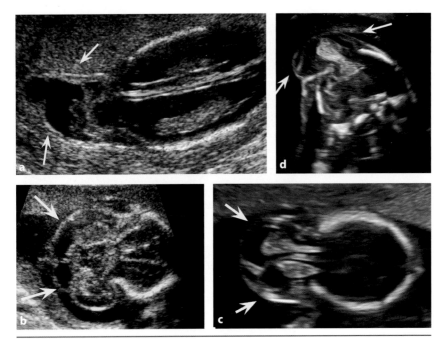

Fig. 6.11 a-d. Encephaloceles (*arrows*) in the fetus. **a** Large posterior meningoencephalocele in Meckel-Gruber syndrome at 19 weeks of gestation. **b** Huge meningoencephalocele containing most of the brain, diagnosed at 18 weeks. **c** Large posterior meningoencephalocele at 18 weeks (*axial view*). **d** The same case as **c**. On the sagittal view it is possible to define the skull margins

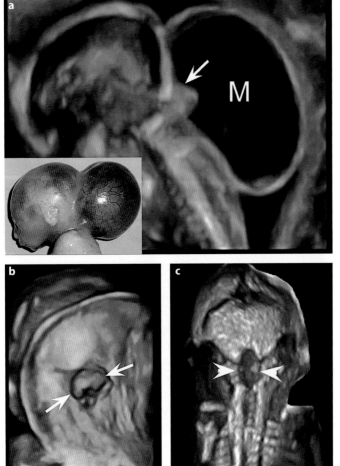

Fig. 6.12 a-c. Chiari III malformation (occipital cephalocele with hernation of the cerebellum) at 19 weeks of gestation. **a** Sagittal three-dimensional rendering showing the cerebellum (*arrow*) herniating through a small occipital defect in the large meningocele (*M*). The inset shows the specimen after termination of pregnancy. **b** Surface-rendering with a posterior approach, showing the cerebellum (*arrows*). **c** Maximum mode rendering highlights the bony components of the calvarium, demonstrating the small occipital defect (*arrowheads*) through which the cerebellum has herniated

celes from are cystic hygroma, teratoma, and hemangioma (Fig. 6.13). The differential diagnosis is easily carried out considering that a cranial vault defect is absent in all but the encephalocele, though a defect of the underlying bony plate has been found in a number of head hemangiomas in the fetus (Fig. 6.13).

- Associated anomalies: In up to 70-80% of the cases, there may be other malformations of the central nervous system (CNS): agenesis of the corpus callosum, ventriculomegaly, holoprosencephaly, microcephaly and spina bifida. Extra-CNS anomalies reported in association with encephaloceles include congenital heart disease and skeletal dysplasias. Of particular importance is the diagnosis of encephaloceles in the context of the Meckel-Gruber syndrome (see below). This is an autosomal recessive inherited condition and, as such, subsequent pregnancies should be monitored as early as possible to rule out recurrence of the syndrome.

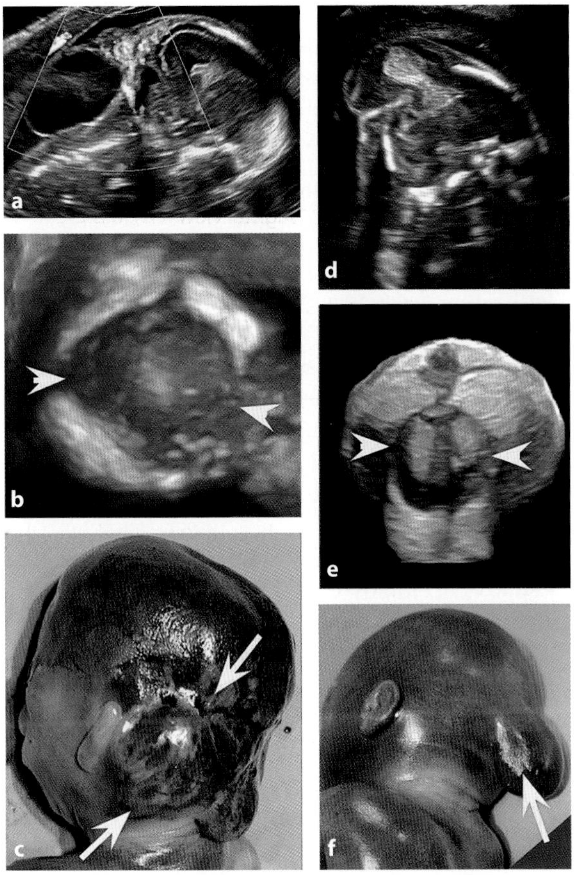

Risk of Chromosomal Anomalies

The risk of chromosomal anomalies is relatively high (7-18%) [8, 9].

Risk of Non-Chromosomal Syndromes

The risk of non-chromosomal syndromes is relatively high. The syndromes possibly associated with encephalocele are [13]:
- Amniotic band syndrome: Encephalocele + amputation of digits or limbs, facial disruptions, and cleft lip/palate;
- Frontonasal dysplasia: Encephalocele + hypertelorism + anterior cranium bifidum occultum, widely set nostrils, median cleft lip/palate [12];
- Meckel-Gruber syndrome: Encephalocele + polydactyly, polycystic kidneys, and other CNS anomalies (e.g., Dandy-Walker) [13];
- Walker-Warburg syndrome: Encephalocele + eye anomalies (microphthalmia and cataract) and other CNS anomalies (ventriculomegaly, midline anomalies, and lissencephaly) [13].

Fig. 6.13 a-f. Occipital hemangioma may sometimes mimic an occipital encephalocele: both share an occipital soft, possibly cystic mass and an underlying bone defect. The only difference is that in an hemangioma there is high vascularization of the mass, whereas in an encephalocele the only vessels are found in the cerebral tissues. Occipital hemangioma at 19 weeks (**a-c**). **a** Sagittal view showing the occipital mainly cystic highly vascularized mass. **b** Three-dimensional rendering of the ample occipital bone defect underlying the mass (*arrowheads*). **c** The specimen after termination, with the highly vascularized occipital mass (*arrows*). Occipital encephalocele at 19 weeks of gestation (**d-f**). **d** Sagittal view of the fetal head showing the high occipital defect with brain herniating through the bone defect. **e** Three-dimensional rendering of the relatively large occipital defect (*arrowheads*). **f** The specimen after termination of pregnancy, showing the occipital skin-covered mass (*arrow*)

Obstetric Management

Whenever an encephalocele is detected in a fetus, a thorough search for possible associated structural anomalies has to be performed, in order to rule out or confirm the presence of one of the syndromic conditions mentioned above. Karyotyping is also indicated, especially if other anomalies are present. Neurosurgical consultation should be sought to give the parents a comprehensive idea of the defect and its possible outcome. In cases continuing until term, delivery by cesarean section is advisable to avoid trauma and infection (through the birth canal) of the exposed brain tissue.

Open Spinal Dysraphisms

Spinal cord malformations are collectively referred to as spinal dysraphisms [14, 15]. They are generated from defects occurring in the early embryologic stages of gastrulation (weeks 2-3), primary neurulation (weeks 3-4), and secondary neurulation (weeks 5-6). Spinal dysraphisms are divided into open spinal dysraphisms (OSD), in which there is exposure of abnormal nervous tissues through a skin defect, and closed spinal dysraphisms (CSD), in which there is complete skin coverage of the underlying malformation. OSD basically includes open spina bifida, with myelomeningocele, and other rare abnormalities such as myelocele and hemimyelo(meningo)cele [14, 15]. CSD will be briefly described at the end of this chapter. With OSD, there is a leakage of cerebrospinal fluid within the amniotic cavity and the ensuing hypotension of subarachoid spaces triggers a cascade of events which eventually results in the Chiari II malformation. In CSD, there is no loss of cerebrospinal fluid and the cranial anatomy is therefore unremarkable.

SPINA BIFIDA

- **Incidence:** 1 in 1,000 at birth. Higher prevalence in Whites and in Hispanics than in African Americans and Asians. Also the birth prevalence of spina bifida is slowly decreasing, though to a lesser extent than that of anencephaly or encephalocele, due to the increased prenatal detection rate
- **Ultrasound diagnosis:** Most cases are detected due to the indirect cerebral signs, including ventriculomegaly, the lemon sign, the banana sign, and effacement of the cisterna magna (Chiari II malformation). Direct signs best detectable on axial planes are C or U shape of the affected vertebra, which is due to the absence of the dorsal arches; interruption of the skin contour with/without a meningocele; splaying of the lateral processes
- **Risk of chromosomal anomalies:** Relatively high: 8-16%
- **Risk of non-chromosomal syndromes:** Low

Definition

The term spina bifida refers to the defective fusion of posterior spinal bony elements in open dysraphism. Myelomeningoceles and myeloceles are characterized by exposure of the placode through a midline defect in the back. In myelomeningoceles, expansion of the underlying subarachnoid space results in elevation of the placode above the cutaneous surface (open spina bifida with dorsal cyst), whereas in myeloceles, the placode is flush with the cutaneous surface.

Etiology and Pathogenesis

Open spinal dysraphism originates from defective closure of the primary neural tube, which leads to the persistence of a segment of non-neurulated placode. The overall majority of cases are located at the lumbosacral level, with the placode being the conus. Since neurulation does not occur, the cutaneous ectoderm does not detach from the neural ectoderm and remains in a lateral position. This results in a midline skin defect. Therefore, the external surface of the placode is directly visible on inspection.

Ultrasound Diagnosis

Until a few decades ago, the prenatal detection rate of spina bifida was relatively low and mostly occurred in those countries, such as USA, where a mass screening program was available. Serum screening was used based on the fact that maternal serum levels, but especially the amniotic fluid levels, of alpha-fetoprotein are very high in all those fetal anomalies in which the cutaneous surface is not intact, such as omphalocele or open spinal dysraphisms. Using this type of approach, employing different screening strategies, detection rates as high as 90% for anencephaly and 80% for spina bifida had been reached [16].

The low detection rate for spina bifida on screening ultrasound was due to the fact that it is often difficult or impossible to obtain a diagnostic view of the fetal spine both in the longitudinal plane (Fig. 6.3) and in the axial one (Figs. 6.4, 6.6): the fetus often lies with its back along the uterine wall and this makes a detailed assessment of the fetal spine often challenging or impossible, especially for the non-experienced sonographer/sonologist. This is why the detection rate of open spinal defects has increased dramatically over the last 20 years following the recognition that indirect cerebral signs, which could be recognized at ultrasound, were present in the overwhelming majority of cases of spina bifida [17].

Indirect Signs

There is a constant association between OSD and the Chiari II malformation. This malformation is characterized by a small posterior fossa associated with downward displacement of a dysmorphic vermis, the brainstem, and the fourth ventricle into the foramen magnum or even into the cervical spinal canal. This cluster of events is determined by the failed closure of the neuropore, which prevents the physiologic accumulation of fluid in the rhombencephalic vesicle responsible for its physiologic dilatation. As a result, the posterior fossa will be too small to accommodate the growing brainstem and cerebellum, which herniates through the cervical canal behind the upper cervical cord. The ultrasound diagnosis of the Chiari II malformation is based upon the recognition of a series of signs including: obliteration of the cisterna

magna (Figs. 6.14a, 6.15); dysmorphic and dysplastic cerebellum featuring an abnormal anterior curvature (banana sign Figs. 6.14a, 6.15); frontal scalloping (Fig. 6.14b), which is responsible for the lemon sign; and moderate to severe ventriculomegaly (Fig. 6.14a, b). The frontal bossing (lemon sign) develops early, is inconstantly present (50% of the cases) and is lost in most cases by 22-24 weeks [18]. On the contrary, obliteration of the cisterna magna and the cerebellar banana sign are the most sensitive features, with the percentage of false positives being close to zero [17-19]. These signs can be found from 16 weeks of gestation until term, though it

Fig. 6.14 a, b. Spina bifida cranial signs (Chiari II malformation). **a** On the transcerebellar view, it is possible to detect the annulment of the cisterna magna (*arrows*) and the banana-shaped hypoplastic cerebellum (*arrowhead*), which characterize the Chiari II malformation. **b** Scalloping of the frontal bones (lemon sign - *arrowheads*) and moderately severe secondary ventriculomegaly (*arrows*)

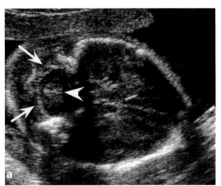
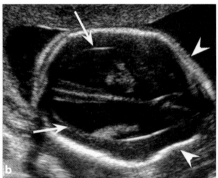

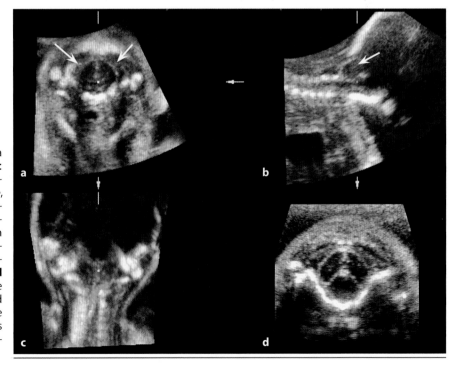

Fig. 6.15 a-d. Spina bifida Chiari II malformation. **a-c** Three-dimensional ultrasound. In multiplanar mode, the degree of herniation (*arrows*) of the cerebellar structures across the foramen magnum is clearly appreciated (*a*: axial plane; *b*: sagittal plane; *c*: coronal plane). **d** Another case in which the hypoplastic cerebellum had herniated so deeply in the vertebral canal that it has reached the level of the clavicles

should be considered that the ultrasound examination of the fetal posterior fossa is severely hampered in the third trimester by the increased calvarial calcification. Ventriculomegaly is a relatively late onset sign. It appears in the late second trimester in most cases (70%), and worsens thereafter (80-90%). As mentioned above, it is due to these indirect cerebral signs that the prenatal detection rate of open spina bifida has reached, in Western countries, figures in the range of 68-90%, with 68% of the diagnoses occurring before 24 weeks of gestation [20, 21].

Direct Signs

Sonographic assessment of the fetal spine is rather difficult even today, being strongly dependent upon the fetal lie. Direct sonographic recognition of the spinal defect requires systematic examination of each neural arch, from the cervical to the sacral regions, in the axial and midsagittal planes. In particular, the midsagittal plane can be used for an adequate evaluation of the cranio-caudal extension of the defect and to assess the dimensions of the myelo-meningocele (Figs. 6.3, 6.16a, d). On axial views, it is possible to detect the interruption of the cutaneous contour at the level of the affected vertebrae, which will therefore show a C or U configuration, due to absence of the dorsal arches (Fig. 6.16b). The coronal planes will demonstrate splaying of the lateral processes (Fig.

6.16c). These three aspects can be simultaneously demonstrated on the same panel of images using the multiplanar display of the three-dimensional ultrasound (Fig. 6.16a-c). It should be emphasized that the direct recognition of the defect is not always so straightforward; in a significant number of cases the spinal lesion is missed on initial evaluation and is diagnosed only because the operator has detected the previously described indirect signs at the level of the fetal head (Fig. 6.17). Fortunately, even small lesions of the spine are associated with these secondary cerebral abnormalities, provided that the spinal defect is an open one. In particular, it has been demonstrated that indirect cranial signs are associated with open spinal defects in more than 99% of the cases [22]. Conversely, closed spinal dysraphism is never associated with cranial signs and can only be recognized on direct inspection of the spine and only in a few circumstances ([22]; see below). In some cases, the spina bifida is complicated by the presence of severe abnormalities of the affected segment; in particular, the lumbo-sacral tract of the spine may be severely distorted, showing acute posterior convexity (Figs. 6.18, 6.19). It should be emphasized that it is possible, by two- and three-dimensional ultrasound, to recognize the level and the extent of the spinal defect very accurately. This has clinical relevance, as the level of the spinal lesion dictates to a certain extent the motor and neurofunctional outcome of the fetus, which is important for antenatal counseling.

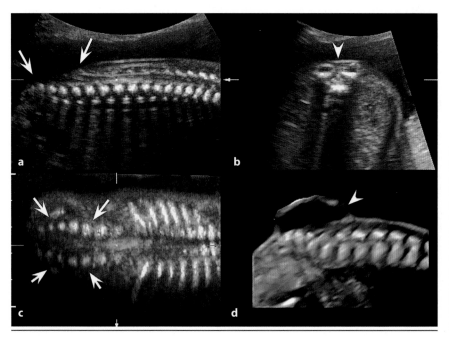

Fig. 6.16 a-d. Open spina bifida at 22 weeks of gestation direct signs on multiplanar imaging of the same case (**a-c**). **a** Sagittal view showing the absence of the posterior processes (*arrows*). **b** Axial view showing the U sign, with the vertebral canal open posteriorly (*arrowhead*). **c** Coronal view, showing splaying of the lateral processes (*arrows*). **d** Another case with a dorsal sac (*arrowhead*)

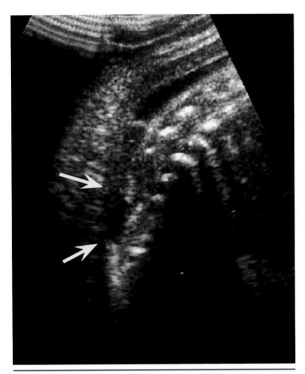

Fig. 6.17. Occasionally small spinal defects can be easily missed (*arrows*). In these cases, the diagnosis is reached due to the ubiquitous presence of cranial signs (Fig. 6.15), always present in open defects

The role of MRI in the prenatal assessment of open spina bifida is rather limited, especially because ultrasound is able to accurately characterize open spinal defects, as mentioned above, and to diagnose the associated cerebral signs and their significance (Figs. 6.14, 6.15). In addition, the prenatal surgical approach to spina bifida is undergoing a phase of critical reappraisal, and this further reduces the role of MRI in this anomaly. On the contrary, it may be speculated that MRI might play a complementary role to ultrasound in the characterization of closed spinal dysraphism (see below).

- Differential diagnosis: This includes sacrococcygeal teratoma, in which the indirect signs related to the posterior cranial fossa are absent and where the absence of a vertebral cleft can be demonstrated on a careful scan of the spine.
- Associated anomalies: Talipes may develop in a significant percentage of cases (Fig. 6.20). Moderate to severe pyelectasis (Fig. 6.18b) and/or bladder distension are rarely seen, and represent signs of neuro-functional damage.

Risk of Chromosomal Anomalies

The risk of chromosomal anomalies is 8-16% [8, 9].

Fig. 6.18 a-d. Complex spina bifida. In some cases, the spinal defect includes abnormal convexity of the affected segment, as in this case (21 weeks of gestation). Multiplanar three-dimensional imaging of the defect. **a** Sagittal view, showing the abnormal spinal convexity at the lumbar level (*arrow*). **b** Axial view, showing the U sign of the open vertebra, the dorsal meningocele, concurrent bilateral pylectasis (*arrowheads*), evidence of neurofunctional compromise. **c** Coronal view, showing the severe vertebral defect. **d** The specimen, after termination of pregnancy

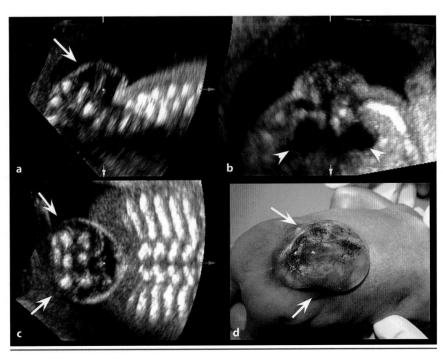

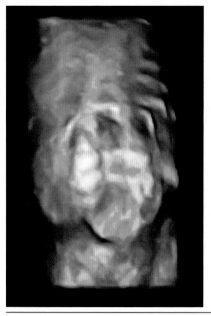
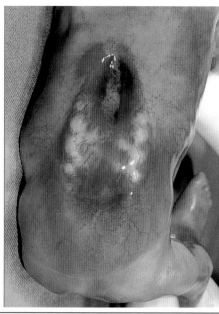

Fig. 6.19. Another case of complex spina bifida, with severe distortion of the thoraco-lumbar tract of the spine. *Left*: three-dimensional imaging; *right*: confirmation after termination of pregnancy

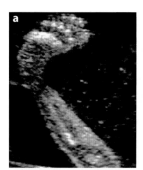
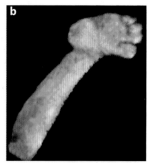
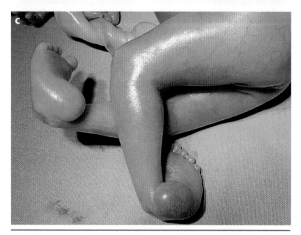

Fig. 6.20 a-c. Talipes can sometimes be seen in utero, and its presence indicates that severe compromise of the neuromotor function of the lower limbs is already developing. **a** Two-dimensional imaging of an equinovarus clubfoot, with the sole of the foot seen on the medial aspect of the leg. **b** Three-dimensional surface rendering. **c** Confirmation after termination of pregnancy

Risk of Non-Chromosomal Anomalies

The risk of non-chromosomal anomalies is low.

Obstetric Management

The occurrence of associated anomalies should be excluded. Fetal karyotyping may be indicated in the presence of associated anomalies. Delivery by cesarean section is recommended to avoid any trauma to, and possible infection of, the myelomeningocele during transit through the birth canal, though this indication is still controversial.

Closed Spinal Dyraphism

Closed spinal dysraphism (CSD) is so named because the spinal defect is covered with skin, and is further categorized based on the association with low spinal subcutaneous masses. CSD with masses are represented by lipomyelocele, lipomyelomeningocele, meningocele, and myelocystocele. CSD without a mass comprise simple dysraphic states and complex dysraphic states. The latter category further comprises defects of midline notochordal integration (basically represented by diastematomyelia) and defects of segmental notochordal formation (represented by caudal agenesis and spinal segmental dysgenesis).

It should be underlined that the prenatal detection rate of CSD is decidedly lower in comparison with that of OSD, due to the absence in the former of the indirect cranial signs [22].

In the following sections, we will briefly review the prenatal diagnosis of some of the above mentioned rare abnormalities. As mentioned earlier, it is likely that MRI might play a significant complementary role in the characterization of these complex lesions: in fact, it should be considered that the possible abnormal communication between the spinal canal and the enteric or urinary tract, which represent a key feature of complex CSD such as split notochord syndrome, often escape prenatal recognition by ultrasound.

Closed Spina Bifida with Meningocele

A posterior meningocele is a skin-covered, CSF-filled mass that is continuous with the CSF in the spinal canal. It may be associated with a tethered cord or hydromyelia, neither of which is detectable antenatally. Its antenatal diagnosis is difficult, as the cranial signs are absent, and relies only on direct evidence of the lesion on the sagittal view of the spine. Therefore, only the largest lesions are usually detected antenatally. They appear as a posterior cystic mass, at the caudal end of the spine (Fig. 6.21). With some attention, the continuity between the cystic mass and the spinal canal may also be seen. By definition, the skin overlying the defect is intact. An associated lipoma (lipomeningocele) occurs occasionally.

Diastematomyelia

Diastematomyelia consists of complete or partial clefting of the spinal cord in a sagittal plane into two symmetric or asymmetric hemicords, usually at the thoraco-lumbar level of the spine. The cord usually reunites more distally. Two subtypes of the lesions are recognized: in type A the two hemicords are contained within a single dural and arachnoid lining without any fibrous or bony dividing spur, whereas in type B each hemicord has its own dural and arachnoid sac and there is a spur or septum separating the two. Cutaneous stigmata (hairy patch, capillary hemangioma, etc.) at the site of the anomaly, cord tethering, and syringo/hydromyelia are commonly associated. Prenatal diagnosis, which has been reported in a few cases [23], relies on the difficult demonstration of the separated cords in type A and on the more straightforward recognition of the bony spur in type B diastematomyelia (Fig. 6.22). This type of diagnosis is made more confidently with three-dimensional imaging (Figs. 6.22b, 6.23).

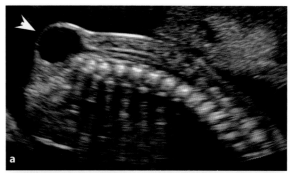

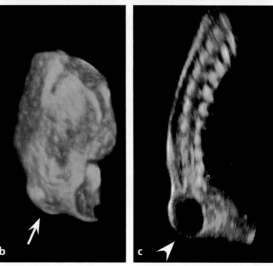

Fig. 6.21 a-c. Closed spina bifida with meningocele, at 22 weeks of gestation. **a** On two-dimensional ultrasound, the cystic mass at the caudal end of the spine is clearly evident (*arrowhead*). The diagnosis of closed defect was made upon the absence of any associated cranial signs. **b** Three-dimensional surface-rendering of the fetal back: the caudal mass deforming the cutaneous contour of the lower back is well evident (*arrow*). **c** Three-dimensional maximum-mode rendering of the fetal spine: the integrity of the vertebrae and the cystic meningocele (*arrowhead*) are easily recognisable on this mid-sagittal view of the fetal spine

---

VATER - Caudal Regression Syndrome, Sirenomelia

- **Incidence:** Rare
- **Etiology:** Unknown. In some cases, maternal insulin-dependent diabetes mellitus is associated
- **Ultrasound signs:** Vertebral anomalies; anal anomalies; cardiac defects; tracheo-esophageal fistula; renal anomalies; limb anomalies (aplasia radii). Caudal regression syndrome and sirenomelia represent extremely severe variants of the VA(C)TER(L)
- **Outcome:** Depends on the severity of the various anomalies
- **Recurrence risk:** Most cases are sporadic

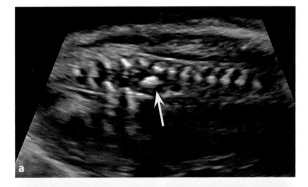

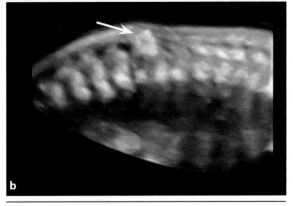

Fig. 6.22 a, b. Diastematomyelia type B (30 weeks of gestatation). **a** Two-dimensional ultrasound: on a coronal plane, the bony spur in the middle of the spinal canal is well evident (*arrow*). **b** Three-dimensional rendering. On a midsagittal view of the spine, the bony spur interrupts the regular contour of the spinous processes (*arrow*)

Definition

In 1972, this malformative cluster involving different organs was defined as VATER/VACTER/VACTERL, according to the different anomalies present at the same time. The original acronym (VATER) included the following malformations: vertebral anomalies (fusion, hemivertebrae, and scoliosis), anal anomalies (anorectal atresia), tracheo-esophageal fistula and renal anomalies (dysplasia, hydronephrosis and ectopia).

Then, the C (for cardiac defects: VSD, tetralogy of Fallot, and transposition of the great arteries) and the L (for limbs: aplasia radii, and polydactyly) were added if necessary.

Caudal regression syndrome is characterized by agenesis of the sacrum and, in some cases, of the lower lumbar part of the spine as well. The extremely rare sirenomelia is the most severe form of caudal regression syndrome, in which the two lower limbs are fused in a single abnormal limb.

Ultrasound Diagnosis

In VATER and its variants, the posterior spinal mass is usually large enough to be detected on screening ultrasound. Once referred, targeted ultrasound performed by skilled sonographers will enable the

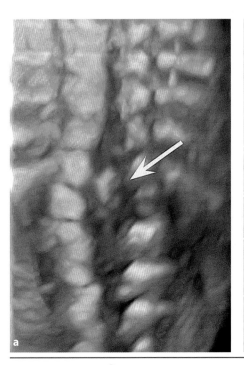

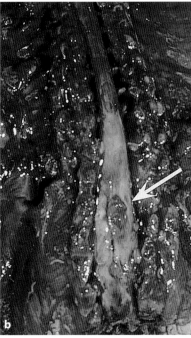

Fig. 6.23 a, b. Diastematomyelia type B (30 weeks of gestatation). **a** Magnified three-dimensional ultrasound. Coronal view showing the bony spur in the middle of the spinal canal (*arrow*). **b** Postmortem image. The posterior processes have been removed to show the cord. Note the bifurcation of the cord into two hemicords at the level of the bony spur (*arrow*)

recognition of the complex spinal defect and the concurrent renal abnormalities, if present (Fig. 6.24). In caudal regression syndrome, the sacral agenesis can be diagnosed on ultrasound, especially when there is involvement of the lumbar segments. The recognition of the most severe form of the caudal regression syndrome, sirenomelia, is straightforward, for in this case the two lower limbs will be fused into one (Fig. 6.25). Renal agenesis or maldevelopment is always associated.

Split Notochord Syndrome

Split notochord syndrome (SNS) represents an extremely rare and pleomorphic form of spinal dysraphism characterized by a wide spinal defect and a persistent communication between endoderm and ectoderm. Basically, SNS consists of a neural tube defect with an endoectodermal fistula opening in the dorsal area, but several variants differing by the type and the site of the associated anomalies, which involve the gastrointestinal tract, the CNS and, less often, the urogenital tract have been described [24]. Considering their overall rarity and their complex anatomy, these lesions are seldom detected antenatally. When the defect is diagnosed antenatally, SNS is suspected on the basis of the as-

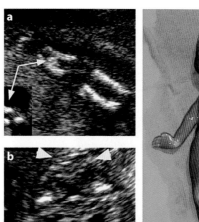
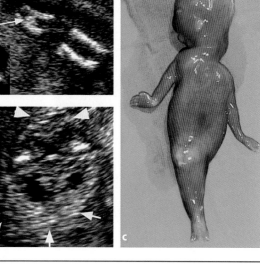
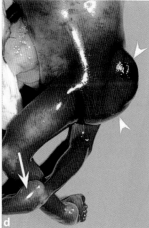

Fig. 6.25 a-c. Sirenomelia at 15 weeks of gestation. **a** Coronal scan of the two legs: there are two separate sets of long bones (fibulae are absent); however, the soft tissues appear fused. The *arrow* demonstrates the abnormal bony remnant of the fibulae, shown also on axial plane (inset). **b** Axial scan of the sacral spine, demonstrating the absence of the sacral vertebrae (*arrowheads*) between the two iliac wings, consistent with a diagnosis of sacral agenesis, and the single dysplastic horseshoe kidney (*arrows*). **c** Confirmation after termination of pregnancy: note that the fusion of the lower limbs is complete, extending to the level of the feet

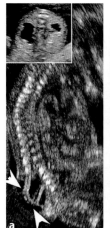
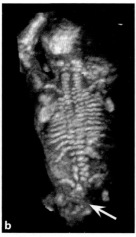
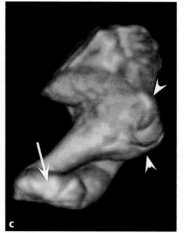
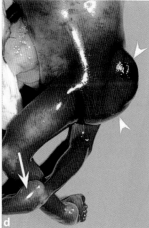

Fig. 6.24 a-d. VATER association at 21 weeks of gestation. **a** Two-dimensional imaging. The *arrowheads* indicate the large spinal defect involving the lumbo-sacral area. The inset shows the associated severe renal dysplasia. **b** Three-dimensional ultrasound showing the sacral agenesis (*arrow*): no vertebrae are visible below the lumbar tract. Note the irregularity of the whole spine. **c** Three-dimensional ultrasound. Surface-rendering showing the large spinal mass (*arrowheads*) and the associated talipes (*arrow*). **d** Confirmation after termination of pregnancy: the spinal mass (*arrowheads*) and the talipes (*arrow*) are evident

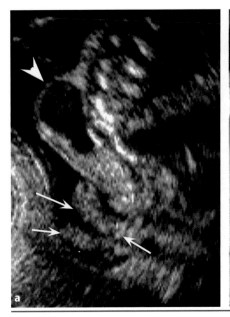
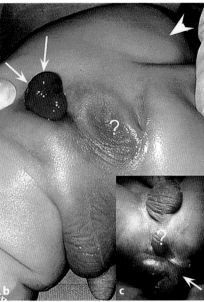

Fig. 6.26 a-c. Split Notocord Syndrome at 22 weeks of gestation. **a** On trans-vaginal ultrasound, the fetal breech contour was altered by the presence of a cystic terminal meningocele (*arrowhead*) and an intestine-like appendix (*arrows*), at the level of the postero-lateral perineal region. **b** After surgery, the presence of the spinal mass, consisting of a lipomeningocele (*arrowhead*) and of an ectopic intestinal loop already partially resected (*arrows*) was confirmed. There was an associated anal atresia (?). **c** Before surgery, the whole length of the ectopic intestinal loop (*arrow*) is evident (?: site of the imperforate anus)

sociation between a sacral spinal mass and additional abnormal findings. In one case described by our group some years ago [25], there was an oblong structure closely resembling an ileal loop protruding from the postero-lateral aspect of the perineum (Fig. 6.26); this rather unusual finding was associated with a cystic spinal mass and the absence of central signs possibly indicative of an open spinal dysraphism. After birth, the presence of a lipo-myelomeningocele, associated with a tethered cord, anal atresia and a vertical cleft below L4 was diagnosed [25].

References

1. ISUOG Education Committee (Chair: Paladini D. Task Force: Malinger G, Monteagudo A, Pilu GL, Timor-Tritsch I, Toi A) (2007) Sonographic examination of the fetal central nervous system: guidelines for performing the basic examination and the fetal neurosonogram. Ultrasound Obstet Gynecol 29:109-116
2. Filly RA, Cardoza JD, Goldstein RB et al (1989) Detection of fetal central nervous system anomalies: a practical level of effort for a routine sonogram. Radiology 172:403-408
3. Paladini D, Volpe P (2007) Ultrasound of congenital fetal anomalies, 1st edn. Informa Healthcare, London
4. Monteagudo A, Timor-Tritsch IE, Mayberry P (2000) Three-dimensional transvaginal neurosonography of the fetal brain: navigating in the volume scan. Ultrasound Obstet Gynecol 16:307-313
5. Becker R, Mende B, Stiemer R et al (2000) Sonographic markers of exencephaly at 9+3 weeks of gestation. Ultrasound Obstet Gynecol 16:582-584
6. Chatzipapas IK, Whitlow BJ, Economides DL (1999) The Mickey Mouse sign and the diagnosis of anencephaly in early pregnancy. Ultrasound Obstet Gynecol 13:196

7. Davis TJ, Nixon A (1976) Congenital malformations associated with anenecephaly. J Med Genet 13:263
8. Kennedy D, Chitayat D, Winsor EJT et al (1998) Prenatally diagnosed neural tube defects: ultrasound, chromosome, and autopsy or postnatal findings in 212 cases. Am J Med Genet 77:317-321
9. Sepulveda W, Corral E, Ayala C et al (2004) Chromosomal abnormalities in fetuses with open neural tube defects: prenatal identification with ultrasound. Ultrasound Obstet Gynecol 23:352-356
10. Jeanty P, Dinesh S, Ulm J et al (1991) Fetal cephalocele. A sonographic spectrum. Am J Perinatol 8:144
11. Zimmer EZ (1991) Transvaginal sonographic follow up on the formation of fetal cephalocele at 13-19 weeks gestation. Obstet Gynecol 78:528
12. Russo R, Agangi A et al (2002) Prenatal ultrasound diagnosis of frontonasal displasia. Prenat Diagn 22:375-379
13. Lyon Jones K (2006) Smiths recognizable patterns of human malformation, 6th edn. W.B. Saunders, Philadelphia
14. Tortori-Donati P, Rossi A, Cama A (2000) Spinal dysraphism: a review of neuroradiological features with

embryological correlations and proposal for a new classification. Neuroradiology 42:471-491

15. Rossi A, Biancheri R, Cama A et al (2004) Imaging in spine and spinal cord malformations. Eur J Radiol 50:177-200

16. Filly RA, Callen PW, Goldstein RB (1993) Alpha-fetoprotein screening programs: what every obstetric sonologist should know. Radiology 188:1-9

17. Nicolaides KH, Campbell S, Gabbe SG et al (1986) Ultrasound screening for spina bifida: cranial and cerebellar signs. Lancet 2:72-74

18. Van den Hof MC, Nicolaides KH, Campbell J et al (1990) Evaluation of the lemon and banana signs in one hundred and thirty fetuses with open spina bifida. Am J Obstet Gynecol 162:322-327

19. Pilu G, Romero R, Reece EA et al (1988) Subnormal cerebellum in fetuses with spina bifida. Am J Obstet Gynecol 158:1052-1056

20. Sebire NJ, Noble PI, Thorpe-Beeston JG et al (1997) Presence of the Lemon sign in fetuses with spina bifida at the 12-14 week scan. Ultrasound Obstet Gynecol 10:403-407

21. Garne E, Loane M, Dolk M et al (2005) Prenatal diagnosis of severe structural congenital malformations in Europe. Ultrasound Obstet Gynecol 25:6-11

22. Ghi T, Pilu GL, Falco P et al (2006) Prenatal diagnosis of open and closed spina bifida. Ultrasound Obstet Gynecol 28:899-903

23. Has R, Yuksel A, Buyukkurt S, Kalelioglu I, Tatli B (2007) Prenatal diagnosis of diastematomyelia: presentation of eight cases and review of the literature. Published Online DOI:10.1002/uog. 4066

24. Byrd SE, Darling CF, McLone DG (1991) Developmental disorders of the pediatric spine. Radiol Clin North Am 29:711-752

25. Agangi A, Paladini D, Bagolan P et al (2005) Split notochord syndrome variant: prenatal findings and neonatal management. Prenat Diagn 25:23-27

CHAPTER 7
The Role of Fetal Neurosurgery in Spina Bifida

Sergio Cavalheiro, Wagner J. Hisaba, Antonio F. Moron, Carlos G. Almodin

The Role of Fetal Neurosurgery in Spina Bifida

Myelomeningocele (MMC) is a nonlethal form of neural tube defect (NTD) that results from failure of the neural tube to fuse during early embryogenesis. The lesion is characterized by protrusion of the meninges through a midline bony defect of the spine, a sac containing cerebrospinal fluid and dysplastic neural tissue not covered by skin. MMC represents an important congenital defect of the brain and spinal cord that affects approximately one in 2,000 live births and about 23% of pregnancies that end in elective abortion [1, 2]. MMC leads to lifelong and significant physical disabilities including paraplegia, hydrocephalus, bladder and fecal incontinence, sexual dysfunction, skeletal deformation and mental impairment [3]. The mortality rate, which can be as high as 47% on long-term followup, is principally attributable to the hindbrain herniation observed in Chiari malformation and to the renal failure observed in neurogenic bladder dysfunction [4].

The cost of treating these patients represents a significant impact on the public health system. The lifetime cost per patient to the United States health care system is more than $340,000 [5], and the annual economic cost of spina bifida is estimated to be nearly $500 million [6].

Evaluation of human pathologic specimens and animal models of MMC have showed that spinal cord injury occurs before birth, secondary to the chemical effects of exposure to the amniotic fluid and meconium [7, 8]. Direct mechanical trauma can affect the neural tissue throughout gestation. This theory leads to a prediction that intrauterine repair of MMC may improve neurologic outcome by preventing damage from environmental factors.

Pathogenesis of Neurological Deficit

Several theories attempt to explain the neurologic defects associated with an open spinal cord defect. The neurologic injury may result from a "two-hit" phenomenon [9]. The first hit is the original defect in neurulation that creates MMC, and the second hit is the secondary trauma to the spinal cord that results from its exposure to the intrauterine environment, such as the amniotic fluid, and from direct trauma in the gestational period, or during labor or delivery. Support for the two-hit hypothesis of spinal cord damage comes from sonographic examinations. Studies have shown leg movements during prenatal ultrasonographic observation and abnormal postnatal leg movements [10, 11]. These movements in the prenatal period could be secondary to spinal arc reflexes or could come from the cerebrum through an intact spinal cord that is damaged secondarily during gestation.

Other support for the theory consists of the neurologic results following a cesarean section prior to labor. Luthy et al. [12] reported 160 cases of infants with MMC and compared their results based on delivery via vaginal or cesarean section routes both prior to the onset of labor and after labor onset. Delivery by cesarean section before the onset of labor resulted in better motor function at 2 years of age. They also observed that delivery by cesarean section after onset of labor but before rupture of membranes resulted in better motor function than cesarean section performed after onset of labor and after rupture of membranes. They conclude that the loss of amniotic fluid with labor, after membrane rupture, may lead to traumatic injury of nerves.

Diagnosis of Myelomeningocele

Prenatal diagnosis of MMC is possible before the twelfth postmenstrual week by noting irregularities on ultrasound of the bony spine or a bulging within the posterior contour of the fetal back in the sagittal view. Meticulous ultrasonography in the axial plane shows the absence of the posterior arches of the vertebrae, with protrusion of a fluid-filled sac. The neural placode, which is scarred in the inner side of the sac, is lifted out of the spinal canal. On coronal section, the affected bony segment shows a divergent configuration instead of the typical parallel lines of the normal vertebral arches [13]. The vertebral level can be assessed in a sagittal plane; the last rib corresponds to T12, the top of the iliac wing to L5/S1. Kollias et al. [14], using this method, reported that the ultrasonographic level correlates with the anatomical level in 64% of the cases.

The diagnostic sensitivities for prenatal sonographic detection of MMC are reported to be 80% and 90% when the examination is performed by a highly qualified sonographer who is carefully evaluating the spine (Fig. 7.1) [15, 16]. In contrast, the sensitivity for detection of a spinal lesion is lower than 50% when ultrasound is performed in a low-risk population, by an inexperienced sonographer, or using less advanced equipment [14, 17].

Indirect signs of MMC are a consequence of the Chiari II malformation. The major features include inferior displacement of the medulla and the fourth ventricle into the upper cervical canal; elongation and thinning of the upper medulla and lower pons; and inferior displacement of the cerebellum (Fig. 7.2) through the foramen magnum ("banana" sign). Ventriculomegaly may result from the hindbrain malformation blocking the flow of cerebrospinal fluid [13]. The changes in the posterior fossa and the hindbrain herniation into the foramen magnum may be seen by ultrafast magnetic resonance imaging (MRI) in the sagittal plane. Ultrasound using axial views is an inadequate substitute for MRI in the evaluation

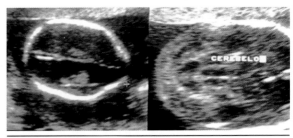

Fig. 7.2. Ultrasound of a fetus at 23 weeks gestation, revealing the lemon and the banana signs

of hindbrain herniation [18]. However, both methods are equally accurate to determine the level of the lesion in fetuses with MMC (Fig. 7.2) [19].

Rationale for Surgery

Almost all children born with MMC have an associated Chiari II malformation, and approximately 85-90% of such babies have hydrocephalus at birth or develop it subsequently, thus requiring a shunt to drain the excess cerebrospinal fluid from the brain into the abdomen, where it is absorbed. Two common problems with shunts are malfunction and infection, and most children with hydrocephalus will require multiple shunt revisions. Shunt dependence carries with it a 1% per year mortality risk [20].

Symptoms related to Chiari II malformation are determined by the degree of descent of the hindbrain and cerebellum down the cervical spine, and include difficulty swallowing, inspiratory stridor, weak cry and insufficient breathing; in severe cases it may lead to death [21].

The level of MMC is an important factor for prediction of the capacity to walk. Patients with lesions at sacral levels are able to ambulate 100% of the time in 93% of cases; 91% of young adults with L5 lesion ambulate 75-100% of the time. However, no patient with a lesion at the level of L3 or above can ambulate most of time without using a wheelchair [22]. Ninety percent of patients with thoracic lesion, 45% with lumbar lesion and 17% with sacral lesions are mobile with the use of crutches or wheelchairs [23].

Most patients with MMC require some form of intermittent catheterization to control urination, with 85% of these patients able to keep dry. Thirty-eight percent of patients use a bowel program and 52% report social continence [22]. About 84% of children with neuropathic bladders have abnormal bowel control and severe chronic constipation [24].

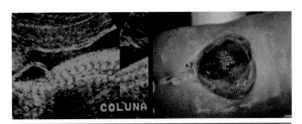

Fig. 7.1. Ultrasound of a fetus at 20 weeks gestation, revealing the myelomeningocele and after birth

Young people with MMC are found to be at greater risk of social isolation, depressive mood, lower self-esteem and suicidal ideation. The quality of their social life is determined by the degree of functional loss (ambulation difficulties, urinary and fecal incontinence) [25].

Significant efforts were made in the past decade to correct MMC in the prenatal period. In an animal model, Michedja [26] performed laminectomies in fetal monkeys. Two groups were created. In one group, the spinal defect was closed immediately, and in the other group no prenatal treatment was performed. After birth, the group without repair developed paraplegia and incontinence, whereas the group with repair showed normal neurological development [26]. Meuli et al. [27] created MMC in fetal sheep, which were all subjected to a laminectomy exposing the spinal cord at 75 days gestation. Again two groups were formed. At 100 days gestation, one group underwent reoperation for repair with a reversed latissimus dorsi flap and in the other group nothing was done until birth. All the sheep were delivered by cesarean section at 140 days of gestation. After birth, the sheep with in utero repair showed nearly normal motor function, normal continence and intact sensation. The control group showed paraplegia and incontinence [27].

These experimental studies showed the importance of protecting the spinal cord from amniotic fluid, and encouraged human fetal surgery for myelomeningocele correction.

Bruner et al. [28] published the first report of in utero coverage of MMC. Four fetuses with MMC underwent endoscopic coverage of the spinal lesion between 22 weeks and 24 weeks of gestation. The fetoscopic surgery involved placing a maternal skin graft over the spinal defect. One fetus was delivered one week after operation and died in the delivery room, from extreme prematurity. Another fetus died intraoperatively from abruptio placentae. In the other two patients, neonatal definitive closure of the spinal lesion was needed, as the skin grafts were not adequate and ventriculoperitoneal shunts had to be placed in both cases [28].

In 1997, direct closure of MMC was performed by hysterotomy at Vanderbilt University (VU) [29] and also at The Children's Hospital of Philadelphia (TCHP) [30]. Opening the uterus for fetal surgery was then a great challenge, and initially was only indicated in fetuses with a high risk of prenatal death. On the contrary, MMC has significant prenatal and postnatal morbidity but the risk of intrauterine death is low. New knowledge of mechanical materials, tocolytic and anesthetic drugs and fetal monitoring were important factors for this management.

Despite different protocols of inclusion and exclusion criteria for surgical candidacy used by these two institutions, more than 200 surgeries have been done, with significant results obtained from their studies.

The most important benefit has been the reduction and sometimes complete reversal of the hindbrain herniation as seen by magnetic resonance imaging [31]. Observation of 104 cases of open fetal surgery from both institutions, followed up for at least one year, revealed that the incidence of shunting occurred in 54% of the cases, compared with 86% in a historical group obtained from The Children's Hospital of Philadelphia, and also that shunting was less common when the surgery was performed prior to 26 weeks gestation (42.7%) [32, 33]. Bruner et al. [34] compared 29 cases of fetal surgery with those of historical controls at Vanderbilt University and observed a decrease in the shunt rate (59% vs. 91%), as well as a decreased incidence of hindbrain herniation (38% vs. 95%) and a decreased incidence of clubfoot (28% vs. 70%).

Despite excellent results in preventing hindbrain herniation, fetal surgery for MMC did not show the same outcome in improving sensorimotor function. Tubbs [35] compared 37 patients who underwent intrauterine procedures at VU with conventionally treated patients at the University of Alabama and, in both groups the average level of leg function roughly approximated the upper level of lesion. It appears that intrauterine correction has little effect on leg function [35]. Johnson et al. [13] questioned the selection criteria of indication at VU. At TCHP the movement of legs and feet observed on ultrasound was an important element to select fetuses for surgery. In their series, 57% had better than predicted leg function at birth in cases of thoracic and lumbar lesion [13, 36]. No improvement in functional bladder outcome was observed at a short follow-up after 1 year of age [37].

Morbidity and perinatal mortality have occurred in cases of open fetal surgery for MMC. The maternal morbidity reported at VU was due to blood transfusion in the postoperative period (2.2%), pulmonary edema (5.1%), bowel obstruction at 33 weeks (0.5%) and uterine dehiscence or rupture from hysterotomy (2.2%). No maternal deaths were noted [38]. Perinatal mortality occurred in 4% of cases at VU and 6% at TCHP and was related to prematurity and infection. In all cases observed, prematurity was the most frequent problem in open fetal surgery, the mean gestational age at delivery being 34 weeks [1].

There are controversies about the real benefits of intrauterine repair of MMC. It is important to consider the effects in a balance where on the one side there is a reduction of MMC defects and on the other side the risk of morbidity due to the surgery and prematurity. Long-term data of the patients submitted to prenatal repair are needed for better comprehension of its real benefits. An initiative called Management of Myelomeningocele Study (MOMS trial) was created in 2002 and consists of a multicentered and randomized trial for a period of 5 years. Three centers have been selected for fetal surgery: Vanderbilt University, The Children's Hospital of Philadelphia and University of California, San Francisco. 100 patients will undergo fetal surgery and 100 patients will be selected to form the control group. George Washington University will collect the data of surgery and follow-up.

Selection of the Patients

The selection criteria for patients to undergo open fetal surgery conform to those of the MOMS trial [39]:
   Inclusion criteria:
a) Gestational age between 19 to 25 weeks and 6 days
b) Maternal age ≥ 18 years
c) Normal fetal karyotype
d) Defect between T1 and S1
e) Atrium < 18 mm
f) Hindbrain herniation seen by magnetic resonance imaging
g) Signed informed consent form
   Exclusion criteria:
a) Multifetal pregnancy
b) Insulin-dependent pregestational diabetes
c) Obesity
d) Fetal kyphosis ≥ 30 degrees
e) Fetal anomaly not related to the myelomeningocele
f) Preterm labor in the current pregnancy
g) Short cervix < 20 mm
h) History of spontaneous delivery < 37 weeks
i) Placenta previa
j) Maternal HIV, hepatitis B and C
k) Uterine anomaly
l) Alloimmunization
m) Contradiction to surgery or anesthesia
n) Mother does not meet psychological criteria

Procedure

Patients are admitted into the surgical room for obstetrical and maternal monitoring and initiation of tocolysis. Thirty minutes prior to surgery the patient receives a rectal indomethacin suppository for initial tocolysis.

Epidural anesthesia, performed with the placement of a catheter (for postoperative control of pain), is followed by general anesthesia with halogenated inhalational agents, with fentanyl providing anesthesia for the fetus. Just after anesthesia induction, the patient receives 3 g of magnesium sulphate as an endovenous tocolytic.

Based on a protocol approved by the Ethics Committee for Research and Protection of Human Subjects, of São Paulo Federal University (UNIFESP – Brazil), we use the data obtained from six patients treated with isolated fetal myelomeningocele, referred for intrauterine repair in conformity with the Vandebilt University surgical criteria slightly modified for our country.

The laparotomy is performed through a 17-20 cm long Pfannenstiel incision made 5-7 cm above the pubic symphysis (Fig. 7.3). The abdominal wall is opened and dissected up to the umbilicus or to the uterine fundus. When the wall is totally open, the uterus is exteriorized (Fig. 7. 4). The MMC, placenta and fetal heart beat are located by ultrasound. As soon as the placenta is found, the uterine incision is defined. Two repair stitches are placed in the uterus with an interval of approximately 2-3 cm between them (Fig. 7.5). The threads are pulled up and an 18G epidural needle is introduced under ultrasonographic guidance. A 1.5 mm guidewire is then inserted through the needle lumen, and the needle is removed.

An aluminum trocar designed by Almodin-Moron (Fig. 7.6) is passed over the guidewire and pushed through the uterine wall under direct ultrasonographic guidance (Fig. 7.7). The Almodin-Moron trocar is a metal version of the Tulipan-Bruner

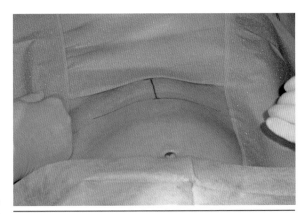

Fig. 7.3. Abdominal Pfannenstiel incision, 7 cm above the pubis

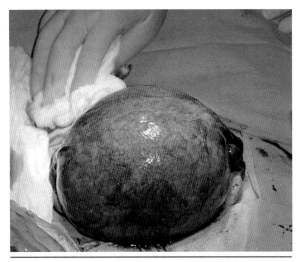

Fig. 7.4. Exposure of the uterus in laparotomy

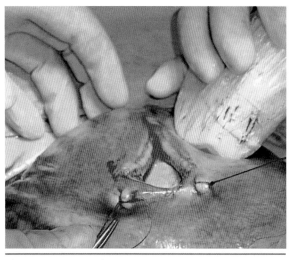

Fig. 7.5. Opening the uterus

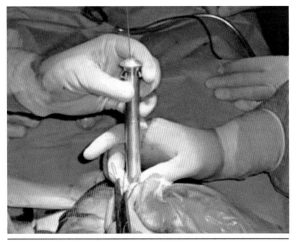

Fig. 7.6. The Almodin-Moron trocar

trocar, which can be sterilized and reused. It consists of a 13.5 cm long, 44 F aluminum central introducer with a blunt tip that tapers for 2 cm into an inner lumen which accepts a 0.9 mm guidewire [40].

Once the guidewire and the introducer are removed, the amniotic fluid is collected through the metal sleeve into a small container, from which it is aspirated with 60 ml syringes and placed onto a double boiler covered with a sterile plastic bag kept at 37°C. A stapling device (U.S. Surgical Premium Poly CS-57; U.S. Surgical Corporation, Norwalk, Conn) [41] is inserted through the slot into the metal sleeve and once it is correctly positioned, the sleeve is removed and the stapler closed. The hysterotomy is created, with the sutured membranes already stapled to the uterine wall.

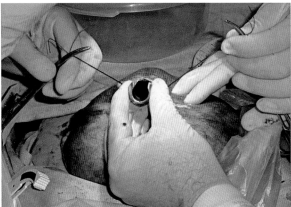

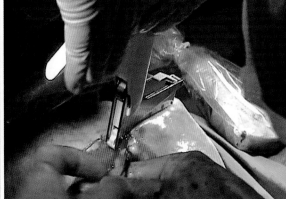

Fig. 7.7. Insertion of the trocar into the uterine cavity and subsequent stapling

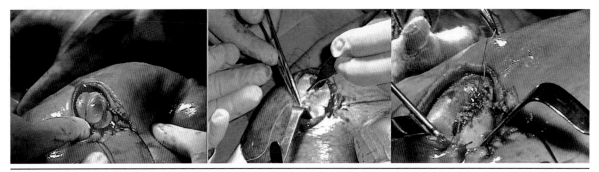

Fig. 7.8. Exposure of MMC and closure

After the lesion is conveniently positioned in the uterine opening, the MMC closure begins. The heart beat is monitored by Doppler throughout the procedure, which is performed under ultrasonographic vision.

Intramuscular fentanyl is injected into the fetal buttock. Compression on the uterine cavity keeps the fetus in a steady position while the myelomeningocele is exposed. The time of fetal exposure must be short, which is why a magnifying lens and not a surgical microscope is used while the defect is being repaired. The placode is isolated and the dura mater broadly exposed. Closure is performed in two layers, using absorbable 6.0 Monocryl thread, and fibrin glue is spread on the suture (Fig. 7.8). The fetus is then returned to the uterine cavity.

In none of our cases was tachycardia observed, implying that the fetus did not suffer from pain during the procedure. Two fetuses had bradycardia after their skin had been closed, due to folding of the umbilical cord, but this condition was soon reverted by changing the position of the fetus in the uterine cavity.

From the neurosurgical point of view, the main difficulty of the closure concerns the fragility of fetal skin. The younger the fetus, the greater the difficulty. The neurosurgeon's position is also awkward during an in utero repair. In all our cases, the approach to the skin was wide enough, but a hermetic closure of the dura mater was not always easy. In none of the surgical procedures, however, did the dura mater closure take more than twenty minutes.

The uterus is closed in two steps. The first continuous suture is performed in the myometrium and does not transfix the uterine wall. The second suture attaches the myometrium to the serosa, and when it is about to reach the end of the incision, a Foley 16 F probe is inserted, through which the amniotic fluid is replaced into the womb, with 500 mg of nafcilin sodium. The probe is then removed and the second suture finished. A biological glue (Baxter's Trombines solution) is spread on the finished suture.

The uterus is returned to the abdominal cavity and the abdominal wall is closed.

Throughout the procedure, magnesium sulphate is given to the mother to prevent uterine contractions for 24 hours.

After surgery, ampicillin and indomethacin are continued until the following day. The fetus and uterine contractions are continuously monitored electronically using ultrasonography. Magnetic resonance imaging is performed 2-3 weeks after surgery to observe the fetal hindbrain herniation.

The amniotic fluid, the ventricular size, the uterine wall and fetal well-being are monitored twice a week until 37 weeks of gestation, when delivery takes place by cesarean section.

Results

In our institution, six patients underwent intrauterine correction of myelomeningocele. In all cases, the gestational age was less than twenty-six weeks. The diagnoses were obtained from ultrasonography and complemented with magnetic resonance imaging. The six fetuses had Chiari type II. Two of them had significant hydrocephalus. In four fetuses the Chiari type II disappeared in utero (Figs. 7.9-7.11) and

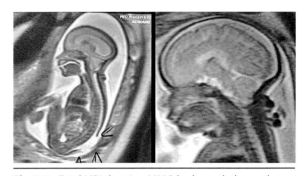

Fig. 7.9. Fetal MRI showing MMC, hydrocephalus, and presence of cerebellar tonsillar herniation

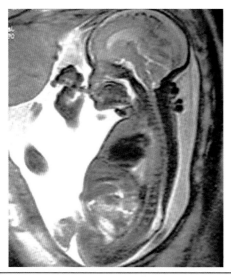

Fig. 7.10. Thirtieth postoperative day follow-up showing closed MMC and no evidence of hydrocephalus or Chiari

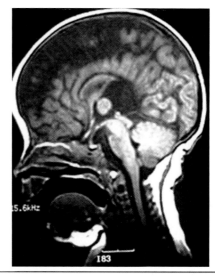

Fig. 7.11. Six month follow-up after intrauterine closure of MMC: absence of Chiari, no hydrocephalus. Prominence of interthalamic adhesion and partial agenesis of corpus callosum

shunting was not needed. The two fetuses with severe hydrocephalus received ventriculoperitoneal shunts. All of the six patients have had excellent cognitive development. Two of them have severe motor deficits and four can walk without difficulty.

Conclusion

Our series is still too small for reliable conclusions to be reached as to whether in utero repair of fetal myelomeningocele is really of great benefit. The procedure is not difficult to perform. For the mother, the risk is almost negligible. The worst hazard is the risk of prematurity. Is it worth taking this risk in order to avoid shunting? Currently, our programme is awaiting the results from MOMS.

References

1. Velie EM, Shaw GM (1996) Impact of prenatal diagnosis and elective termination on prevalence and risks estimates of neural tube defects in California. 1989-1991. Am J Epidemiol 144:473-479
2. Copp AJ (1993) Neural tube defects. Trends Neurosci 16:381-383
3. Hunt GM, Poulton A (1995) Open spina bifida: a complete cohort reviewed 25 years after closure. Dev Med Child Neurol 37:19-29
4. Center for Disease Control and Prevention (1992) Economic costs of birth defects and cerebral palsy – United States. MMWR 1995; 44:694-699
5. National Institute of Child Health and Human Development. Management of Myelomeningocele study. Available at http://www.spinabifidamoms.com
6. Correia-Pinto J, Reis JL, Hutchins GM (2002) In utero meconuim exposure increases spinal cord necrosis in a rat model of myelomeningocele. J Pedriatr Surg 37:488-492
7. Petzold A, Stiefel D, Copp AJ (2005) Amniotic fluid brain-specific proteins are biomarkers for spinal cord injury in experimental myelomeningocele. J Neurochem 95:594-598
8. Lemire RJ (1975) In: Normal and abnormal development of the human nervous system. Harper & Row, New York, pp 1-421
9. Hirose S, Meuli-Simmen C, Meuli M (2003) Fetal surgery for myelomeningocele: panacea or peril? World J Surg 27:87-94
10. Koremromp MJ, Van Good JD, Bruinesse HW et al (1986) Early fetal movements in myelomeningocele. Lancet 1:917-918
11. Sival DA, Begger JH, Staal-Schreinemachers AL et al (1997) Perinatal motor behaviour and neurological outcome in spina bifida aperta. Erly Human Dev 50:27-37
12. Luthy DA, Wardinsky T, Shurtleff DB et al (1991) Cesarean section before the onset of labor and subsequent

motor function in infants with myelomeningocele diagnosed antenatally. N Engl J Med 324:662-68

13. Jonhson MP, Sutton L, Rintoul N et al (2003) Fetal myelomeningocele repair: short term clinical outcomes. Am J Obstet Gynecol 189:482-487

14. Kollias SS, Goldstein RB, Cogen PH et al (1992) Prenatally detected myelomeningocele: sonographic accuracy in estimation of the spinal level. Radiology 185:109-112

15. Nicolaides KH, Campbell S, Gabbe, SG et al (1986) Ultrasound screening for spina bifida: cranial and cerebellar signs. Lancet 2:72-74

16. Thiagarajah S, Henke J, Hogge A et al (1987) Early diagnosis of spina bifida: the value of cranial ultrasound markers. Obstet Gynecol 70:247-250

17. Nyberg DA, Mack LA, Hirsch J et al (1988) Abnormalities of fetal cranial contour in sonographic detection of spina bifida: evaluation of the "lemon" sign. Radiology 167:387-392

18. Mangels KJ, Tulipan N, Tsao LY et al (2002). Fetal MRI in the evaluation of intrauterine myelomeningocele. Pediatr Neurosurg 32:124-131

19. Aaronson OS, Hernnz-Schulman, Bruner JP et al (2003) Myelomeningocele: prenatal evaluation – comparison between transabdominal US and MR imaging. Radiology 227:839-843

20. Iskandar BJ, Tubbs S, Mapstone TB et al (1998) Death in shunted hydrocephalic children in 1900s. Pediatric Neurosurg 28:173-176

21. Northrup H, Volcik KA (2000) Spina bifida and other neural tube defects. Curr Probl Pediatr 30:313-340

22. Bowman RM, McLone DG, Grant JA et al (2001) Spina bifida outcome. A 25-year prospective. Pediatr Neurosurg 34:114-120

23. Cochrane DD (1996) Prenatal spinal evaluation and functional outcome of patients born with myelomeningocele: information for improved prenatal counselling and outcome prediction. Fetal Diagn Ther 11:159-168

24. Skobejo-Wlodarska (2002) Treatment of neuropathic urinary and faecal incontinence. Eur J Pedriat Surg 12:318-321

25. Cate IMP, Kennedy C, Stevenson J (2002) Disability and quality of life in spina bifida and hydrocephalus. Dev Med Child Neurol 44:317-322

26. Michejda M (1984) Intrauterine treatment of spina bifida: primate model. Z Kinderchir 39:259-261

27. Meuli M, Meuli-Simmen C, Yingling C et al (1995) In utero surgery rescues neurological function at birth in sheep. Nat Med 1:342-347

28. Bruner JP, Richards WO, Tulipan N et al (1999) Endoscopic coverage of fetal myelomeningocele in utero. Am J Obstet Gynecol 180:153-158

29. Tulipan N, Bruner JP (1998) Myelomeningocele repair in utero: a report of three cases. Pediatr Neurosurg 28:177-180

30. Adzick NS, Sutton L, Crombleholme T et al (1998) Successful fetal surgery for spina bifida. Lancet 352:1675-1676

31. Sutton L, Adzik NS, Johnson MP (2003) Fetal surgery of myelomeningocele. Childs Nerv Syst 19:587-591

32. Tulipan N, Sutton L, Bruner JP et al (2003) The effect of intrauterine myelomeningocele repair on the incidence of shunt dependent hydrocephalus. Pediatr Neurosurg 38:27-33

33. Tulipan N (2003) Intrauterine myelomeningocele repair. Clin Perinatol 30:521-530

34. Bruner JP, Tulipan N, Paschall RL et al (1999) Fetal surgery for myelomeningocele and the incidence of shunt-dependent hydrocephalus. JAMA 282:1819-1825

35. Tubbs RS, Chamber MR, Smyth MD et al (2003) Late gestational intrauterine repair does not improve lower extremity function. Pediatr Neurosurg 38:128-132

36. Sutton L, Adzick N, Bilaniuk L et al (1999) Improvement in hindbrain herniation demonstrated by serial fetal magnetic resonance imaging following fetal surgery for myelomeningocele. JAMA 282:1826-1831

37. Holzbeierlein J, Pope JI, Adams MC et al (2000) The urodynamic profile of myelodysplasia in childhood with spinal closure during gestation. J Urol 164:1336-1339

38. Bruner JP, Tulipan N (2005) Intrauterine repair of spina bifida. Clin Obstet Gynecol 48:942-955

39. Werler MM, Louik C, Shapiro S et al (1996) Prepregnant weight in relation to risk of neural tube defects. JAMA 275:1089-1092

40. Almodin CG, Moron AF, Cavalheiro S (2006) The Almodin-Moron trocar for uterine entry during fetal surgery. Fetal Diagn Ther 21:414-417

41. Bruner JP, Boehm FH, Tulipan N (1999) The Tulipan-Bruner trocar for uterine entry during fetal surgery. Am J Obstet Gynecol 181:1188-1191

Section III
INITIAL MANAGEMENT

CHAPTER 8
Preoperative Care of the Newborn with Myelomeningocele

M. Memet Özek

Children with spina bifida comprise one of the largest groups of patients for whom pediatric neurosurgeons care. Management of these children is extraordinarily complex and may require the integrated efforts of caregivers from many disciplines.

Delivery Room Assessment and Immediate Concerns

If available, the maternal history should be reviewed specifically with respect to the results of amniocentesis and prenatal ultrasounds. Pediatric Neurosurgery should be notified of the expected delivery and the pediatric team should be present in the delivery room.

Although somewhat controversial, the majority of studies support the delivery of babies with spina bifida by planned cesarean section, allowing a more careful delivery of the baby in order to protect the spinal cord from injury and to prevent possible rupture of the meningeal sac (Fig. 8.1). Some experts believe that cesarean delivery before the onset of labor may be associated with better motor function [1-3].

Infants with myelomeningocele (MMC) have challenges related to thermoregulation and fluid management and are at risk of infection. In addition to supplies routinely needed in the delivery room, sterile gauze, warm saline and nonpermeable coverings for the dressing should be provided.

Infants with open spinal dysraphism are at risk of latex allergy [4]. Though the precise etiology of this allergy is not well understood, repetitive exposure to latex through bladder catheterization and surgical procedures may be contributing factors. This allergy is an IgE-mediated reaction. It may be mild, with urticaria, or severe, with bronchospasm, laryngeal edema and systemic anaphylaxis. The prevalence of clinical allergic reactions may be as high as 20-30% [5]. In a recent study, 48% of pa-

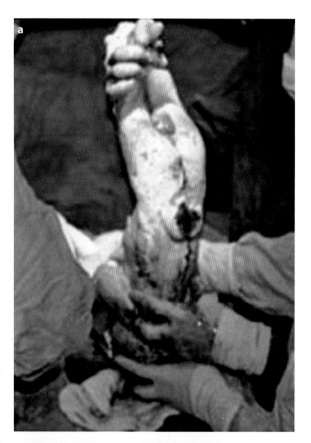

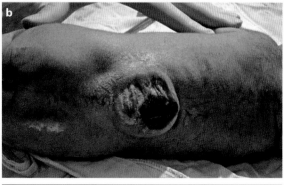

Fig. 8.1 a, b. a Abdominal delivery of a baby with myelomeningocele. **b** Avoid positioning the infant on the lesion in the delivery room

tients with MMC showed a latex sensitization with specific IgE > 0.7 kU/l while 15% were allergic to latex (specific IgE > 0.7kU/l with clinical manifestations). The introduction of a formidable predisposing factor to latex sensitization due to the contact of gloves with the meninges is an issue to consider since repeated intra-abdominal measures do not carry the same risk of sensitization [6]. The association of hydrocephalus causes a rise in the occurrence of latex sensitization among myelodysplastic patients because of the significant number of neurosurgical procedures they undergo as a result of shunt malfunction [6-8].

These results underline the importance of avoiding latex exposure [9]. All diagnostic and therapeutic procedures therefore should be conducted in latex free environments. The baby should be handled with sterile, non-latex gloves and with sterile clothing and sheets.

In the delivery room, the steps in newborn resuscitation are followed as described in the Neonatal Resuscitation Program (NRP) [10]. The infant is placed on its side while suctioning, drying, and evaluating its respiratory effort. Respiratory insufficiency is anticipated in high thoracic lesions. If the infant must be placed supine for any reason, a foam mattress with a cut-out area is used to prevent pressure on the lesion. Protracted supine positioning may predispose the infant to increased neurological sequelae from pressure on exposed nervous tissue. Infants with open spinal dysraphism are kept in a prone or lateral recumbent position to protect the neural tissue.

For the protection of the nervous tissue and the prevention of the fluid loss, a sterile non-adhesive dressing that is soaked in Ringer's lactate solution or in warm normal saline is placed over the open lesion in the delivery room. [11].

A logical approach would be to place a nonpermeable covering over the moist gauze in order to minimize evaporative heat loss, prevent drying of the lesion and fecal contamination of the site, thus minimizing the risk of infection (Fig. 8.2). The sterile dressing should be moistened every 4 hours with 3-5 ml sterile saline with the help of a feeding tube port.

Thermoregulation is of prime importance. Moist dressings with warmed saline limit this heat loss. Affected infants have decreased movement of the lower limbs and a decreased ability to generate heat from muscle movement. To regulate the temperature, the infant is kept in an incubator or under a radiant warmer [12].

Once the infant is stabilized, the defect is protected and thermoregulatory needs are met, a complete physical and neurological assessment is done.

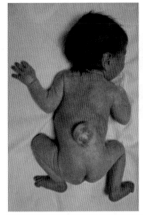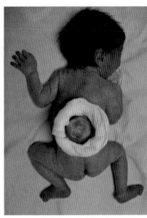

Fig. 8.2. Place a "donut" on the skin surrounding the lesion and prevent drying

Preoperative Evaluation

The neonatal pediatric and neurosurgical assessment of a newborn suffering from a MMC is the initial step prior to any surgical procedure planning [13]. Shortly after birth, with the infant stabilized, a thorough pediatric evaluation is conducted with the aim of obtaining necessary information about the cardiovascular, respiratory, gastro-intestinal and genito-urinary systems, as well as any other condition that may hinder general anesthesia, and influence both the surgical procedure and the post-operative course. Other than determining the lesion's level, the neurosurgical evaluation aims to identify the site, extension and characteristics of the spinal malformation along with ruling out any other linked spine deformity (namely severe kyphosis and/or scoliosis, hemimyelocele, split cord malformation, etc.) that may have an impact on the surgical planning (Fig. 8.3) [14]. In a similar fashion, ascertaining the presence of hydrocephalus during neurosurgical assessment is crucial for ensuring the correct order of surgical interventions.

Closure of a MMC within 24-48 hours is customary. Withholding surgery is only considered in the face of severe abnormality of the central nervous system and associated complex life-threatening birth defects (e.g., cardiac, trisomy 13 and 18) [15].

Evaluation of the cardiac, gastrointestinal, and genitourinary system is undertaken. These systems are formed concurrently with or adjacent to the malformed neurologic system. Echocardiogram should be performed on all patients prior to surgery. Preterm newborns with MMC are more likely to have congenital heart disease and a syndromic origin than term newborns [12].

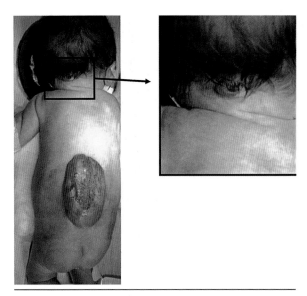

Fig. 8.3. A large lumbar myelomeningocele associated with a high cervical neural tube defect

Ultrasound examination of the kidneys, ureters, and bladder is performed but is usually normal in the neonatal period. Most infants void in the first 24 hours of life. Lack of urination or abdominal distension may be a sign of urinary retention. Dribbling of the urine suggests the possibility of a neurogenic bladder. Intermittent catheterization may be needed to ensure bladder decompression [16].

As many as 85-90% of infants with open spinal defects either have hydrocephalus at birth or develop it soon after [17]. The higher the level of lesion, the greater the incidence of hydrocephalus. Hydrocephalus usually becomes clinically apparent within the first 2 weeks of life. For the baby with MMC, a head ultrasound is performed immediately to clarify ventricular size. The vast majority of patients with spina bifida exhibit some degree of Chiari type II malformation. Approximately one-third of babies with MMC develop symptomatic Chiari II malformation [17, 18]. MRI is used to define the craniocervical junction and the anatomy of the Chiari malformation, with direct visualization of the extent of hindbrain displacement and compression in the cervical canal [5]. Lower brain-stem symptoms in newborns include difficulty in swallowing, repeated aspirations, apnea, inspiratory stridor, weak or poor cry, and sustained arching of the head. When severe, these symptoms result in insufficient breathing. The need to follow these findings necessitates continuous cardiorespiratory monitoring of these infants during their stay in the neonatal intensive care unit (NICU) [1].

Magnetic resonance imaging (MRI) of the entire spine may be necessary if symptoms suggest the presence of spinal malformations. In MMC, detailed imaging prior to closure is usually not required, but after repair imaging may be performed to identify other associated malformations.

These patients may also have coexisting conditions of the craniocervical junction, such as basilar invagination, atlantoaxial instability, or segmentation anomalies that should be evaluated with plain-film radiographs and computed tomography (CT) [5].

The preparation of the neonate for surgery is usually not difficult. Though there are no guidelines regarding the need for coagulation studies on newborns before surgery, coagulation studies such as prothrombin time and partial thromboplastin time should be considered prior to surgery. The hemoglobin level is usually kept above 13 g/dl. Fluid electrolyte balance and biochemical stability (normal blood glucose level, liver and kidney function tests) should be established. Most of the newborn babies have high hematocrit levels and an adequate intravascular volume, therefore fluid resuscitation is usually not necessary. The most notable perioperative complications include hypoglycemia and hypothermia, both of which are preventable.

In our center, surface culture of the lesion is usually obtained and the use of broad-spectrum antibiotic prophylaxis (Penicillin/Ampicillin + Gentamicin) from the first 24 hours of life to the time of surgery is a routine practice, as in many other units [1, 19, 20].

Examination of the Baby Born with a Myelomeningocele

The examination of the lesion includes noting its circumference, shape, the placode, skin integrity, and the extent of the cutaneous and epithelialized layers (Fig 8.4). The spinal column is examined for evidence of early scoliosis, kyphosis, and visible and palpable prominent laminae at the lateral margin of the lesion. Orthopedic deformities of hips, knees, ankles, and feet are noted and give further clues of the functional neurologic level. Early orthopedic consultation may be needed for evaluation of foot deformities and possible early casting. The presence of dysmorphic features may indicate a syndromic cause of MMC [12].

It is crucial to evaluate the neurological function and determine the level of spinal involvement. Progressive spinal neurological deficit in patients suffering from spina bifida is a very common clinical phe-

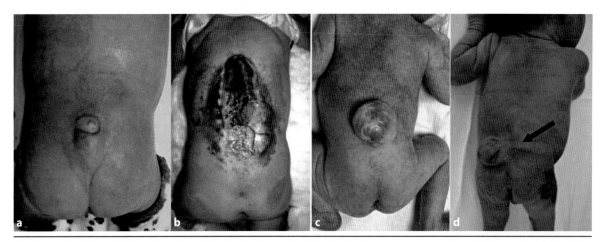

Fig. 8.4 a-d. A detailed examination of the lesion is needed for the further treatment. **a** A small contaminated and infected myelomeningocele. **b** A huge difficult-to-close defect. **c** A typical midline myelomeningocele. **d** Asymetrically localized myelomeningocele typical for hemimyelomeningocele (*black arrow*)

nomenon. The patient's neurological status should be carefully followed, paying particular attention to the spinal level of neurological function. Various scoring systems have been applied in this field for children with spina bifida [21-23]. The Spina Bifida Neurological Scale (SBNS) is a commonly used scoring system and is very useful in both the evaluation of patients' clinical status and the quantitative analysis of chronologic ages in their neurological status [21]. This scale is based on motor function, reflexes, bladder and bowel function. The scoring system can be applied to neonates and infants and may be used to foresee their daily activities in the future (Tables 8.1-8.3) [21].

The most common and important clinical problems related to the primary lesion in spina bifida patients are (1) standing, (2) ambulation, and (3) voluntary control of bladder and bowel function. These functions are linked with the level of spinal involvement. Consequently, the assessment of residual function is through the assessment of motor func-

Table 8.1. Scoring scale for motor function. Reproduced from [21]

Functioning	C-Th	L1	L2	L3	L4	L5	S1
Nonfunctioning	L2		L3	L4	L5	S1	S2
Hip							
Flexion	–		±	+	+	+	+
Extension	–		–	–	–	–	±
Adduction	–		±	+	+	+	+
Abduction	–		–	–	–	+	+
Knee							
Extension	–		±	+	+	+	+
Flexion	–		–	–	–	±	+
Ankle							
Dorsiflexion	–		–	–	±	+	+
Plantarflexion	–		–	–	–	–	±
Inversion	–		–	–	±	+	+
Eversion	–		–	–	–	–	–
SBNS motor (worse side)	1		2	3	4	5	6

–, complete paresis; ±, incomplete paresis; +, intact; *SBNS*, Spina bifida neurological scale

Table 8.2. Scoring scale for preserved reflexes. Reproduced from [21]

Functioning	C-Th ~L2	L3	L4	L5	S1	S2	S3
Nonfunctioning	L3	L4	L5	S1	S2	S3	S4
Patellar reflex	–	±	+	+	+	+	+
Achilles reflex	–	–	–	±	+	+	+
Anal reflex	–	–	–	–	–	±	±
SBNS reflex (worse side)	1	2		3		4	

–, absent; ±, diminished; +, intact

Table 8.3. Scoring scale for bladder and bowel function. Reproduced from [21]

Functioning	C.Th L. S1	S2						S3
Nonfunctioning	S2	S3						S4
Bladder control	–	–	±	+	±	+	+	+
Bowel control	–	±	–	±	+	±	+	+
SBNS BB control	1	2		3		4		5

–, uncontrollable; ±, partially controllable; +, controllable; *BB*, Bladder and bowel function scale

tion, reflexes, and bladder and bowel function. Impairment of sensation is also a major symptom of spina bifida, but its assessment is difficult in newborns and infants.

The motor examination can be conducted with pinpricks over the baby's torso or upper extremities. A newborn with a lesion at T12 or above has flail legs. Hip flexion requires L1 to L3 function while knee extension involves L2 to L4 function. Knee flexion signifies a L5 to S1 function. Plantar flexion demands function at S1-2 [24].

Spontaneous movements are best assessed by suspending the infant in the prone position and examining for spontaneous movements of the feet, legs, and hips [25]. All stimulation is best restricted to the shoulders since stimulation of paralysed lower limbs and trunk may result in reflex movements, giving a false impression.

Reflex testing is important as an intact reflex arch confirms both afferent (sensory) and efferent (motor) neural function. Commonly evaluated reflexes include the patellar tendon reflex (femoral nerve, L2-4), Achilles tendon reflex (tibial nerve, S1-2), and anal reflex (pudendal nerve, S3-4) [21]. The sensory level can be determined by the stimulation of the distal to proximal dermatomal segments with pinpricks. The sensory level is usually one or two segments higher than the anticipated motor level [24].

Judgement of the functional level of the lesion makes certain the reasonable estimates of potential future capacities. Most patients with lesions below S1 have the ability to walk without an aid. Infants with lesions above L2 often depend on a wheelchair for the majority of activities. Patients with intermediate lesions show similar degrees of wheelchair dependency (L3) or will be primarily ambulatory with braces or other devices (L4, L5) [1]. Variability is possible between subsequent ambulatory status and apparent neurological segmental level with midlumbar lesions [26]. Good strength of iliopsoas (hip flexion) and quadriceps (knee extension) is important for predicting ambulatory potential. Segmental level is also necessary in determining the scoliosis development. Most patients with lesions above L2 exhibit significant scoliosis, while it is not very common in patients with lesions below S1 [1].

The bladder problems connected with spina bifida are almost always of the lower motor neuron type with neurological flaccidity of the bladder due to a lesion of the sacral portion (S2-4) of the cord of cauda equina. Thus, bladder and bowel control evaluation measures the spinal levels below those evaluat-

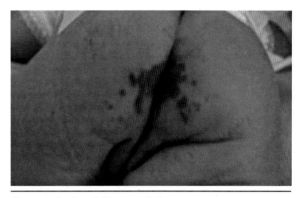

Fig. 8.5. Perianal skin excoriation

ed by motor function testing. Until infants and neonates develop voluntary voiding, the voiding status cannot be clinically evaluated [21].

Sphincter function is evaluated through observation of the anal tone and observing whether urine dribbles continuously from the urethra. Infants with a positive anocutaneous reflex have a better prognosis for urinary continence.

Anal and urethral mucosae may prolapse in severely paralyzed cases [27, 28]. Very early diaper dermatitis may also be a sign of incontinence (Fig. 8.5).

Discussion with Parents

Clearly, the parents always make the final decision concerning surgery, but it is the neurosurgeon's responsibility to provide current factual data on the natural history if left untreated and the prognosis with aggressive prompt management.

Parents of babies with spinal dysraphism may experience feelings of crisis, shock, confusion, helplessness, disappointment, anxiety, stress, denial, fear and lowered self esteem (see Chapter 33). The initial approach of the neurosurgeon and pediatrician is extremely important. In the preoperative period, the pediatric neurosurgeon should spend adequate time with the family explaining the diagnosis, treatment, complications and outcome expectations. In order to make rational decisions, parents need accurate prognostic information. Overly optimistic or pessimistic explanations should be avoided. In a recent study, it has been argued that parental hope is an important determinant of health-related quality of life [29]. The importance of hope should be recognized by physicians caring for children with spina bifida.

References

1. Volpe J (2001) Neural tube formation and prosencephalic development. In: Volpe J (ed) Neurology of the newborn. WB Saunders, Philadelphia, pp 3-44
2. Elias ER, Hobbs N (1998) Spina Bifida: Sorting out the complexities of care. Contemp Pediatr 15:156-171
3. Lewis D, Tolosa JE, Kaufmann M et al (2004) Elective cesarean delivery and long term motor function or ambulation status in infants with meningomyelocele. Obstet Gynecol 103:469-473
4. Martinez JF, Molto MA, Pagan JA (2001) Latex allergy in patients with spina bifida and treatment. Neurocirugia 12(1):36-42
5. Kaufman B (2004) Neural tube defects. Pediatr Clin N Am 51:389-419
6. Buck D, Michael T, Wahn U et al (2000) Ventricular shunts and the prevalence of sensitization and clinically relevant allergy to latex in patients with spina bifida. Pediatr Allergy Immunol 11:111-115
7. Degenhardt P, Golla S, Wahn F et al (2001) Latex allergy is dependent on repeated operations in the first year of life. J Pediatr Surg 36:1535-1539
8. Obojski A, Chodorski J, Barg W et al (2002) Latex allergy and sensitization in children with spina bifida. Pediatr Neursurg 37:262-266
9. Rendeli C, Nucera E, Ausili E et al (2006) Latex sensitization and allergy in children with myelomeningocele. Childs Nerv Syst 22:28-32
10. Kattwinkel J (2006) Textbook of neonatal resuscitation, 5th edn. American Association of Pediatrics/American Heart Association, Illinois
11. Lynam L, Verklan MT (2004) Neurologic disorders. In: Verklan MT, Walden M (eds) Core curriculum for neonatal intensive care. Saunders Elsevier, St Louis, pp 821-857
12. Brand MC (2006) Examining the newborn with an open spinal dysraphism. Adv Neonatal Care 6(4):181-196
13. Cohen AR, Robinson S (2001) Early management of myelomeningocele. In: McLone DG (ed) Pediatric neurosurgery. WB Saunders, Philadelphia, pp 241-258
14. Dias MS (1999) Myelomeningocele. In: Choux M, Di Rocco C, Hockley AD, Walker ML (eds) Pediatric neurosurgery. Churchill Livingstone, London, pp 33-59
15. Punt J (2001) Surgical management of neural tube defects. In: Levene MI, Chervenak FA, Whittle MJ (eds) Fetal and neonatal neurology and neurosurgery. Churchill Livingstone, London, Edinburgh, New York, pp 753-773
16. Snodgrass WT, Adams R (2004) Initial urologic management of myelomeningocele. Urol Clin N Am 31:427-434
17. Northrup H, Volcik K (2000) Spina bifida and other neural tube defects. Curr Probl Pediatr 30:317-332
18. Griebe ML, Oakes WJ, Worley G (1991) The Chiari Malformation associated with myelomeningocele. In: Rekate HL (ed) Comprehensive management of spina bifida. CRC Press, Boston
19. McLone D (1998) Care of the neonate with a myelomeningocele. Neurosurg Clin North Am 9:111-120
20. Clark RH, Bloom BT, Spitzer AR et al (2006) Empiric use of Ampicillin and Cefotaxime, compared with Ampicillin and Gentamicin, for neonates at risk for sepsis is associated with an increased risk of neonatal death. Pediatrics 117:67-74
21. Oi S, Matsumoto S (1992) A proposed grading and scoring system for spina bifida : Spina bifida neurological scale. Childs Nerv Syst 8:337-342
22. Glard Y, Launay F, Viehweger E et al (2007) Neurological classification in myelomeningocele as a spine deformity predictor. J Pediatr Orthop 16:287-292
23. Bartonek A, Saraste H, Knutson LM (1999) Comparison of different systems to classify the neurological level of lesion in patients with myelomeningocele. Dev Med Child Neurol 41:796-805
24. Hahn YS (1995) Open myelomeningocele. Neurosurg Clin North Am 9:231-241
25. Sival DA, Brouwer JL, Bruggink JS et al (2006) Movement analysis in neonates with spina bifida aperta. Early Hum Dev 82:227-234
26. McDonald CM, Jaffe KM, Mosca VS et al (1991) Ambulatory outcome of children with myelomeningocele. Dev Med Child Neurol 33:482-490
27. Sanders C, Driver CP, Rickwood AM (2002) The anocutaneous reflex and urinary continence in children with myelomeningocele. BJU Int 89:720-721
28. Punt J (2001) Surgical management of neural tube defects. In: Levene MI, Chervenak FA, Whittle MJ (eds) Fetal and neonatal neurology and neurosurgery. Churchill Livingstone, London, Edinburgh, New York, pp 753-773
29. Kirpalani HM, Parkin PC, Willan AR et al (2000) Quality of life in spina bifida: importance of parental hope. Arch Dis Child 83:293-297

CHAPTER 9
Radiological Evaluation of Myelomeningocele – Chiari II Malformation

Charles Raybaud, Elka Miller

Introduction

Myelomeningocele (MMC) is a malformation characterized by the failure of closure of the neural tube, usually (but not only) at the lumbo-sacral level. Synonyms are spina bifida aperta, open spinal dysraphism, and Chiari II malformation complex. MMC is typically associated with a metamerically consistent paraplegia, a posterior fossa deformity known as the Chiari II malformation, hydrocephalus, and a constellation of central nervous system (CNS) dysplasias. It is the most common malformation of the CNS worldwide, with an incidence evaluated at 0.4-1 per 1000 live births, and is one of the leading causes of infantile paralysis in the world today. In developed countries incidence is decreasing thanks to antenatal screening procedures, as well as dietary supplementation with folic acid to the women at risk prior to and during pregnancy [1, 2].

Neural Tube Defects

A neural tube defect (NTD) occurs when the neural tube fails to close. Depending on the location of the defect along the closure line, different subtypes of malformation may result. At the anterior neuropore, it is termed exencephaly, which itself tends to evolve into anencephaly through a process of necrosis. It may be minimal, and present with the features of the atretic parietal encephalocele. At the level of the cranio-cervical junction, it is termed the Chiari III malformation. In the spinal region, it is the typical myelo(meningo)cele, usually terminal lumbosacral, but possibly also segmental lumbar, thoracic or rarely cervical [3, 4]. The occipital meningoencephalocele and the basal or fronto-nasal meningoencephaloceles are likely different from the dysraphic NTDs, with different pathophysiologies and mechanisms.

In patients with MMC the neural folds do not fuse on the midline to form the neural tube. Several explanations have been proposed for this: failure of the initial steps of neurulation, disruption of the neural plate bending and secondary re-opening of the neural tube from hydrocephalus. The convincing hypothesis has been proposed of a ventral neural over-growth or over-differentiation that locally prevents the normal apposition of the neural folds [5-7]. The ectoderm adjacent to the neural plate has also been shown to play a role in neurulation [7]. Whatever the mechanism, the neural tube remains open and the flat terminal neural plate remains continuous with the skin (non-disjunction). If the meningeal sac protrudes together with the neural tissue, it forms a sac called MMC; if it remains flat and even to the skin, it is called a myelocele. This unclosed portion of the spinal cord exposed at the dorsal surface of the patient usually is referred to as the neural placode. The dysplastic portion of the cord is therefore open like a book. The exposed dorsal surface corresponds to what should have been the ependymal aspect of the placode. It is covered by the medullovascular zone, a rich network of primitive vessels. It is also partially epithelialized at the periphery, forming the membranoepithelial zone. The pia-covered ventral surface of the placode should have been the external aspect of the cord. It is facing the spinal canal and the arachnoid; ventral (medial) and dorsal (lateral) roots emerge from it on a sagittal plane, and radiate from the placode and the adjacent cord as they course rostrally, laterally and caudally to their respective neural foramina. The lack of separation of the placode from the adjacent cutaneous ectoderm prevents the normal interposition of the mesenchyme posterior to the neural ectoderm. The vertebral pedicles and lamina remain postero-lateral, and the spinal canal presents with a fusiform enlargement throughout the extent of the spina bifida. There is no fat to cover the placode under the epithelial layer.

Basis for Differential Diagnosis: Classification of Spinal Dysraphisms

For lack of clear genetic correlation, the malformations of the spine and cord are classified according to the assumed embryological sequence, and to the pathological-radiological findings.

Abnormal development of the notochordal process leads to notochordal dysraphism. A persistent communication of the notochordal canal with the ventral endoderm results in the rare neuroenteric canals and/or neuroenteric cysts. Duplication of the notochord leads to a tentative duplication of the spine and a partial duplication of the cord, and results in the diastematomyelia (which rarely may be associated with a MMC). The skin is intact but a characteristic patch of hair is commonly present.

Failed closure of the spinal cord causes the open spinal dysraphism and its topographic variants: spinal MMC, Chiari III and exencephaly-anencephaly. Spinal MMC occurs frequently at the lumbosacral level, but also at the thoracic and cervical levels (often confused with non-terminal myelocystoceles). It is usually isolated but may sometimes be found in association with diplomyelia (hemi-myelomeningocele), lipomas, and epidermoid/dermoid cysts. It is essentially always associated with the Chiari II malformation of the hindbrain in a small posterior fossa. It may occur as a familial disorder, and can be prevented by the administration of folic acid.

The neural tube may close properly but remain attached to the skin, which then is pulled upward into the spinal canal during the relative upward ascent of the cord. The resulting dermal tract/dermal cyst abnormality extends from the skin to the neural tube across the neural arches/ligaments and the meninges. The tract/cyst becomes progressively filled with dermal secretions and expands; as it is open to the environment, in two-thirds of cases it becomes infected. Usually lumbosacral, it may be observed anywhere along the dorsal midline, especially at the cervico-thoracic junction and in the posterior fossa. Except for the dermal pit the skin is intact but may present a flat angioma with some hair. The nasal dermal tract is different: the skin is pulled in by the anterobasal dura of the foramen caecum instead, and does not extend to the nervous tissue.

The lipomyelomeningocele (LMMC, or spinal lipoma) is assumed to result from the accidental trapping of mesenchymal cells in the central canal at the time of the separation from the skin, with a subsequent lipomatous dysplasia. Actually the process may be more complex, as the lipomatous mass is often multitissular. The lipoma is typically sacral at the level of the low lying caudal cord, and always involves the posterior aspect of the cord. It is typically continuous with the subcutaneous fat through a bony defect of the neural arches, and it blends with the adjacent dura. The cerebrospinal fluid (CSF)-filled meningeal sac may bulge through the bone defect, often asymmetrically. The cord remains low, tethered to the lipoma. A syringomyelia may develop. A Chiari II malformation is never associated with a LMMC (the neural tube is not open). The subcutaneous fat is often thickened; the skin covering is intact but a flat cutaneous angioma is typically present. In other topographic variants, the lipoma may be found in the cord above the conus, or below it in the filum terminale; usually it is then strictly subpial, although it may sometimes be attached to the dorsal dura.

The "simple" meningocele is a rare malformation of unknown mechanism. It is a CSF-filled meningeal sac, always covered with skin (sometimes dystrophic) but not by fat. By definition it should not contain neural elements, but it may contain some secondarily herniated neural tissue, dystrophic filum or nerve roots. The conus is in a normal location. A Chiari II malformation is never associated but because of a hydrodynamic imbalance with exaggerated compliance of the dural sac, a Chiari I deformity and hydrosyringomyelia may develop.

The uncommon myelocystocele is typically terminal (sacral), but it may be found anywhere along the spine (non-terminal myelocystocele). It is often confused with classical spinal MMC. Its mechanism is unknown. It corresponds to a hydromyelic sac protruding out of the cord into a bulging dorsal meningeal sac. The skin is intact, the subcutaneous fat is present. There is no Chiari II malformation, but for hydrodynamic reasons a Chiari I deformity may develop. It may be associated with pelvic and abdominal malformations.

The anterior sacral meningocele may be simple and isolated, or associated with a tethered cord, a lipoma, or a dermoid/teratoma (Currarino triad). It is extruded anteriorly within the posterior pelvic cavity through an anterior sacral defect. This is typically associated with a "scimitar" sacral deformity. It is never associated with a Chiari II malformation.

Imaging Tools

The optimal modalities with which to investigate MMC and the Chiari II malformation are magnetic resonance (MR) imaging above all, computed tomography (CT) for the bony abnormalities, and ultrasonography (US) for a non-invasive bedside evaluation of pathology in an infant or a fetus. However, at birth, the diagnosis is a clinical one, and assessing cardiac or urologic anomalies is more important than assessing the malformation itself.

MR imaging produces a good depiction of the spinal and cranial morphological abnormalities, and a precise identification of the normal and dysplastic tissues. Generally assumed to be more innocuous than CT (no ionizing radiation), MR is, however, not fully non-invasive in the young child as sedation or general anesthesia are needed. Specifically in a newborn with MMC, it is important to examine the infant lying on the side, to avoid compression of the meningeal sac. The quality of imaging may be suboptimal as compared to that in older children because of the high water and low myelin content in the neonate, and because of the small size of the subjects. On the contrary, from the age of a few months MR imaging yields spectacular results with which the repaired MMC, the dysplasia of the hindbrain and its sinovenous surroundings, and the midbrain and forebrain dysplasia can be assessed. Hydrocephalus also can be precisely evaluated. Coronal imaging of the scoliotic bony spine may also be helpful. In utero, MR is extremely useful as a complement to US for the diagnosis of MMC/Chiari II. It can be performed in utero, at or even before 20 weeks; i.e., well before the limit of legal termination in most countries, and before the limit of fetal surgery at 25 weeks. It depicts the level and extent of the spinal defect and better than US, the Chiari II malformation, the ventriculomegaly and the dysplastic hemispheres, which are important features if fetal surgery is contemplated.

CT can be useful to evaluate the spine and the skull anomalies, using low dose imaging, but it is not really useful for analysing the malformation itself. It is obviously not used for diagnosis in utero. It is a simple way to follow-up shunted hydrocephalus however, if MR is not readily available.

A comment must be made about latex allergy, which is a problem particular to the children with MMC/Chiari II. Up to two-thirds of patients may be affected. This high incidence is thought to be related to the repetition of surgical interventions [8, 9]. Consequently, every care should be taken to avoid the use of and any contact with latex gloves while preparing the patients for sedation, anesthesia, or placement of a venous line. The technicians, physicians and nurses involved in pediatric imaging should be well aware of the risks, and ideally,

given the relatively large number of MMC patients, any pediatric radiology setting should be kept latex-free.

Prenatal Imaging

In addition to biology, prenatal imaging is extremely important for the diagnosis of NTDs, for several reasons. The first is that it makes the morphologic diagnosis clear. The second is that it identifies the features that help to prognosticate the disorder (level and extent of the defect, mobility of the lower limbs, severity of the posterior fossa changes, degree of ventriculomegaly/hydrocephalus). The third reason is that, together with the personal, affective, familial, religious and legal contexts, it helps in decision-making: to do nothing or, on the contrary, terminate the pregnancy; to prepare for delivery by caesarean section, and for early perinatal care; to perform fetal surgery where available. Early fetal surgery (before 25 weeks) is performed in a few, highly specialized centres. It is not free of complications (retethering, epidermoids, increased perinatal mortality [10]). However, it has led to rapid reversal (within three weeks) of the Chiari II malformation [11-13]. Hydrocephalus is less common, and develops later: patients with a ventricular size less than 14 mm at the atrium and a defect at or below L4 are less likely to require eventual ventriculo-peritoneal shunting [14, 15]. When leg motion is present, it seems to grant a somewhat better long-term neurological function compared with that expected in conventionally treated patients [10, 16-18], presumably by avoiding the noxious effect of prolonged contact of the neural placode with the amniotic fluid [10, 19]. Early imaging is therefore of utmost importance in making such significant choices. It is easily done with US, and it may take more effort with MR imaging (small fetal size, fetal/maternal motion). US is sufficient for the diagnosis of MMC itself, but MR is more useful for a global assessment of the CNS. MR can be performed, and be fully diagnostic as early as 18 gestational weeks; i.e., well before the end of the surgical window (25 weeks), and before the end of the legal period for termination in most countries.

Ultrasound

US is the standard screening method for detection of the spine defect in the fetus and is discussed in Chapter 6.

Fetal MR Imaging

Transabdominal US has been the mainstay of prenatal imaging for more than 25 years. However, there remain circumstances in which US data are limited or technically difficult to obtain (maternal obesity, oligo-hydramnios, unfavorable position of the fetus). It is also limited by the fact that it only shows interfaces. For years now, technical developments have led to an increased use of MR imaging for the evaluation of the fetal CNS [20]. Fetal MRI offers the advantage of providing superior anatomic resolution, regardless of maternal body habitus or the position of the fetus in the uterus, and better tissular definition. It displays images that are more comprehensible to the patient and many physicians. One of the problems of fetal MR is that artifacts from fetal motion and maternal breathing can degrade the images, especially with younger fetuses: this can be partly compensated by the use of morphologically satisfying ultrafast T2 sequences (HASTE) that provide an image of each slice in less than one second. Another limitation is spatial definition, related to the small size of the fetal brain (about 80 g at 20 weeks), and fetal MR imaging cannot routinely be used before 20, and at best 18, gestational weeks. As it is, however, MR imaging is a natural and helpful complement to US in case of intracranial and spinal malformations [21, 22].

The diagnosis is simple when the spinal bony defect and the (bulging) myelomeningocele are demonstrated (Fig. 9.1). MR may not be better than US in identifying the vertebral level and the extent of the defect [23, 24]. However, fetal MR is useful in identifying dysraphisms that are not MMC, such as a terminal myelocystocele [25] or a lipomeningocele (Fig. 9.2) [26], which carry a different prognosis and do not need early treatment. Fetal MR recognizes the craniocervical abnormalities of Chiari II malformation and better assesses a dysgenetic ventriculomegaly versus hydrocephalus (Fig. 9.2). It may also better demonstrate the specific dysplastic features that may influence prognosis, such as a commissural agenesis/dysgenesis or periventricular heterotopias (Fig. 9.1) [27].

Prenatal Diagnosis

Ultrasound is a good screening method
    Best imaging clue:
- Spine defect.
- Chiari II: "lemon", "banana" signs (as early as 12 weeks).
- Ventriculomegaly.
    Fetal MRI is a complementary technique.

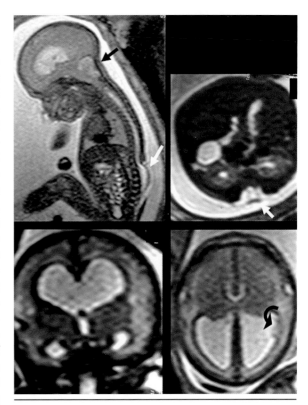

Fig. 9.1. MR, 22 weeks fetus, MMC-Chiari II. *Upper left*, sagittal: large posterior lumbosacral defect (*white arrow*), small posterior fossa with Chiari II malformation (*black arrow*). *Upper right*, axial: posterior spine defect with exposed placode (*white arrow*). *Lower left*, coronal: moderate ventriculomegaly. *Lower right*, axial: posterior colpocephaly with periventricular heterotopia (*curved black arrow*)

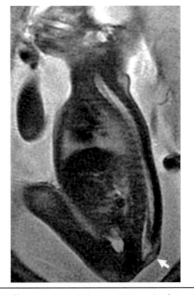

Fig. 9.2. Differential: LMMC. MR, 25 weeks fetus: low posterior spine defect, closed with a thick covering of fatty tissue, and the dark lining of the skin (*white arrow*)

Neonatal Imaging and Post-surgical Follow-up

MMC is usually diagnosed by prenatal ultrasound or MR. When continuation of pregnancy is chosen, an elective caesarean delivery is planned. Unexpected MMC are uncommon, and concern mostly low, small, non-bulging myeloceles. Optimally, the delivery should be scheduled in a center where a neurosurgeon specialized in the care of children is available. At birth, the diagnosis of MMC is confirmed by visual examination, and imaging the MMC is, as a rule, unnecessary. On the contrary, imaging studies are mandatory to assess associated conditions, such as pulmonary or cardiac abnormalities, which might affect prognosis and hence the decision to go to surgery. Cranial and renal sonograms are also important, but need not delay surgical intervention; they can be performed after surgery. Spinal films are not essential. The timing of surgery, usually in the first 48 hours after birth, is important because an increased infection rate is associated with delayed surgery [28]. The MMC is usually located in the lumbosacral area. In rare instances, it may be located higher; it is not clear whether the mechanism of the high spinal MMC is the same as that of the low MMC. Cervical MMC seem to have a better long-term neurological prognosis than low spinal MMC [29, 30]. The information, however, is compounded by the fact that there may be some confusion in the literature between true MMC and non-terminal myelocystocele [31], which seems to carry a poor motor prognosis [32].

If the neonate presents with brainstem-related clinical features, it is important to carefully investigate the anatomic status of the cranio-vertebral junction (bone, dura, venous sinuses and effluents) and of the lower hindbrain with MR. As part of the brainstem dysfunction can be related to degenerative, rather than dysplastic lesions, an early decompressive surgery may be indicated to correct them [33].

Non-CNS Investigations

Clinically, apart from the known limb paresis and CNS anomalies, patients with myelomeningoceles are at risk of renal failure in adolescence or adult life, secondary to neuropathic bladder-sphincter dysfunction. Sometimes the urodynamic changes may precede the neurological deficit related to cord tethering or progressive hydrosyringomyelia. In MMC, detrusor sphincter dyssynergia creates the functional obstruction of the bladder outlet that causes an upper urinary tract dilatation and high-pressure vesico-ureteral reflux in 50% of affected patients. Incomplete bladder emptying adds recurrent urinary tract infections. Urodynamic studies in children with MMC assess the detrusor muscle and urethral sphincter functions during bladder filling and emptying, and better identify the disorder as incontinence or obstruction. A voiding cysto-urethrogram should be performed simultaneously to assess the degree of vesico-ureteral reflux. In the first years of life US evaluation of the renal parenchyma is also important as these children are at high risk of infection [34, 35].

US Imaging

The use of US in MMC/Chiari II malformation is obviously limited to the newborn and young infant, when the cranial and spinal acoustic windows are still accessible.

Cranial US

US is a safe investigating modality that can be used bedside. The primary indication for performing cranial sonography in the newborn with a neural tube defect is to determine the ventricular size. Hydrocephalus that is associated with MMC is commonly mild in utero, and tends to becomes more severe after birth and especially after the surgical closure of the MMC, presumably because surgery reduces the compliance of the dural sac and interrupts the CSF leakage. It may also result from the association of multiple anatomical causes, such as compression of the aqueduct by the upwardly herniated cerebellum, the compression of the fourth ventricle or the obstruction of its outlet, and the crowding of the posterior fossa and foramen magnum. Beside hydrocephalus, the forebrain often presents a characteristic ventriculomegaly with small pointed frontal horns and disproportionately large posterior atria (colpocephaly). This is typically associated with a dysplastic corpus callosum and it points to a developmental defect of the white matter. The coronal images may demonstrate widening of the interhemispheric fissure and gyral interdigitation. The third ventricle is often expanded and the large massa intermedia may be noted filling the ventricle in the coronal images. The fourth ventricle is not often visualized because it is compressed, elongated and displaced toward the upper spinal canal. The posterior fossa and cerebellum are small [36-38].

Cranial Sonographic Findings in Chiari II Malformation

- Inferomedial pointing of frontal horns, colpocephalic atria.
- Partial absence of corpus callosum and septum pellucidum.
- Prominent interhemispheric fissure.
- Large massa intermedia.
- Effaced fourth ventricle.

Spinal US

US is not needed on the exposed neural placode but occasionally, if the placode is well epithelialized it may be helpful to tell the difference between a MMC and a meningocele or a lipomyelomeningocele. Nerve roots can be seen extending between the sac and dysraphic spinal canal in the MMC, whereas meningocele appears as an empty sac, or a sac containing only strands of thin, randomly oriented lacelike membranes [39]. Scanning over the sac must be performed gently and carefully, so as not to disrupt or contaminate it, and when no skin is covering the defect, a plastic wrap or drape may be used [38]. If ultrasound is performed in the neonate before surgery the remainder of the cord should be imaged in search of associated anomalies: hydrosyringomyelia, lipoma, etc. [40-42]. The cervical canal in the newborn can be imaged by US through the posterior aspect of the neck. In contrast to the free cisterns seen in normal newborns, the newborn with MMC will typically demonstrate echogenic soft tissue dorsal to the upper cervical cord, and the cord oscillation is dampened when the herniation is severe [43].

CT imaging has no place at this stage as the information needed can be easily obtained from US or from MR when it is performed.

MR imaging may be requested when the clinical features or the dysraphism are atypical, or when it is difficult to make a surgical decision. MR imaging is the procedure of choice that provides the most detailed picture of the spinal malformation and of the associated intracranial abnormalities. When the MMC is bulging, the patient should be lying on the side to avoid the discomfort of compressing the sac and increasing the CSF pressure. Multiplanar T1 and T2 weighted sequences should be used for the spine and the brain; given the diagnostic importance of fat tissue, sequences without fat saturation should always be obtained. No contrast agent is needed at this stage.

Pre-Surgical Spinal MR Imaging

The quality of spinal imaging is usually lower in newborns than at later ages because of the high water content of all tissues in the newborn and because of exaggerated CSF flow artifacts. However, it may still provide useful information. The MR diagnosis of MMC rests upon the presence of a posterior spinal bone defect, usually low lumbar and sacral, with the CSF-filled sac bulging posteriorly (Fig. 9.3). The stretched cord can be seen attached to the posterior wall of the sac where it blends into the neural placode. No mesenchymal tissue, and especially no fat, is seen overlying the placode, which by definition is exposed neural tissue on the child's back. The fat reappears at the junction line between the placode and the surrounding normal ectoderm (Fig. 9.3). Anterior to the placode, the nerve roots sometimes are seen cours-

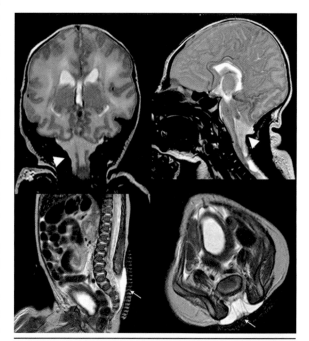

Fig. 9.3. MR, neonate, MMC-Chiari II. *Lower left*, sagittal: large posterior spinal defect (*arrow*) with no fat covering. *Lower right*, axial: good demonstration of the neural placode, with the lateral sensory and the medial motor roots emerging from it anteriorly; the meningocele is bulging mildly; the placode is limited laterally by the subcutaneous fat. *Upper left*, coronal and *right*, sagittal midline: typical Chiari II malformation with a very small posterior fossa and T2-hyperintense hindbrain herniated in upper cervical canal; note the encysted tela choroidea bulging below the cerebellum; no hydrocephalus, the pericerebral spaces are attenuated because of the leak of CSF. Cerebellar hyperdensity likely edematous, possibly early stage of "vanishing cerebellum"

ing toward the neural foramina (Fig. 9.3). The anterior motor roots are located medially, and the lateral sensory roots are located laterally. The cord usually ends at the MMC; but when the MMC involves the upper lumbar, the thoracic or the cervical segments, the lower cord continues below the malformation.

Associated abnormalities should be looked for, although usually these do not modify the surgical approach at this stage. The classical diplomyelia is better depicted on axial planes. Other possible abnormalities may include an associated lipoma, an (epi)dermoid cyst, a dermal tract, and a compressive arachnoid cyst. At this age, the spine is often not grossly abnormal, although the lumbar lordosis may be lost. However, a congenital kyphosis, or segmentation disorders (from the simple hemivertebra to the mosaic-type vertebral column) may be present, both fixed and typically associated with short-radius kyphoscoliosis. The vertebral abnormalities are best demonstrated on sagittal and coronal T2-weighted sequences with fat saturation.

Differential diagnosis includes the group of spinal dysraphisms. The lipomyelomeningocele (LMMC, spinal lipoma) is characterized by a fatty mass dorsal to the tethered cord (Fig. 9.4). The myelocystocele (MCC) is a herniated syrinx protruding out of the spine into a fat covered meningocele (Fig. 9.5). The anterior sacral myelomeningocele, which is usually discovered later in childhood, develops into the pelvic cavity, typically associated

with a teratoid mass and a tethered cord to form the Currarino triad (Fig. 9.6). The dorsal spinal meningocele is devoid of neural elements. Chiari II is not a feature of any of these entities.

Diplomyelia/diastematomyelia may be associated with the MMC.

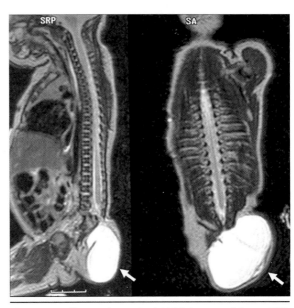

Fig. 9.5. Differential, terminal MCC. Low cord, huge CSF-filled sac herniated trough the dorsal sacrum, comprising both an extruded syrinx and a meningocele. The sac is skin- and fat-covered. No Chiari II malformation

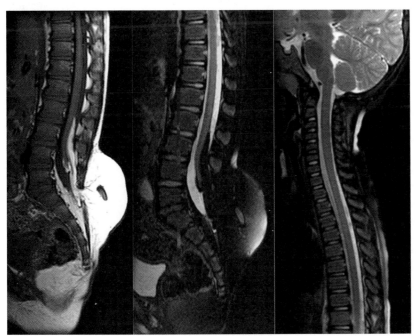

Fig. 9.4. Differential: LMMC. Huge fatty mass blending with the dorsal lower cord, and continuous with the hypertrophied subcutaneous fat through a posterior spine defect. *Left*: T1 imaging; *center*: T2 fat saturated imaging; *right*: note the absence of Chiari II malformation

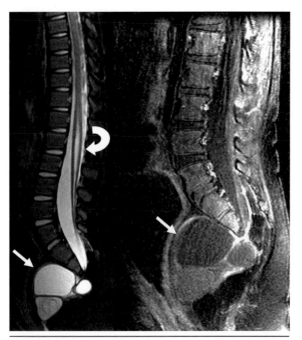

Fig. 9.6. Differential, anterior sacral meningocele. CSF-filled sac extruded through an anterior sacral defect into the pelvic cavity (*white arrow*), together with multiple, partly enhanced teratoid components; the cord is tethered to the sac (Currarino syndrome); caudal hydrosyringomyelia (*curved arrow*)

congenital hydrocephalus. Congenital hydrocephalus has been related to a combination of factors: compression of the aqueduct of Sylvius by the transtentorial cerebellar herniation, compression of the fourth ventricular outlet, and/or crowding of the posterior fossa and foramen magnum. This is suggested by a dilatation of the third ventricle, and a bowing and stretching of the corpus callosum, often with a dehiscent septum pellucidum (Fig. 9.7). Nonhydrocephalic ventriculomegaly, however, is a characteristic feature of Chiari II (Fig. 9.8), with the so-called colpocephaly (predominantly posterior ventricular dilatation), as well as the downward pointing of the rounded, enlarged frontal horns. Together with the commonly associated callosal dysgenesis, extensive white matter maldevelopment is suggested. A large, sometimes duplicate massa intermedia is a prominent feature in the third ventricle. Stenogyria (numerous serrated small gyri with an otherwise normal-looking cortical ribbon and global sulcal pattern) is already apparent in infants, and is typically predominant in the posterior medial aspect of the hemispheres. Periventricular heterotopia points to a significant cortical dysgenesis and may indicate a less-than-optimal brain function.

Pre-surgical Cranial MR Imaging

The second step of MR imaging is the cranium. At this age, a possible dysplastic CNS may be less apparent than when the maturation is complete. However, the morphology of the cerebellum (from normal – rarely – to almost non-existent), its descent into the cervical spine, the crowding of the posterior fossa and upper cervical spine are significant features that should be assessed (Fig. 9.3). The cerebellum may be mechanically compromised and this may be the first step toward the so-called "vanishing cerebellum" (Fig. 9.3) [44, 45]. The morphology of the posterior fossa and tentorium is also important; MR venography demonstrates the location and size of the dural sinuses well. This is especially important when assessing whether the infant presents with brainstem-related symptoms, and when early surgery is contemplated to correct these and prevent further deterioration [33]. As the head circumference is typically small, it is usually considered that hydrocephalus is not present at birth, but when the ventricles are markedly dilated it is difficult to recognize whether this relates to poor white matter development or to

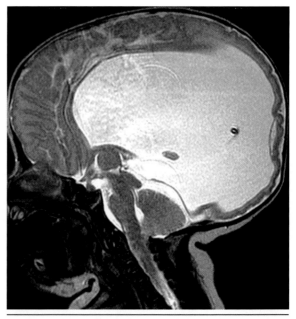

Fig. 9.7. MMC-Chiari II, neonate (same patient as Fig. 9.13). Congenital hydrocephalus: huge ventricular dilatation associated with a Chiari II malformation; the aqueduct seems not to be patent. Note the large massa intermedia in the third ventricle

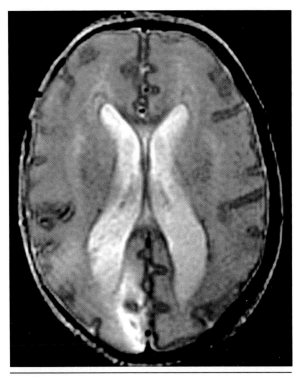

Fig. 9.8. MMC-Chiari II, premature neonate, 32 weeks. Mild ventriculomegaly. The pericerebral spaces are attenuated (leaking CSF). Incidental cortical hemorrhage

The pericerebral CSF-spaces are effaced in Chiari II before the MMC is surgically closed (Fig. 9.8) and the calvarium is poorly expanded and dysplastic with multiple lacunae (craniolacunia, "Lückenschädel", or lacunar skull). The clivus is short and concave. The foramen magnum is very large (it is always normal or narrow in Chiari I). The occipital squama may be flattened or even convex superiorly; this may be related to the low insertion of the tentorium below the nuchal muscular line.

MRI Findings of MMC (Open Spinal Dysraphism)

- Widely open spinal canal, CSF sac closed by neural placode, no fat.
- Tethered cord and lower roots embedded in placode.
- Chiari II malformation.

Differential Diagnosis of MMC

- No Chiari II malformation.
- Lipomyelomeningocele: cord lipoma through posterior bony defect.

- Simple meningocele: no attached neural element, no fat covering.
- Myelocystocele: ependymal cyst into meningocele, normal fat covering.
- Anterior sacral meningocele: pelvic, through anterior sacral defect.

Early Post-Surgical Imaging

Schematically stated, surgery of the MMC consists of the dissection of the neural placode from the surrounding ectoderm, reconstitution of a neural tube, and closure of the dural sac and of the more superficial layers, including the skin. If there is no surgical complication, there is no need for post-surgical imaging. Should it be performed, it is to check that a satisfactory anatomical result has been obtained.

The viscera should be imaged (typically by US) in the early post-surgical period because surgery has to be performed quickly after birth to avoid infectious complications. It is also the time when hydrocephalus develops because the closure of the MMC reduces the compliance of the meninges and stops the leakage of the CSF. A close surveillance therefore should be kept during the subsequent weeks. In infants, the ventricles may dilate before any significant increase in head circumference appears. Transcranial US performed every few days is the easiest, most efficient and least invasive way to detect this dilation. If the hydrocephalic process is confirmed (increasing size of the ventricles between two examinations), the choice for surgical treatment is between shunt placement and endoscopic third ventriculostomy (ETV) [46]. MR best appreciates the status of the third ventricular floor and interpeduncular cistern. In a case where cerebellar descent into the cervical canal compromises the function of the medulla, upper cord and low cranial nerves, MR with MR venography again is most appropriate to evaluate the anatomy, especially venous, of the surroundings structures of the cranio-vertebral junction.

Late Post-Surgical Complications

Following MMC repair, infants typically have neurological deficits that are stable: sensory-motor deficits of the lower limbs, bowel and bladder incontinence, brainstem, upper cord and low cranial nerve dysfunction, psycho-intellectual delay. If further neurological deterioration develops, scoliosis worsens quickly, a discrepancy appears between the neurological level and the level of the MMC or a gross asymmetry of the neurologic function of the lower limbs develops, MR of the spine is indicated. There are diverse mechanisms proposed to explain a clinical worsening, including re-tethering of the cord, constriction of the dural sac, focal compression from an (epi)dermoid cyst or an arachnoid loculation, and evolving hydrosyringomyelia and/or hydrocephalus.

Years ago, great efforts were made to prevent the so-called cord re-tethering, and correlatively to show whether the cord was free or not, by conventional imaging, by performing MR in the supine position, or by studying the cord motion by phase contrast imaging [47-49]. This did not prove to be very productive, and today it is widely accepted that the cord remains tethered at the surgical site in every child with repaired MMC [50], whereas only 10-30% of patients will deteriorate neurologically. Causes other than re-tethering therefore should be considered to explain this deterioration.

Compression of the reconstructed distal cord may be due to a post-surgical dural constriction: progressive sclerosis at and around the reconstituted dural sac may result in progressive narrowing of the spaces around the cord and, either directly because of the acquired stenosis or indirectly because of a vascular involvement, generate a progressive myelopathy. This dural stenosis can easily be recognized with MR, without or with intravenous contrast.

Another possible meningeal cause for compression is an arachnoid cyst or loculation. Spinal arachnoid cysts have been reported to be relatively common in MMC patients [51], particularly when positive contrast myelogram or myelo-CT were performed. They can become compressive with time, at any level within the spinal canal. In addition, surgery at and around the MMC, with the attempted reconstruction of a pia-covered neural tube and of a closed dural canal, may result in the development of arachnoid loculations that can also expand and become compressive with time. This has also been observed after decompression of the cranio-cervical junction [52]. Either developmental or acquired, these arachnoid cysts contain pure CSF and are difficult to diagnose on MR. The best clue is the local mass effect they exert on the cord and/or the roots: displacement and compression. They do not enhance with contrast.

A third cause for compression of the cord and roots is a developing (epi)dermoid cyst (Fig. 9.9). It may develop as an intrinsic association with the MMC, or it may result from inclusion of a skin fragment in the wound at the time of surgery. This especially seems to occur in the context of fetal MMC surgery [53]. Developmental or acquired, (epi)der-

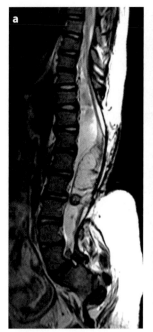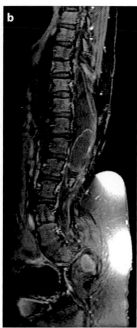

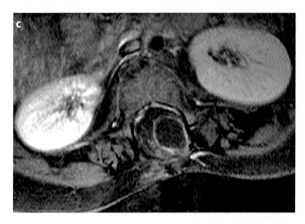

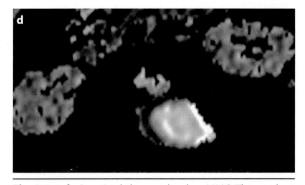

Fig. 9.9 a-d. Repaired thoraco-lumbar MMC. The cord remains tethered to the dorsal dural sac. **a** Two masses are demonstrated, one with high, the other below with low T2 signals. **b**, **c** Both masses enhance (T1FS C+ sagittal and axial), the largest one at the periphery only. **d** Axial diffusion imaging shows restriction in the larger mass, consistent with an epidermoid cyst

moid cysts accumulate desquamation and secretion products, expand slowly and may compress the cord. The diagnosis may be missed on T1 and T2 weighted imaging, even with contrast, because the signal of the cysts may be close to that of the CSF; the use of FLAIR or diffusion sequences (Fig. 9.9d) is necessary to locate and recognize them.

Finally, major causes of neurological deterioration of MMC patients are expanding hydrosyringomyelia and hydrocephalus, singly or in association. Both are easily diagnosed on MR, and even on CT. As they are not related in any way to the surgery, but are both typical complications of the Chiari II malformation, they will be described later in this chapter.

Imaging the Chronic Changes in MMC/Chiari II

Imaging of the Spine: Congenital and Acquired Scoliotic Changes

Imaging of the MMC depends upon MR, but imaging of the orthopedic spine over the years primarily depends upon plain X-ray (Fig. 9.10), occasionally complemented with spinal CT (with triplanar and 3D reformats) (Fig. 9.11) or, when depiction of the spinal content is needed, with MR, typically triplanar T2 with

fat saturation sequence. Spine imaging is made necessary by the common association of spinal deformities with MMC. Indeed, 90% of MMC patients present with orthopedic deformities [54, 55] combining kyphosis, scoliosis, and hyperlordosis. These defor-

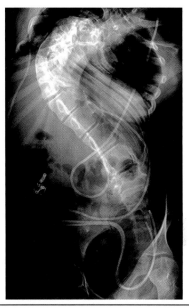

Fig. 9.10. MMC, scoliosis. Plain X-ray of a severe thoracic large-radius, kyphoscoliosis

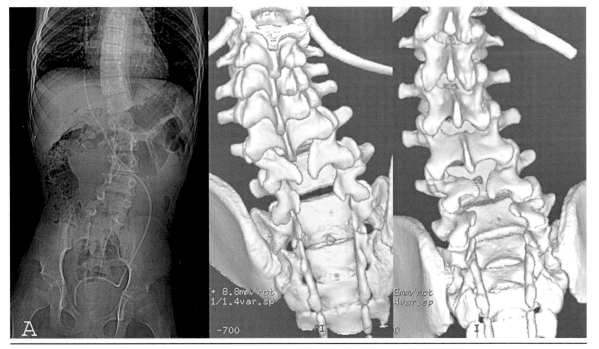

Fig. 9.11. MMC, spinal features. Plain X-ray (*left*) and CT 3D-volume rendering (*center, right*) of a mild MMC-related scoliosis. Good depiction of the defect of the lumbosacral neural arches with the laminar eversion developing from L4 downwards

mities may be developmental, acquired early in utero, or acquired later during childhood because of muscular inbalance and/or neurological deterioration [56, 57].

Developmental changes are seen in 30% of patients. They are best illustrated by coronal T2 with fat saturation (Fig. 9.12). They include vertebral body abnormalities ranging from single hemivertebrae to a jumbled mass of malsegmented vertebral components or spurs; at the thoracic level, ribs may be absent or fused. Malformative scolioses have a short radius, are often rigid, and may keep progressing in early childhood.

Acquired curves are more frequent (65%), usually caused by mechanical imbalance due to paralysis of the extensor muscles and/or to their anterior dislocation related to the eversion of the laminae. Congenital kyphosis affects less than 10% of patients with MMC but it is the most severe spinal deformity. It develops in utero and is fixed and rigid. The curve is most likely secondary to the action of the unopposed abdominal musculature in utero, as the posterior musculature, attached to the anteriorly everted laminae, pulls in the same direction. The apex of the curve is usually upper lumbar, the vertebral body at the apex is wedged, "bullet shaped" [58], with deficient posterior elements (Fig. 9.13). The vertebral body may be slipped posteriorly, and then compress the cord. Associated vertebral fusion is occasionally found. The kyphosis tends to compress the

abdominal viscera and compromises the pulmonary function, and surgical correction with spinal wedge osteotomy is necessary [56, 59].

Acquired kyphosis may also develop later in childhood and early adolescence in patients with MMC. About 95% of patients with a thoracic or upper lumbar level paralysis and 40% of patients with lower lumbar paralysis will develop a kyphoscoliosis (Figs. 9.10 and 9.11). Again, the cause is typically a muscular imbalance between the strong spinal flexor muscles and either the weak extensors, or their dislocated pull. They have a large radius, and tend to be less rigid than the congenital curves [56]. In 20% of patients they may possibly also be secondary to uneven skeletal growth. Classically, when large radius scoliosis develops secondarily, especially with increased distal neurological deficit and spasticity, hydrosyringomyelia is considered, and an MRI of the spine with sagittal, coronal and axial T2 images should be performed (Fig. 9.14); however, the role of hydrosyringomyelia as a cause of scoliosis is controversial [55]. Re-tethering has been reported to be another cause of progressive scoliosis, particularly in young children, and frequently in association with marked lumbar lordosis. As tethering is the rule rather than the exception, every other possible cause should be excluded first before considering such a diagnosis [56].

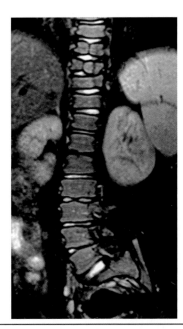

Fig. 9.12. Lumbosacral MMC, segmentation abnormalities. MR coronal T2w with fat saturation demonstrating abnormal vertebral bodies T7-8, T12-L1 block and severe lumbosacral scoliosis

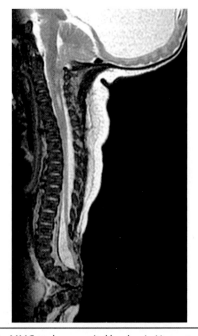

Fig. 9.13. MMC and congenital kyphosis. Neonate. Thoracolumbar MMC with T11-L5 posterior spine defect with severe lumbar, fixed, short-radius kyphosis

Hyperlordosis is actually the most common abnormal developmental curve seen in patients with MMC; it may possibly be compensatory for a pelvic instability or dislocation (Fig. 9.14).

Other orthopedic disorders are worth mentioning here: subluxation and dislocation of the hip, coxa valga, contractures of the hip, and femoral torsion; knee deformities; rotational abnormalities of the lower extremity and external and internal torsion; ankle and foot abnormalities such as ankle valgus, calcaneus foot, congenital vertical talus (rocker-bottom deformity), and talipes equinovarus; and metaphyseal, diaphyseal, and physeal fractures.

Plain Skull Imaging

The head is small at birth, and tends to increase in size after closure of the MMC; obviously more so in the case of hydrocephalus. Conversely, in older children with shunted hydrocephalus, the calvarium may be strikingly thickened. Irregular dysplastic lacunae of the inner and outer surfaces of the skull, described as craniolacunia, lacunar skull or "Lückenschädel" are present in at least 85% of patients with MMC/Chiari II malformation at birth, but tend to disappear with age (Fig. 9.15) [58, 60].

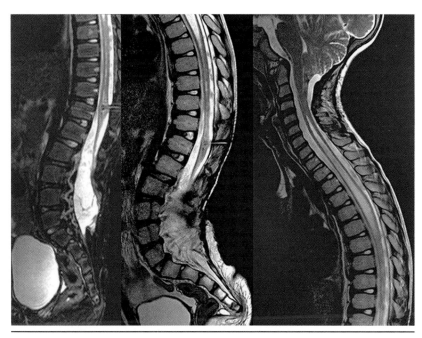

Fig. 9.14. Repaired MMC-Chiari II. T2 fat saturation early (*left*) and T2 late imaging (*center*), midline sagittal. Lumbo-sacral hyperlordosis and thoracic kyphosis have developed in the interval. Note wide spinal canal at the level of MMC with thick predural fat (saturated), the cord tethered to the scar, the radiating course of the nerve roots and the shunted syrinx. Hydrosyringomyelia, Chiari II, and arachnoid cyst or loculation behind the medulla and lower cerebellum (*right*)

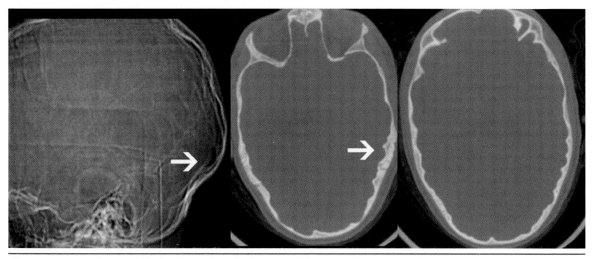

Fig. 9.15. MMC-Chiari II, skull dysplasia. Plain skull X-ray and bone CT demonstrate the classical lacunar skull

These lacunae correspond to an intrinsic mesenchymal defect, and are not an effect of an increased intracranial pressure. They are also different from the normal digital markings of the growing child. Of marginal diagnostic importance, a plain skull X-ray is not justfied, as the lacunae can be clearly seen on bone windows of a cranial CT. The lateral view of the cranio-cervical junction demonstrates a large foramen magnum and a short, concave (scalloped) clivus. The inion may be low and the occipital squama may be flat or convex upwards, possibly because of the low attachment of the tentorium. The related sinovenous markings are low. The upper cervical canal is enlarged, mostly due to the Chiari II malformation. The neural arch of C1 is incomplete in 70% of the cases. C2 is usually intact. There is typically no basilar impression or invagination [61].

Radiographic Findings in Chiari II Malformation

- Lacunar skull or "Lückenschädel".
- Small posterior fossa with scalloped clivus.
- Widened upper cervical canal.

Computed Tomography (CT)

Spinal CT may be used to delineate the spinal dysraphism, with the CSF-filled meningeal sac with the attached cord herniated through the bony defect, but a better delineation of the placode is obtained with MR imaging. The defect is usually located in the lumbosacral region and is associated with fusiform widening of the spinal canal because the laminae are everted (Fig. 9.16). The posterior lumbar muscular masses are dislocated antero-laterally. Atrophy or fat degeneration of the muscles may be seen. The quality of axial imaging of the spine is often poor because of the abnormal spinal curvatures. Use of three-dimensional (3D) surface rendering and of different planar reformats is therefore recommended for evaluation of the bony defects and scoliosis if orthopedic imaging of the spine is needed (Fig. 9.11). Should complete diastematomyelia be present, the location of the spur is easily identified with CT.

Cranial CT is mostly useful for the surveillance of hydrocephalus, and for post-surgical control after shunting or shunt replacement. On bone windows, it may show the lacunar skull (Fig. 9.15). The posterior fossa is small with a large tentorial incisura and a large foramen magnum. Flattening (10%) or frank concave scalloping (80%) of the petrous pyramids

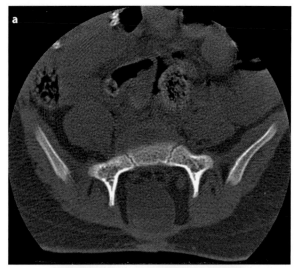

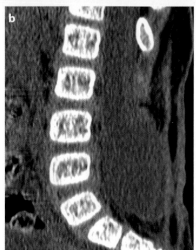

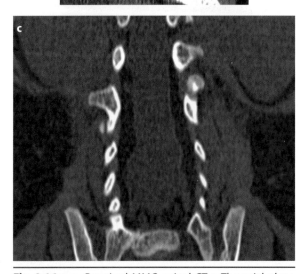

Fig. 9.16 a-c. Repaired MMC, spinal CT. **a** The axial plane demonstrates the laminae everted on each side of the repaired MMC, with muscular masses dislocated laterally. **b** Sagittal reformat showing the extent of the posterior bone defect. **c** Coronal reformat showing widened canal between everted laminae

is common. The internal auditory canals usually are short. The diameter of C1 is much less than that of the foramen magnum, its neural arch often is incomplete (70%). C2 is always intact and basilar impression is not a common finding [61].

CT is not very useful in depicting the brain malformation itself and typically is not needed for the diagnosis. Still, it presents an extremely characteristic appearance [60-63], but is now performed for long-term surveillance only. It shows crowding of the posterior fossa with a large tentorial incisura (the tentorium is hypoplastic in 95% of Chiari II patients studied at necropsy) [60, 64] and upward towering of the cerebellum, deformity of the hemispheres secondary to the white matter and especially the callosal dysplasia, and a hypoplastic falx with gyral interdigitation across the midline [60].

Imaging the Cord

The only efficient way to image the cord is MR, using T1 and T2 with fat saturation sequences, in sagittal and axial planes. Typically, beyond the neonatal period, the MMC itself presents a stable postsurgical appearance with the fibrous tissue of the scar present on the dorsal aspect of the lumbosacral malformation. The cord is essentially always tethered to the scar after neonatal repair [47, 48, 50], and it is typically impossible to differentiate the cord reconstituted from the neural placode, from the scar to which it is attached (Fig. 9.14). The spinal canal is enlarged at the level of the former MMC, with some hyperlordosis and horizontalization of the sacrum. The anterior epidural fat is usually prominent in MMC patients, thicker, and extends farther cranially than in normal individuals where it would only cover the posterior aspect of L5 and mildly the posterior aspect of L4. The nerve roots are seen crossing the subarachnoid space in a radiating fashion, toward their neural foramina (Fig. 9.14). Other post-operative changes such as compressive arachnoid loculations and fibrous dural stenosis may be seen. Masses such as lipomas and (epi)dermoid cysts may be present. When the MMC is located high in the lumbar or thoracic segment, an often lowlying cord continues in the lower lumbar levels. Exceptionally, associated MMC, or encephalocele (Fig. 9.17), or multiple "atretic MMC" may be observed above the level of the main lesion. The cord is typically flat, thin in its anterior-posterior diameter but transversely widened (Fig. 9.18). There may be a partial clefting or a duplication of the central canal, as some degree of diplomyelia is commonly

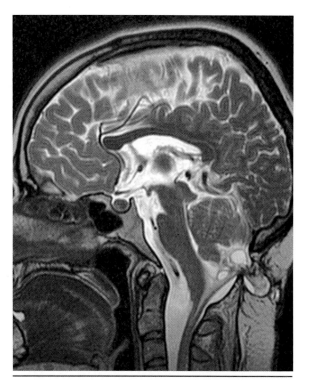

Fig. 9.17. Posterior fossa meningo-encephalocele (truly Chiari III), found in association with classical lumbosacral MMC

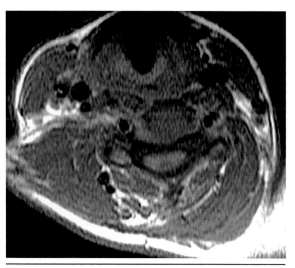

Fig. 9.18. MMC-Chiari II, cord dysplasia. Flattened cervicothoracic cord (same patient as Fig. 9.19)

found in association with MMC (Fig. 9.19) [65-68], if only histologically. Previous pathological studies of children with MMC have revealed a 36% incidence of associated split cord malformation (SCM), typically within one to two vertebral levels of the MMC. On the other hand, the term hemimyelocele

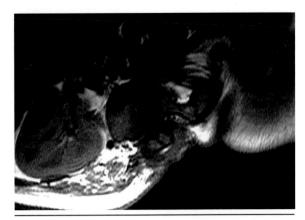

Fig. 9.19. MMC-Chiari II, cord dysplasia. Divided cord (diplomyelia) just above the neural placode (same patient as Fig. 9.18)

describes a variant of diplomyelia or diastematomyelia in which one of the two hemicords exhibits a small MMC on one side, off the midline, whereas the other hemicord is either normal, or tethered by a thickened filum terminale or with another MMC at a different level [69, 70]. Clinical series of patients with SCM have shown this association to be quite common, present in between 33-39% of patients [71, 72]. In general, affected patients have more impaired neurological function on the side of the hemimyelocele but normal or nearly normal function of the normal side.

Hydrosyringomyelia is an active distension of the central ependymal canal with expansion of the cord (Fig. 9.14). It should not be confused with the image of so-called prominent central canal, with no cystic expansion. In normal individuals, the central ependymal canal is virtual, histologically identified only by its ependymal lining. In patients with MMC the central canal remains open, as a part of the malformation [65], perhaps because the persistent leakage of the ventricular CSF during the late embryonic and the fetal stages maintained its patency, but not necessarily dilated. When present, hydrosyringomyelia may affect the whole cord, or only one or two of its segments. Longstanding hydrosyringomyelia may enlarge the spinal canal and produce thinning of the vertebral bodies and neural arches. While modern understanding of CSF dynamics suggests that common hydrosyringomyelia result from the obstruction of the foramen magnum (e.g., Chiari I), in Chiari II with MMC it may result from hydrocephalus because of a persistent communication between the cerebral ventricles and the abnormally patent central canal, through the obex. However, the mechanism of a syrinx restricted to the lower cord is more uncertain.

Spinal arachnoid cysts are not unusual in MMC/Chiari II, as a primary feature or after surgery [51, 52]. As they are CSF-filled, they can be recognized only by the mass effect they exert on the cord and the roots (Fig. 9.14).

Imaging the Hindbrain: the Chiari II Malformation

MMC/Chiari II is a complex, diffuse dysplasia of the entire CNS. The malformation of the hindbrain known as the Chiari II malformation represents its most spectacular expression. The specific features are the small posterior fossa and the dislocation of a significant portion of the brainstem, fourth ventricle and cerebellum into the upper cervical canal with, as a consequence, a large foramen magnum and large upper cervical canal (Figs. 9.20 and 9.21). Chiari II is always part of an NTD, and is observed in at least 98% of MMCs. Its mechanism has long been debated (traction by the tethered cord, expulsion by overlying hydrocephalus, different rate of growth of the CNS and spine, primary failure of development, abnormal pontine flexure, excessive dorsalization by dysregulation of the corresponding gene of development) [65]. There is a general agreement now with the hypothesis of McLone and Knepper who, from

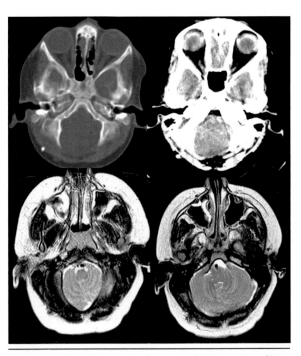

Fig. 9.20. Chiari II, posterior fossa. Axial CT (*upper*) and T2w MR (*lower*) imaging. Large foramen magnum, crowded with cerebellar tissue. The anterior cerebellum wraps around the brainstem

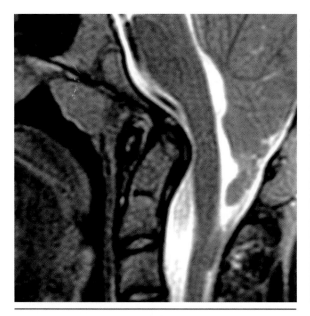

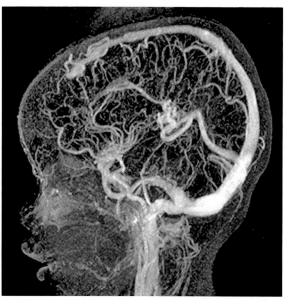

Fig. 9.21. Chiari II, posterior fossa. Sagittal T2w MR. Scalloping of clivus, large foramen magnum and wide upper cervical canal. Exaggerated occipito-cervical flexure. Elongated, bilocular fourth ventricle and cerebellum herniated through foramen magnum, and deformity of the posterior aspect of the upper cord

Fig. 9.22. Chiari II, venous abnormalities. MR venography. Very low transverse sinuses, elongated vein of Galen with prominent affluent veins

animal experimental evidence, postulate that because of the CSF venting through the unclosed neural tube, the rhombencephalic vesicle, and therefore the bony posterior fossa, do not enlarge properly; it is therefore unable to accommodate the subsequent cerebellar growth [73]. Data from fetal imaging and fetal surgery support this hypothesis: the pericerebral spaces are effaced in the MMC fetus, while they are prominent in normal fetuses; surgery of MMC in utero before week 25 causes reversal of the Chiari II herniation, which therefore has to be secondary to the MMC [11-13]. The pathology of MMC/Chiari II has been extensively studied over the years [64, 65, 68, 69, 74-82], and modern imaging therefore is based on a wide body of anatomic data.

The brain CT images of patients with MMC/Chiari II are relatively specific and may be useful [60-63, 83]. Still, MRI is the best imaging modality to investigate these patients fully, given its high sensitivity to tissular changes and its high-resolution multiplanar display of anatomy [84]. Beside the usual T1 and T2 weighted sequences, high definition 3D-T2 acquisition and MR venography are useful for a better structural assessment (Fig. 9.22). The most eloquent imaging plane is the sagittal plane. It shows the small posterior fossa with a short, concave clivus (scalloping) (Fig. 9.23), the low attachment of the

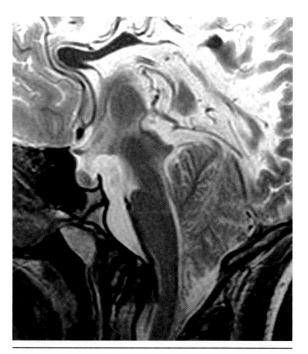

Fig. 9.23. Chiari II, posterior fossa. Sagittal T2w. Scalloping of the clivus, small posterior fossa and tentorium, descent of the brainstem and cerebellum, effaced fourth ventricle, verticalized primary fissure, atrophy of lower cerebellum. Note also tectal beaking, large massa intermedia, low and small anterior commissure, dysplastic posterior corpus callosum

hypoplastic tentorium (Figs. 9.3, 9.7 and 9.23-9.26), the elongated vein of Galen that joins the short straight sinus and the low transverse sinuses close to the enlarged foramen magnum (Fig. 9.22). Anteriorly the pons is narrow, flattened and elongated, located close or even across the foramen magnum (Figs. 9.21, 9.23, 9.24 and 9.26c); the ponto-medullary sulcus may be effaced (Figs. 9.23, 9.24 and 9.26c). The fourth ventricle is flattened and stretched inferiorly (Figs. 9.3, 9.21, 9.23 and 9.26b, c); it may present a bilocular appearance resulting from the encroachment of the vermis. The fastigial point may be effaced (Figs. 9.21, 9.23 and 9.26b). On occasions, the tela choroidea of the fourth ventricle bulges inferiorly below the cerebellum, forming a cyst (Fig. 9.3), perhaps a sign of failed opening of ventricular roof, and a risk of encysted fourth ventricle if the aqueduct is also occluded. When contrast agent is given, the enhanced choroid plexus can be seen lining the bulging cyst. Behind the ventricle, the cerebellum itself protrudes superiorly through the large incisura, often indented by the free edge of the tentorium. It mostly herniates downwards through the foramen magnum behind the pons, medulla and fourth ventricle, to a variable extent (Figs. 9.21 and 9.23-9.25). All degrees of Chiari II malformation can be seen (Figs. 9.3 and 9.26). Rarely (2% at most), the small hindbrain maintains a normal relationship with the small posterior fossa (Fig. 9.25a). In other instances, only a small tongue of cerebellar tissue is seen protruding inferiorly, and the cisterna magna can even be recognized. Typically, the descent of the hindbrain is significant and the medulla appears compressed and indented by the cerebellum. In the most severe cases, the medulla is fully dislocated behind the upper cord, which still remains tethered to C1 by the dentate ligament. This results in the complex cervico-medullary kink of the brainstem within the upper cervical canal, located just caudal to the level of the gracile and cuneate nuclei [65, 85]. A complex malformative pattern associates, from the front to the back, the cord anteriorly, the displaced medulla behind it, the lumen of the fourth ventricle and posteriorly, the deformed cerebellum. All these elements are bound together by fibrous meningeal adhesions [65].

The cerebellum is indented superiorly by the tentorium and inferiorly by the foramen magnum. The portion of cerebellum above the tentorium assumes the general configuration of the incisura and acts like an extra-axial mass called "pseudotumor of the tentorium" [83] or "cerebellar towering"; the base of the temporo-occipital lobes is elevated and displaced laterally (Fig. 9.25). The ascent of the cerebellum may be associated with a large pool of CSF, which is designated as the peri-cerebellar cistern [62]. The cerebellum typically also wraps around the brainstem into the peri-pontine and peri-medullary cisterns, behind the scalloped petrous pyramids (Fig. 9.20). This is referred to as the triple peaked appearance [61, 62]. It may cover the cranial nerves so that they emerge between the cerebellar folia. The cerebellar hemispheres may even coalesce on the anterior midline and cover the basilar artery. Due to downward displacement of the medulla and pons, the upper cranial nerves typically follow a longer intracranial course between the caudally displaced brain stem and their exit foramina, and the lower cranial nerves actually ascend through the cervical spinal canal and foramen magnum to enter the skull before turning toward their normal exit foramina. The cervical spinal cord is also abnormal in 96% of Chiari II patients with ascending roots.

Hindbrain herniation may result in parenchymal damage. Microscopically, the cerebellar tissue shows depletion of Purkinje and granule cells, and poor myelination; cortical dysplasia and heterotopia can be found; the pontine nuclei, the olivary nuclei and the nuclei of the cranial nerves may be dysgenetic [65, 82]. These abnormalities may be primarily dysgenetic, or secondarily destructive. An extreme form of damage has been described as the "vanishing cerebellum" [44, 45]. This may sometimes be

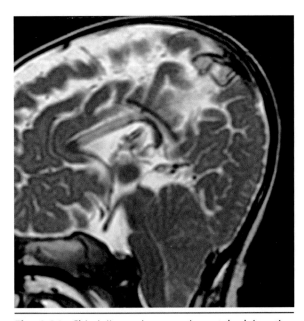

Fig. 9.24. Chiari II, previous cranio-vertebral junction surgery. Very small and packed posterior fossa, huge upwards towering of cerebellum, packed foramen magnum and upper cervical canal

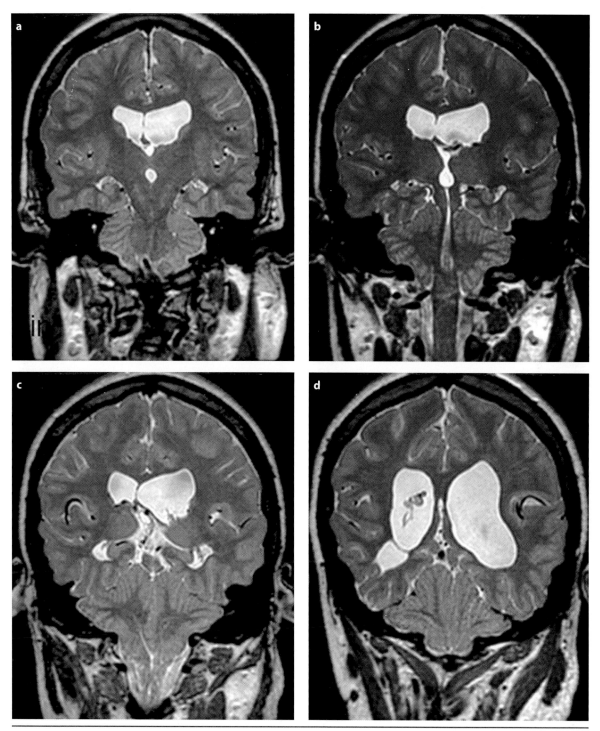

Fig. 9.25 a-d. Chiari II, posterior fossa and limbic. Coronal T2. **a-d** Small posterior fossa with extremely hypoplastic tentorium, **b** compressed but patent aqueduct and dislocated medial temporal lobes, **c** vermis buried between the hemispheres, **d** verticalized cerebellar sulci. Note also the abnormal limbic structures with outward rotation of mesial temporal lobes (everted hippocampi, parahippocampal gyri displaced supero-medially); unusual sulcal pattern: the collateral sulcus in particular cannot be identified with certainty

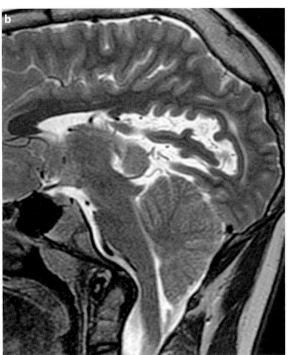

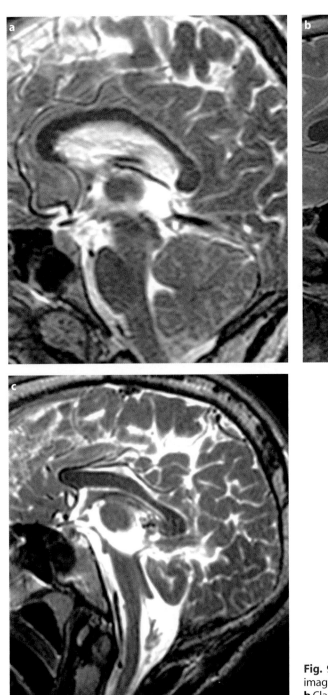

Fig. 9.26 a-c. Spectrum of Chiari II malformations. T2w imaging. **a** Hindbrain close to normal in small posterior fossa. **b** Classical Chiari II appearance. **c** "Vanished" or agenetic cerebellum in extremely small posterior fossa: note the atrophy of the pons

detected in utero by ultrasound or MRI, and diffuse cerebellar edema may be observed at birth (Fig. 9.3). Primary cerebellar agenesis can be distinguished from the vanishing cerebellum by the presence of a relatively normal-sized posterior fossa, the identification of symmetrical remnants of the anterior quadrangular lobules, the lack of scattered remnants of cerebellar tissue and the presence of a normal brain and spine. Common to both conditions is a small brainstem with loss of the normal pontine configuration [44, 45]. The vermis herniated into the cervical spinal canal is often poorly differentiated from the cerebellar hemispheres [61]. Variend [78] and Variend and Emery [79, 81] pathologically reviewed the lobular pattern of the herniated portion of the cerebellum in 100 children with MMC. They found that in addition to the vermis, a wide range of cerebellar deformity can be found: in 10% of patients there is no cerebellar herniation or displacement of the tonsils; at the maximum, the horizontal fissure was displaced below the foramen magnum so that the superior surface of the cerebellum was dislocated in the upper cervical canal [80]. A recent study has described a proportionately larger mid-sagittal vermis in 68 Chiari II patients, likely related to mechanical pressure that squeezes the vermis toward the midline [86].

From 300 autopsies of children with MMC/Chiari II malformation, Emery and Mackenzie [76] grouped the cervico-medullary deformities into different grades of severity. In the mildest form, the fourth ventricle had not descended through the foramen magnum, and the only evidence of the abnormality was the upward angle at which the first and second cervical nerve roots exit the cord. In the most severe form, the fourth ventricle herniates through the foramen magnum with a pronounced medullary kink or spur in the upper cervical canal, in association with a cystic cavity, contiguous with and arising from the dorso-caudal aspect of the fourth ventricle. They also reported that the severity of the hindbrain malformation was directly related to the number of spinal segments involved in the MMC and inversely proportional to the length of the dentate ligaments in the upper cervical region.

The complexity of the hindbrain abnormalities in Chiari II malformation makes it easy to differentiate it from the classical Chiari I deformity, which is characterized by the descent of the cerebellar tonsils only, with the brainstem, fourth ventricle and most of the cerebellum being otherwise normal; moreover, the foramen magnum and the ring of C1 are small and not enlarged. Other tonsillar prolapses may be mechanically explained by a mass effect, a bony skull hypertrophy, a venous congestion, or an increased compliance of the spinal dural sac. The Chiari III malformation is a neural tube defect located in the posterior fossa at the craniocervical junction (Fig. 9.17 illustrates a Chiari III malformation that was associated with a MMC).

Posterior Fossa Features of Chiari II Malformation

- Small posterior fossa, concave clivus, low hypoplastic tentorium.
- Global descent of hindbrain.
- Anterior brainstem "wrapping" by cerebellar hemispheres.

- "Towering cerebellum" through incisura.
- Pons and 4th ventricle elongated and dislocated Cervico-medullary kink.

Differential Diagnosis of Chiari II Malformation

Chiari III: occipito-cervical hindbrain encephalocele
Chiari I: isolated tonsillar descent, normal (small?) posterior fossa
- Mechanical tonsillar herniation.
- Mass effect in posterior fossa.
- Bone dysplasia/hypertrophy.
- Venous congestion/venous outlet stenosis.
- Intracranial hypotension (dural changes).
- Lumboperitoneal shunting.

Imaging the Midbrain

Characteristic of MMC/Chiari II patients is the inferior beaking of the tectal plate with fusion of the inferior colliculi (Figs. 9.27-9.29) [65]. The midbrain itself typically appears elongated antero-posteriorly, and transversely narrowed, presumably because of the compression from the surrounding herniated cerebellar hemispheres. The aqueduct may be occluded or narrowed, but not always; this is considered one of the possible causes for hydrocephalus. In a study of 100 brains from children dying with hydrocephalus and MMC, Emery found that the aqueduct was always anatomically patent [77] but that there was evidence of severe overall shortening of the aqueduct by pressure from the temporo-occipital lobes on the brainstem [77, 87, 88].

Imaging the Forebrain

The Third Ventricle

The third ventricle is usually small in Chiari II patients [84]. A large massa intermedia is commonly found (Figs. 9.3, 9.22, 9.23a, b, 9.25a-c, 9.27a, 9.28 and 9.29a, c); it may sometimes be duplicated (Fig. 9.27b). All this may limit the use of third ventriculostomy [2, 89]. The lamina terminalis is sometimes thick [90]. The anterior commissure may be absent (or at least not found on triplanar imaging), or very thin. Usually located at the anterior-inferior margin of the interventricular foramina of Monro, it may sometimes be seen in a low, aberrant position about halfway between the foramina of Monro and the optic chiasm [90]. A small transverse structure connecting the lateral walls of the anterior-inferior

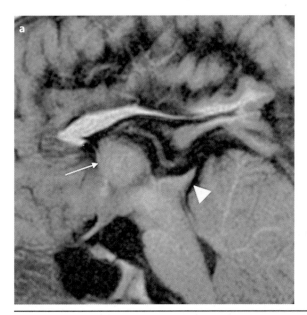

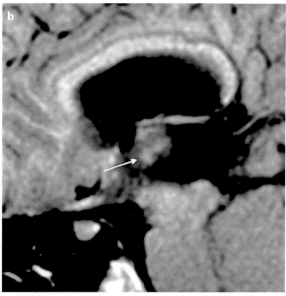

Fig. 9.27 a, b. Chiari II, midbrain and diencephalic dysplasia. T1w imaging. **a** Beaking of the tectal plate (*arrowhead*); large massa intermedia (*arrow*); note the low anterior commissure also, and the dysplastic posterior corpus callosum. **b** Duplication of the massa intermedia

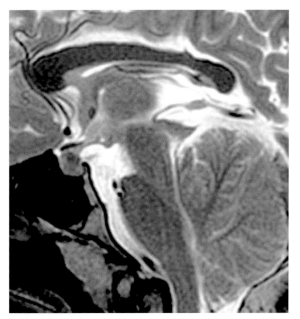

Fig. 9.28. Chiari II, diencephalic dysplasia. T2w imaging. The anterior commissure is located below the large massa intermedia, halfway between the foramen of Monro and the optic chiasm (normally, it forms the anterior inferior margin of the foramen of Monro). Note the tectal beaking

third ventricle is commonly found; as it appears to be made of gray matter on MR, it can be properly described as a hypothalamic adhesion in reference to thalamic adhesion, the other name of the massa intermedia (Fig. 9.29a, b). Only histology can tell whether this unusual structure contains commissural fibers [90]. It suggests that some degree of hypothalamic dysplasia may also exist in Chiari II (Fig. 9.29c). The pineal gland may be normal, absent, or dysplastic, located at a distance from the posterior and habenular commissures and imbedded in the sometimes hugely distended posterior ventricular wall of the ventricle [90].

The Interhemispheric Structures

The interhemispheric commissural plate comprises the corpus callosum and, posteriorly attached on its inferior aspect, the hippocampal commissure. The anterior commissural abnormalities are better described with the third ventricle. Abnormalities of the corpus callosum are common, seen in 33-90% of patients, but complete agenesis is rare [84]. The

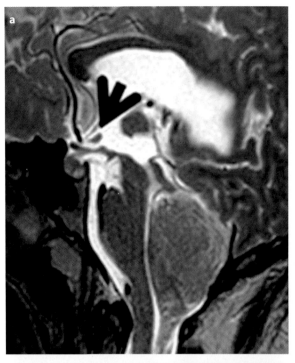

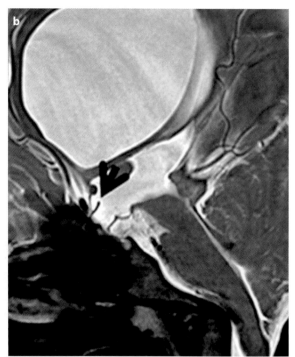

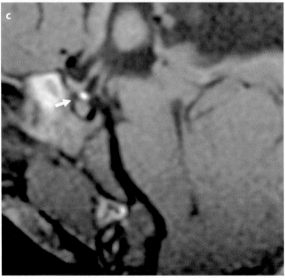

Fig. 9.29 a-c. Chiari II, diencephalic dysplasia. T2w imaging. The "hypothalamic adhesion" is a supernumerary structure crossing the anterior inferior portion of the third ventricle to join the lateral hypothalami; it is usually attached to the lower part of the lamina terminalis. Its visibility is independent of whether the patient presents with **a** shunted or **b** active hydrocephalus, and therefore does not correspond to an apposition of the ventricular walls due to ventricular collapse. It may be similar to the hypertrophy of the massa intermedia, and reflect a diencephalic dysplasia. **c** This ectopic posterior pituitary (*arrow*) may be part of the dysplasia as well

deformity obviously may be related to hydrocephalus when the corpus callosum appears stretched around the actively dilated lateral ventricles. A straight but otherwise complete commissural plate might also be consistent with a previous, presently shunted hydrocephalus [90]. Beside these, real dysplasia of the corpus callosum (and hippocampal commissure) is common: global or segmental hypoplasia, thinning, tapering, posterior agenesis and folding may be observed in various combinations (Fig. 9.30) [90]. These abnormalities are morphologically different

from the description of the classical forms of commissural agenesis [91], and a Probst bundle is never observed in Chiari II patients [90]. Typically, the callosal defects can be correlated with the ventricular morphology and are in keeping with a global developmental defect of the white matter in Chiari II patients [90]. A particular feature is a callosal ridge, commonly seen coursing over the corpus callosum. It is a bundle of white matter, triangular in section, broad or thin depending on the patient, running obliquely from the back to the front and from one

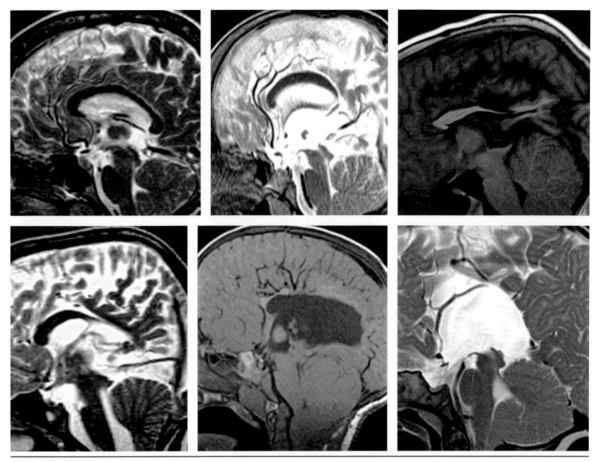

Fig. 9.30. Chiari II, hemispheric dysplasia. The spectrum of malformations of the dysplastic corpus callosum range from near to normal (*upper left*) to nearly non-existent (*lower right*)

side to the other on the superior aspect of the corpus callosum (Fig. 9.31) [90]. It is consistent with what has been described by Hori and Stan [92, 93] histologically in non-Chiari II patients as a possible heterotopic cingulum, and radiologically proven to be a heterotopic cingulum by Vachha et al. [94] in Chiari II patients, using diffusion-tensor imaging (DTI).

The septum pellucidum contains the cinguloseptal fibers, and it develops simultaneously with the commissures [95, 96]. A septal dehiscence may be explained by hydrocephalus, as it is commonly observed in congenital hydrocephalus and may be caused by shunt placement. However, when the septum pellucidum is grossly hypoplastic or dysplastic, often in association with callosal dysplasia, it has to be considered developmental [90].

The lateral ventricles also are commonly abnormal in Chiari II. It is a subject of endless debate as to whether the abnormality is intrinsic, developmental, or secondary to hydrocephalus. Loss of white matter is a usual complication of hydrocephalus.

However, there are good reasons to believe that the white matter abnormalities in Chiari II may be primary defects [91]. Abnormal rounded frontal horns pointing antero-medially are a classical feature of Chiari II [84]. The ventriculomegaly may be observed already in utero, even in the absence of any sign of active hydrocephalus (it is often associated with microcephaly) (Fig. 9.1). The morphology of the ventricles is often particular, with disproportionate dilation of their posterior portion (so-called colpocephaly); the lack of white matter predominates on the postero-medial aspect of the hemisphere (explaining the peculiar aspect of posterior dilatation of the interhemispheric cistern after shunting, not seen in other forms of hydrocephalus) (Figs. 9.1 and 9.7). The common occurrence of partial posterior callosal agenesis also points to a lack of posterior fibers. Finally, the cortex is abnormal in Chiari II patients and neuronal migration anomalies are found [82]; this also may be associated with, and explain, a defective white matter.

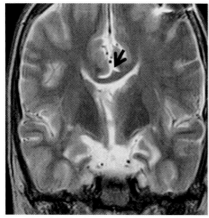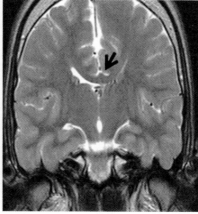

Fig. 9.31. Chiari II, hemispheric dysplasia. Coronal T2w imaging in two different patients. The "callosal ridge" is a triangular bundle of white matter that runs on the superior aspect of the corpus callosum. It has been identified as an aberrant cingular bundle crossing the midline in a study on Chiari II limbic abnormalities, using DTI [94]

The Cortex

The nature of the cortical abnormalities has also been debated. The most characteristic abnormality is a cortical overfolding, with closely packed gyri which respect the general organization of the brain (different in this respect from polymicrogyria in which the normal sulcation is lost). It predominates in the posteromedial cortex, and is observed in about 50% of patients with Chiari II malformation [82, 97]. This special pattern has been called stenogyria (Fig. 9.32). It can be observed in a neonate without, or before the development of, hydrocephalus (Fig. 9.33). Other unusual cortical findings include the gyral interhemispheric interdigitations (commonly attributed – without proof – to the hypoplasia of the falx) (Fig. 9.34), sometimes forming the so-called "accessory lobes" that may protrude from the medial parieto-occipital cortex into the interhemispheric fissure (Figs. 9.32b and 9.35).

Periventricular heterotopia can be also seen, focally (Fig. 9.36) or diffusely (Fig. 9.37). In an autopsy report, the cortex was found to be abnormal in 92% of severe cases of patients with MMC who died before the age of 2 years. True polymicrogyria (40%), subcortical neuronal heterotopia (44%), disordered lamination (24%), immature cortical development (24%), and polygyria with irregular cortex (16%)

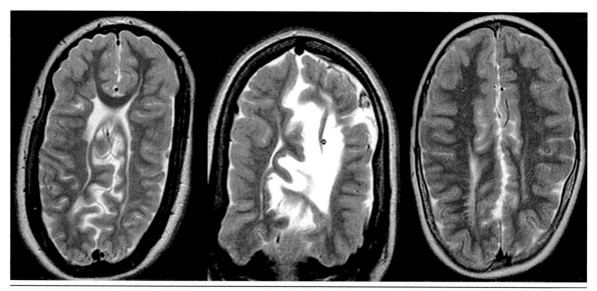

Fig. 9.32. Chiari II, hemispheric dysplasia. Three different patterns of abnormal cortical and white matter patterns: interdigitation with posterior callosal dysplasia (*left*); "accessory lobes" protruding into a dilated posterior interhemispheric cistern with hypoplasia of the postero-medial hemispheric wall, especially on the left (*center*); medial parietal stenogyria with its serrated appearance (*right*)

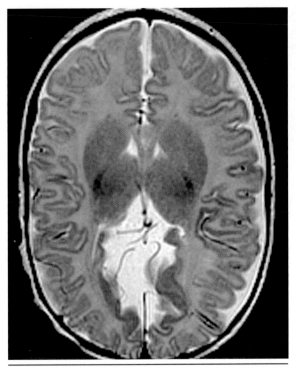

Fig. 9.33. Chiari II, hemispheric dysplasia. Infant, shunted hydrocephalus. Abnormal appearance of the posterior medial temporo-occipital cortex

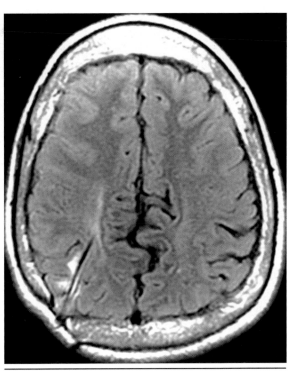

Fig. 9.34. Chiari II, hemispheric dysplasia. Gyral interdigitation across the midline. Note the calvarial thickening (shunted hydrocephalus)

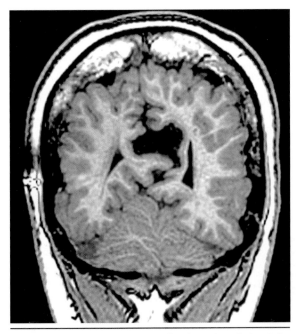

Fig. 9.35. Chiari II, hemispheric dysplasia. Dysplasia of the medial hemispheric walls with "accessory lobe". Note the bone apposition on the thickened calvarium (shunted hydrocephalus)

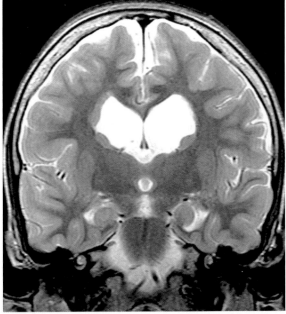

Fig. 9.36. Chiari II, hemispheric dysplasia. Ventriculomegaly with frontal subependymal gray matter heterotopia on the right side (neuronal migration disorder). Note also the paucity of temporomesial white matter (cingular bundle)

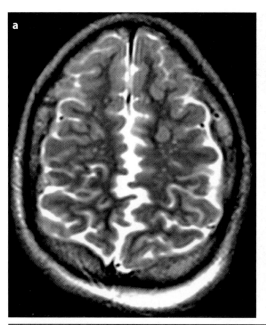 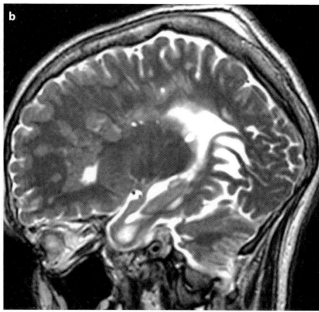

Fig. 9.37 a, b. Chiari II, hemispheric dysplasia. **a** Diffuse subcortical and **b** subependymal heterotopia, expressing a major neuronal migration disorder

were found [82]. This again indicates that beside the effects of hydrocephalus, the brain in Chiari II presents with multiple and diffuse dysplastic changes.

There are also specific changes affecting the limbic structures: the hippocampi frequently are small, verticalized, everted laterally, and the adjacent parahippocampal white matter (cingulum) is poor (Fig. 9.24) [90]. The posterior limbic lobe, including the posterior cingulate and the posterior parahippocampal gyri, is commonly disorganized, often in association with posterior callosal dysgenesis [90]. This, as well as abnormalities of the fornix, was demonstrated by DTI in a small series of Chiari II patients, and a clear correlation with non-verbal recall deficit was found [94].

Imaging the Meninges

The falx cerebri is frequently fenestrated, short, partially absent or hypoplastic; this is best appreciated on coronal images on MRI (or CT). It is assumed to be the cause of the cortical interdigitation across the interhemispheric fissure [60]. In shunted patients, the collapse of the ventricles pulls the poorly developed postero-medial wall, and this results in the characteristic widening of the posterior portion of the interhemispheric fissure. The tentorium is also hy-

poplastic, with an elongated vein of Galen coursing through the dilated cistern to join the straight sinus. It is not clear whether this has any relation to the redundant deep venous pattern that is sometimes observed. As noted in the description of the posterior fossa abnormalities, the tentorium is attached low on the occipital squama, in close relation with the foramen magnum, making the surgical approach to the herniated brain perilous because of the proximity of the transverse sinuses.

Supratentorial Anomalies in Chiari II Malformation

Third ventricle
- Large massa intermedia.
- Dislocated anterior commissure.
- Hypothalamic adhesion.
- Dysplastic pineal.

Interhemispheric midline
- Dysplastic corpus callosum and septum pellucidum.

Hemispheres
- Hypoplastic white matter.
- Stenogyria, gyral interdigitation, "accessory lobes".
- Periventricular heterotopia.
- Dysplastic limbic structures.
- Hypoplastic falx and tentorium.

The Long-Term Complications of MMC/Chiari II

Hydrocephalus

Hydrocephalus is common in MMC/Chiari II, presumably related to posterior fossa crowding and aqueductal compression. As it typically develops shortly after the surgical MMC closure in the neonatal period (that reduces the compliance of the meninges and stops the CSF leakage), it is usually dealt with in the first weeks or months after MMC repair. The early surveillance is done with US; it has to be done with CT or MR after closure of the fontanels. Like any patient with chronic hydrocephalus, the child is exposed to late complications, and to repeated imaging. Therefore, one should be aware of the normal appearance of the brain in this context. CT is commonly used, and is efficient; due to the potential hazard of ionizing radiation, MR would be the modality of choice, but in young children, it requires sedation or general anaesthetic, more than CT. The use of the ultrafast MR T2 weighted sequences used in fetal imaging has been advocated to avoid sedation, but although they show the size and morphology of the brain and ventricles, the resulting images are less than optimal, with a poor signal specificity. Therefore CT still is considered necessary in many centers, especially since good axial and coronal reformats may be obtained. Whatever the modality used, current studies should always be compared with previous ones.

The large majority of children and adolescents with chronic Chiari II have been classically treated with a ventriculo-peritoneal (VP) shunt. The morphological appearance of the brain is characteristic on axial image in those children. The shunted ventricles are commonly larger posteriorly than anteriorly. When the cerebral mantle is deficient, the collapse of the shunted ventricles results in a significant widening of the subarachnoid spaces. This is usually not apparent over the convexity because the often major thickening of the calvarium effaces the subarachnoid spaces (Figs. 9.23b, 9.24, 9.25 a-c and 9.34-9.37). However, it is conspicuous in the region of the posterior midline where a short dysplastic corpus callosum, a deficient cerebral mantle postero-medially, and a large pericerebellar cistern between the laterally displaced temporal lobes and the hypoplastic tentorium act to exaggerate it (Figs. 9.33, 9.38 and 9.39). On the floor of this dilated cistern, the towering cerebellum is seen. The elongated midbrain with tectal beaking is seen in front of it. The posterior fossa is

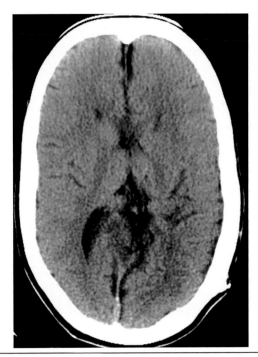

Fig. 9.38. Chiari II, follow-up of hydrocephalus. Characteristic CT appearance. Small ventricles, mild enlargement of the ambient cistern, related to the dysplasia of posterior medial hemisphere

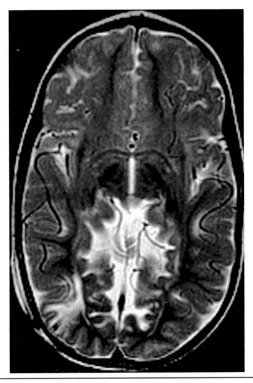

Fig. 9.39. Chiari II, follow-up of hydrocephalus. Characteristic MR appearance. Markedly enlarged posterior interhemispheric spaces due to the medial hemispheric dysplasia

usually crowded, with a deformed folial pattern of the cerebellar hemispheres, a buried vermis, wrapping of the brainstem by the cerebellum, and the herniated hindbrain filling the large foramen magnum. The fourth ventricle is not usually seen.

When the shunt is not patent, and when the child presents with hydrocephalus, the lateral ventricles become prominent, effacing the subarachnoid spaces. Periventricular interstitial edema is uncommon. Rarely, the fourth ventricle may be trapped and therefore become prominent. Then the risks of compression of the brainstem in an already packed posterior fossa are high. Disconnection of the shunt may sometimes be demonstrated on appropriately windowed images of the soft tissue of the upper neck. The lower segments of the device are routinely examined with plain films. In case of peritoneal encystment, abdominal US is indicated.

Findings are the same on axial MR images if MR is used. A better description of the various brain dysplasias is obtained from the sagittal and coronal planes.

Increasingly in recent years, endoscopic third ventriculostomy (ETV) has been performed in infants [46]. This requires a precise presurgical MR assessment of the anterior third ventricle and of the interpeduncular cistern to plan the procedure as, depending on the severity of the Chiari II malformation, the cistern may be effaced or packed with cerebellar tissue. Typically after the procedure the ventricles remain much larger than after placement of a VP shunt [98], and the diagnosis of developing chronic hydrocephalus may be difficult to make on imaging alone. Careful comparison with previous studies may help, together with the assessment of the clinical features.

Finally, a VP shunt may be removed and replaced by an ETV. Again, a presurgical assessment is needed, and the lateral ventricles are expected to remain large after the procedure, more than after the VP shunt placement.

Rarely, other complications of shunted hydrocephalus may occur. The morphological abnormalities behind the "slit ventricle syndrome" are difficult to assess, as the CSF pressure increase develops in an essentially non-expandable ventricle. Rare conditions such as subdural collections and infections need the appropriate imaging.

Hydrosyringomyelia

Pathology studies of the cord have shown that the central canal of the cord remains dilated in patients with MMC [65]. A prominent central canal is therefore commonly seen on MR images of patients with MMC,

the incidence being evaluated in 40-95% of cases. The dilation sometimes becomes significant and appears as a real hydrosyringomyelia, either focal, segmental or diffuse. Short segments of hydromyelia may be seen just below the Chiari II malformation in the cervical cord, or just above the MMC in the terminal cord; they are typically asymptomatic. It is uncertain how they form. In general, hydrosyringomyelia, usually associated with Chiari I deformities, can be explained by a hydrodynamic imbalance of the CSF above and below the obstructed foramen magnum. A similar mechanism might be involved in Chiari II malformation. However, the persistent patency of the central ependymal canal and its communication with the cerebral ventricles through the obex might explain the classical association of hydrosyringomyelia with hydrocephalus in the MMC patients [54, 61, 85, 99]. This is the explanation of the clinical rule that hydrocephalus should be ruled out and the VP shunt patency should be checked when hydrosyringomyelia develops in a MMC/Chiari II patient.

Hydrosyringomyelia should be considered when a patient presents with a secondary neurological deterioration, such as a new spasticity. Classically, scoliosis also is considered a manifestation of hydrosyringomyelia, but this assumption has recently been challenged [55]. Although axial CT of the spine can show the cystic appearance of the cord, MR is the modality of choice, mostly T2 weighted sagittal and axial planes [100]. It demonstrates the enlarged cord effacing the subarachnoid spaces around it, the elongated CSF-filled expanding cyst within the cord and its level and extent cranially and caudally. The usual horizontal septations are thought to represent more resistant planes of decussation. MR should be extended to the brain to look for hydrocephalus, or for a trapped fourth ventricle with signs of compression of the brainstem. The classical syringobulbia (rupture of the dilated central canal and CSF leakage forming a syrinx in the medulla) is, at most, exceptional, and it is the Chiari II malformation, rather than this hypothetical syringobulbia, that usually explains the occasional development of low brainstem symptoms.

Conclusion

The myelomeningocele and Chiari II malformation are early (fourth embryonic week), complex malformations of the entire central nervous system. If the MMC is at birth the most striking morphological and neurological disorder, modern imaging, beyond the MMC, demonstrates major abnormalities of the cord (e.g., diplomyelia), hindbrain (e.g., Chiari II malformation, although this is potentially partially regressive), midbrain (e.g., tectal plate), diencephalon (e.g., massa intermedia, hypothalamic adhesion) and hemispheres (e.g., white matter and cortical defects, heterotopia). Imaging plays a major role in the diagnosis and surveillance of the surgical abnormalities

(repaired MMC and shunted hydrocephalus). It may now play an essential role also in the assessment of the multiple dysplasias, from midgestation to adolescence, and therefore help to predict the psycho-intellectual potential of the affected patients, beyond their neurological impairment.

References

1. Smithells RW, Sheppard S (1980) Possible prevention of neural-tube defects by periconceptional vitamin supplementation. Lancet 1:647
2. McLone DG, Dias MS (2003) The Chiari II malformation: cause and impact. Childs Nerv Syst 19:540-550
3. Pang D, Dias MS (1993) Cervical myelomeningoceles. Neurosurgery 33:363-372; discussion 372-373
4. Nishio S, Morioka T, Hikino S, Fukui M (2001) Cervical (myelo)meningocele: report of two cases. J Clin Neurosci 8:586-587
5. Greene ND, Gerrelli D, Van Straaten HW, Copp AJ (1998) Abnormalities of floor plate, notochord and somite differentiation in the loop-tail (Lp) mouse: a model of severe neural tube defects. Mech Dev 73:59-72
6. Rogner UC, Spyropoulos DD, Le Novere N (2000) Control of neurulation by the nucleosome assembly protein-1-like 2. Nat Genet 25:431-435
7. Cai W, Zhao H, Guo J, Li Y (2007) Retinoic acid-induced lumbosacral neural tube defects: myeloschisis and hamartoma. Childs Nerv Syst 23:549-554
8. Estornell Moragues F, Nieto Garcia A, Mazon Ramos A et al (1997) [Latex allergy in children with myelomeningocele. Incidence and associated factors]. Actas Urol Esp 21:227-235
9. Rendeli C, Nucera E, Ausili E et al (2006) Latex sensitisation and allergy in children with myelomeningocele. Childs Nerv Syst 22:28-32
10. Sutton LN, Adzick NS, Johnson MP (2003) Fetal surgery for myelomeningocele. Childs Nerv Syst 2003,19:587-591
11. Tulipan N, Hernanz-Schulman M, Bruner JP (1998) Reduced hindbrain herniation after intrauterine myelomeningocele repair: A report of four cases. Pediatr Neurosurg 29:274-278
12. Tulipan N, Hernanz-Schulman M, Lowe LH, Bruner JP (1999) Intrauterine myelomeningocele repair reverses preexisting hindbrain herniation. Pediatr Neurosurg 31:137-142
13. Bouchard S, Davey MG, Rintoul NE (2003) Correction of hindbrain herniation and anatomy of the vermis after in utero repair of myelomeningocele in sheep. J Pediatr Surg 38:451-458; discussion 451-458
14. Bruner JP, Tulipan N, Paschall RL et al (1999) Fetal surgery for myelomen-ingocele and the incidence of shunt-dependent hydrocephalus. JAMA 282:1819-1825
15. Bruner JP, Tulipan N, Reed G (2004) Intrauterine repair of spina bifida: preoperative predictors of shunt-dependent hydrocephalus. Am J Obstet Gynecol 190:1305-1312
16. Tulipan N, Bruner JP, Hernanz-Schulman M et al (1999) Effect of intrauterine myelomeningocele repair on central nervous system structure and function. Pediatr Neurosurg 31:183-188
17. Tulipan N, Bruner JP (1999) Fetal surgery for spina bifida. Lancet 353:406; author reply 407
18. Sutton LN, Sun P, Adzick NS (2001) Fetal neurosurgery. Neurosurgery 48:124-142; discussion 142-124
19. Hutchins GM, Meuli M, Meuli-Simmen C (1996) Acquired spinal cord injury in human fetuses with myelomeningocele. Pediatr Pathol Lab Med 16:701-712
20. Girard N, Raybaud C, d'Ercole C (1993) In vivo magnetic resonance imaging of the fetal brain. Neuroradiology 35:431-436
21. Simon EM (2004) MRI of the fetal spine. Pediatr Radiol 34:712-719
22. von Koch CS, Glenn OA, Goldstein RB, Barkovich AJ (2005) Fetal magnetic resonance imaging enhances detection of spinal cord anomalies in patients with sonographically detected bony anomalies of the spine. J Ultrasound Med 24:781-789
23. Aaronson OS, Hernanz-Schulman M, Bruner JP et al (2003) Myelomeningocele: Prenatal evaluation – Comparison between transabdominal US and MR imaging. Radiology 227:839-843
24. Bruner JP, Tulipan N, Dabrowiak ME et al (2004) Upper level of the spina bifida defect: How good are we? Ultrasound Obstet Gynecol 24:612-617
25. Midrio P, Silberstein HJ, Bilaniuk LT et al (2002) Prenatal diagnosis of terminal myelocystocele in the fetal surgery era: case report. Neurosurgery 50:1152-1154; discussion 1154-1155
26. Leung EC, Sgouros S, Williams S, Johnson K (2002) Spinal lipoma misinterpreted as a meningomyelocele on antenatal MRI scan in a baby girl. Childs Nerv Syst 18:361-363
27. Mangels KJ, Tulipan N, Tsao LY (2000) Fetal MRI in the evaluation of intrauterine myelomeningocele. Pediatr Neurosurg 32:124-131
28. Gaskill SJ (2004) Primary closure of open myelomeningocele. Neurosurg Focus 16:E3
29. Meyer-Heim AD, Klein A, Boltshauser E (2003) Cervical myelomeningocele – follow-up of five patients. Eur J Paediatr Neurol 7:407-412

30. Habibi Z, Nejat F, Kazmi SS, Kajbafzadeh AM (2006) Cervical myelomen-ingocele. Neurosurgery 58:1168-1175

31. Arts MP, de Jong TH (2004) Thoracic meningocele, meningomyelocele or myelocystocele? Diagnostic difficulties, consequent implications and treatment. Pediatr Neurosurg 40:75-79

32. Sun JC, Steinbok P, Cochrane DD (2000) Cervical myelocystoceles and meningoceles: long-term follow-up. Pediatr Neurosurg 33:118-122

33. Pollack IF, Kinnunen D, Albright AL (1996) The effect of early cranio-cerebral decompression on functional outcome in neonates and young infants with myelodysplasia and symptomatic Chiari II malformations: results from a prospective series. Neurosurgery 38:703-710; discussion 710

34. van Gool JD, Dik P, de Jong TP (2001) Bladder-sphincter dysfunction in myelomeningocele. Eur J Pediatr 160:414-420

35. Rickwood AM (2002) Assessment and conservative management of the neuropathic bladder. Semin Pediatr Surg 11:108-119

36. Babcock DS, Han BK (1981) Caffey award: cranial sonographic findings in meningomyelocele. AJR Am J Roentgenol 136:563-569

37. Byrd SE, Osborn RE, Radkowski MA et al (1988) Disorders of midline structures: holoprosencephaly, absence of corpus callosum, and Chiari malformations. Semin Ultrasound CT MR 9:201-215

38. Rumack C, Wilson S, Charboneau JW, Johnson JA (2004) Diagnostic ultrasound. Mosby, London

39. Jacobs NM, Grant EG, Dagi TF, Richardson JD (1984) Ultrasound identification of neural elements in myelomeningocele. J Clin Ultrasound 12:51-53

40. Zieger M, Dorr U (1988) Pediatric spinal sonography. Part I: Anatomy and examination technique. Pediatr Radiol 18:9-13

41. Zieger M, Dorr U, Schulz RD (1988) Pediatric spinal sonography. Part II: Malformations and mass lesions. Pediatr Radiol 18:105-111

42. Glasier CM, Chadduck WM, Leithiser RE et al (1990) Screening spinal ultrasound in newborns with neural tube defects. J Ultrasound Med 9:339-343

43. Cramer BC, Jequier S, O'Gorman AM (1986) Sonography of the neonatal craniocervical junction. AJR Am J Roentgenol 147:133-139

44. Sener RN (1995) Cerebellar agenesis versus vanishing cerebellum in Chiari II malformation. Comput Med Imag and Graph 19:491-494

45. Boltshauser E, Schneider J, Kollias S et al (2002) Vanishing cerebellum in myelomeningocele. Eur J Paediatr Neurol 6:109-113

46. Gorayeb RP, Cavalheiro S, Zymberg ST (2004) Endoscopic third ventriculoscopy in children younger than 1 year of age. J Neurosurg 100 (Supl Pediatrics):427-429

47. Just M, Ermert J, Higer HP et al (1987) Magnetic resonance imaging of postrepair-myelomeningocele-findings in 31 children and adolescents. Neurosurg Rev 10:47-52

48. Tamaki N, Shirataki K, Kojima N et al (1988) Tethered cord syndrome of delayed onset following repair of myelomeningocele. J Neurosurg 69:393-398

49. Levy LM, Di Chiro G, McCullough DC et al (1988) Fixed spinal cord: diagnosis with MR imaging. Radiology 169:773-778

50. Hudgins RJ, Gilreath CL (2004) Tethered spinal cord following repair of myelomeningocele. Neurosurg Focus 16:E7

51. Rabb CH, McComb JG, Raffel C, Kennedy JG (1992) Spinal arachnoid cysts in the pediatric age group: an association with neural tube defects. J Neurosurg 77:369-372

52. Jean WC, Keene CD, Haines SJ (1998) Cervical arachnoid cysts after craniocervical decompression for Chiari II malformations: report of three cases. Neurosurgery 43:941-944; discussion 944-945

53. Mazzola CA, Albright AL, Sutton LN et al (2002) Dermoid inclusion cysts and early spinal cord tethering after fetal surgery for myelomeningocele. N Engl J Med 347:256-259

54. Nelson MD Jr, Bracchi M, Naidich TP, McLone DG (1988) The natural history of repaired myelomeningocele. Radiographics 8:695-706

55. Dias MS (2005) Neurosurgical causes of scoliosis in patients with myelom-eningocele: an evidence-based literature review. J Neurosurg 103 (1 Suppl):24-35

56. Westcott MA, Dynes MC, Remer EM et al (1992) Congenital and acquired orthopedic abnormalities in patients with myelomeningocele. Radiographics 12:1155-1173

57. Guille JT, Sarwark JF, Sherk HH, Kumar SJ (2006) Congenital and developmental deformities of the spine in children with myelomeningocele. J Am Acad Orthop Surg 14:294-302

58. Harwood-Nash DC, Fitz CR (1976) Neuroradiology in infants and children. CV Mosby Company, Saint Louis

59. Shimode M, Kojima T, Sowa K (2002) Spinal wedge osteotomy by a single posterior approach for correction of severe and rigid kyphosis or kyphoscoliosis. Spine 15:2260-2267

60. Naidich TP, Pudlowski RM, Naidich JB et al (1980) Computed tomographic signs of the Chiari II malformation. Part I: Skull and dural partitions. Radiology 134:65-71

61. Naidich TP, McLone DG, Fulling KH (1983) The Chiari II malformation: Part IV. The hindbrain deformity. Neuroradiology 25:179-197

62. Naidich TP, Pudlowski RM, Naidich JB (1980) Computed tomographic signs of Chiari II malformation. II: Midbrain and cerebellum. Radiology 134:391-398

63. Naidich TP, Pudlowski RM, Naidich JB (1980) Computed tomographic signs of the Chiari II malformation. III: Ventricles and cisterns. Radiology 134:657-663

64. Peach B (1965) Arnold-Chiari malformation. Anatomic features of 20 cases. Arch Neurol 12:613-621

65. Harding BN, Copp AJ (2002) Malformations. In: Graham DI, Lantos PL (eds) Greenfield's neuropathology, 7th edn. Arnold, London, New-York, New-Delhi

66. Breningstall GN, Marker SM, Tubman DE (1992) Hydrosyringomyelia and diastematomyelia detected by MRI in myelomeningocele. Pediatr Neurol 8:267-271
67. Jaeger HJ, Schmitz-Stolbrink A, Mathias KD (1997) Cervical diastematomyelia and syringohydromyelia in a myelomeningocele patient. Eur Radiol 7:477-479
68. Iskandar BJ, McLaughlin C, Oakes WJ (2000) Split cord malformations in myelomeningocele patients. Br J Neurosurg 14:200-203
69. Emery JL, Lendon RG (1973) The local cord lesion in neurospinal dysraphism (meningomyelocele). J Pathol 110:83-96
70. Campbell LR, Dayton DH, Sohal GS (1986) Neural tube defects: a review of human and animal studies on the etiology of neural tube defects. Teratology 34:171-187
71. Rokos J (1975) Pathogenesis of diastematomyelia and spina bifida. J Pathol 117:155-161
72. Kumar R, Bansal KK, Chhabra DK (2002) Occurrence of split cord malformation in meningomyelocele: complex spina bifida. Pediatr Neurosurg 36:119-127
73. McLone DG, Knepper PA (1989) The cause of Chiari II malformation: a unified theory. Pediatr Neurosci 15:1-12
74. Daniel PM, Strich SJ (1958) Some observations on the congenital deformity of the central nervous system known as the Arnold-Chiari malformation. J Neuropathol Exp Neurol 17:255-266
75. Blaauw G (1970) The dural sinuses and the veins in the midline of the brain in myelomeningocele. Dev Med Child Neurol Suppl 22:12-27
76. Emery JL, MacKenzie N (1973) Medullo-cervical dislocation deformity (Chiari II deformity) related to neurospinal dysraphism (meningomyelocele). Brain 96:155-162
77. Emery JL (1974) Deformity of the aqueduct of sylvius in children with hydrocephalus and myelomeningocele. Dev Med Child Neurol 16:40-48
78. Variend S (1974) Proceedings: deformity of the lateral cerebellar lobes in children with meningomyelocele. Arch Dis Child 49:495-496
79. Variend S, Emery JL (1974) The pathology of the central lobes of the cerebellum in children with myelomeningocele. Dev Med Child Neurol 16 (Suppl 32):99-106
80. Variend S, Emery JL (1976) Cervical dislocation of the cerebellum in children with meningomyelocele. Teratology 13:281-290
81. Variend S, Emery JL (1979) The superior surface lesion of the cerebellum in children with myelomeningocele. Z Kinderchir Grenzgeb 28:228-235
82. Gilbert JN, Jones KL, Rorke LB et al (1986) Central nervous system anomalies associated with meningomyelocele, hydrocephalus, and the Arnold-Chiari malformation: reappraisal of theories regarding the pathogenesis of posterior neural tube closure defects. Neurosurgery 18:559-564
83. Zimmerman RD, Breckbill D, Dennis MW, Davis DO (1979) Cranial CT findings in patients with meningomyelocele. AJR Am J Roentgenol 132:623-629
84. Wolpert SM, Anderson M, Scott RM et al (1987) Chiari II malformation: MR imaging evaluation. AJR Am J Roentgenol 149:1033-1042
85. El Gammal T, Mark EK, Brooks BS (1988) MR imaging of Chiari II malformation. AJR Am J Roentgenol 150:163-170
86. Salman MS, Blaser SE, Sharpe JA, Dennis M (2006) Cerebellar vermis morphology in children with spina bifida and Chiari type II malformation. Childs Nerv Syst 22:385-393
87. Masters CL (1978) Pathogenesis of the Arnold-Chiari malformation: the significance of hydrocephalus and aqueduct stenosis. J Neuropathol Exp Neurol 37:56-74
88. Yamada H, Nakamura S, Tanaka Y et al (1982) Ventriculography and cisternography with water-soluble contrast media in infants with myelomeningocele. Radiology 143:75-83
89. Marlin AE (2004) Management of hydrocephalus in the patient with myelomeningocele: an argument against third ventriculostomy. Neurosurg Focus 16:E4
90. Miller E, Widjaja E, Blaser S, Raybaud C. Supratentorial MR findings in Chiari II malformation (in preparation)
91. Raybaud C, Girard N (2005) Malformations of the telencephalic commissures. Callosal agenesis and related disorders. In: Tortori-Donati P (ed) Pediatric neuroradiology. Springer, Berlin Heidelberg
92. Hori A, Stan AC (2004) Supracallosal longitudinal fiber bundle: heterotopic cingulum, dorsal fornix or Probst bundle? Neuropathology 24:56-59
93. Hori A, Stan AC (2004) Letter to the editor: heterotopic cingulum. Neuropathology 24:266
94. Vachha B, Adams RC, Rollins NK (2006) Limbic tract anomalies in pediatric myelomeningocele and Chiari II malformation: anatomic correlation with memory and learning – Initial investigation. Radiology 240:194-206
95. Hankin MH, Silver J (1988) Development of intersecting CNS fiber tarcts: the corpus callosum and its perforating fiber pathway. J Comp Neurol 272:177-190
96. Shu T, Shen WB, Richards LJ (2001) Development of the perforating pathway: an ipsilateral projecting pathway between the medial septum/diagonal band of Broca and the cingulated cortex that intersects the corpus callosum. J Comp Neurol 436:411-422
97. Muller J (1983) Congenital malformation of the brain. The clinical neuroscience, vol 3. Churchill, New York
98. Nowoslawska E, Polis L, Kaniewska D et al (2004) Influence of neuroendoscopic third ventriculoscopy on the size of ventricles in chronic hydrocephalus. J Child Neurol 19:579-585
99. Batnitzky S, Hall PV, Lindseth RE, Wellman HN (1976) Meningomyelocele and syringohydromyelia. Some radiological aspects. Radiology 120:351-357
100. Samuelsson L, Bergström K, Thuomas KA et al (1987) MR imaging of syringomyelia and Chiari malformations in myelomeningocele patients with scoliosis. AJNR Am J Neuroradiol 8:539-546

CHAPTER 10
Myelomeningocele Primary Repair Surgical Technique

Massimo Caldarelli, Concezio Di Rocco

Introduction

A clear understanding of the pathologic anatomy of the spinal malformation is a fundamental prerequisite of the pre-operative work-up in spina bifida patients [1]. The malformed spinal cord or primitive neural plaque (placode) presents as a flat tongue of neural tissue with its borders merging into the contiguous malformed meningeal coverings. As an effect of the failed neurulation process, both ventral and dorsal spinal roots exit from the ventral aspect of the placode, the dorsal roots exiting laterally to the ventral ones, and corresponding to the boundary between the placode and the arachnoid membrane (junctional zone). The presence of an intact subarachnoid space ventral to the placode confirms the lesion as a myelomeningocele (MMC) (Fig. 10.1), whereas its absence confirms it to be a myelocele, which more closely resembles the deranged anatomy of failed neurulation (Fig. 10.2).

The residual function of the placode has been much debated [2]. Spontaneous movements are present in many myelodysplastic newborns, as well as in response to intraoperative electrical stimulation of the placode [3]. Likewise, somatosensory evoked potentials can be elicited within the placode by means of peripheral nerve stimulation. Cortical evoked responses can be recorded after placode electrical stimulation [2]. Furthermore, even in the absence of cortical control, the placode may still maintain intact local spinal reflexes that may contribute to bowel and bladder function [4]. All of the above considerations make it plausible that some residual functional neural elements are still present in the placode; these con-

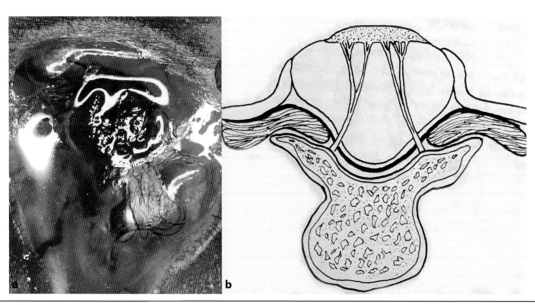

Fig. 10.1 a, b. Clinical appearance of a lumbar myelomeningocele (**a**) and schematic drawing (**b**) of the malformation, demonstrating the relationship of the placode with the subarachnoid space and cutaneous layers, and the exit and course of the spinal roots within the malformed sac

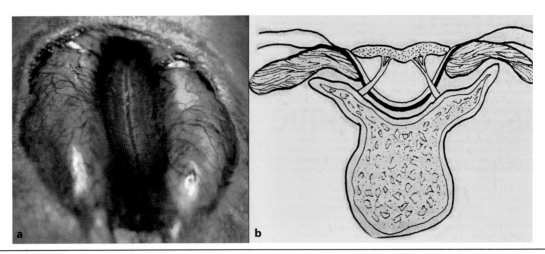

Fig. 10.2 a, b. Clinical appearance of a lumbar myelocele (**a**) and schematic drawing (**b**) of the malformation, demonstrating its relationship with the surrounding meningeal and cutaneous layers

sequently deserve special attention and care. From a practical point of view the placode must be handled with care to minimize the risk of harming that residual functional nervous tissue, and be protected from dehydration by covering it with a gauze dressing soaked in a sterile saline solution. The application of a plastic wrap over the gauze will help to keep the placode adequately moistened [5, 6]. The usefulness of systemic antibiotic therapy to prevent cerebrospinal fluid (CSF) infection is debated; conversely, local antibiotics or iodine-containing medications are to be avoided for their potentially adverse effect on the placode [5, 6].

Timing of Surgery

MMC repair should be performed soon after birth provided that the newborn's general condition is good and signs of meningeal infection are absent. According to the literature the operation is usually performed within the first 48 hours of life [2, 5-9]. Such delay, whilst not deleterious for neurological function nor for increasing the risk of CSF infection, allows the neurosurgeon to obtain more comprehensive information on the child's clinical condition (including thorough neuroradiological investigation), and for the parents to become better acquainted with the problems related to the malformation in order to give adequately informed surgical consent [10, 11]. Surgery should not be delayed beyond 72 hours of life, as it has been demonstrated that after this time there is a 37% risk of ventriculitis, compared to only 7% when operated upon

in a more timely fashion [5, 9]. A delay in surgical repair also exposes the myelodysplastic newborn to the risk of deterioration in neurological and bladder function [12].

At present, surgical repair is generally performed at an early stage. Since MMC is detected prenatally in up to 90% of cases, the spina bifida team has usually already been alerted prior to birth, and the parents usually sufficiently informed of the various clinical and surgical aspects of the spinal malformation, as to make their consent to surgery readily available soon after birth [2, 5-8, 11]. Due to prenatal diagnosis and counseling, the birth of a child affected by MMC is a planned event in the vast majority of cases (Fig. 10.3). There is still enduring debate as to the best means to deliver a child with myelomeningocele, namely, whether a cesarean section reduces the risk of neurological dysfunction [13-15]. Without addressing specific obstetric issues, these children are usually delivered at term, or slightly before term, after reaching pulmonary maturity, by means of a planned pre-labor cesarean section [11, 12, 15]. As the team responsible for the initial care of the myelodysplastic newborn (neonatal intensivist, anesthesiologist, neurosurgeon) has already been mobilized prior to delivery, the time interval to surgical repair is presently much shorter than previously necessary. At our institution, cesarean section is the modality of choice to deliver a fetus with a prenatal diagnosis of open spinal dysraphism, even in cases theoretically amenable to vaginal delivery [16]. Consequently, when a fetus with MMC reaches term, a cesarean section is planned to be performed early in the morning in order to have the

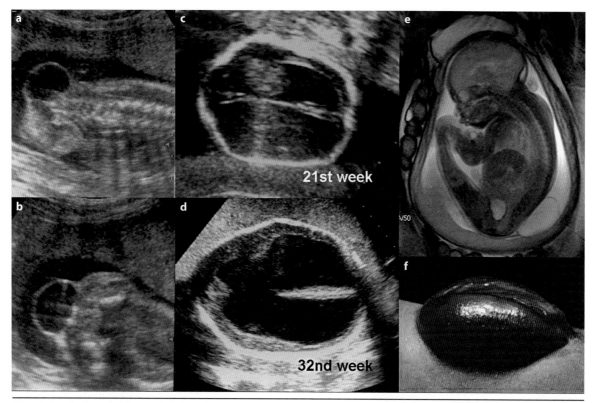

Fig. 10.3 a-f. Prenatal diagnosis of myelomeningocele. **a, b** Ultrasound demonstration of the spinal defect (AP and lateral views) **c, d** and evolution of the ventriculomegaly from the 21st to the 32nd gestational week. **e** T2-weighted fetal MRI demonstrating the spinal malformation; note the absence of ventricular dilatation at this stage. **f** Clinical appearance of the malformation at birth

newborn ready for neurosurgical closure early in the afternoon, as long as the newborn's general condition does not require further investigation. Under such circumstances the spinal defect is repaired within the first 6-12 hours of life, i.e., much earlier than as described in the literature.

On the other hand there are still cases, fortunately increasingly rare, of children affected by MMC who are delivered without a prenatal diagnosis and who are consequently sent to a tertiary hospital only hours or days after birth. In these circumstances, mobilizing the team, acquiring all clinical data as well as giving the parents adequate information and obtaining their consent to the operation, may require more time.

Whenever the operation is delayed beyond 72 hours of life, either due to delayed parental consent or to delayed referral from a peripheral hospital, it seems appropriate to obtain CSF cultures prior to undergoing surgical repair. When these are positive the newborn should be treated with antibiotic therapy and definitive closure delayed until the infection is cleared.

Early Management of Hydrocephalus

Hydrocephalus is so frequently associated with MMC (85-90%) as to be considered part of the malformation. As largely debated in the literature, many factors may contribute to its occurrence, namely aqueduct stenosis, fourth ventricle outlet obstruction, and obliteration of the posterior fossa subarachnoid spaces or their obstruction at the tentorial notch (Fig. 10.4) [17, 18]. It is this great variety of pathogenesis that accounts for the different modalities of clinical presentation and their different ages of onset. In fact, in less than 15% of the cases hydrocephalus is already overt at birth, manifesting with the classical signs of raised intracranial pressure (ICP) (split sutures, tense anterior fontanel, sunsetting eyes, vomiting, etc.) or even with the life-threatening signs of brainstem dysfunction (poor feeding; poor sucking and swallowing; nasal regurgitation; repeated coughing; weak or high-pitched cry; stridor; apneic spells; pneumonia, etc.), secondary to the impaction of neural

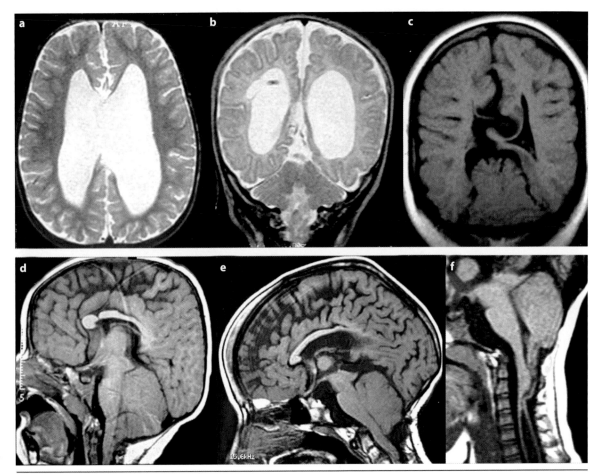

Fig. 10.4 a-f. Radiological features of hydrocephalus associated with myelomeningocele. **a** T2-weighted axial and **b** T2-weighted coronal views demonstrate a huge ventricular dilatation with disproportionately enlarged occipital horns. **c** Post-operative T1-weighted coronal view shows the reduction in ventricular volume and the abnormal shape of the midline cerebral cortex. **d-f** T1-weighted sagittal images demonstrate the small posterior fossa and the descent of the cerebellar tonsils and inferior vermis into the spinal canal, as well as the upward herniation of the superior vermis associated with other typical aspects of the Chiari II malformation (beaking of the tectum; thinned and malformed corpus callosum; large massa intermedia; stenogyric appearance of the occipital cortex; etc). **f** Note also the associated hydromyelia

structures within the small posterior fossa (due to the Chiari II malformation). This particular subset of myelodysplastic newborns with significant hydrocephalus warrants early surgical treatment [2, 7].

Among the presently available surgical modalities for treating hydrocephalus, ventriculo-peritoneal (VP) shunting remains the treatment of choice. Standard VP shunting not only ensures immediate relief of intracranial hypertension but is also beneficial to spinal wound healing by avoiding CSF pooling and leakage at the site of surgical repair [2, 5, 7, 8]. There has been some debate in the literature as to the best site for positioning the ventricular catheter, i.e., frontal or occipital. Authors almost equally suggest either frontal [19] or occipital [20, 21] positioning as associated with a lower percentage of mechani-

cal shunt malfunctions. We utilize the occipital route almost exclusively. The main reason for our choice is the asymmetrical ventricular dilatation, with disproportionally large occipital horns and relatively small frontal horns, which is typical of the hydrocephalus associated with MMC. This asymmetrical enlargement also minimizes the risk of the ventricular catheter coming in contact with and becoming occluded by the choroid plexus. Furthermore, tunneling of the shunt system to the parietal region is easier and the maneuver requires fewer skin incisions than placing the ventricular catheter frontally.

There is no general agreement as to the most appropriate timing of the two surgical procedures (MMC repair and VP shunt), should they need to be performed at the same stage. The question is obviously limited to the small percentage of myelodysplastic newborns that require immediate treatment of the associated hydrocephalus; in fact, in the vast majority (more than 85% of cases) treatment of hydrocephalus is usually postponed for weeks to months following MMC repair. When the hydrocephalus requires urgent treatment, many reports in the literature underline the advantages of unifying MMC repair and VP shunting at the same procedure [22-24]. Usually the newborn undergoes insertion of the VP shunt first, and then MMC repair. The advantages derived from combining the two operations are the rapid relief of intracranial hypertension and its beneficial effect on spinal wound healing. One study indicates that there is no significant difference in the infection rate between patients undergoing the two operations at the same stage or separately, provided that they are performed within the first 48 hours of life [25]. We too have adopted that policy on occasions; however, in our experience the association of MMC repair and CSF shunting in the same surgical procedure has been marked by a higher incidence of infectious shunt complications, compared to the cases where the two operations were performed separately [26]. This result has caused us to be more cautious and frankly reluctant to combine the two procedures. In addition, the problem seems overestimated as, in our experience, cases of hydrocephalus requiring such immediate treatment are quite rare. Given that most of the observed infectious complications in our patients were demonstrated to be due to a preexisting CSF sub-clinical infection, in the limited number of patients with significant hydrocephalus requiring prompt neurosurgical treatment, we have adopted the policy of performing temporary external ventricular drainage contemporaneously to MMC repair. In patients where CSF infection is confirmed, the same route can also be utilized to administer intraventricular antibiotics until resolution of the infection. In conclusion, our present position is to no longer treat hydrocephalus and spinal dysraphism at the same stage, but rather to perform MMC repair first as an independent procedure. As soon as clinical signs of intracranial hypertension occur, or if there is local pooling of CSF at the site of the spinal wound, we proceed to VP shunting. In our experience, postponing VP shunting in this manner neither increases the risk of infection nor alters the final neurological outcome.

Recent reports in the literature have proposed endoscopic third ventriculostomy (ETV) as an alternative to VP shunting in children affected by MMC [27-29]. However, these same reports, whilst indicating a relatively high success rate in cases of "secondary" ETV (i.e., in those myelodysplastic children presenting with VP shunt malfunction), underline a poor success rate in cases of "primary" ETV. Furthermore, the young age of the patient, which is typically a contraindication to ETV, acts as a further adverse factor in myelodysplastic newborns [27, 29]. The only report dealing with a significantly high population of myelodysplastic patients reflects the same considerations, i.e., only 29% success in cases of "primary" ETV and 12.5% success rate in children less than 6 months old [27]. We perform ETV in myelodysplastic children as either a primary or secondary procedure. Our preliminary results [30] have been more positive than those previously reported in the literature, with a significantly higher success rate of "primary" ETV in myelodysplastic newborns. However, further investigation is warranted.

Myelomeningocele Repair

Aims of the surgical treatment of MMC are: (1) to remove the malformed sac; (2) to prevent central nervous system infection by creating a barrier between the spinal canal and the exterior; and (3) to restore the normal CSF environment around the malformed spinal cord, thus preserving its residual motor and sensory functions. These results may be obtained by means of reconstruction of the placode, and multilayer closure of the meningeal, fascial, subcutaneous and skin layers; in other words, surgical repair should complete the interrupted neurulation process [2, 6, 7, 31, 32].

Contemporary surgery of MMC requires magnification (both operative microscope and loupes); with optional laser and intraoperative electrical stimulation [31, 32]. Utilization of the operative microscope enables the neurosurgeon to perform the surgery in a safer way than previously possible, especially during neural structure manipulation. Such technical tools have allowed neurosurgeons to obtain better functional results as demonstrated by the frequent observation of postoperative neurological improvement [6].

As myelodysplastic children are prone to develop latex allergy it is appropriate when planning the surgical repair to utilize a latex-free setting, if such a dedicated facility is already available in the hospital, or to prepare a similar surgical environment by sterilizing the operating room with regard to latex proteins and by utilizing only latex-free products [33].

Anesthesia and Positioning of the Patient

Although local anesthesia associated with mild sedation has been utilized in the past, at present the operation is performed only under general anesthesia with orotracheal intubation [34]. During pre-operative anesthetic procedures (positioning of venous and arterial lines, bladder catheterization, orotracheal intubation) the newborn is positioned supine over a gauze or jelly donut to protect the spinal malformation. After completing the anesthetic work-up, the newborn is positioned prone on firm chest rolls to allow optimal thoracic expansion; pads are positioned on all pressure points to avoid pressure sores. We usually place the newborn in an inverted position, with his/her back in front of the operator. A mild Trendelenburg position is suggested to avoid CSF escape from the spinal canal and the risk of pneumocephalus. During these procedures the body temperature must be strictly regulated, to avoid the deleterious effects of hypothermia.

Skin Preparation and Draping

An adequate amount of the skin surface around the spinal defect is bordered with plastic wraps, proportional to the diameter of the malformation and to the amount of skin to be presumably mobilized to optimize skin closure. Such initial definition of the surgical field reduces the surface to be prepared and consequently reduces heat loss. It also assures a separation of the anal and perineal regions from the surgical field, thereby minimizing the risk of infectious complications. Subsequently the skin is cleansed with Povidone iodine solution, paying particular attention to avoid any contact with the placode. After completing the skin preparation, the placode is simply cleaned with saline or Ringer's solution.

The operative field is subsequently covered in the usual fashion with an adhesive plastic drape in which a central hole corresponding to the inner part of the malformation has been fashioned and then bordered with drapes, again paying attention to leave an adequate amount of skin around the malformation (Fig. 10.5) [35].

Planning the Surgical Procedure

As with any other surgical procedure, MMC repair should be accurately planned, with the specific characteristics of the affected child taken into consideration. Inspection of the spinal malformation allows the appreciation of the site, extension and characteristics of the lesion, as well detection of any associated spine deformity that may influence surgical management [2, 6-8]. For example, kyphosis that is present at birth in about 15% of the affected chil-

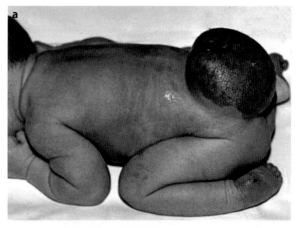

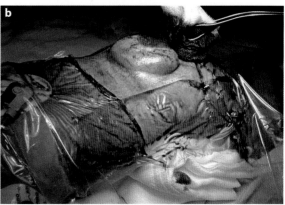

Fig. 10.5 a, b. Newborn infant with a large lumbar myelomeningocele. **a** Patient positioning for surgical correction. Definition of the surgical field by means of adhesive drapes and skin preparation with respect to the placode

dren may prevent, although very rarely, perfect closure of the spinal malformation and thus require correction at the same time as the MMC repair [36]. Similarly, severe kyphoscoliosis associated with significant asymmetry of the lower limbs suggests an associated split cord malformation that may alter the surgical strategy [37, 38].

A further fundamental aspect of pre-operative neurosurgical evaluation is appreciation of the quality and amount of the skin available for reconstruction. In fact, skin closure may be, on some occasions, the most difficult aspect of the surgical procedure. For example, in large lumbosacral myeloceles where the skin defect is significant, and the subcutaneous tissue scarce, reconstruction of the superficial layers is almost impossible, and plastic surgical reconstruction becomes necessary. On the other hand, a large lumbar MMC with redundant skin covering the defect poses no problem, but the excess tissue needs to be removed. In these cases it is advisable to delay the sacrifice of the redundant skin until all the other cutaneous layers are closed.

Apart from these considerations, a perfect knowledge of the pathologic anatomy of the spinal malformation is mandatory in order to correctly manipulate the placode during dissection and reconstruction (Figs. 10.1 and 10.2) [1]. It is known that the placode retraces the primitive neural plaque, with its edges continuing into the contiguous arachnoidal and dural coverings (junctional zone). As an effect of the failed neurulation, both ventral and dorsal spinal nerve roots exit from the ventral aspect of the placode (the dorsal roots exiting laterally to the ventral ones), at the border between the placode and the adjacent arachnoid layer. It is important to recognize this region in order to avoid injury to the nerve roots during the initial dissection.

Skin Incision

A limited midline linear skin incision is performed at the upper limit of the malformation, over the spinous processes of the first two normal vertebrae rostral to the spinal defect. Thereafter the incision is brought along the border between the dystrophic skin and the arachnoid that surrounds the malformation (Fig. 10.6), and circumferentially until the entire placode (with its incomplete arachnoid margin) is completely freed; thus saving all available skin so that it can be utilized for the final reconstruction of the superficial layers. Finally a further midline linear incision is performed at the lower extremity of the spinal defect. These two supplementary vertical incisions help to identify the normal elements rostral and caudal to the malformation. Identification of nor-

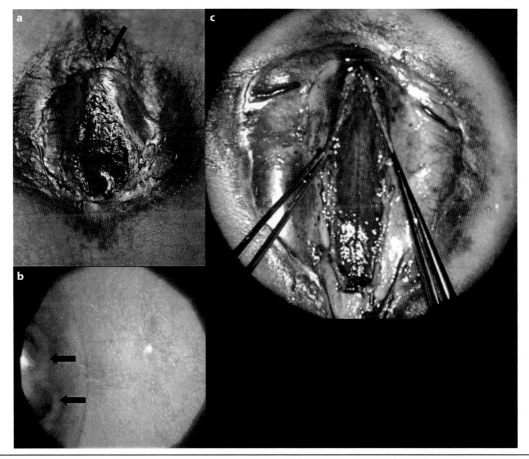

Fig. 10.6 a-c. Initial steps in the surgical repair of the myelomeningocele (under microscope magnification). **a** The placode with its arachnoid membrane is circumferentially connected to the cutaneous layers; the arrow indicates the site of the initial incision. **b** Under further magnification the site of the initial incision is indicated (*arrows*) at the edge of the arachnoid membrane (junctional zone). **c** After completing placode dissection, the margins of the malformation can be approximated in the midline

mal dura rostral to the malformation is fundamental for the safe dissection of neural structures. The scalpel is preferred to the Colorado needle for the skin incision. The latter, which is so helpful in minimizing blood loss in many surgical procedures, should be avoided as it may necrotize the already dystrophic skin margins, thus interfering with the healing process.

Placode Dissection

After completing the skin incision, the placode is dissected free from the surrounding arachnoid remnants along the junctional zone under microscope (or loupe) magnification [6, 32, 39, 40]. Dissection usually begins at the upper limit of the malformation, where the placode fuses with the normal spinal cord, and proceeds circumferentially along its borders. As already underlined, the dorsal root entry zone is immediately adjacent to the border of the spinal malformation. This relationship places them at risk of inadvertent injury; and care must be taken when manipulating the border of the placode. Any dystrophic arachnoid remnants should be meticulously removed, utilizing wherever possible sharp dissection, as they may contribute to late tethering of the spinal cord [2, 5, 7, 41-43]. Likewise, the accurate removal of any epidermal or dermal remnants is extremely important since they are potentially responsible for delayed dermoid/epidermoid cyst formation [40, 41, 44]. These maneuvers are best performed with microdissectors and microscissors, which allow more delicate manipulation of the neural structures (Fig. 10.6). Bipolar coagulation should be as limited as much as possible during this step of the surgical repair.

After completing the circumferential dissection, the filum terminale is usually identified beneath the most caudal portion of the placode. Section of the filum terminale (whenever clearly identifiable) is an integral part of the procedure as doing so minimizes the risk of secondary tethering [2, 5, 7, 8, 31, 40-42]. Notably, there are other anatomical variants that favor late tethering of the spinal cord, namely anomalies in the shape and length of the spinal roots, which cannot be surgically corrected [43].

Inspection of the inner aspect of the open dural sac often reveals the presence of aberrant nerve roots that terminate in the dural sac; these neural elements are devoid of any functional activity and can be divided without the risk of harming the neurological status of the child.

Frequently, relatively large vessels are encountered that enter the ventral aspect of the placode. These vessels must be manipulated carefully and dissected free from arachnoid adhesions in order to optimize their mobilization during the following phase of placode "tubulization". It is essential that any injury or coagulation of these vessels is avoided as their thrombosis may interfere with placode vascularization and viability, thus resulting in further neurological damage [40, 41]. As indicated above, coagulation should be avoided; and as such, hemostasis should preferably be obtained by local application of Spongostan or Flo-seal.

Before proceeding with the following steps, an accurate inspection of the intradural space should rule out any other associated malformations such as lipomas or dermoids that also deserve surgical treatment.

Neural Tube Reconstruction

Once dissection has been completed, the placode will lie at the bottom of the widely open dural sac, continuing rostrally with the intact spinal cord, and with the spinal roots emerging ventrally to it. The following step of surgical repair is represented, whenever possible, by an attempt to "reconstruct" the spinal cord. To this end the lateral edges of the placode are approximated in the midline, and their pia-arachnoid borders are sutured under microscope magnification, with a 7.0 non-absorbable monofilament (Fig. 10.7) [6, 31, 32]. This maneuver will transform the malformed placode into a structure resembling the primitive neural tube, completely invested by normal leptomeningeal coverings, thus completing the failed neurulation process. Care should be taken during this phase to avoid any compression to the neural structures originating from an excessively tight closure. Should the placode be too bulky to allow its "tubulization", it is advisable to abandon this part of the surgical procedure. We are aware that placode reconstruction is potentially devoid of any beneficial effect on the child's neurological outcome; nevertheless, it usually facilitates dural closure and minimizes the arachnoid scar by reducing the area of dorsal adhesion. It is widely accepted, and it is also our experience that pia-arachnoid suture significantly reduces the occurrence of symptomatic late tethering [6, 10, 31, 40, 43].

Unfortunately, too large a placode or too flat a spinal canal may risk compression of the reconstructed spinal cord at the time of dural closure. In these cases utilization of a dural patch for dural repair will usually resolve the problem.

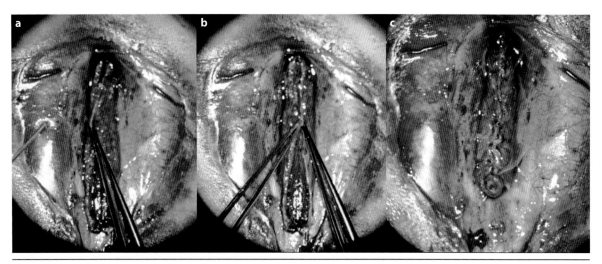

Fig. 10.7 a-c. Surgical repair of myelomeningocele: closure of the placode. **a, b** Under microscope magnification the placode has been detached from the surrounding arachnoid and cutaneous layers, and its margins approximated in the midline to allow **c** a pial-to-pial suture of its dorsal aspect with a 7.0 monofilament

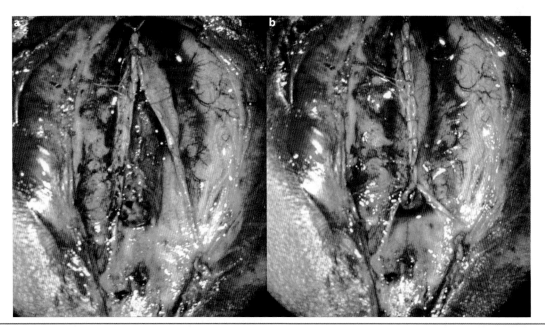

Fig. 10.8 a, b. Surgical repair of myelomeningocele: dural closure. **a** Two dural sheets have been sharply separated from the underlying lumbar fascia under microscope magnification, and approximated in the midline. **b** The dural edges are being sutured on the midline paying attention to avoid tension on the underlying neural structures

Dural Dissection and Closure

The following step of surgical repair consists of reconstruction of the dural sac. The intact meningeal coverings must first be identified at the upper extremity of the malformation, just beneath the first normal vertebra, where the malformed dura continues into the normal dural sac. Starting from this point the dural layer is dissected circumferentially along the borders of the defect, proceeding centripetally from the periphery to the midline (Fig. 10.8a). Although preferable, sharp dissection alone does not always enable the development of a dural layer. Isolation of the dura is more difficult at the edges of the defect where the dura fuses with the thoracolumbar fascia. Dissection, therefore, should start close to the midline where a true epidural space is already present and the small amount of epidural fat facilitates dissection in the correct plane. We recommend using a scalpel for the initial circumferential incision, and subsequent sharp dissection for completing the development of the bilateral dural flaps utilized for dural sac reconstruction.

The newly developed dural sheets are then approximated on the midline and sutured with either 5.0 silk suture or monofilament (Fig. 10.8b). Occasionally dural flaps may be so large as to permit a double layer suture. Continuous suture is generally preferable as it assures better impermeability of the reconstructed dural sac; occasionally interrupted sutures may be used when the size of the meningeal flap is insufficient.

As in the previous surgical step, dural closure should avoid any compression to the underlying neural structures. In fact, too tight a dural closure may compromise the blood supply to the reconstructed placode and facilitate its adhesion from its dorsal aspect to the dural envelope, representing the basis for secondary re-tethering. To avoid this potential complication, a dural patch should be used when the dural sheets appear insufficient.

Dural patching may be performed using various dural substitutes, the most physiologic being autologous tissues, such as muscle and fascia. In this case a sufficient amount of thoracolumbar fascia is dissected over the child's back and separated from the underlying muscles by sharp dissection. The newly developed fascial flap is then interposed between the insufficient dural sheets and sutured to cover the dural defect. The patient's anatomy may not allow for such autologous grafting, thus making it necessary to utilize allografts such as cadaveric dura or bovine pericardium [45]. Unfortunately, these substitutes share the same adverse effect, i.e., the development of arachnoiditis resulting in late tethering. Synthetic materials such as silicone have similar adverse effects. A recent innovation is the new dural substitute composed only of colloidal collagen (TissuDura), which acts as a non-porous biomatrix for dural regeneration by triggering the formation of new extracellular collagen and rapid fibroblast migration. One of the most positive aspects of this material is the limited host inflammatory response [46, 47]. We have been using TissuDura over the last 3 years and have found that the patch ensures adequate dural closure and protection against CSF leak [48].

Dural closure should be water-tight to avoid postoperative CSF leak or even CSF pooling at the surgical site, which retards healing of the spinal wound

[49] and exposes the newborn to the risk of infectious complications. To verify water-tightness a Valsalva maneuver should be performed after completing the dural suture. The presence of even a minimal CSF leak warrants further sutures or the use of dural glues.

Dural closure should be reinforced, whenever possible, by suturing the thoracolumbar fascia over the reconstructed dural sac. To this end the fascial borders are approximated and sutured over the midline defect, with the aid where necessary of lateral relaxing incisions (Fig. 10.9). Frequently this is not possible due to the width of the spinal defect; in this case, two fascial flaps are dissected from the underlying thoracolumbar muscles in the same fashion as for the dural flap, starting from the posterior iliac crest (or even more medially if less amount of tissue is needed). Of note, the sacral attachment of the fascia should not be incised [31]. Occasionally these fascial flaps can be integrated with periosteal flaps by dissecting the periosteum from the lumbar pedicles and transverse processes [50]. These fascial flaps are then approximated and sutured in the midline to protect the neural structures.

Subcutaneous Dissection and Skin Closure

The following step of MMC repair is the development of the subcutaneous layer and skin closure. Dissection of the superficial layers from the fascial plane is performed by simply undermining the skin (often solely utilizing digital dissection) all around the just closed spinal defect. Attention must be paid to avoid excessive coagulation of perforator vessels to the skin that may compromise the blood supply of the cuta-

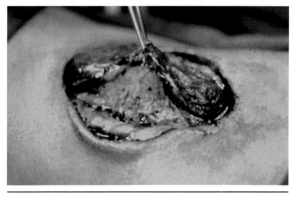

Fig. 10.9. Surgical repair of myelomeningocele: dissection and suture of the fascia. Two fascial flaps have been dissected and approximated in the midline to provide further protection to the dural suture

neous coverings [51-53]. The subcutaneous layer is usually minimal at the border of the malformation, becoming thicker beneath the junctional zone. For this reason, we place subcutaneous sutures at this level, to approximate the suture margins without excessive tension. Alternatively, in children with very large defects, sutures are placed 2-3 cm away from the skin edge and anchored to the underlying fascia with the same result of approximating the suture margins while reducing tension at the suture site. These "stay sutures" facilitate subsequent skin closure. The interposition of an adequate subcutaneous layer beneath the superficial skin layers is very important to reduce the incidence of unpleasant and potentially deleterious retracting scars. Initially, following closure, the skin may be blanched as a sign of tension. Such initial discoloration usually improves rapidly and wound dehiscence rarely occurs. A nitroglycerine ointment has been suggested to be helpful in some cases [54].

While perfect approximation of suture edges is always possible in cases of well-epithelized MMC with redundant skin, this is not the case when the surgeon is faced with large flat myeloceles with deficient cutaneous layers that will require a more complex plastic surgery reconstruction.

Once the subcutaneous layer has been reconstructed, the skin margins are debrided and closed in the habitual fashion with the non-absorbable sutures generally preferred when there is residual skin tension. Skin closure should be performed in a midline vertical fashion, where possible, with skin edges having little or no tension (Fig. 10.10). Occasionally a horizontal or oblique suture may be needed.

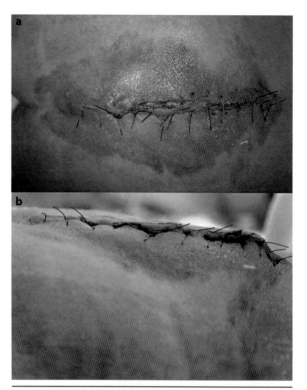

Fig. 10.10 a, b. Surgical repair of myelomeningocele: skin suture. The skin has been undermined circumferentially, approximated in the midline and sutured in a linear fashion

Myocutaneous and Cutaneous Flaps

As already mentioned, the skin defect and adverse patient anatomy may prohibit skin closure in the usual fashion [55]. The kind of skin closure performed is determined by the width of the spinal defect, with one study suggesting that an area of skin deficit larger than 20-25 square centimeters is an indication for plastic surgical reconstruction [56]. In such cases, a variety of cutaneous and myocutaneous flaps have been designed to ensure adequate protection to the neural structures. They are discussed in Chapter 15.

Tissue expansion has been proposed to enable sufficient skin harvesting for MMC closure [57, 58], particularly in cases of delayed referral and closure. This has less applicability to newborns with MMC [59].

The various modifications of both cutaneous and myocutaneous flaps that can be found in the litera-

ture suggest that an ideal solution to the problem of skin coverage in MMC surgery is still lacking. Moreover, there is no general agreement on the true necessity for these sophisticated techniques. In general, neurosurgeons tend to perform direct skin closure, whereas pediatric surgeons are more prone to utilize plastic/reconstructive techniques. Some experienced pediatric neurosurgeons [31] refute the necessity for plastic/reconstructive techniques even in large defects. Our personal experience is in favor of this point of view, as only two out of more than 600 cases operated over a 30-year period required plastic surgery.

Postoperative Course

After completing skin closure, the wound is cleansed again and covered with sterile gauze. The anus and perineal area are kept separated from the wound dressing by the interposition of an adhesive plastic drape that limits the contact of the wound with urine or fecal material. The newborn is usually observed in the neonatal ICU for the first 1-2 postoperative days, for apnea and/or any other sign of brainstem dysfunction. The child is maintained prone with the lower back slightly elevated above the level of the head to reduce the risk of CSF leak from the wound. Should CSF pool beneath the wound or leak through the suture, immediate management of hydrocephalus should be undertaken. Prophylactic intravenous antibiotics are given either for the first 24 hours postoperatively or for a longer time (in our experience 5 days or more if there is significant risk of infection). The wound dressing is changed every 48 hours, or anytime it is soiled. If non-absorbable sutures have been used we remove these on the tenth postoperative day, a little later than is usual for other neurosurgical procedures.

Operative mortality is practically absent while morbidity may be significant [41, 42]. The most frequent complication is wound breakdown usually secondary to CSF leak, which is known to be an adverse factor for wound healing [49]. Conversely, wound infection is a much rarer complication of MMC repair, occurring in less than 2% of procedures [42]. It is managed by changing wound dressing and intravenous antibiotics. The most severe, though rare, complication of MMC surgery is meningitis with sepsis, which remains the main cause of death in these newborn children. Intravenous antibiotics are the treatment of choice, and ultimately CSF shunt removal if already implanted.

References

1. Amacher L (1978) The microsurgical anatomy of lumbar rachischisis. Adv Ophthalmol 37. Karger, Basel, pp 197-202
2. Dias MS (1999) Myelomeningocele. In: Choux M, Di Rocco C, Hockley AD, Walker ML (eds) Pediatric neurosurgery. Churchill Livingstone, London, pp 33-59
3. Reigel DH, Dallmann DE, Scarff TB, Woodford J (1976) Intra-operative evoked potential studies of newborn infants with myelomeningocele. Dev Med Child Neurol 37(suppl):42-49
4. McGlaughlin TP, Banta JV, Gahm NH, Raycroft JF (1986) Intraspinal rhizotomy and distal cordectomy in patients with myelomeningocele. J Bone Joint Surg 68A:88-94
5. McLone DG (1998) Care of the neonate with a myelomeningocele. Neurosurg Clin North Am 9:111-120
6. McLone DG (2005) Spinal dysraphism: impact of technique and technology on expectations. Clin Neurosurg 52:261-264
7. Park T (1999) Myelomeningocele. In: Albright L, Pollack I, Adelson D (eds) Principles and practice of pediatric neurosurgery. Thieme, New York, pp 291-320
8. Cohen AR, Robinson S (2001) Early management of myelomeningocele. In: McLone DG (ed) Pediatric neurosurgery. Saunders, Philadelphia, pp 241-258
9. Charney E, Walker S, Sutton L et al (1985) Management of the newborn with myelomeningocele. Time for a decision-making process. Pediatrics 75:58-64
10. McLone DG (1983) Results of treatment of children born with a myelomeningocele. Clin Neurosurg 30:407-412
11. Shurtleff D, Lemire R (1995) Epidemiology, etiologic factors, and prenatal diagnosis of open spinal dysraphism. Neurosurg Clin North Am 6:183-193
12. Tarcan T, Onol FF, Ilker Y et al (2006) The timing of primary neurosurgical repair significantly affects neurogenic bladder prognosis in children with myelomeningocele. J Urol 176(3):1161-1165
13. Luthy DA, Wardinsky T, Shurtleff DB (1991) Cesarean section before the onset of labor and subsequent motor function in infants with meningomyelocele diagnosed antenatally. N Engl J Med 324:662-666
14. Cochrane D, Aronyk K, Sawatzky B et al (1991) The effects of labor and delivery on spinal cord function and ambulation in patients with meningomyelocele. Childs Nerv Syst 7:312-315
15. Merrill DC, Goodwin P, Burson JM et al (1998) The optimal route of delivery for fetal meningomyelocele. Am J Obstet Gynecol 179:235-240
16. Masini L, De Santis M, Noia G et al (2002) Spina bifida: prenatal diagnosis ultrasonographic diagnosis and long-term follow-up in 127 cases. Ultrasound Obstet Gynecol 20 (suppl):17
17. Di Rocco C, Caldarelli M, Ceddia A, Rende M (1989) Hydrocephalus and Chiari malformation. In: Gjerris F, Borgesen SE, Sorensen PS (eds) Outflow of cerebrospinal fluid. Munksgaard, Copenhagen, pp 106-118
18. Dias MS, McLone DG (1993) Hydrocephalus in the child with dysraphism. Neurosurg Clin N Am 4:715-726
19. Albright AL, Haines SJ, Taylor FH (1988) Function of parietal and frontal shunts in childhood hydrocephalus. J Neurosurg 69:883-886
20. Bierbrauer KS, Storrs BB, McLone DG et al (1990-91) A prospective, randomized study of shunt function and infections as a function of shunt placement. Pediatr Neurosurg 16:287-291
21. Sainte-Rose C, Piatt JH, Renier D et al (1991-92) Mechanical complications in shunts. Pediatr Neurosurg 17:2-9
22. Chadduck W, Reding D (1988) Experience with simultaneous ventriculoperitoneal shunt placement and myelomeningocele repair. J Pediatr Surg 23:913-916
23. Parent AD, McMillan T (1995) Contemporaneous shunting with repair of myelomeningocele. Pediatr Neurosurg 22:132-135
24. Miller PD, Pollack IF, Pang D, Albright AL (1996) Comparison of simultaneous versus delayed ventriculoperitoneal shunt insertion in children undergoing myelomeningocele repair. J Child Neurol 11:370-372

25. Gamache F (1995) Treatment of hydrocephalus in patients with meningomyelocele or encephalocele. A recent series. Childs Nerv Syst 11:487-488

26. Caldarelli M, Di Rocco C, La Marca F (1996) Shunt complications in the first postoperative year in children with meningomyelocele. Childs Nerv Syst 12:748-754

27. Teo C, Jones R (1996) Management of hydrocephalus by endoscopic third ventriculostomy in patients with myelomeningocele. Pediatr Neurosurg 25:57-63

28. Fritsch MJ, Mehdorn HM (2003) Indication and controversies for endoscopic third ventriculostomy in children. Childs Nerv Syst 19:706-707

29. Walker DG, Coyne TJ, Kahler RJ, Tomlinson FH (2003) Failure of endoscopic third ventriculostomy in myelomeningocele patients: preoperative clinical and radiological features. Childs Nerv Syst 19:707-708

30. Tamburrini G, Caldarelli M, Massimi L et al (2004) Primary and secondary endoscopic third ventriculostomy in children with hydrocephalus and myelomeningocele. Childs Nerv Syst 20:666

31. Reigel DH, McLone DG (1987) Myelomeningocele: Operative treatment and results. Karger, Basel

32. McLone DG (1990) Technique for closure of myelomeningocele. Childs Nerv Syst 6:66-73

33. Rendeli C, Nucera E, Ausili E et al (2006) Latex sensitisation and allergy in children with myelomeningocele. Childs Nerv Syst 22:28-32

34. Conran AM, Kahana M (1998) Anesthetic considerations in neonatal neurosurgical patients. Neurosurg Clin N Am 9:181-185

35. Haddad FS (1997) Draping an infant for repair of meningomyelocele. Surg Neurol 48:530

36. Reigel DH (1979) Kyphectomy and myelomeningocele repair. Modern techniques in surgery. Neurosurgery 13:1-9

37. Iskander BJ, McLaughlin C, Oakes WJ (2000) Split cord malformations in myelomeningocele patients. Br J Neurosurg 14:200-203

38. Kumar R, Bansal KK, Chhabra DK (2002) Occurrence of split cord malformation in meningomyelocele: complex spina bifida. Pediatr Neurosurg 36:119-127

39. Venes JL (1985) Surgical considerations in the initial repair of meningomyelocele and the introduction of a technical modification. Neurosurgery 17:111-113

40. McCullough DC, Johnson DL (1994) Myelomeningocele repair: technical considerations and complications. 1988. Pediatr Neurosurg 21:83-90

41. McLone DG, Dias MS (1991-92) Complications of myelomeningocele closure. Pediatr Neurosurg 17:267-273

42. Pang D (1995) Surgical complications of open spinal dysraphism. Neurosurg Clin North Am 6:243-257

43. Caldarelli M, Di Rocco C, Colosimo C Jr et al (1995) Surgical treatment of late neurological deterioration in children with myelodysplasia. Acta Neurochir (Wien) 137:199-206

44. Scott RM, Wolpert SM, Bartoshesky LE et al (1986) Dermoid tumors occurring at the site of previous myelomeningocele repair. J Neurosurg 65:779-783

45. Park TS, Delashaw JB, Broaddus WC, Vollmer DG (1985-86) Lyophilized cadaver dura mater for primary repair of myelomeningoceles. Pediatr Neurosci 12:315-319

46. Laquerriere A, Yun J, Tiollier J et al (1993) Experimental evaluation of bilayered human collagen as a dural substitute. J Neurosurg 78:487-491

47. Knopp U, Christmann F, Reusche E, Sepehrnia A (2005) A new collagen biomatrix of equine origin versus a cadaveric dura graft for the repair of dural defects – a comparative animal experimental study. Acta Neurochir (Wien) 147:877-887

48. Pettorini B, Tamburrini G, Massimi L et al (2006) The use of a collagen foil dura mater substitute in pediatric neurosurgical procedures. Childs Nerv Syst 22:1044-1045

49. Babuccu O, Kalayci M, Peksoy I et al (2004) Effect of cerebrospinal fluid leakage on wound healing in flap surgery: histological evaluation. Pediatr Neurosurg 40:101-106

50. Fiala TG, Buchman SR, Muraszko KM (1996) Use of lumbar periosteal turnover flaps in myelomeningocele closure. Neurosurgery 39:522-525

51. Lanigan MW (1993) Surgical repair of myelomeningocele. Ann Plast Surg 31:514-521

52. Lehrman A, Owen MP (1984) Surgical repair of large meningomyeloceles. Ann Plast Surg 12:501-507

53. Perry VL, Albright AL, Adelson PD (2002) Operative nuances of myelomeningocele closure. Neurosurgery 51:719-723

54. Lehman RA, Page RB, Saggers GC, Manders EK (1985) Technical note: the use of nitroglycerin ointment after precarious neurosurgical wound closure. Neurosurgery 16:701-702

55. Ozveren MF, Erol FS, Topsakal C et al (2002) The significance of the percentage of the defect size in spina bifida cystica in determination of the surgical technique. Childs Nerv Syst 18:614-620

56. de Chalain TM, Cohen SR, Burstein FD et al (1995) Decision making in primary surgical repair of myelomeningocele. Ann Plast Surg 35:272-278

57. Mowatt DJ, Thomson DN, Dunaway DJ (2005) Tissue expansion for the delayed closure of large myelomeningoceles. J Neurosurg 103 (suppl 6):544-548

58. Arnell K (2006) Primary and secondary tissue expansion gives high quality skin and subcutaneous coverage in children with a large myelomeningocele and kyphosis. Acta Neurochir (Wien) 148:293-297

59. Ersahin Y, Yurtseven T (2004) Delayed repair of large myelomeningoceles. Childs Nerv Syst 20:427-429

CHAPTER 11
Anesthesiology of the Newborn with Spina Bifida

Nigar Baykan

Introduction

Neural tube malformations involving the spinal cord and vertebral arches are referred to as spina bifida and present as a spectrum of malformations with protrusion of the spinal cord and/or meninges through a defect in the vertebral arch at the most severe end. Neural tube defects do not appear to be associated with other congenital syndromes; however, cardiac and renal anomalies which may not be apparent at birth may co-exist, prompting an in-depth assessment of these children. Additionally, children with spina bifida often have hydrocephalus and the Chiari type II malformation in association.

Since infection is the primary risk associated with myelomeningocele, most neurosurgeons repair the defect within the first days of life. The Chiari malformation, a developmental anomaly frequently associated with myelomeningocele, involves a downward displacement of the inferior cerebellar structures into the upper cervical spinal canal [1]. The accompanying elongation of the medulla and fourth ventricle causes obstructive hydrocephalus, which may require early ventriculostomy or the placement of a ventriculoperitoneal shunt [2]. Children with spina bifida will therefore be exposed to anesthetics in the first week of life and/or several times thereafter [3]. An understanding of newborn physiology, the pathophysiology and the interactions of anesthetic drugs being provided, along with full preparation for and anticipation of likely problems ensures the best possible outcome in the management of these children.

The most significant physiological transition in the newborn occurs in the first 24-72 hours after birth. All systems of the body are involved in this process; however, the most important to the anesthesiologist are the circulatory, pulmonary, hepatic and renal systems.

Circulatory Changes at Birth

Significant anatomic, physiologic and functional differences exist between the fetal and newborn circulations. The fetal circulation is characterized by high pulmonary and low systemic vascular resistance. In utero, most of the cardiac output is directed from the placenta across the foramen ovale into the ascending aorta, whereas superior vena cava blood is directed to both the pulmonary artery and the ductus arteriosus. At birth, clamping of the umbilical cord and aeration of the lungs produce enormous circulatory changes in the newborn. The transition of the alveoli from a fluid-filled to an air-filled state results in a reduced compression of the pulmonary alveolar capillaries, with a reduction in pulmonary vascular resistance and an increase in pulmonary blood flow. Increasing blood return to the heart via the pulmonary veins raises the pressure of the left atrium above that of the right, causing a functional closure of the foramen ovale. Both shunts (the ductus arteriosus and foramen ovale) usually close permanently in the first few months of life. During this critical period many factors (hypoxia, hypercarbia, and anesthesia-induced changes in peripheral vascular tone) can affect this precarious balance and result in a sudden return to the fetal circulation [4].

In the systemic circulation, the arterial pressure during the first days of life is about 70/45 mmHg. It rises gradually in the first week to approximately 90/50 mmHg. The ability of the infant to maintain its blood pressure in response to various circulatory stresses is therefore more difficult to assess than it is in older children and adults. The response to hemorrhage, for example, produces little increase in heart rate or change in total peripheral resistance since the neonatal baroreflex activity is impaired.

Transition of the Pulmonary System

The neonate has limited respiratory reserve. During the first 5-10 minutes of extrauterine life, normal ventilatory volumes develop and normal tidal ventilation is established. Ventilation is essentially diaphragmatic. Abdominal distention may cause splinting of the diaphragm leading to respiratory failure. It is important to remember that the tidal volume for a newborn in mL/kg is the same as it is in adults; however, the oxygen consumption is three times greater, resulting in alveolar ventilation that is also three times greater. Due to higher metabolic rate and alveolar minute volume in infants, volatile agents achieve a more rapid induction and emergence than they do in adults. The alveolar arterial oxygen tension gradient is greater in neonates than it is in adults, which reflects the fact that infants operate very near to closing volume during tidal breathing [5]. Alveolar minute volume is therefore rate dependent. The resting respiratory rate and oxygen consumption in neonates are approximately double than that in adults. Tidal volume and dead space have comparable adult values by the end of the first week of life.

Renal Considerations

Renal function is markedly diminished in neonates. Renal blood flow is reduced due to high renal vascular resistance. The neonatal renal tubules also have a decreased ability to absorb sodium, bicarbonate, glucose, amino acids, and phosphates [6]. All of these factors contribute to the potential for overhydration, dehydration, metabolic acidosis, and hyponatremia.

The Liver

At term, the functional maturity of the liver is somewhat incomplete. Metabolic enzyme systems have matured by the 12th week, but some drugs are metabolized more slowly and others are metabolized by enzyme pathways different from those in adults [7]. The action of barbiturates, benzodiazepines, and opioids in the neonate is therefore prolonged and enhanced.

The normal-term neonate in the fed state shows a decline in blood glucose from maternal levels to 50 mg/dL at 2 hours of age, rising to about 70 mg/dL by the third day of life. Carbohydrate reserves are low in neonates; hence the sick or stressed neonate is vulnerable to hypoglycemia. In the case of hypoglycemia, a glucose level below 36 mg/dL may lead to grave ischemic damage if left untreated [8].

Anesthetics can mask the symptoms and signs of hypoglycemia, such as irritability and seizures. Apnea due to hypoglycemia obviously does not occur in patients who are intubated and mechanically ventilated. The only signs of hypoglycemia may be changes in heart rate or blood pressure caused by sympathetic arousal or substrate depletion. The preferred method of administration of intravenous dextrose for neonates is 0.5-1.0 g/kg given as a 10% solution. 50% dextrose is not used in neonates because of its extremely high osmolality (about 2800 mOsm/L), which may cause significant local tissue damage.

Thermoregulation

The surface area of a normal child's head represents 18% of the total body surface area; double that of an adult. In general, children have a much larger surface area-to-weight ratio than adults, and also have much less subcutaneous fat. The vasoconstrictor response is limited and the minimal ability to shiver during the first three months of life makes cellular thermogenesis (i.e., metabolism of brown adipose tissue) the principal method of heat production.

General anesthetics depress the thermoregulatory response in children and adults; heat is lost from the core to the cooler peripheral tissues, particularly in non-shivering thermogenetic neonates [9]. This problem is compounded by cold operating rooms, wound exposure, cold intravenous fluid and blood administration, or dry anesthetic gases. Prolonged hypothermia can lead to a profound acidosis and impaired perfusion, which have been associated with delayed awakening from anesthesia, cardiac irritability, respiratory depression, increased pulmonary vascular resistance and altered drug responses.

Loss of heat during anesthesia and surgery can be prevented by several simple measures such as raising operating room temperature to 28-30°C, wrapping the extremities and head with cotton blankets, cloth and paper operating room drapes, and administering warm infusion solutions and blood. Inhaled anesthetic gases should also be heated and humidified.

Fluid Balance

In neonates, 80% of the total body weight is water. Neonatal insensible losses vary greatly due to factors such as radiant warmers, increased ambient temperature, fever and decreased humidity; as a consequence the turnover of water is more than double that of an adult. A small increase in loss or reduction in intake of fluid can rapidly lead to dehydration. Fluid maintenance, calculated from the calorie requirement, depends directly on metabolic demand: 100 mL water is required for each 100 calories of expended metabolism. Maintenance requirements for neonates can be determined using the 4-2-1 regime – 4 mL/kg/h for each of the first 10 kg, 2 mL/kg/h for the second 10 kg, and 1 mL/kg/h for each subsequent kg (Table 11.1) [10].

In addition to a maintenance infusion, any preoperative fluid deficits should be replaced. The deficit amount should be administrated with hourly maintenance in aliquots of 50% in the first hour, and 25% in the second and third hours. Third space losses are replenished according to the surgical procedures [11].

A balanced salt solution (e.g., lactated Ringer's and/or 5% dextrose in 0.45% normal saline) is usually the initial fluid of choice. In the first several days of life, 10% glucose solution can be used until glucose values are stabilized in newborns to prevent hypoglycemia. An infusion pump should be used to prevent overhydration and/or hyperglycemia. The neonate requires 3-5 mg/kg/min of glucose to maintain euglycemia.

Hematological Considerations

In general, blood volume is approximately 100-120 mL/kg for premature neonates, 90 mL/kg for full-term neonates and 80 mL/kg for infants. An initial hematocrit of 55% in the full-term neonate gradually falls to as low as 30% in the three month-old infant before rising up to 35% within six months. Hemoglobin type is also changing during this period.

The predominant hemoglobin type at term is HbF (80-90%) which falls to 10-15% and has been replaced by HbA.

Blood loss is extremely difficult to measure in the neonate and infant. The use of blood products in pediatric patients has diminished greatly. Hematocrit values, in the low 40% range within prematures and neonates, and within the 20% range in older children, are generally well-tolerated. Ideally, when these values are out of these ranges, blood transfusion is required; fresh blood must be supplied.

Factors for Anesthesiological Risk Evaluation

Neurosurgery in the neonatal period is usually performed to repair the myelomeningocele or encephalocele. Early surgery is indicated to close the defects where there is a flimsy dural sac, which can easily become damaged or infected, leading to meningitis. In routine practice, broad spectrum antibiotics must therefore be initiated within the first 24 hours of life and continued until surgery. Spina bifida children often have associated neurologic deficits, hydrocephalus and Chiari malformation and these and any other causes of increased intracranial pressure may result in bilateral vocal card paralysis. For the anesthesiologist, the major concerns in a child with a myelomeningocele are positioning for tracheal intubation, volume and electrolyte problems, and blood loss. Additionally, the anesthesiologist caring for a neonatal patient must be prepared for the unexpected. The neonate has unique requirements for equipment, intravenous access, fluid and drug therapy, anesthetic dosage, heat loss, and environmental control.

Preoperative Assessment

Preparing the neonatal patient for anesthesia begins with the history and physical examination. The preoperative evaluation includes attention to age, body weight, associated neurological and systematic problems, medication, neonatal history, and family history of adverse reactions to anesthetics and allergies.

The physical examination should focus upon airway anatomy, head size, dural sac, vital signs, hydration status, and coexisting disease. The spina bifida neonate needs a preoperative laboratory examination, which should include a recent hematocrit, glucose, and

Table 11.1. Maintenance fluid requirements for pediatric patients

Weight (kg)	Hourly Fluid (ml)
<10	4 ml/kg
11-20	40 ml+2 ml/kg >10
>20	60 ml+1 ml/kg >20

urine tests. It is essential that the blood samples are taken by qualified personnel. Excessive blood sampling will decrease the already low blood volume of the neonate. It is advised that all patients be cross-matched.

Preoperative hemoglobin less than 10 g/dL is abnormal and should be investigated. The physiological anemia of infancy varies between 10 to 12 g/dL. If blood transfusion is required, it has to be completed within the preoperative period. For patients without a history of prior blood transfusions, blood samples may be obtained when the intravenous line is inserted, if the laboratory is able to return the results in a timely manner [12].

Hydration status may be assessed by skin turgor, mucous membranes, fontanel fullness and urine output. If hypovolemia is diagnosed, it should be treated preoperatively.

Speaking to the parents directly and treating the child as the center of attention is very important since this will help the parents understand that your focus is on their child. The more information one can provide to the child and the family, particularly about monitoring and safety, the greater will be the reduction in anxiety [13].

Preoperative Fasting

Infants and young children have a higher metabolic rate and a larger body surface area to weight ratio than adults do; hence they become dehydrated more easily. With the avoidance of a prolonged fasting period there is less potential for intra-operative hypoglycemia. Several studies demonstrate that there is no difference in gastric residual volume or pH between standard fasting and shortened fasting periods [14-16]. Depending on age, regular formula feeding or solid foods are continued until 4-8 hours before surgery. Breast milk is cleared from the stomach more rapidly than formula milk in infants, and both have shorter transit times than solid food. Clear fluids are offered until 2-3 hours, breast or formula milk up to 4 hours before induction; while solid food requires a minimal 6 hours fasting (Table 11.2).

Table 11.2. Fasting guidelines for children

Age	Fasting Time	(Hours)
	Solids, milk, formula, breast milk	Clear Liquids
< 1 month	4	2
6-36 months	6	2-3
>36 months	6-8	2-3

Premedication

Neonates and infants under six months of age should not require preoperative sedative medication. The use of premedication in the older infant should be considered to facilitate smooth induction and to decrease agitation. Oral midazolam (0.5 mg/kg – max. dose 10 mg) can be very effective in these patients if intravenous access is not available prior to induction (Table 11.3).

Anticholinergic drugs can be used to decrease the likelihood of bradycardia during induction. Atropine (0.02 mg/kg oral or intramuscular) reduces the incidence of anesthetic-induced hypotension in children less than six months of age [4]. Atropine can also prevent accumulation of secretions.

Intravenous (IV) Line

Neonates often have good superficial veins on the hands or on the wrists. When choosing the location for catheter placement in a pediatric patient, one should consider the child's age, development, mobility, and hand dominance [17]. Factors such as good lighting, a competent anesthetist and assistant, and selection of correct catheter size and material make the insertion easier. An alternative to a peripheral site on the hand or wrist is the cephalic and median vein of the forearm and/or antecubital area. Veins of the lower extremity and external jugular vein are not preferred for the prone position. After successful cannulation, the catheter is stabilized and the extension set is attached to the catheter hub. Subsequently, the patency of the catheter should be rechecked after taping. Infusion pumps should be used to ensure an appropriate rate of flow of intravenous fluids.

A central venous catheter is not indicated in spina bifida surgery. When peripheral venous cannulation is not possible, a central venous catheter may be preferred over venous cut down. The femoral, internal jugular, external jugular, antecubital and subclavian veins are commonly used for central venous catheterization. Complications of central venous catheters such as bleeding, pneumothorax, thrombosis, infection, and perforation should also be taken into account.

Arterial catheterizations are not indicated in spina bifida, unlike Arnold-Chiari operations. However, if the neonate needs arterial blood gas examination and continuous monitoring of systematic arterial blood pressure, then an arterial catheter should be inserted. The most commonly used location is the radial artery, with other choices being the brachial dorsalis pedis, posterior tibial and femoral arteries.

Table 11.3. Pediatric drug dosage

Premedication			
Atropine	0.01-0.02 mg/kg	IV or IM	
Midazolam	0.5 mg/kg	oral administration	
Induction			
Thiopental	4-6 mg/kg		
– Neonates	2-4 mg/kg		
Propofol	2-3 mg/kg		
Muscle Relaxants			
Succinylcholine	1-2 mg/kg		
Atracurium	0.5 mg/kg		
Cis-atracurium	0.2-0.4 mg/kg		
Mivacurium	0.1-0.2 mg/kg		
Pancuronium	0.1 mg/kg		
Vecuronium	0.1 mg/kg		
Opioids			
Alfentanil	30-50 mcg/kg as slow bolus	0.5-1 mcg/kg/min infusion	
Fentanyl	1-3 mcg/kg bolus		
Remifentanil	1-2 mcg/kg bolus	0.1-2 mcg/kg/min infusion	
Morphine	0.05-0.1 mg/kg		
Reversl and Antagonists			
Glycopyrolate	10 mcg/kg		
Neostigmine	50 mc/kg		
Naloxone	5-10 mcg/kg	(IV incrementally)	
Flumazenil	10-20 mcg/kg	(repeat if necessary)	
Postop. Analgesia			
Codeine	0.5-1.0 mg/kg	IM, PO, PR	6 hourly
Meperidine	0.5 mg/kg	IV or IM	6 hourly
Acetaminophen	20-40 mg/kg	PR	6 hourly

Intubation

The airway of the infant and neonate is different than that of the teenager or adult. The neonatal head is proportionately larger than the adult one, with a shorter neck and smaller mandible. The tongue in neonates is relatively larger in size compared to the oropharynx. This may cause technical difficulties during laryngoscopy.

The larynx is located anterior and higher in the neck (C_3 in neonates, C_{3-4} in infants, C_{5-6} in adults). When straight blades are used, the laryngeal inlet may be more easily seen by raising the epiglottis.

Contrary to adults, the endotracheal tube in neonates usually passes easily through the vocal cords, but its passage may be blocked at the cricoid cartilage where the airway is the narrowest.

The head should be in a neutral position and the shoulders should be supported if necessary. Gentle cricoid pressure is often helpful. Tracheal intubation in the supine neonate with myelomeningocele ne-cessitates the use of padding, which will prevent contact of the myelomeningocele with the operating table.

If the dural sac is in the neck, intubation and laryngoscopy may be difficult in the supine position and alternatively, the lateral position may be used.

In neonates or infants with hydrocephalus and raised intracranial pressure, vomiting may cause cardio-respiratory compromise. The Chiari malformation may also be associated with bradycardia and stridor secondary to unilateral or bilateral vocal cord paresis. These children should therefore be carefully monitored during intubation.

Pediatric endotracheal tubes should be uncuffed until at least six years of age. A correctly sized tube allows adequate ventilation with a small audible leak of air present when positive pressure is applied at 20 cmH$_2$O [18].

Tracheal tube positioning must avoid endobronchial intubation resulting in overinflation of the lung, alveolar rupture and interstitial emphysema and/or hypoventilation with atelectasis. The length of the trachea in neonates and infants is short, leaving little margin for error. It is important to remember therefore that during head-neck extension and/or pre-positioning, the tracheal tube may come to lie in the subglottic region or the patient may be inadvertently extubated [19, 20].

Recently, a new cuffed pediatric tracheal tube with a high volume-low pressure cuff has been introduced [21]. This kind of cuffed pediatric tube appears to be useful to guarantee adequate tracheal tube placement with a cuff-free subglottic region of the tube shaft and a sufficient margin for preventing inadvertent endobronchial intubation, or tracheal extubation [22, 23].

Monitoring of Patients

Routine monitoring will include cardiac rate and rhythm by electrocardiogram (ECG), blood pressure (non-invasive and/or invasive), pulse oximetry, capnography, and full gas monitoring with a ventilatory alarm, esophageal stethoscope, nasopharyngeal or tympanic temperature and intermittent measurement of arterial blood gases, hematocrit, serum electrolytes, and osmolality and urinary output. Detection of venous air embolism is accomplished with the use of the precordial ultrasonic Doppler in the surgery of Chiari malformation.

Induction of Anesthesia

Induction of anesthesia is commonly performed by facemask. Most of the inhalational anesthetics currently used, including halothane, isoflurane, sevoflurane, and desflurane, have been successfully utilized in the maintenance of pediatric anesthesia, but not all children have the same susceptibility to each agent. The phase of induction is the most dangerous period since it is very easy to misjudge the depth of anesthesia and cause cardiac depression. Volatile agents depress myocardial contractibility and cause vasodilatation, reduce heart rate and depress the compensatory reflex mechanisms [24]. During induction by volatile anesthetics, it is vital to maintain the inspired concentration, which may rapidly rise up to critical levels, until an intravenous line is in place. Neonates and premature infants have lower anesthetic requirements than older infants and children. The minimal alveolar concentration (MAC) of volatile agents is lower in neonates and higher in children relative to adult values [25]. The neonate has an immature central nervous system with attenuated responses to nociceptive cutaneous stimuli.

Inhalational Anesthetics

Halothane has long been the mainstay of pediatric anesthesia. It is non-irritating to the airway, it has a relatively pleasant odor, and it is well-suited for inducing anesthesia via facemask.

Sevoflurane has many features of an ideal inhalational agent; its low blood-gas solubility and non-pungent smell suggest a smooth, uncomplicated and rapid induction and emergence from anesthesia [26]. Sevoflurane is associated with the emergence of delirium in the early recovery period [27, 47].

Sevoflurane is more stable hemodynamically than halothane, but bradycardia and apnea have both been reported at high concentrations [48, 49].

Desflurane and isoflurane are more pungent than halothane or sevoflorane and are associated with more coughing, breath holding, and laryngospasm during inhalational induction.

In view of the fact that inhalational anesthetics cause a decrease in heart rate and systolic blood pressure, atropine 0.02 mg/kg IV must be included at induction.

Intravenous Anesthetics

Intravenous induction of anesthesia is the most reliable and rapid technique if the patient is brought to the operating room with an intravenous line (Table 11.3). Thiopental is still in common use in pediatric practice. It is indicated for neonatal induction but at a reduced dose of 2 mg/kg in the first week of life.

Propofol is an intravenous drug useful for both induction of anesthesia as a bolus and for maintenance when administered as a continuous infusion for children over one month of age. Induction and recovery times are generally rapid, and the depth of anesthesia is readily titratable. Since hypotension occurred in 50% of the cases [50], it may be reasonable to provide intravenous fluid replacement of the calculated deficit in an effort to decrease the incidence of hypotension.

Remifentanil hydrochloride is a short-acting opioid, which is widely used in pediatric anesthesia [51-53]. It is known to cause bradycardia and hypotension [54]. It can be used continuously in neonates. The cardiovascular side-effects of remifentanil appear to be similar to those of other opioids (such as fentanyl and alfentanil), although the degree of bradycardia with remifentanil seems greater than that of the other opioids. The decrease in blood pressure induced by remifentanil in children during sevoflurane anesthesia was mainly due to a fall in cardiac index. Although atropine is able to reduce the fall in heart rate, it did not completely prevent the reduction in cardiac index [55].

Muscle Relaxants

Neuromuscular transmission is immature at birth but it reaches adult levels of maturity by two to three months of age (Table 11.3) [56].

Succinylcholine is characterized by rapid onset of muscle relaxation providing optimal conditions for intubation. It has received much attention, however, due to the severity of its possible complications and its routine use in pediatric patients is no longer recommended.

The choice of non-depolarizing muscle relaxant depends on the side effects and the duration of muscle relaxation required. Clinically, neonates and infants appear to be more sensitive to non-depolarizing muscle relaxants and their response varies to a greater degree [57].

The doses of long acting muscle relaxants used for neonates should be titrated carefully due to the extreme variability in response.

Neuromuscular blockade should be reversed in all neonates and infants, since any increase in the work of breathing may cause fatigue and respiratory failure.

Alternatively, propofol and remifentanil combinations could be used without a muscle relaxant to facilitate tracheal intubation in children [58-60].

Position

The patient should be positioned with the sac of the meningocele or occipital encephalocele in a 'doughnut' head ring, where the remainder of the baby is supported on a folded towel providing a neutral supine position for intubation without damaging the flimsy dural sac (Fig. 11.1).

The operations are carried out prone and great care must be taken with positioning; not only to produce a free abdomen for easy ventilation, but also to reduce blood loss by avoiding inferior vena cava compression and increased paraspinal venous pressure.

Careful positioning is paramount to avoid complications arising from poor positioning, including dislodging or kinking of the endotracheal tube, corneal abrasion or perioperative neuropathy.

Many types of padding materials are advocated to protect exposed body parts. They often consist of cotton, foam sponges, and gel pads. There are no data suggesting that any of these materials is more effective than any other, or that they are better than no padding at all (Fig. 11.2).

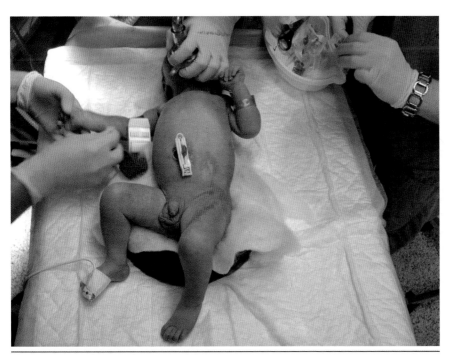

Fig. 11.1. Anesthesia induction position

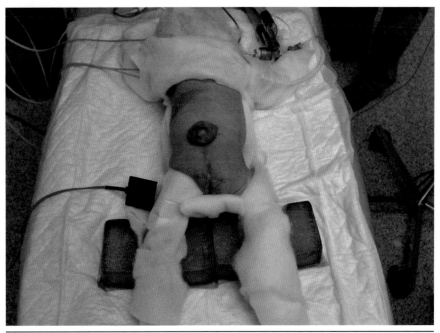

Fig. 11.2. Surgical position

Awakening

At the end of the surgery, the neonate should be warm, well-saturated, normocarbic, and pain-free. A cold acidotic neonate will not breathe post-operatively.

The criteria for extubation include intact cough and gag, a negative inspiratory force of 15-30 cmH$_2$O, a force vital capacity breath in excess of 10 mL/kg, an air leak around the tube with inflation pressures less than 25 cmH$_2$O as well as the maintenance of acceptable oxygenation and ventilation on minimal ventilatory support. Adequate reversal of neuromuscular blockade is demonstrated by either a sustained arm lift or leg lift. Extubation is performed only when the child is awake and breathing well.

The immediate complications after extubation include laryngospasm, bronchospasm and post-extubation croup. Post-extubation croup is associated with early childhood (1-4 years old), repeated intubation attempts, size of the endotracheal tube, duration of surgery, head and neck procedures, and excessive movement of tube (coughing with the tube in place, moving the patient's head, prone position). Symptoms include hoarseness, stridor, and a 'croupy' cough with or without inspiratory retraction. Treatment of post-extubation croup includes cool mist or humidified oxygen, racemic epinephrine and corticosteroids.

Apnea is a common post-operative problem in preterm neonates [61, 62]. It is significant if the episode exceeds 15 seconds or if cyanosis or bradycardia occur.

The anemic neonate (hemoglobin < 10 g/dL) is particularly at risk [63]. Caffeine given intravenously (10 mg/kg) has been recommended [64].

All babies under 46 weeks must be monitored with an apnea alarm.

Post-Operative Analgesia

The fear of side effects and addiction has limited the use of narcotic agents in neonates. Opiates including codeine phosphate are only given to babies over 5 kg during the surgery and post-operatively, due to respiratory depression and dose-related cardiovascular effects (Table 11.3) [65].

Acetaminophen is widely used in neonates and infants. The recommended loading dose of rectal acetaminofen is 20-40 mg/kg at the beginning of the surgical procedure [66].

Single injections of local anesthetics for infiltration in subcutaneous tissues and muscles surrounding the operative site provide adequate analgesia. For this purpose, 0.25% bupivacaine in the form of 2 mg/kg applications is recommended [67].

Latex Allergy

Spina bifida patients represent a group with the highest risk for latex sensitization and allergy with life-threatening symptoms, mostly during surgery [28-32].

From the initial surgical repair of the myelomeningocele, children with spina bifida are submitted to multiple surgeries due to neurological, orthopedic, and urological problems [33, 34].

The importance of an accurate and detailed patient history has been emphasized. It has been shown that atopic subjects are more likely to develop an allergy to latex. It is important therefore to obtain an accurate history from the spina bifida patient and their parents as to whether there has been any unusual, idiopathic, or perioperative allergic reactions in the past [35, 36]. Direct IgE mediation appears to be the pathogenesis of the anaphylactic response to latex. Although preoperative diagnosis of latex allergy with skin or radioallergosorbent (RAST) testing may be desirable, concern remains about sensitivity, specificity and safety of such testing [37-42].

Patients with a positive history of rubber allergy may be pre-treated before surgery with a protocol suggested for the prevention of anaphylactoid reactions (Table 11.4) [36]. Latex allergy in infants younger than one year-old is unusual, but given time and recurrent exposure, a significant number of these infants surely will experience the reaction [43, 44]. A latex-avoidance protocol should be established regularly in these patients, because even very young children with spina bifida might be sensitized to latex.

The prevalence of latex sensitization can be significantly reduced by using protocols for primary latex allergy prophylaxis during surgery, and even in the high-risk group of spina bifida patents in anesthesia and pediatric wards [32]. Sensitized patients continue to have severe life-threatening reactions despite pharmacologic prophylaxis as well as avoidance of latex products. Preoperative prophylaxis is recommended with corticosteroids (methylprednisolone) and antihistamines (diphenhydramine, cimetidine) the night before and morning of the surgery [28, 45, 46].

Onset of anaphylaxis is normally delayed by 20-60 minutes following exposure to the antigen and progressively worsens over 5-10 minutes. The reaction presents with hypotension, tachycardia, rash, increased peak airway pressures, and arterial desaturation. It may be difficult to exclude anaphylaxis from anesthetic drugs since it presents in a similar manner and is treated in the same way. Cardiopulmonary resuscitation is performed with the administration of epinephrine, fluids, steroids, histamine blockers, and in some cases the surgical procedure must be stopped. It should be considered that the doses of epinephrine recommended for resuscitation during cardiac arrest are not the same as those required for the treatment of anaphylaxis.

The surgery, nursing, and anesthesia teams must work closely together and communicate before bringing the patient into the operating room so that the entire staff is aware of avoiding exposure to latex, rather than trying to rigidly fit a program for the patient according to a prevention and treatment protocol. Coordination with the post-anesthesia care unit and nurses in charge should be carried out so that the patient care area is clearly marked and all personnel are familiar with the patient's intolerance to latex products.

Table 11.4. Latex-avoidance protocol. Reproduced from [36], with permission

- Use of non-latex gloves by surgical, anesthesia, and nursing personnel
- Avoidance of any known latex product in the sterile field by the surgeon
- Use of plastic anesthesia face mask for pre-oxygenation and positive-pressure ventilation
- Use of non-latex anesthetic reservoir bag for positive-pressure ventilation
- Use of non-latex tourniquet for intravenous catheter placement
- Use of non-latex blood pressure cuff/tubing, electrocardiogram leads, stethoscope
- Use of non-latex tape
- Intravenous injection via stopcock rather than rubber injection port

References

1. Northrup H, Volcik KA (2000) Spina bifida and other neural tube defects. Curr Probl Pediatr 30:312-332
2. Steinbok P, Irvine B, Cochrane DD, Irwin BJ (1992) Long-term outcome and complications of children born with myelomeningocele. Child Nerv Syst 8:92-96
3. Oakeshott P, Hunt GM (2003) Long-term outcome in open spina bifida. Br J General Practice 53:632-636
4. Cote CJ (2005) Pediatric anesthesia. In: Miller RD (ed) Miller's anesthesia, vol 60, 6th edn. Elsevier Churchill Livingstone, Philadelphia, pp 2367-2407
5. Hillier SC, Krishna G, Brasoveanu E (2004) Neonatal anesthesia. Seminars in Pediatric Surgery 13:142-151
6. Drukker A, Guignard JP (2002) Renal aspects of the term and preterm infant: A selective update. Curr Opin Pediatr 14:175-182

7. Gow PJ, Ghabrial H, Smallwood RA et al (2001) Neonatal hepatic drug elimination. Pharmacol Toxicol 88:3-15

8. Berry FA (1996) Neonatal anesthesia. In: Barash PG, Cullen BF, Stoelting RK (eds) Clin Anesthesia, vol 43, 3rd edn. Lippincott-Raven, Philadelphia, pp 1091-1114

9. Sessler DI (2005) Temperature monitoring. In: Miller RD (ed) Miller's anesthesia, vol 40, 6th edn. Elsevier Churchill Livingstone, Philadelphia, pp 1571-1597

10. Morgan GE, Mikhail MS, Murray MJ, Larson CP (2002) Pediatric anesthesia: Clin Anesthesiology, vol 44, 3th edn. McGraw-Hill, New York, pp 849-874

11. Rice HE, Caty MG, Glick PL (1998) Fluid therapy for pediatric surgical patient. Pediatr Clin North Am 45:719-727

12. Cote CJ, Zaslavsky A, Downes JJ et al (1995) Postoperative apnea in former preterm infants after inguinal herniorrhaphy. A combined analysis. Anesthesiology 82:809-822

13. Kain ZN, Caranico LA, Mayes LC et al (1998) Preoperative preparation programs in children: a comparative examination. Anesth Analg 87:1249-1255

14. Nicolson SC, Dorsey AT, Schreiner MS (1992) Shortened preanesthetic fasting interval in pediatric cardiac surgical patients. Anesth Analg 74:694-697

15. Fasting S, Soreide E, Raeder JC (1998) Changing preoperative fasting policies. Impact of a national consensus. Anaesthesiol Scand 42:1188-1191

16. Green CR, Pandit SK, Schork MA (1996) Preoperative fasting time: is the traditional policy changing? Results of a national survey. Anesth Analg 83:123-128

17. Webster PA, Salassi-Scotter MR (1997) Peripheral vascular access. In: Dieckmann RA, Fiser DH, Selbst SM (eds) Pediatric emergency and critical care procedures, vol 30. Mosby-Year Book, St Louis, pp 187-195

18. Motoyama EK (1990) Endotracheal intubation. In: Motoyama EK, Davis PJ (eds). Anesthesia for infants and children, 5th edn. Mosby Company, St Louis, pp 272-275

19. Hartrey RM, Kestin IG (1995) Movement of oral and nasal tracheal tubes as a result of changes in head and neck position. Anesthesia 50:682-687

20. Weiss M, Knirsch W, Kretschemer O et al (2006) Tracheal tube-tip displacement in children during head-neck movement – a radiological assessment. Br J Anaesth 96:486-491

21. Goel S, Lim SL (2003) The intubation depth marker: the confusion of the black line. Paediatr Anaesth 13:579-583

22. Weiss M, Gerber AC, Dullenkopf (2005) Appropriate placement of intubation depth marks in a new cuffed paediatric tracheal tube. Br J Anesth 94:80-87

23. Weiss M, Balmer C, Dullenkopf A et al (2005) Intubation depth markings allow an improved positioning of endotracheal tubes in children. Can J of Anesth 52:721-726

24. Lerman J, Burrows FA, Oyston JP et al (1990) The minimum alveolar concentration (MAC) and cardio-vascular effects of halothane isoflurane and sevoflurane in newborn swine. Anesthesiology 73:717-721

25. Taylor RH, Lerman J (1991) Minimum alveolar concentration of desflurane and hemodynamic responses in neonates, infants and children. Anesthesiology 75:975-979

26. Lerman J, Sikich N, Kleinman S, Yentis S (1994) The pharmacology of sevoflurane in adults and children. Anesthesiology 80:814-824

27. Walker SM, Haugen RD, Richards A (1997) A comparison of sevoflorane and halothane in paediatric day care surgery. Anest Intense Care 25:643-649

28. Setlock MA, Cotter TP, Rosner D (1993) Latex allergy: Failure of prophylaxis to prevent severe reaction. Anest Analg 76:650-652

29. Porri F, Pradal M, Lemiere C et al (1997) Association between latex sensitization and repeated latex exposure in children. Anesthesiology 86:599-602

30. Bowman RM, McLane DG, Grant JA et al (2001) Spina bifida outcome: a 25-year prospective. Pediatr Neurosurg 34:114-120

31. Degenhardt P, Golla S, Wahn F, Niggemann B (2001) Latex allergy in pediatric surgery is dependent on repeated operations in the first year of life. J Pediatr Surg 36:1535-1539

32. Cremer R, Diepenbruck UK, Hering F, Holschneider AM (2002) Reduction of latex sensitization in spina bifida patients by a primary prophylaxis programme (five years experience). Eur J Pediatr Surg 12:19-21

33. Cremer R, Hoppe A, Korsch E et al (1998) Natural rubber latex allergy: prevalence and risk factors in patients with spina bifida compared with atopic children and controls. Eur J Pediatr 157:13-16

34. Niggemann B, Kulig M, Bergmann R, Wahn U (1998) Development of latex allergy in children up to 5 years of age – a retrospective analysis of risk factors. Pediatr Allergy Immunal 9:36-39

35. Liebke C, Niggemann B, Wahn U (1996) Sensitivity and allergy to latex in atopic and non-atopic children. Pediatr Allergy Immunal 7:103-107

36. Birmingham PK, Dsida RM, Grayhack SS, Han J et al (1996) Do latex precautions in children with myelodysplasia reduce intraoperative allergic reactions? Journal of Pediatric Orthopaedics 16:799-802

37. Monaret-Vautrin DA, Laxenaire MC, Bavoux F (1990) Allergic shock to latex and ethylene oxide during surgery for spina bifida. Anesthesiology 73:556-558

38. Slater JE, Mostello LA (1991) Routine testing for latex allergy in patients with spina bifida is not recommended (letter). Anesthesiology 74:391

39. Ellsworth PJ, Merguerian PA, Klein RB, Rozycki AA (1993) Evaluation and risk factors of latex allergy in spina bifida patients: is it preventable? J Urol 150:691-693

40. Slater JE (1993) Latex allergy. Ann Allergy 70:1-2

41. Kelly KJ, Kurup VP, Reijula KE, Fink JN (1994) The diagnosis of natural rubber latex allergy. J Allergy Clin Immunol 93:813-816

42. Nieta A, Mazon A, Pamies R et al (2002) Efficacy of latex avoidance for primary prevention of latex sensitization in children with spina bifida. J Pediatr 140:370-372

43. Slater JE, Mostello LA, Shaer C (1991) Rubber-specific IgE in children with spina bifida. J Urol 146:578-579

44. Kimato H (2004) Latex allergy in infants younger than 1 year. Clin Exp Allergy 34:1910-1915

45. McKinstry LJ, Fenton WJ, Barrett P (1992) Anaesthesia and the patient with latex allergy. Can J Anaesth 39:587-589

46. Halzman RS (1993) Latex allergy: An emerging operating room problem. Anesth Analg 76:635-641

47. Moore JK, Moore EW, Elliott RA et al (2003) Propofol and halothane versus sevoflurane in paediatric day-case surgery: induction and recovery characteristics. Br J Anaesth 90:461-466

48. Holzman RS, Van der Velde ME, Kaus SJ et al (1996) Sevoflorane depresses myocardial contractility less than halothane during induction of anesthesia in children. Anesthesiology 85:1260-1267

49. Russel JA, Miller Hance WC, Gregory G et al (2001) The safety and efficacy of sevoflorane anesthesia in infants and children with congenital heart disease. Anesth Analg 92:1152-1158

50. Hertzag JH, Dalton HJ, Anderson BD et al (2000) Prospective evaluation of propofol anesthesia in the pediatric intensive care unit for elective oncology procedures in ambulatory and hospitalized children. Pediatrics 106:742-747

51. Wee LH, Moriarty A, Cranstan A, Bagshaw O (1999) Remifentanil infusion for major abdominal surgery in small infants. Paediatr Anaesth 9:415-418

52. Prys-Roberts C, Lerman J, Murat I et al (2000) Comparison of remifentanil versus regional anaesthesia in children anaesthetized with isoflurane / nitrous oxide. International remifentanil paediatric anaesthesia study group. Anaesthesia 55:870-876

53. Ross AK, Davis PJ, Dear GL et al (2001) Pharmacokinetics of remifentanil in anesthetized pediatric patients undergoing elective surgery or diagnostic procedures. Anest Analg 93:1393-1401

54. De Souza G, Lewis MC, Ter Riet MF (1997) Severe bradicardia after remifentanil. Anesthesiology 87:1019-1020

55. Chanavaz C, Tirel O, Wodey E et al (2004) Haemodynamic effects of remifentanil in children with and without intravenous atropine. An echocardiographic study. Br J Anaesth 94:74-79

56. Goudsouzian NG, Standaert FG (1986) The infant and the myoneural junction. Anesth Analg 65:1208-1217

57. Meakin GH (2001) Recent advances in myorelaxant therapy. Paediatr Anaesth 11:523-531

58. Klemola UM, Hiller A (2000) Tracheal intubation after induction of anesthesia in children with propofol-remifentanil or propofol-recuronium. Can J Anaesth 47:854-859

59. Batra YK, Alquattan AR, Ali SS et al (2004) Assessment of tracheal intubating conditions in children using remifentanil and propofol without muscle relaxant. Pediatric Anesthesia 14:452-456

60. Crawford MW, Hayes J, Tan JM (2005) Dose-response of remifentanil for tracheal intubation in infants. Anesth Analg 100:1599-1604

61. Kurth CD, LeBard SE (1991) Association of postoperative apnea, airway obstruction, and hypoxemia in former premature infants. Anesthesiology 75:22-26

62. Cote CJ, Zaslavsky A, Downes JJ et al (1995) Postoperative apnea in former preterm infants after inguinal herniorrhaphy. A combined analysis. Anesthesiology 82:809-822

63. Welborn LG, Hannallah RS, Luban NLC et al (1991) Anemia and postoperative apnea in former preterm infants. Anesthesiology 74:1003-1006

64. Welborn LG, Hannallah RS, Fink R et al (1989) High-dose caffeine suppresses postoperative apnea in former preterm infants. Anesthesiology 71:347-349

65. Callahan JM (1997) Pharmacologic Apends, vol 12. In: Dieckmann RA, Fiser DH, Selbst SM (eds) Pediatric emergency and critical care procedures. Mosby Year Book, St Louis, pp 53-67

66. Birmingham PK, Tobin MJ, Honthoin TK et al (1997) 24-hour pharmacokinetics of rectal acetaminophen in children: An old drug with new recommendations. Anesthesiology 87:244-252

67. Gunter JB (2002) Benefit and risks of local anesthetics in infants and children. Pediatr Drugs 4:649-672

CHAPTER 12
Postoperative Care of the Newborn with Myelomeningocele

Eren Özek, Roger F. Soll

Failure of the neural tube to close is potentially one of the most devastating and severely disabling congenital malformations of the newborn. Of these lesions, myelomeningocele (MMC) comprises 98.8% of open spinal dysraphism [1]. Myelomeningocele has been described as "the most complex treatable, congenital anomaly consistent with life" [2]. This squarely places the onus of successful treatment onto the multidisciplinary team of caregivers who will manage the diagnosis, repair, postoperative care and follow-up of children with MMC. Management of neonates with MMC is multifaceted. Various organ systems including the skeletal, muscular, urological, respiratory, skin and central nervous system are involved. This involvement of so many different organ systems results in interrelated problems requiring immediate and long-term consultation from a variety of different medical specialties. Compared with the treatment of older children, neurosurgical treatment of these neonates is extraordinarily complex. The neonate has limited pulmonary, cardiac, renal, nutritional and thermoregulatory reserves, is more susceptible to infection and has an altered metabolic response to operative stress [3].

Many families and caregivers are aware of the diagnosis of MMC prior to birth due to routine ultrasound and prenatal screening. Therefore case management can be planned prior to delivery. Although controversial, most studies support the delivery of infants with spina bifida by planned cesarean section, allowing a more careful delivery of the infant to protect the spinal cord from injury [4, 5].

Once an infant with a myelomeningocele is delivered, it is necessary to repair the defect within 24 to 48 hours in order to reduce the risk of infection [6]. When the infant arrives in the neonatal intensive care unit (NICU) after the operation, it is essential for the neonatologist and neurosurgeon to spend adequate time with the family relaying information about the operation, explaining the clinical condition of the infant, describing the care the infant will receive in intensive care, and addressing the parent's perceptions and expectations.

Immediate Postoperative Considerations

Much of postoperative care is a continuation of the care that began in the delivery room and follows the routine practices utilized for all critically ill newborns. Careful attention to these practices will lead to an optimal outcome.

Thermoregulation

Thermoregulation is of prime importance. This is true both before and after operative repair. Maintaining a normal core body temperature in the operating room is difficult. In the operating room, surfaces are uncovered to allow access to the surgical site and for monitoring. Evaporative heat loss can result from the open skin lesion and other exposed surfaces [7].

Infants with MMC often have decreased movement of the lower limbs limiting the potential to generate heat from muscle movement. Newborn infants rely on the chemical thermogenesis of brown fat metabolism for heat production [8]. Anesthesia may induce peripheral vasodilatation and inhibit brown fat thermogenesis. In particular, fentanyl has been shown to inhibit heat production in the liver and can cause hypothermia [9]. Hypothermia in the neonate in turn causes a rise in the metabolic rate due to brown fat breakdown with a threefold to fourfold increase in oxygen consumption. Metabolic breakdown products accumulate with the development of acidosis. Aggressive efforts must be made to prevent hypothermia in the operating room. After the operation, the infant should be kept under radiant warmer in the neonatal unit in a thermoneutral environment. The infant's head and extremities should be wrapped, all intravenous solutions (including blood and crystalloid solutions) warmed, and agents for inhalation warmed and humidified [7, 10].

Nursing Implications

Routine neonatal care is undertaken postoperatively. In cases with an uncomplicated postoperative course, feeding and handling by parents should be encouraged. However, the baby must be nursed prone in a way that minimizes soiling of the wound until the wound is well healed in 7-10 days [6]. Meticulous care is needed to keep stool off the wound. Careful hand hygiene is essential to avoid contaminating the wound with coliform bacteria. The infant should be observed for skin integrity over pressure points. Pressure on the suture lines should be avoided until wound healing is complete.

Dribbling of urine suggests the possibility of a neurogenic bladder. Strict measurement of intake and output is important as urinary retention is common and predisposes the infant to urinary tract infection. Intermittent catheterization for residual urine (every 4-6 hours) may be needed to assure bladder decompression [11]. In addition, infants with MMC are at risk for neurogenic bowel that can result in incontinence. Continuous soiling and anal excoriation is suggestive of a neurogenic bowel [12]. Perianal skin excoriation is prevented with meticulous skin care and frequent diaper changes. Emollient ointments may be effective in promoting perianal skin integrity [1].

Pain Management

Pain management is an important consideration in the postoperative period. In the first hours after surgery, the infant's expression of pain may be temporarily blunted. However, as the anesthetic agents used in surgery wear off, the infant may experience pain. The amount of pain an infant experiences depends on the type, extent and location of the incision and the amount of tissue injury involved. The severity of the surgical procedure may not always predict the intensity of pain after surgery [13]. Postoperative pain instruments for preverbal infants (Neonatal Infant Pain Scale, Modified Infant Pain Scale, etc.) can be employed for the assessment of observed pain and are essential for an appropriate approach to pain management [14]. Pain can result in a higher heart rate, a higher blood pressure, an increase in pulmonary vascular resistance, an increase

in intracranial pressure, and lower oxygen saturation. In infants with pain, catecholamine and cortisol levels rise dramatically and are abolished with appropriate analgesia [15].

In the postoperative period, systemic narcotics may be safely employed for pain relief. Narcotic treatment will blunt the physiologic effects of pain and stress [16]. Morphine and fentanyl are used most commonly. These drugs should be carefully dosed and the infant should be followed closely on a cardiorespiratory monitor. It has been shown that continuous infusion of fentanyl in postoperative neonates is associated with fewer episodes of apnea in comparison with bolus dosing of the same amount of fentanyl [17]. For patients with MMC, it is important to note that opioid analgesics can produce a decrease in intestinal peristalsis resulting in constipation and ileus. These drugs can also cause bladder spasm and urinary retention [16].

For moderate pain, acetaminophen is safe in full term and preterm neonates postoperatively and can be administered orally and rectally [18].

Postoperative Cardiorespiratory Monitoring

A neonate can be extubated at the end of the operative procedure if the infant is vigorous, well oxygenated, hemodynamically stable and normothermic. The infant should remain intubated and ventilated until stabilized. Airway obstruction from relaxation of soft tissues, laryngospasm, subglottic edema or secretions is an important postoperative hazard [7, 19]. In the postoperative period, apnea can occur as a result of a decreased respiratory drive from anesthesia and narcotic pain medications. Cardiorespiratory monitoring is essential during the immediate postanesthesia recovery period. Neonates are especially prone to respiratory and cardiovascular complications at this time [20].

Close monitoring for apnea, hypoxia, heart rate and blood pressure abnormalities should be done during the stay in NICU. Postoperatively, attention must be directed to the oxygen saturation of the infant. Hypoxia in the immediate postoperative period may be related to hypoventilation or transient diminution in functional residual capacity with ventilation perfusion imbalance [7, 21].

Hormonal and Metabolic Response to Stress

During surgery, neonates exhibit elevations in serum catecholamine levels as well as insulin and growth hormone resistance [7, 22]. Postoperatively, there may be prolonged hyperglycemia necessitating insulin administration. Serum lactate, pyruvate, free fatty acids, glycerol, ketone bodies and corticosteroids may be elevated. Full term babies are able to mount a response of increased insulin levels postoperatively in response to hyperglycemia [23]. Levels of cytokines are elevated due to metabolic, endocrine and immunologic response to injury. These inhibit visceral protein synthesis and divert the liver to produce acute phase reactants that have immunologic and repair functions [24].

Serum cortisol levels are increased in response to surgical stress. The hypercatabolic state is characterized by the breakdown of carbohydrates, proteins and fats. Given the limited nutritional reserves of neonates, this may be detrimental. Particularly in preterm babies, surgical stress can produce hyperglycemia and may lead to osmotic diuresis, dehydration and intraventricular hemorrhage [7]. Neonates undergoing surgery are predisposed to both hypoglycemia and hyperglycemia and, therefore, the serum glucose level must be carefully monitored. Hepatic glycogen stores are limited in newborns, especially if they are under stress or have low birth weight. Therefore glucose must be supplied to prevent hypoglycemia, which can result in apnea, bradycardia, hypotension, convulsions and brain damage [22].

Fluid and Electrolyte Management

Reliable vascular access should be achieved before beginning the operative procedure. Postoperatively, the position of the central venous line and the function of any peripheral line should be assessed on infants returning to the nursery.

In the newborn period the glomerular filtration rate is only 25% of that in adults and the infant's renal medulla has a relatively low concentration of urea [25]. Therefore, the neonatal kidney has a limited ability to concentrate the urine. Although this is of little consequence in infants receiving appropriate amounts of water, it can become clinically important in infants receiving high osmotic loads. Neonates are also less capable of excreting excess sodium. As a consequence, the kidneys cannot be relied on to correct for any significant error in fluid management [7, 26]. Before surgery it is essential that intravascular volume is restored. In addition to maintenance fluids, the postoperative neonate may require additional volume and sodium to compensate for the third space shifts of flu-

id secondary to the trauma of the operative procedure. In the postoperative period, the neonate cannot tolerate either hypovolemia or fluid overload [7, 25]. It is vital that the fluid status be reassessed at 8 to 12 hour intervals to allow for accurate replacement of fluid needs. Urine output should exceed 1.5-2 ml/kg/hr. Routine monitoring of the weight of the infant, blood pressure and electrolyte status are essential to appropriate fluid and electrolyte management [7]. The most common cause of hypotension or oliguria in the postoperative period is hypovolemia. This may not be associated with obvious clinical findings of dehydration. The neonate may even exhibit edema because of the third space accumulation of fluid. Postoperative hypovolemia must be promptly recognized and corrected. The maintenance fluids can be increased or a bolus of 10-20 ml/kg of isotonic fluid given [7, 27]. It is controversial whether there is also an inherent tendency for increased postoperative sodium and water retention [28].

Multisystem organ failure may occur in the neonate who undergoes major surgery [7]. Persistent capillary leakage may be the first sign of multisystem organ failure followed by renal, hepatic, hematologic, lung and myocardial failure. Unexplained weight gain and edema may be early warning signs of multisystem organ failure, and careful investigations should be initiated to detect the cause, such as infection [7, 29]. Hypocalcemia is potentiated by stress, hypothermia and infection, all of which occur in neonates undergoing surgery. Ionized calcium levels must be monitored and calcium administered as needed.

Nutrition

Adequate nutrition is key to postoperative recovery. Nutrition must be started as soon as possible after surgery. Enteral nutrition is usually preferred. The safety of initiating enteral feeds depends on several factors, including recovery of the gastrointestinal tract from anesthesia, hemodynamic and respiratory stability. Evidence that gastrointestinal function has returned includes diminished output from the nasogastric tube, resolution of abdominal distention, and passage of stool [7]. The overall energy expenditure of neonates may not increase after uncomplicated surgery. These infants are often sedated and exhibit limited activity in a thermoneutral environment [30].

Infants who are well, sucking and swallowing effectively may be breastfed like healthy infants. Infants with Chiari II malformation may have swallowing difficulties and are at risk of aspiration. Disorders of swallowing, caused by disordered lower cranial nerve or brainstem dysfunction, are the most common clinical manifestations and may include choking on liquids, nasal regurgitation during drinking, and frequent vomiting or significant gastroesophageal reflux [31]. A nasogastric tube can be inserted for gavage feeding. When gastric emptying is impaired and gastroesophageal reflux is a concern, a soft transpyloric feeding tube can be placed under radiographic guidance and small quantities of enteral feedings administered and increased as tolerated. A gastrostomy tube is useful if prolonged tube feeding is required. If significant reflux is identified, fundoplication is considered at the time of gastrostomy [32]. Management of the nutritional needs of these infants should be carried out in consultation with a nutritionist and gastroenterologist. Nutrition support helps to avert complications of aspiration, pneumonia, or sepsis, which can further complicate the deleterious effects of this disease.

Hemoglobin and Coagulation

Although there is limited data to support the practice, traditionally the hemoglobin levels of babies undergoing major surgery are kept above 10-13 g/dl for full term infants and 13 g/dl for preterm infants [33]. Neonates have limited capacity to compensate for low hemoglobin levels and they are unable to increase their stroke volumes. Fetal hemoglobin restricts oxygen extraction at tissue level. Indications for consideration of maintaining a higher hemoglobin level indicate critical illness, prematurity, hypoxia and undergoing an operative procedure in which significant blood loss is anticipated [7, 26].

There are no guidelines regarding the need for coagulation studies on newborns before surgery [7]. Coagulation studies such as platelet count, prothrombin time and partial thromboplastin time should be considered prior to surgery. Vitamin K is administered to all newborns to prevent hemolytic disease of the newborn. Despite having received vitamin K at birth, the coagulation activity of neonates may remain low for days. In particular, prematurity is associated with coagulation deficiencies [34]. Neonates can also develop thrombocytopenia with or without disseminated intravascular coagulation secondary to sepsis or perinatal asphyxia. Neonates who have received large volume of transfusions and those with abnormal coagulation studies are at risk of postoperative bleeding [35].

Infection

The open neural tube is continuous with the surface of the skin. For this reason, infants with open spinal dysraphism are at high risk for bacterial meningitis. Leak of cerebrospinal fluid is commonly observed. The major indication for early operative repair (within 24-48 hours) is the prevention of infection [6, 36].

In a previous study, only 1 of 73 infants (1%) receiving preoperative prophylactic broad-spectrum antibiotic therapy developed ventriculitis compared with 5 of 27 (19%) who did not receive antibiotics [37]. The use of prophylactic broad spectrum antibiotics (ampicillin and gentamicin) from the first 24 hours of life to the time of surgery is routinely practiced. Although perioperative antibiotics should be used, there is no evidence that prophylactic postoperative antibiotics prevent meningitis or ventriculitis. The occurrence of ventriculitis may relate more to wound breakdown and cerebrospinal fluid (CSF) fistulation at the site of closure than the actual delay in closure [6, 38].

During postoperative care, the wound is observed daily for signs of infection, CSF leak, or wound breakdown. Evidence of wound infection includes erythema, swelling, tenderness and purulent discharge. Such wounds should be drained, specimens obtained for culture and gram stain and systemic broad spectrum antibiotics administered [6, 39].

The onset of meningitis is accompanied by identical signs of illness as observed in infants with sepsis. In addition to the physical findings observed in infants with meningitis, fluid and electrolyte abnormalities associated with inappropriate antidiuretic hormone secretion, including hyponatremia, decreased urine output, and increased weight gain, may also be evident. Occasionally, the onset of meningitis has been followed by a transient or persistent diabetes insipidus [39].

Interpretation of CSF values in the newborn may be difficult. The cell content and chemistry of the CSF of healthy newborns differ from those of older infants. The values vary widely during the first weeks of life. CSF parameters observed in a healthy term neonate can overlap with those observed in an infant with meningitis [40, 41]. A Gram-stain smear of CSF should be examined and appropriate media should be inoculated with the CSF specimen. Microorganisms can be isolated from CSF that has normal white blood cell and chemistry values [39].

In the initial management of meningitis, ampicillin and an aminoglycoside are commonly used. Cefotaxime has superior in vitro and in vivo bactericidal activity against many microorganisms. Until results of susceptibility testing are known, treatment of enteric gram-negative bacillary meningitis should include cefotaxime and an aminoglycoside [42]. Meningitis caused by gram-negative enteric bacilli can cause serious management problems. Eradication of the pathogen often is delayed and serious complications can occur [39]. Concern regarding the persistence of gram negative bacilli in the CSF despite bactericidal levels of antimicrobial drug led to the evaluation of intraventricular gentamicin. The study of intraventricular gentamicin was stopped early because of the high mortality in the group of infants treated with parenteral plus intraventricular gentamicin therapy [43]. In infants who have been in the nursery for a prolonged period or in a neonate who had previous courses of antimicrobial therapy, alternative empirical antibiotic regimens should be considered. A combination of vancomycin, an aminoglycoside, and cefotaxime may be appropriate for enterococci and resistant gram-negative enteric bacilli. Other antibiotics (meropenem, ciprofloxacin etc.) may be necessary for the treatment of highly resistant organisms [39, 44, 45]. The increased use of antibiotics can result in alterations in antimicrobial susceptibility patterns of bacteria necessitating changes in initial empirical treatment. The hospital laboratory must regularly monitor isolates to assist the physician in choosing the most appropriate treatment [39].

Associated Anomalies: Presentation, Diagnosis and Management

Infants with a congenital malformation have a higher risk for additional abnormalities and further studies should be considered. In babies with MMC, evaluation of the cardiac, gastrointestinal and genitourinary systems should be undertaken as these systems formed concurrently or adjacent to the malformed neurological system [12]. Portable ultrasound examinations of the head and urinary system should be obtained and an echocardiogram should be performed on all patients before surgery [1]. Cardiology consultation should be requested early if an anomaly is present.

MMC is rarely an isolated malformation; it is usually accompanied by other clinically significant central nervous system (CNS) abnormalities. Of major importance is hydrocephalus, which is frequently associated with the Chiari II malformation [36].

Approximately 85-90% of babies with spina bifida either have hydrocephalus at birth or develop it

soon after [1]. Hydrocephalus usually becomes clinically apparent within the first two weeks of life. The confirmation of hydrocephalus requires the demonstration of enlargement of the ventricular system and excessive head enlargement. Head circumference should be measured around the largest part of the occiput and the midfrontal area of the brow. The head circumference must be plotted on a percentile chart that is appropriate for the gestational age, postnatal age, sex and ethnic group of the infant. In full term infants, an increase in the occipital-frontal circumference of the head (OFC) > 1 cm per week may be indicative of hydrocephalus [1, 36]. It is of prime importance to obtain a cranial ultrasound in premature infants, since the brain is more compliant and the ventricles may expand with little change in head size. Cranial ultrasound is the quickest, least expensive, and most convenient method of demonstrating ventricular enlargement [38]. Ventricular width is measured from the midline to the lateral border of the lateral ventricle in the mid-coronal view. Percentiles for postmenstrual age have been developed. Ventricular width 4 mm over the 97th centile is a useful criterion to define ventricular dilatation severe enough to consider treatment [46].

The patient with spina bifida should be observed for the signs and symptoms of progressive hydrocephalus. These signs include apnea, bradycardia, decreased activity, poor feeding, projectile emesis, irritability or lethargy, an increase in the head circumference, bulging fontanel, split cranial sutures or tenseness of the spinal repair. If hydrocephalus develops, the patient is evaluated for signs of infection. If no infection is identified, a shunt is placed [46, 47].

Approximately one third of infants who are born with MMC develop symptomatic Chiari malformation [6, 36]. As hydrocephalus develops, compromise of the hindbrain related to the Chiari II malformation escalates. Early recognition and intervention is essential as hindbrain dysfunction is associated with high morbidity. The first symptoms are progressive slowing of the infant's feeding with nasal regurgitation and a change in the pitch of the infant's cry. The principal clinical abnormalities of brainstem dysfunction are vocal cord paralysis with stridor, abnormalities of ventilation (both obstructive and central), cyanotic spells, swallowing difficulties, recurrent aspiration pneumonia, and sustained arching of the head. The need to follow these findings necessitates continuous monitoring of these infants during their stay in NICU [47]. If the infant presents with cardiorespiratory distress, apnea, bradycardia, laryngeal stridor or aspiration with swallowing, an evaluation for Chiari II malformation (blood gases, oximetry, magnetic resonance imaging (MRI) of the brainstem, sleep study, videofluoroscopy of swallowing) is justified. Although the symptoms resolve for most patients, a third of those who remain symptomatic will die [36].

The other important central nervous system anomaly seen in babies with MMC is abnormality of cerebral cortical development. The occurrence of seizures in approximately 25% of children with MMC might be accounted for in part by cortical dysgenesis. Caregivers should be aware of the risk of seizures in these babies. MRI is the study of choice for imaging neural tissue and for identifying specific defects [38].

Many infants will have deformities of the foot, knee and hip requiring orthopedic consultation, though rarely on an emergent basis [1].

Poor bladder emptying immediately after neural tube defect (NTD) closure may be temporary ('spinal shock') and improvement of bladder function may be observed up to 6 weeks after repair. However, most infants with MMC will have a neurogenic bladder and will need urologic consultation during the initial hospitalization [1, 11]. Disordered innervation adversely affects bladder function and potentially threatens the upper urinary tract. These infants are at risk for secondary damage from neurogenic bladder based on increased intravesical pressure. Elevated pressure places these infants at risk for hydronephrosis, reflux and urosepsis [48]. Early treatment protects the bladder from additional damage. Many patients initially require intermittent catheterization at frequent intervals to avoid bladder overdistention. Some of these infants are still in need of intermittent catheterization when discharged home [1].

A renal ultrasound and a voiding cysto-urethrogram will show whether there is hydronephrosis, retention of urine, trabeculation in the bladder and/or ureteric reflux. Other renal defects, such as single kidney, horseshoe kidneys, pelvic kidney and double pelvis and ureters are ten times more common than in infants without neural tube defects [48]. Nevertheless, the initial urological care of newborns with MMC is rarely emergent.

Latex Allergy

Infants with spina bifida are at greater risk than the general population for developing latex allergies. The risk of developing latex IgE antibodies rises with multiple operations [49]. Infants with spina bifida have a high degree of exposure to latex products as a consequence of repeated surgical procedures, implantation of latex containing materials and catheterization. Previous reports indicate a prevalence of latex allergy in patients with spina bifida ranging between 10% and 73% [50]. The prevalence of clinical allergic reactions may be as high as 20-30% [12]. This allergy is an IgE-mediated reaction that may be mild with urticaria or severe with bronchospasm, laryngeal edema, and systemic anaphylaxis. In one report, the serologic evidence of sensitivity was 40% [51]. Several reports indicate that latex allergy in spina bifida children is related to age, to the number of operations and perhaps to a genetic predisposition. Intraoperative anaphylaxis to latex involves cutaneous, respiratory and circulatory changes that may be fatal if not promptly recognized and treated [52]. Any allergic history in children with MMC should alert the clinician to the possibility that severe anaphylactic reactions may occur, especially when large mucosal surfaces are exposed [49]. All diagnostic and therapeutic procedures should be conducted in latex-free environments.

Discharge Plan

Parent education (beginning early in the hospitalization) and organization of a discharge plan for parents is essential prior to discharge. The parents are overwhelmed with the complexity of the disorder and frequently confused. Accordingly, it is important to present an accurate picture, the likely sequelae, and the outlook for intellectual, urinary, sensorimotor, and sexual function.

Children with open neural tube defects need comprehensive follow-up in a multidisciplinary setting involving neonatology, pediatric neurosurgery, pediatric neurology, pediatric orthopedics, urology and physical therapy [1]. Developmental specialists and social workers should also participate in the infants' care. Prior to discharge, arrangement should be made for the patient to be enrolled in a Spina Bifida Clinic. Clinic appointments need to be tailored to the needs of each infant and family.

Before discharge, every infant should have a nutrition consult, immunization plan and neonatal hearing evaluation [53]. Appointment for hip ultrasound should be arranged. Hip dislocation or subluxation is usually evident within the first year of life, especially in patients with midlumbar MMC [54].

Genetic counseling is suggested in view of the 2-4% recurrence risk of neural tube defects in subsequent siblings and the risk of chromosomal abnormalities that have been associated with neural tube defects [6, 55].

References

1. Brand MC (2006) Examining the newborn with an open spinal dysraphism. Adv Neonatal Care 6:181-196
2. Bunch WH (1972) Modern management of myelomeningocele. WH Green, St Louis, pp 168-174
3. Wang KS, Ford HR, Upperman JS (2006) Metabolic response to stress in the neonate who has surgery. Neo Reviews 7:410
4. Elias ER, Hobbs N (1998) Spina Bifida: sorting out the complexities of care. Contemp Pediatr 15:156-171
5. Lewis D, Tolosa JE, Kaufmann M et al (2004) Elective cesarean delivery and long term motor function or ambulation status in infants with meningomyelocele. Obstet Gynecol 103:469-473
6. Punt J (2001) Surgical management of neural tube defects. In: Levene MI, Chervenak FA, Whittle MJ (eds) Fetal and neonatal neurology and neurosurgery. Churchill Livingstone, London, Edinburgh, New York, pp 753-773
7. Katz AL, Wolfson P (2005) General surgical considerations. In: Spitzer AR (ed) Intensive care of the fetus and neonate. Elsevier Mosby, Philadelphia, pp 1353-1368
8. Chandra S, Baumgart S (2005) Fetal and neonatal thermal regulation. In: Spitzer AR (ed) Intensive care of the fetus and neonate. Elsevier Mosby, Philadelphia, pp 495-513
9. Okada Y, Powis M, Ewan A et al (1998) Fentanyl analgesia increases the incidence of postoperative hypothermia in neonates. Pediatr Surg Int 13:508-511
10. Krishne G, Emhardt JD (1992) Anesthesia for the newborn and ex-preterm infant. Semin Pediatr Surg 1:32-44
11. Snodgrass WT, Adams R (2004) Initial urologic management of myelomeningocele. Urol Clin N Am 31:427-434
12. Kaufman BA (2004) Neural tube defects. Pediatr Clin N Am 51:389-419
13. Beyer JE, Bournaki M (1989) Assessment and management of postoperative pain in children. Pediatrician 16:30-38
14. Dijk M, Peters JWB, Bouwmeester N et al (2002) Are postoperative pain instruments useful for specific group of vulnerable infants? Clin Perinatol 29:469-491
15. Anand KJS, Phil D, Hickey PR (1987) Pain and its effects in the human neonate and fetus. N Engl J Med 317:1321-1325
16. Taddio A (2002) Opoid analgesia for infants in the neonatal intensive care unit. Clin Perinatol 29:493-509
17. Vaughn PR, Townsend SF, Thilo EH et al (1996) Comparison of continuous infusion of fentanyl to bolus dosing in neonates after surgery. J Pediatr Surg 31:1616-1622
18. Van lingen RA, Simons SHP, Anderson BJ et al (2002) The effects of analgesia in the vulnerable infant during perinatal period. Clin Perinatol 29:511-534
19. Bryant LD, Dierdorf SF (1992) Postanesthesia recovery. Semin Pediatr Surg 1:45-54
20. Kurth CD, Spitzer AR, Broennle AM et al (1987) Postoperative apnea in preterm infants. Anesthesiology 66:483-488
21. Montoyama EK, Glazener CH (1986) Hypoxemia after general anesthesia in children. Anesth Analg 65:267-272
22. Chawls WJ (1998) Metabolic considerations. In: O'Neill JA, Rowe MI, Grosfeld JL (eds) Pediatric surgery. CV Mosby, St Louis, pp 57-70
23. Anand KJS, Brown MJ, Bloom SR et al (1985) Studies on the hormonal regulation of fuel metabolism in the human newborn infant undergoing anesthesia and surgery. Horm Res 22:115-128
24. Tsang TM, Tam PKH (1994) Cytokine response of neonates to surgery. J Pediatr Surg 29:794-797
25. Brooker PD, Bush GH (1990) Neonatal physiology and its effect on pre- and postoperative management. In: Lister J, Irwing M (eds) Neonatal surgery. Butterworths, London, pp 18-27
26. Presson RG, Hiller SC (1992) Perioperative fluid and transfusion management. Semin Pediatr Surg 1:22-31
27. Winthrop AL, Jones PJH, Schoeller DA et al (1987) Changes in the body composition of the surgical infant in the early postoperative period. J Pediatr Surg 22:546-549
28. Krummel TM, Lloyd DA, Rowe MI (1985) The postoperative response of the term and preterm newborn infant to sodium administration. J Pediatr Surg 20:803-809
29. Smith SD, Tagge EP, Hannakan C et al (1991) Characterization of neonatal multisystem organ failure in the surgical newborn. J Pediatr Surg 26:494-497
30. Pereira GR, Ziegler MM (1989) Nutritional care of the surgical neonate. Clin Perinatol 16:233-253
31. Lynam L, Verklan MT (2004) Neurologic disorders. In: Verklan MT, Walden M (eds) Core curriculum for neonatal intensive care. Elsevier Saunders, St Louis, pp 821-857
32. Reming VM, Romero FC (2003) Medical nutrition therapy for neurologic disorders. In: Mahan KL, Stump SE (eds) Food nutrition, diet therapy. Elsevier, WB Saunders, Philadelphia, pp 1081-1120
33. Seashore JH, Touloukian RJ, Kopf GS (1983) Major surgery in infants weighing less than 1500 grams. Am J Surg 145:483-487
34. Najmaldin A, Francis J, Postle A et al (1993) Vitamin K coagulation status in surgical newborns and the risk of bleeding. J Pediatr Surg 28:138-143
35. Sola MC, Vecchio A, Rimsza LM (2000) Evaluation and treatment of thrombocytopenia in the neonatal intensive care unit. Clin Perinatol 27:655-679
36. Northrup H, Volcik KA (2000) Spina bifida and other neural tube defects. Curr Probl Pediatr 30:317-332
37. Charney EB, Melchionni JB, Antonucci DL (1991) Ventriculitis in newborns with myelomeningocele. Am J Dis Child 145:287-290

38. Volpe J (2001) Neural tube formation and prosencephalic development. In: Volpe J (ed) Neurology of the newborn. WB Saunders, Philadelphia, pp 3-44

39. Palazzi DL, Klein JO, Baker CJ (2006) Bacterial sepsis and meningitis. In: Remington JS, Klein JO, Wilson CB, Baker CB (eds) Infectious diseases of the fetus and newborn infant. Elsevier Saunders, Philadelphia, pp 247-295

40. Ahmed A, Hickey SM, Ehrett S et al (1996) Cerebrospinal fluid values in the term neonate. Pediatr Infect Dis J 15:298-302

41. Sarff LD, Platt LH, MacCracken GH (1976) Cerebrospinal fluid evaluation in neonates: comparison of high risk infants with and without meningitis. J Pediatr 88:473-476

42. Feigin RD, MacCracken GH, Klein JO (1992) Diagnosis and management of meningitis. Pediatr Infect Dis J 11:785

43. McCracken GH, Mize SG, Threlkeld N (1980) Intraventricular gentamicin therapy in gram-negative bacillary meningitis of infancy. Lancet 1:787-791

44. Köksal N, Hacımustafaoğlu M, Bağcı S et al (2001) Meropenem in neonatal severe infections due to multiresistant gram negative bacteria. Ind J Pediatr 68:15-18

45. Khaneja M, Naprawa J, Kumar A et al (1999) Successful treatment of late onset infection due to resistant Klebsiella pneumoniae in an extremely low birthweight infant using ciprofloxacin. J Perinatol 19:311-313

46. Whitelaw A (2001) Neonatal hydrocephalus – clinical assessment and non-surgical treatment. In: Levene IM, Chernevak AF, Whittle MJ (eds) Fetal and neonatal neurology and neurosurgery. Churchill Livingstone, London, Edinburgh, New York, pp 739-761

47. Dias MS (2005) Neurosurgical management of myelomeningocele. Pediatrics in Review 26:50-60

48. Weindling AM, Rennie JM (2005) Central nervous system malformations. In: Rennie JM (ed) Roberton's textbook of neonatology. Elsevier Churchill Livingstone, pp 1186-1203

49. Rendelli C, Nucera E, Ausili E et al (2006) Latex sensitization and allergy in children with myelomeningocele. Childs Nerv Syst 22(1):28-32

50. Martinez JF, Molto MA, Pagan JA (2001) Latex allergy in patients with spina bifida and treatment. Neurocirugia 12(1):36-42

51. Tosi LL, Slater JE, Shaer C et al (1993) Latex allergy in spina bifida patients : prevalence and surgical implications. J Pediatr Orthop 13:709-712

52. Banta JV, Bonanni C, Prebluda J (1993) Latex anaphylaxis during spinal surgery in children with myelomeningocele. Dev Med Child Neurol 35(6):543-548

53. Wolraich ML, Hesz N (1988) Meningomyelocele. Assessment and management. Pediatrician 15:21-28

54. Witt C (2003) Detecting developmental dysplasia of the hip. Adv Neonatal Care 3:65-75

55. Mitchell LE, Adzick NS, Melchionne J et al (2004) Spina Bifida. Lancet 364:1885-1895

CHAPTER 13
Early Surgical Complications of Spina Bifida

M. Memet Özek

In our daily practice, most myelomeningoceles are closed within 48 hours of birth. In case of an unstable child, closure may be safely delayed for up to 72 hours without an increase in complications [1-3]. Early postoperative mortality for myelomeningocele repair is near zero; however, the morbidity due to complications of the repair can be significant [2, 4-8]. These complications may affect the patient's quality of life and are usually due to faulty techniques that are by and large preventable.

Wound Healing Problems

Newborns who have had myelomeningocele surgery have nutritional issues that include, but are not limited to, body weight, nitrogen balance, serum protein, and total lymphocyte count. These are markers of the fact that these neonates have passed through a period of significant catabolic changes. Spontaneous recovery from this state does not occur until up to one month after the surgical procedure [2]. This innate catabolic response is due to the alterations of the hormonal milieu stimulated by general anesthesia, severe stress of surgery and blood transfusions. They include rises in circulating levels of adrenocorticotropic hormone (ACTH), cortisol, free thyroxine, growth hormone, and antidiuretic hormones [9]. During this stage, the nitrogen balance remains constantly negative; the resistance to infection is diminished; and all anabolic processes such as wound healing, are momentarily slowed.

This period occurs at the same time as potential feeding problems related to hydrocephalus, postoperative ileus, Chiari malformation, and prematurity. Consequently, wound dehiscence is the single most widespread complication that is observed during the first postoperative week.

To avoid wound breakdown the skin should be sutured in triple layers (muscle, subcutaneous tissue, and skin) so that there is good coverage over the dur-al closure and adding extra protection against cerebrospinal fluid (CSF) leak [2, 3, 10].

Local factors also play a part in wound dehiscence. A large skin defect corresponds to higher tension at the suture line, which should be avoided [10, 11]. A linear, midsagittal closure is the most satisfactory and recommended procedure [3, 5, 6]. It provides easy access to the placode, should later detethering or spinal stabilization procedures become necessary. In large myelomeningoceles a few different surgical techniques have been developed to minimize suture line tension over the defect (Chapter 15) [12]. Tension on the suture line will affect the local blood supply and cytobiologic activities at this area (Fig. 13.1).

An untreated kyphus contributes a vertical vector to the stretching of the wound and intensifies the ischemia further (Fig. 13.2). When a prominent kyphus is present, it should be resected at the time of sac closure to eliminate the vertical pressure on the suture line if there are no contraindicating factors to this procedure [13, 14].

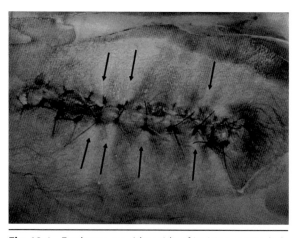

Fig. 13.1. Erythema on either side of incision, particularly in areas of high tension

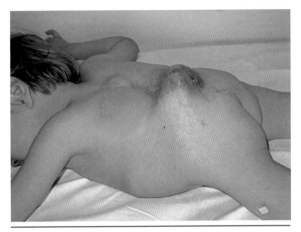

Fig. 13.2. Kyphosis can lead to skin breakdown

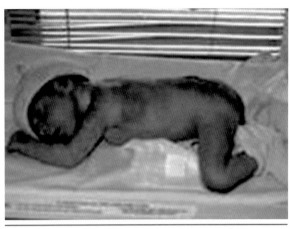

Fig. 13.4. Avoid incorrect positions

All preventive measures should be taken to avoid any blood or serum collection under the flap. A seroma or hematoma aggravates the tension of the skin and prevents the flap from attaching to the underlying tissues from which neovascularization for the flap arises (Fig. 13.3) [2, 11].

The wound should be inspected every day by a physician and maintained with a light nonadhesive dressing so that it can be easily lifted for inspection. Any additional external pressure on the incision caused by a tight bandage should be avoided. Wound management with antibiotic-embedded petrolatum dressings provides both an antibacterial protective layer and keeps the wound moist; thus providing an optimal environment for wound epithelization.

For the first 7-10 days, the infant is to be nursed lying face down at all times [3]. Incorrect positioning of the patient will interfere with the healing of the surgical field (Fig. 13.4). A plastic drape may be placed between the wound and the anus to prevent feculent contamination of the wound.

Skin Flap Necrosis

Necrosis after myelomeningocele repair occurs due to ischemia of the skin tissue. It happens as a result of either insufficient blood supply or tension on the suture line (Fig. 13.5). In small areas, sloughing of the epidermis layer entails only simple dressing

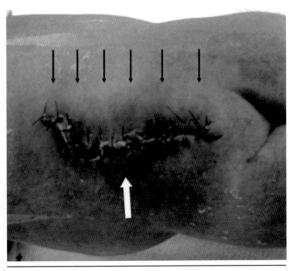

Fig. 13.3. Subcutaneous collection with tension on the suture line

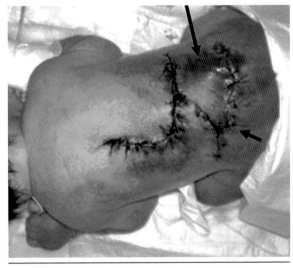

Fig. 13.5. The flap looks deep red as a result of venous stasis (*long arrow*). Necrosis at the tip (*short arrow*)

changes since the wound ultimately epithelializes over the underlying dermal and subdermal layers. Skin grafting is not obligatory [2, 12]. If the skin necrosis is full thickness but there is a healthy muscled layer beneath it, the wound should be debrided carefully until it is moderately clean and a healthy bleeding surface becomes visible. It may be left for healing by secondary intention (Fig. 13.6). This procedure will take time since the new epithelium can grow only from the edges. Therefore, the prevention of a superficial infection may be difficult. As such, the use of partial-thickness skin grafting, which will remain intact with a vascularized base, is a wise solution. Management of full thickness skin necrosis depends on the defect size (Fig. 13.7) [12]. Defects less than a centimeter square can still be followed up with expectant therapy but larger defects definitely need debridement and reconstruction with flaps.

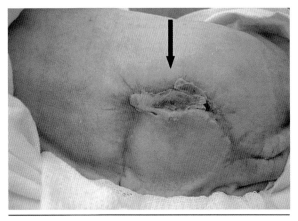

Fig. 13.6. Partial thickness skin loss may be managed only by secondary intention (*arrow*)

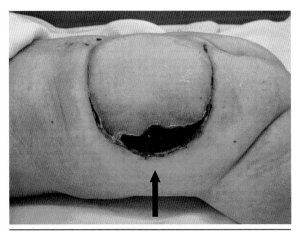

Fig. 13.7. Full thickness necrosis with demarcation (*arrow*)

Wound Infection

The surgical infection rate of meningomyelocele surgery is reported to be about 1 to 12% [2, 6, 8]. This low infection rate is surprising considering that, in a significant number of patients, the exposed neural placode is contaminated.

The extended catabolic phase after surgery interferes with white blood cell functions, weakening the newborn's cellular immunity against infections [1]. The capability of immunoglobin (Ig) formation is poor during the first 3 months and the infant is dependent on transplacentally acquired maternal antibodies. As IgA cannot cross the placenta well, a common problem is infection from enteric bacteria. As expected, prematurity is a factor that increases this vulnerability [1].

Infection can be intradural or extradural. Intradural infection pathogens are virulent gram-negative enteric bacteria [9]. Systemic signs of sepsis are most commonly in attendance within 3 days and occasionally even within the first 24 hours of surgical treatment. In neonates, these early signs are more likely to be nonspecific and not obvious. The infant displays poor feeding, intermittent lethargy and an alternately ashen complexion and mottled blotches over the trunk. Hypothermia is more widespread than pyrexia, and the white blood count often falls below 4000 cells/mm3 even though the band cell count may be excessively high [9].

If the dural sac is well covered with vascularized skin or myocutaneous flaps, an intradural abscess develops with almost no signs of infection in the back wound. Thus, a ventricular tap to acquire CSF for bacteriologic examination must be performed where infants show early signs of unapparent sepsis during the first 3 days after myelomeningocele closure [14]. The presence of CSF infection eventually leads to intractable seizures and obtundation. However, the long term prognosis of gram-negative ventriculitis in the newborn relies almost always on the swiftness of diagnosis and treatment alone. If an intradural infection is confirmed on CSF examination, specifically in cases where the back wound appears tense, the dural closure should be explored in the operating room for an intradural swelling. The purulent material should be removed carefully without causing damage to the placode or nerve roots, which may be heavily coated with fibrinous exudate. The area should be widely irrigated with antibiotic solution and a new watertight dural closure obtained. The patient should be placed on a broad-spectrum, CSF-penetrating antibiotic (third generation cephalosporins)

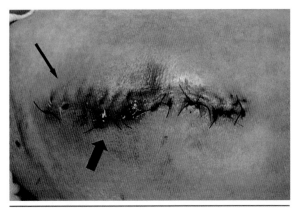

Fig. 13.8. Infected wound with drainage of purulent material (*short arrow*). One or more sutures could be taken out for drainage (*long arrow*)

and an antibiotic specific for the *Staphylococcus* species endemic to the hospital.

Initially, if the infection is confined to the extradural space, erythema, fluctuance and calor occur at the operative site around day 5-7 after surgery [15]. The swelling should be aspirated for purulent material and cultured for aerobic and anaerobic bacteria. Opening of one or two sutures may also allow draining of purulent material, which will continue to drain during the following days until the infection resolves (Fig. 13.8). The open part of the wound may be left to close through secondary intention. At this stage the infant continues to feed and remains alert. However, left untreated, subcutaneous infections ultimately enter into the CSF as the newborn dura is not a strong barrier against virulent organisms.

Cerebrospinal Fluid Leak

CSF leak is one of the major complications of myelomeningocele closure. Its incidence is reported to be as high as 17% [5, 16]. It arises from:
1. Insufficient closure of the dura or through suture holes at closure
2. Inappropriate closure of the anatomical layers
3. Increased CSF pressure

A small amount of transdural CSF leak is likely to occur in most cases of myelomeningocele closure. Keeping in mind the thinness of the newborn dura, even the suture holes may serve as a source of minor leaks for a short time until healing occurs. During the first few postoperative days therefore, an insignificant increase in fluctuance under the skin flaps is most likely a combination of CSF as well as a serosanguinous ooze [2]. Most commonly at day 5-6 after closure, a large transdural leak presents as a rapid accumulation of a bulging fluctuant mass in the wound.

If closure of the layers is strong enough to prevent outward leak of CSF, the small transdural seepage is self-limiting, the subcutaneous collection spontaneously resorbs and there is no risk of infection or fistula. If the layers are not intact, CSF will accumulate in the subcutaneous space. Eventually, the skin suture line and the integrity of the flap may be under threat as a result of the progressive increase in the subcutaneous accumulation. Ultimately, this accumulation causes a fistula or a pseudomeningocele to occur. It has also been shown that CSF leakage itself has effects on wound healing [10].

Since 85% of all myelomeningoceles are associated with hydrocephalus, the increased CSF pressure poses an additional risk for postoperative CSF leak [1, 5, 14]. Despite the high percentage of patients that ultimately need a shunt, fewer than 25% of the patients are born with an unusually large head and gross ventriculomegaly [14, 16]. The reservoir effect of the expandable lumbosacral sac allows absorption of most of the forces, tending to distend the ventricles until the sac is surgically closed. However, many surgeons have noted that hydrocephalus is exacerbated by and becomes symptomatic after the myelomeningocele is closed [5, 17-19].

The timing of the progressively increasing CSF pressure coincides with the weakening of a tenuous suture line, and hence CSF leak most likely occurs on day 4-8 post repair [2, 5]. Such a delayed leak will not stop spontaneously.

When CSF does break through the skin, the risk of gram negative infection rapidly climbs and treatment must be instituted rapidly. Difficulty arises when there is minor skin incision dehiscence after 5 or 6 days, exposing a small amount of subcutaneous tissue from which drains thin, pale yellow fluid. This is reminiscent of xanthochromic CSF, but more often represents an innocuous exudate from fat necrosis. The wound should be watched for 1 or 2 days: a late CSF leak, after formation of an external fistula, almost always increases in amount and the drainage accordingly becomes more copious, clear, and watery [2, 5]. On the contrary, an exudate from fat necrosis gradually turns milky and after a couple of days dries up.

Finally, even the best dural or myocutaneous closure is not expected to resist high CSF pressures when progressive hydrocephalus occurs. Good judgment emphasizes the importance of the prompt treatment of progressive hydrocephalus, in the first 2 weeks after birth, with a shunt or an external ventricular drain (EVD), not only for protection of the brain, but also of the fragile suture lines.

A shunt is effective in preventing CSF leak, but is not recommended after the leak has breached the skin closure [9, 20]. In case of large subcutaneous collections, the shunt will not be helpful. The resistance of a medium pressure shunt is much higher than the pressure on the skin tissue, which is slightly higher than atmospheric pressure. Therefore the preferential route for CSF egress out of the subcutaneous region is still into the back wound and not the shunt. If a CSF leak perseveres in the presence of a shunt, the latter eventually becomes infected.

An external ventricular drain is a much better decompression system when a substantial leak is present. The drainage pressure can be adjusted through positioning the external ventricular drain chamber relative to the external auditory meatus in the supine patient. Dropping the chamber below this level enables CSF to drain away from the back wound at negative pressures. With cessation of active leakage, the probability of infection is significantly reduced. Everyday CSF samples should be sent to the laboratory for cells, protein and glucose content, and cultured for aerobic and anaerobic bacteria.

Exploration of the wound is indicated if the CSF leak persists despite all measures, or recurs after the external ventricular drain chamber is elevated. In this instance most patients will have a dural defect that should be closed followed by meticulous closure of all the more superficial layers.

Meningitis

The treatment of meningitis is discussed in Chapter 12.

Detoriation of Neurological Function

Worsening of neurological function after closure is by and large preventable and is reported to occur in about 9.5% of patients [7, 8].

During the transfer of the baby to the operating room, meticulous care should be taken to avoid mechanical injury to the placode. The anesthesiology team should be experienced enough not to damage the placode area during their intubation and preparation for the surgery (see Chapter 11).

During the sterile preparation, povidone iodine solution, which is toxic to neural tissues, is used only on the skin and membranous part of the sac. It should not be splashed on to the placode. The placode itself should be cleansed with warm jets of bacitracin-saline solution and not subjected to any mechanical scrubbing [1].

The placode should always be handled gently, as described in Chapter 10.

If the placode is very thick, mechanical trauma may occur when reconstituting the neural tube. The blood supply of the placode may also be limited.

During placode manipulation, pulling too hard on the placode against the proximal spinal cord guarantees aggravation of the neurologic deficit. Even when the initial examination fails to demonstrate movement of muscles innervated by the placode, the placode should still be considered functional, as over one-third of these children will subsequently gain motor function not previously detected [6, 15].

Great care should be conducted while separating the edge of the placode from the contiguous cutaneous epithelium (Chapter 10) [1, 21]. Retained fragments, even as small as a single cell, may produce an inclusion dermoid if imbricated within the closure. These additional dermoids not only produce tumors, but associated desquamative debris may also incite an intense arachnoiditis (Fig. 13.9). As a result of this, tethered cord release in the face of the scar produced by this inflammatory process can be challenging.

When it comes to the dural closure, most pediatric neurosurgeons advocate a watertight closure. Nevertheless, there should be a wide enough CSF space for the cord. It makes little sense to preserve the placode through careful dissection and then to strangulate it with a tight, constricting dural closure [6]. In routine practice, the dura is limited most of the time. On the other hand, to put tight sutures on the newborn's dura will cause a fistula to occur. Therefore it is advisable to use dural grafts.

The fascia lata or the fascia of paravertebral muscles is the most suitable graft material. It is not only because it is autologous, but also because it is closest in uniformity and thickness to newborn dura [5].

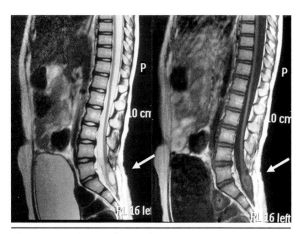

Fig. 13.9. Inclusion dermoid (*arrow*)

Postoperative Ileus

Paralytic ileus, which occurs after the myocutaneous flaps are used to close large defects, is a rare complication in the immediate postoperative period. Deep dissection and extensive mobilization of the latissimus dorsi and erector spinae muscles that results from inadvertent puncture of the posterior peritoneum may result in reflex ileus [2]. On the contrary, the autonomic nerves in the retroperitoneum may be injured as a result of disturbance of the quadratus lumborum and may cause neurogenic ileus [2].

Some of the symptoms include, but are not limited to feeding intolerance with increased gastric residuals, vomiting, abdominal distention and diminished bowel sounds. Abdominal x-rays usually show distended bowel loops [2].

The process is usually self-limiting. Bowel rest with nasogastric suction is performed. In cases where enteral feeding cannot be carried on after a few days, total parenteral nutrition should be considered.

Postoperative Pneumothorax

Deep dissection of the upper reaches of the latissimus dorsi tendon may puncture the posterior pleura and result in a postoperative pneumothorax [2], which can be diagnosed through clinical signs, physical examination, arterial blood gases, transillumination, and radiography.

Clinical presentation of pneumothorax includes grunting, hypotension, retractions, cyanosis, decreased breath sounds over the affected side, shift in cardiac point of maximal impulse and tachypnea [22]. It is essential to diagnose promptly. Radiographic evidence is confirmatory, but delay is inherent. Fiberoptic transillumination, showing extensive 'lighting up' of the affected side has proven useful for diagnosis when radiography is delayed [23].

During the preparation of the patient for chest tube placement, needle aspiration may be palliative. Chest tube drainage, specifically in infants receiving positive pressure ventilation, is necessary for continuous drainage of pneumothoraces [24].

Necrotizing Enterocolitis

Necrotizing enterocolitis (NEC) occurs in 1-3 per 1000 live born babies. Although 10% of all cases of NEC occur in term infants, it is more commonly seen in preterm infants and particularly those with birth weights less than 1000 grams. The incidence in this group of babies is approximately 5-10%. NEC is the most commonly occurring gastrointestinal emergency in preterm infants. It accounts for up to 5% of admissions to neonatal intensive care units [9, 25, 26].

NEC is defined as inflammation of the bowel wall with or without necrosis. The etiology of this disease is complex. Bowel hypoxia or hypoperfusion, bacterial invasion, feedings or substrate in the bowel, interventions, immunological and nonimmunological host defense mechanisms interact to produce the clinical picture [27].

NEC occurs in epidemics. A wide variety of organisms have been associated with these outbreaks including *Klebsiella pneumoniae*, *Escherichia coli*, *Clostridia*, coagulase-negative-*staphylococci* and rotavirus [28].

NEC has been shown to affect babies with myelomeningocele slightly more often than the normal population [9]. Hypotension secondary to blood loss from the myelomeningocele closure, anoxia secondary to hydrocephalus or the Chiari malformation, and umbilical arterial lines have been implicated in the etiology of NEC in this group of patients [4]. Umbilical arterial catheters may pose a serious risk to the intestinal vasculature. It has been suggested that embolization of catheters may result in embolization of mesenteric arteries [25].

Most infants present initially with nonspecific signs of sepsis as reflected by temperature instability, apnea, lethargy, hypotension and feeding intolerance. Abdominal distention, bilious drainage from feeding tubes, and hematochezia usually follow. Abdominal signs initially may be limited to distention and tenderness and then may progress to palpable loops of bowel, fixed mass and abdominal wall erythema. As the disease progresses, neutropenia, thrombocytopenia, acidosis and coagulopathy may develop [26].

The age at onset of NEC is inversely related to gestational age, with a mean age of 3-4 days for term infants and 3-4 weeks for infants born at less than 28 weeks of gestation [29]. The more immature the infant, the later the onset of disease.

Diagnosis is usually confirmed by an abdominal x-ray that may show free air, pneumatosis intestinalis and air in the portal venous tree [25].

Most infants recover with conservative treatment. Antibiotics and bowel rest are the mainstay of the treatment. The length of treatment is largely empirical and depends on certainty of diagnosis, severity of disease and clinical progress. Most units continue for 7-14 days, or until the abdomen appears normal and bowel function returns [26].

The generally accepted indications for surgical intervention are pneumoperitoneum, intestinal obstruction, fixed intestinal loops on plain film, progressive peritonitis and uncontrolled sepsis [29]. The mortality of NEC is still high, approaching 30-50% [30].

References

1. McLone DG (1998) Care of the neonate with a meningomyelocele. Neurosurg Clin N Am 9:111-120
2. Pang D (1995) Surgical complications of open spinal dysraphism. Neurosurg Clin N Am 6:243-257
3. Sutton L (2005) Spinal dysraphism. In: Rengachary SS, Ellenbogen RG (eds) Principles of neurosurgery. Elsevier Mosby, Edinburgh, pp 99-115
4. Cohen AR, Robinson S (2001) Early management of myelomeningocele. In: McLone D (ed) Pediatric neurosurgery. WB Saunders Company, Philadelphia, London, New York, pp 241-259
5. Hahn YS (1995) Open meningomyelocele. Neurosurg Clin N Am 6:231-241
6. McLone OC, Dias MS (1991-92) Complications of myelomeningocele closure. Pediatr Neurosurg 17:267-293
7. Mirzai H, Ersahin Y, Mutluer S et al (1998) Outcome of patients with meningomyelocele. Childs Nerv Syst 14:120-123
8. Gross HR, Cox A, Tatyrek R et al (1983) Early management and decision making for the treatment of meningomyelocele. Pediatrics 72:450-458
9. Cohen AR, Robinson S (2001) Early management of meningomyelocele. In: McLone DG (ed) Pediatric neurosurgery. Surgery of the developing nervous system. WB Saunders Company, Philadelphia, pp 241-259
10. Babuccu O, Kalaycı M, Peksoy I et al (2004) Effect of cerebrospinal fluid leakage on wound healing in flap surgery: Histological evaluation. Pediatr Neurosurg 40:101-106
11. McLone D (1980) Technique for closure of myelomeningocele. Childs Brain 6:65-73
12. Ramasastry SS, Cohen M (1995) Soft tissue closure and plastic surgical aspects of large open myelomeningoceles. Neurosurg Clin N Am 6:279-291
13. Hoppenfeld S (1967) Congenital kyphosis in meningomyelocele. J Bone Joint Surg Br 49:276-280
14. Dias MS, McLone DG (2008) Meningomyelocele. In: Albright AL, Pollack IF, Adelson PD (eds) Principles and practice of pediatric neurosurgery. Thieme, New York, pp 338-366
15. McLone D (1983) Results of treatment of children born with a myelomeningocele. Clin Neurosurg 30:407-412
16. Reigel DH, McLone DG (1988) Meningomyelocele. Operative treatment and results. In: Marlin AE (ed) Concepts in pediatric neurosurgery, Vol 8. Karger, Basel, pp 41-50
17. Parent AD, McMillan T (1995) Contemporaneous shunting with repair of meningomyelocele. Pediatr Neurosurg 22:132-135
18. Epstein F (1983) Meningomyelocele: "pitfalls" in early and late management. Clin Neurosurg 30:366-384
19. Wakhlu A, Ansari NA (2004) The prediction of postoperative hydrocephalus in patients with spina bifida. Childs Nerv Syst 20(2):104-106
20. Gamache F (1995) Treatment of hydrocephalus in patients with myelomeningocele or encephalocele: A recent series. Childs Nerv System 11:487-488
21. Mazolla C, Albright AL, Sutton L et al (2002) Dermoid inclusion cysts and early spinal cord tethering after fetal surgery for meningomyelocele. N Eng J Med 347:256-259
22. Donn SM, Baker FC (2006) Thoracic airleaks. In: Donn SM, Sinha SK (eds) Manual of neonatal respiratory care. Mosby Elsevier, Philadelphia, pp 445-451
23. Cabatu EE, Brown EG (1979) Thoracic transillumination: Aid in the diagnosis and treatment of pneumopericardium. Pediatrics 64:958-960
24. Donn SM, Engmann C (2003) Neonatal resuscitation: Special procedures. In: Donn SM (ed) The Michigan manual of neonatal intensive care. Hanley & Belfus, Philadelphia, pp 33-41
25. Hunt MN (2006) The acute abdomen in the newborn. Seminars in fetal and neonatal medicine 11:191-197
26. Newell SJ (2005) Gastrointestinal disorders. In: Rennie JM (ed) Roberton's textbook of neonatology. Elsevier-Churchill-Livingstone, Philadelphia, pp 692-710
27. Beeby PJ, Jeffrey H (1992) Risk factors for necrotizing enterocolitis. Arch Dis Child 67:432-435
28. Lawrence G, Bates J, Gaul A (1982) Pathogenesis of neonatal necrotizing enterocolitis. Lancet 1:137-139
29. Srinivasan P, Burdjalov V (2005) Necrotizing enterocolitis. In: Spitzer AR (ed) Intensive care of the fetus and neonate. Elsevier Mosby, Philadelphia, pp 1027-1045
30. Pokorni WJ, Garcia JA, Barry YN (1986) Necrotizing enterocolitis: incidence, operative care, and outcome. J Pediatr Surg 21:1149-1154

CHAPTER 14
Vertebral Anomalies and Spinal Malformations in Myelomeningocele

M. Memet Özek, Muhittin Belirgen

Congenital Vertebral Anomalies in Myelomeningocele

Associated spinal cord anomalies and vertebral anomalies significantly affect the prognosis of children with myelomeningocoele. The problem is that vertebral anomalies will eventually lead to skeletal deformities that increase the complexity of the clinical picture. The presence of spinal cord malformations either complicate the primary surgery or lead to tethered cord in the long term. It is therefore important to evaluate these patients from this perspective and identify these associated anomalies.

Skeletal deformity in myelomeningocele may occur for three reasons: (1) unequal skeletal growth caused by congenital malformations of the spine; (2) mechanical instability caused by absence or deficiency of posterior elements of the spine or by paralysis, and (3) neurological abnormalities caused by hydromyelia and tethered cord.

Embryological Aspects

In order to understand developmental anomalies of the spine, it is necessary to understand the normal embryological development of the vertebral axis. A complex interrelationship exists between the neural elements of the spine and the mesenchymal elements that protect and support it.

Development of the vertebra and spinal column begins in the third embryonic week and is completed around 20 years of age [1]. Development occurs through the processes of membrane formation, chondrification and ossification in the fetal and postnatal periods. The embryonic cellular tissue organization proceeds in an exact sequential manner. As it proceeds in cephalocaudal sequence, a congenital malformation is induced in the upper (cephalic side) vertebra with early exposure to teratogenic factors, and in the lower (caudal) parts with late exposure [2]. Exposure to an effective teratogenic factor causes predictable types of vertebral anomalies specific to each temporal period: (1) disorders of notochord, (2) disorders of the unsegmented mesoderm, (3) disorders of segmentation and (4) disorders of sclerotome differentiation [1].

As the process of neurulation takes place dorsally, the notochord is assisting the formation of the structural or mesenchymal elements of the spine [3]. On both sides of the notochord, the mesoderm differentiates into three main areas: paraxial, intermediate and lateral mesoderm (Fig. 14.1) [4, 5]. At the same time, the notochord induces the mesoderm to differentiate longtitudinal segmentation into somites [6-8]. Development of the somites occurs in a craniocaudal fashion and will eventually help in forming the bones of the head, vertebrae and other bony structures of the thorax and associated musculature. Each somite develops into two parts: a medial sclerotome and a lateral dermatomyotome (Fig. 14.2). The cells of the sclerotome are responsible for the formation of the spine, and the dermatomyotomes form muscle cells and the overlying dermis of the skin [4]. Scle-

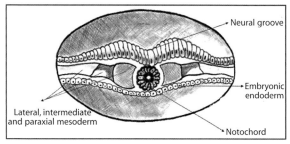

Fig. 14.1. Approximately day 17 of the developing embryo – the notochordal plate folds itself and forms the notochord. Mesodermal tissue around it differentiates into paraxial, intermediate and lateral mesoderms. These mesodermal tissues subsequently further differentiate into the somites. Modified from [5b], with permission from Elsevier

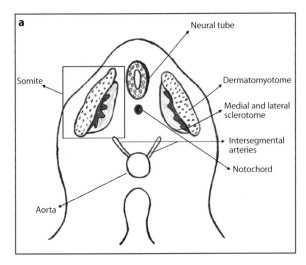

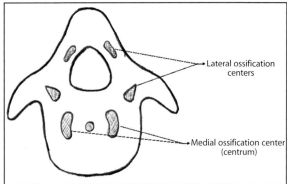

Fig. 14.3. Vertebral ossification centers. Modified from [5]

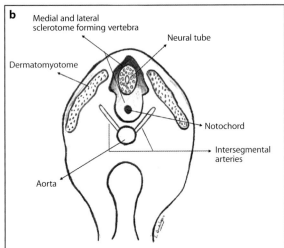

Fig. 14.2 a, b. Cross section of the developing embryo on **a** the 22nd and **b** 28th days of embryogenesis

rotomes are also subdivided into medial and lateral segments. Medial sclerotomes form the vertebral body (bone, cartilage, intervertebral disc, and meninges) while the lateral sclerotomes migrate posteriorly between the cutanenous ectoderm and the fused neural tube to form the posterior elements of the spinal canal. Associated dermatomyotomes migrate in a similar fashion and form the paraspinal musculature and dermis. Each vertebral segment arises from a corresponding notochordal segment. Failure of this longitidunal segmentation results in fusion anomalies such as failure of segmentation anomalies.

During the sixth week of the fetus' life, the vertebral bodies begin chondrification from two lateral centers that are separated by the notochordal sheath [5, 9]. After the fusion of the chondrified centers, the intervening notochordal part is extrudes into the intervertebral disk. The merged vertebral body chon-

drification centers connect with the lateral chondrification centers, which are fused posteriorly in the midline. Three different ossification centers are observable in the neonatal spine: the centrum and two lateral centers (Fig. 14.3). The bulk of the vertebral body consists of the centrum, while the posterior lateral portion results from the lateral ossification centers. The ossification centers blend and the intervening notochordal element is consequently extruded into the intervertebral disk. The centrum begins to solidify during week 9. Disorders during the fusion of ossification centers may cause problems such as hemivertebra, butterfly vertebra, sagittal or coronal cleft, and absence of the vertebral body. During the preliminary stages of ossification, the centrum is separated into an anterior segment and a posterior segment through a transitory plate that clearly elucidates the incidence of coronal clefts. These clefts correspond to the demonstration of incomplete fusion of anterior and posterior compartments of the centrum, not of persistence of the notochord. Coronal clefts are not usually visible after the first few months of life. Sagittal clefts are secondary to centers of ossification developing from each chondrification center. Sagittal clefts, similar to coronal clefts, are not usually found after the first few months of life. Persistent sagittal clefts give rise to butterfly vertebra.

Due to the closure of the neural tube, the neural tissue does not split from the cutanenous ectoderm (nondisjunction) in myelomeningocele; it remains fused to the skin along the lateral surface of the placode. Lack of separation of the placode from the cutanenous ectoderm disables the mesenchyme from moving posterior to the neural ectoderm and thus is forced to stay anterolateral to the nervous tissue. The pedicles and the lamina that are created from this mesenchyme are everted, facing posterolateraly instead of posteromedialy. As a result of the rotation of the lamina and pedicles, the spinal canal undergoes a fusiform extension throughout the spina bifida. The maximum enlargement of the canal takes place when the laminae are in the sagittal plane. Additional rotation of the lamina reduces the canal's size [10]. The vertebral bodies can either function almost normally or have anomalies of segmentation varying from single hemivertebrae to malsegmented vertebral components. Since the vertebra and the neural axis develop in parallel, the presence of vertebral anomalies indicates the presence of neural anomalies in a large percentage of affected children. Secondary problems with subsequent primary neurulation may result in associated myelomeningoceles through a failure of segmental neurulation, which comprise skin-covered variants of spina bifida, as well as meningocele, lipomas, lipomyelomeningoceles and dermal sinus tracts due to an abnormality of cutaneous ectodermal separation [11].

The embryological insult in humans is not known. In animal models it is known that maternal hypoxia at the critical time of gestation can induce congenital vertebral deformities [12].

Classification of Congenital Vertebral Anomalies

Vertebral anomalies are classified into segmentation, formation, or mixed problems that can occur at any part in the vertebral ring (anterior, anterolateral, lateral, posterolateral, or posterior). As in the other types of congenital deformities of the spine, the deformity may be attributed to any of these embryological causes (Table 14.1, Fig. 14.4).

Table 14.1. Classification of congenital vertebral anomalies

Congenital vertebral bony anomalies can be classified as:

1. Failure of formation
   a) Wedge vertebrae
   b) Hemivertebrae
   c) Butterfly vertebrae
   d) Missing vertebrae
2. Failure of segmentation
   a) Block vertebrae
   b) Unsegmented bars
3. Mixed type (failure of formation and segmentation)
4. Other anomalies such as:
   a) Absence of the spinous processes and lamina (rachischisis) or rudimentary vertebrae
   b) Reduction in the anteroposterior size of vertebral body
   c) Increase in the interpeduncular distance
   d) Decreased height of the pedicle
   e) Laterally extended transverse processes
   f) Midline osseous or fibrocartilagenous spurs (split cord malformations)

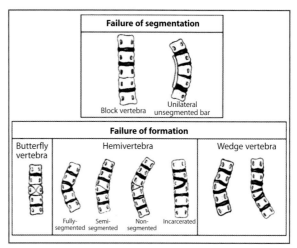

Fig. 14.4. Schematic representation of vertebral anomalies. Modified from [5b], with permission from Elsevier

Failure of Formation

Failure of formation arises due to the absence of structural elements of a vertebra. Any region of the vertebral ring may be affected: anterior, anterolateral, posterior, posterolateral or lateral. Failure of formation may be partial or complete with wedge vertebra representing the partial form and hemivertebra, butterfly vertebra and vertebral aplasia representing complete types of failure of formation.

Hemivertebra

Hemivertebra is one of the most common vertebral anomalies. It results from failure of a vertebra to form on one side with half a vertebral body, a single pedicle, and hemilamina. It represents a complete unilateral failure of vertebral formation. A hemivertebra is not an extra vertebra, but rather the remainder of the vertebra that did not form. It is this absent bone that gives rise to the deformity with absent growth potential in the area of the anomaly, and resultant growth in the remainder of the vertebral ring.

Hemivertebra may be fully segmented (65%), semisegmented (22%), or incarcerated (12%) (Fig. 14.5) [13]. Fully segmented hemivertebra have a normal disk superior and inferior to the involved vertebral anomaly (Fig. 14.6). Semisegmented hemivertebra are fused to the neighboring vertebrae on one side and with one open disk space on the opposite side. Nonsegmented spaces may also occur and are represented as superior or inferior hemivertebra fused to both vertebrae with no interval disk attached to the involved vertebral anomaly. When both the cranial and

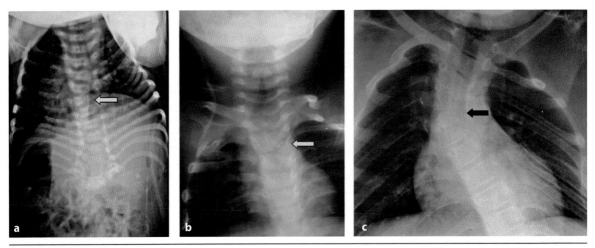

Fig. 14.5 a-c. Anteroposterior spinal X-rays showing **a** segmented, **b** incarcerated and **c** semisegmented hemivertebrae (*arrows*) associated with MMC

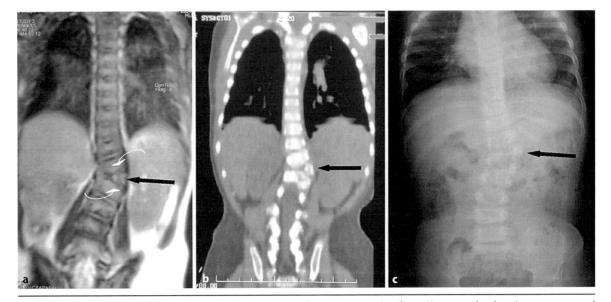

Fig. 14.6 a-c. **a** Coronal MRI, **b** coronal reconstruction CT and **c** anteroposterior direct X-ray graphs showing a segmented hemivertebra of a MMC patient (*black arrows*). Note also the intervertebral discs both above and below the hemivertebra (*white arrows*)

caudal vertebrae conform in shape to make room for the hemivertebra, the anomalous vertebra is referred to as incarcerated. Incarcerated hemivertebrae may not affect the shape of the spine. The pedicles of an incarcerated hemivertebra are in line with the curve created by the pedicle cranial and caudal to it.

Hemivertebra occur mostly in the thoracic spine. Tsoe et al. [14] proposed that this anomaly is the result of a pairing defect of sclerotomic cells with asynchronous development of the hemimetameric pair. The most common mechanism of hemivertebra formation is believed to consist of paired somite derivatives that are not in the same developmental phase by the time mid-

line fusion occurs. The tardy side may shift one segment caudad (solitary hemivertebra). If two asynchronous pairs deploy tardy hemimetamers on contralateral sides, double balanced hemivertebra will develop.

Wedge Vertebra

A wedge vertebra results from dysplastic formation of a vertebral body on one side where the pedicles are still present. It usually involves a unilateral partial failure of formation of one of the chondrification centers (Fig. 14.7).

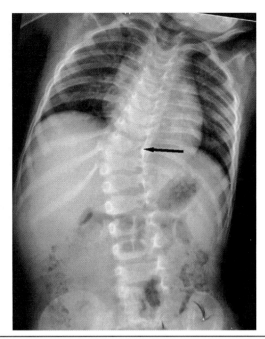

Fig. 14.7. A wedge vertebra (*arrow*) in a MMC patient

happens centrally, probably after incomplete fusion of two chondral centers with hypoplasia at the junctional site. Butterfly vertebra can result from a developmental abnormality leading to regression of the cauda dorsalis and formation of sagittal clefts in the vertebral body. A funnel-like defect divides the vertebra into right and left halves. There are usually no symptoms. Butterfly vertebrae of normal height do not necessarily result in a deviation of the spinal column axis.

Missing Vertebra (Vertebral Aplasia)

Total aplasia of a vertebral body may also occur. The condition will most likely lead to kyphosis. The embryologic insult which leads to this abnormality is still unclear, but it may occur during the late chondrification or early ossification phase of formation of the vertebral body centrum. As the remainder of the spinal segment develops from separate chondrification centers, these portions are usually not affected. Rarely the entire vertebral body segment may fail to develop or the vertebral maldevelopment may occur at multiple levels.

Butterfly Vertebra

Butterfly vertebra results from separate bilateral ossification centers that fail to unite (Fig. 14.8) and resemble a bilateral hemivertebra with a central cleft. Butterfly vertebrae have a cleft through the body of the vertebrae and a funnel shape at the ends. This gives the appearance of a butterfly on X-ray. It is caused by persistence of the notochord (which usually only remains as the center of the interverebral disc) during vertebrae formation. Constriction of the vertebral body

Failure of Segmentation

These anomalies are vertebral column malformations resulting from deranged embryological development of normal segmentation. If two adjacent somites or their associated mesenchyme do not separate properly, a segmentation defect will occur. This failure of segmentation is more commonly observed in the cervical or lumbar spines [1]. Examples of failure of segmentation are unilateral unsegmented bar and block vertebra.

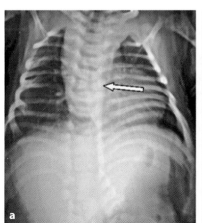
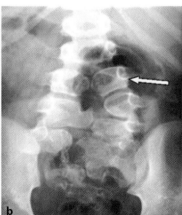
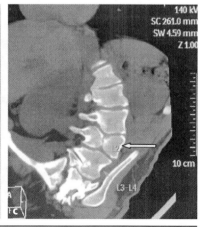

Fig. 14.8 a-c. Butterfly vertebrae (*arrows*) associated with MMC. **a** Simple and **b** associated with complex hemivertebra deformity. **c** Coronal Tri-D CT of another MMC patient

Block Vertebra

Block vertebra is caused by a bilateral failure of segmentation with fusion of the disk between the involved vertebrae (Fig. 14.9). It may result from nonsegmentation of vertebral somites. It can be seen as a congenital abnormality in the cervical, thoracic or lumbar regions of the spine. Usually only two ver-

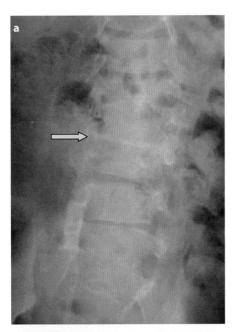

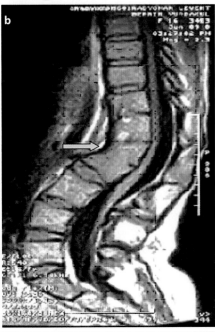

Fig. 14.9 a, b. Block vertebrae (*arrows*) associated with MMC. **a** X-ray showing a lumbar block vertebra and **b** late MRI scans in a patient operated for MMC

tebrae are affected, and the patient is asymptomatic. Any or all parts of the vertebrae may be involved (vertebral body, vertebral arches, and/or spinous processes). The intervertebral discs may be missing or are represented by rudimentary calcified structures. An hourglass appearance is often seen owing to the presence of a waist-like constriction of the fused vertebral bodies at the level of the intervertebral disc. This indicates the lack of full development of endplates. The block vertebrae may be of the same length as the number of involved vertebrae or may be shorter and result in an abnormal angulation of the spine.

Unilateral Unsegmented Bar

The unilateral unsegmented bar anomaly is the second most commonly seen congenital vertebral anomaly. It represents a unilateral failure of vertebral segmentation affecting two or more vertebrae, usually over three vertebrae. It is a vertebral bar fusing both disks and facets on one side. Rib fusions are frequently present on the same side as the bar. The unsegmented bar does not contain growth plates and does not grow longitudinally. It acts as an asymmetric rigid tether to normal growth.

Mixed Anomalies

Mixed anomalies are represented by combinations of both segmentation and formation failures (e.g., a unilateral unsegmented bar with congenital hemivertebra). Defects of formation and segmentation are not necessarily mutually exclusive. Often, an individual case is a mixture of a failure of formation and a failure of segmentation, creating complex structural abnormalities.

Rachischisis and Other Posterior Arch Anomalies

Rachischisis is the absence or nonfusion of the spinous process, with or without accompanying laminal defects (Fig. 14.10). It can occur anywhere along the vertebral axis. Involvement of the entire spine is found in cases of complete neural tube dysraphism and a gradation of less severe involvement occurs with isolated myeloschisis. Rachischisis of multiple vertebra is a common finding in both anencephaly [15] and myelomeningocele [16]. In addition, in myelomeningocele, vertebral arches show lack of fusion or they are absent. There is lateral broadening of vertebrae, lateral displacement of pedicles and a widened spinal canal.

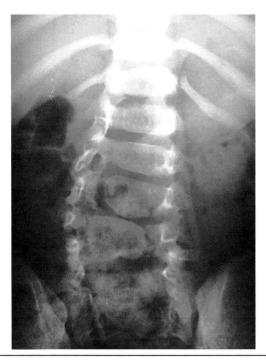

Fig. 14.10. X-rays showing the absence of posterior bony structures and wide interpeduncular distance in a MMC patient

Demographics and Etiology

There is not clear data regarding the incidence of the association of myelomeningocele and congenital vertebral anomalies, but it can be said that the presence of multifocal complex anomalies is related to an increased risk of neural tube defects [17]. The overall incidence is unknown but is increasing, with a more aggressive multidisciplinary approach to the care of these patients leading to increased patient longevity and increased diagnosis of these anomalies. The etiopathogenesis of hemivertebra and other hypoplastic vertebral anomalies is still obscure. Isolated anomalies (hemivertebrae) are sporadic with no familial or genetic tendencies [18]. Other authors, however, have suggested a role for hereditary factors, such as in a report of monozygotic twins [19], or familial episodes in several generations [20].

Patient Evaluation

Since the majority of the meningomyelocele patients diagnosed in the antenatal period are operated within 36 hours of birth it is not always possible to have a detailed preoperative examination. For these pa-

tients postsurgery, and for those diagnosed later, presurgical radiologic evaluations are essential. Baseline radiographs of the entire spine should be completed in the anteroposterior and lateral planes with attention paid to the relative positions of the radiographs such as the supine, sitting, or standing position. Other than the low lumbar and sacral level patients who can stand autonomously, radiographs are usually made with the patient in the sitting position. Verification regarding the deformity, associated congenital anomalies and the level of the spinal dysraphism should be documented. Serial radiographs should be carried out every 6 months so that curve stability or progression can be easily documented. The convex growth is significant and thus the quality of the bone and disk spaces on the convexity must be visualized and inspected precisely. If the disk spaces are present and clearly defined and the convex pedicles are visibly formed, there is a possibility of convex growth and the prognosis is poor. If the convex disks are not clearly formed and the convex pedicles are poorly demarcated, the convex growth potential is less and the prognosis is better. In the first few years of life, cartilage forms a significant part of the vertebra and consequently at this stage prognostication is not as exact as in an older child. Routine coronal and sagittal views are attained primarily to understand the deformity in both planes, with successive examinations required, depending on the deformity that exists. It is important to visualize the whole spine from the skull to the sacrum on both views since multiple anomalies that may occur on opposite ends of the spine are possible (e.g., one cervical and one lumbosacral). Accurate vertebral landmarks should be selected on the end vertebrae of the curves measured; exactly the same landmarks are utilized for subsequent radiographs, guaranteeing the consistency of the evaluation. For congenital anomalies, careful choice of these landmarks is crucial since the normal anatomy is distorted, disabling the accurate curve measurement. This difficulty results in a greater measurement error in these cases. Magnetic resonance imaging (MRI) study of the brain and spinal canal should be used within the first 2 years of life for baseline purposes studies and should be repeated where clinically indicated.

Clinical Course

Vertebral anomalies progress to scoliosis, kyphosis, lordosis or mixed skeletal anomaly causing clinical symptoms and signs. Certain anomalies constantly progress (the unilateral unsegmented bar). This occurs to the extent that the patient with this anomaly should have an immediate fusion, without waiting for radiological progression. The unilateral segmented bar results in the total lack of growth on the concave side of the curve, and if growth continues on the reverse side, a severe deformity occurs as an outcome. Once it is formed, this deformity is extremely rigid and almost impossible to correct other than through complex surgery. Consequently, it is wiser to prevent an increase in the deformity in the beginning than to correct it after it has become severe.

Hemivertebrae may be single, multiple and balanced or unbalanced. Contralateral hemivertebrae, if balanced, may not progress and as a result do not need treatment. When it is separated by several segments, a double curve is formed and both of these curves may progress and necessitate fusion. A single hemivertebra, which is the most common anomaly, may or may not cause a progressive deformity. Due to this ambiguity, the patient with this problem should be carefully followed, and when deformity occurs, fusion should be performed. A single hemivertebra at the lumbosacral level produces significant decompensation since there is no space underneath the hemivertebra for natural compensation to occur. Another area where the vertebral anomalies cause decompensation is the cervicothoracic area due to the restricted ability of the cervical spine to balance the cervicothoracic curve.

Asymmetric growth results in variable rates of deformity, disabling the ability to predict the natural history of these deformations. If anomalies have clinical or radiological deterioration, this continues until skeletal maturity with the highest risk periods being the first 2 years of life and adolescence [21], even though rapid change may occur at any time. Owing to this, close follow-up is needed throughout the life of these patients [22]. The prognosis depends upon both the type and the site of the anomaly. Guidelines concerning the risk of progression for each type of vertebral anomaly with median yearly rates of progression are as follows: unilateral unsegmented bar with contralateral hemivertebra (5-10 degrees per year), unilateral unsegmented bar (3-9 degrees per year), two unilateral fly segmented hemivertebra (1-3 degrees per year). Wedge vertebra may get worse relatively slowly. Block vertebra have no growth potential and hence remain stable. A standard progression per patient is 5 degrees per year [22]. The prognosis becomes poorer when the anomaly is located in the lower thoracic spine, thoracolumbar spine, or in lumbosacral junction with an oblique take-off. Despite the fact that age at diagnosis is not a strong predictor of prognosis, it is not uncommon that those diagnosed earlier in life have a worse prognosis compared to those diagnosed later in life.

Additional Spinal Malformations

Spinal cord anomalies associated with myelomeningocele include tight filum terminale, split cord malformation (SCM), hemimyelomeningocele, dermoid/epidermoid tumors, teratoma and defective myelinization [23]. In a study of Gilbert et al. [24], these concomitant anomalies were found in 88% of 25 autopsy cases.

Tight and/or Fatty Filum Terminale

The tight filum terminale is characterized by a short and hypertrophic filum terminale that tethers the spinal cord and impairs the ascent of the conus medullaris. It is thought to occur as a disorder of secondary neurulation [25]. Generally, a low-lying conus medullaris is associated with this anomaly but a normal position of the conus is also possible. In at least 80% of cases, the tip of the conus lies inferior to the L2 vertebra [26]. The fatty filum is characterized by a thickened fibrolipomatous filum terminale. Like the tight filum, it is also an anomaly of secondary neurulation and can also tether the spinal cord [27]. The exact incidence of the association of tight and/or fatty filum and myelomeningocele is not known. If the tight and/or fatty filum terminale are seen during surgery for a myelomeningocele, they should be sectioned so that possible future tethering is reduced.

Split Cord Malformation

Delayed tethering of the spinal cord in myelomeningocele patients is usually caused by scarring of the placode to surrounding tissues [28, 29]. However, another less frequent cause is the concomitant presence of a SCM with the myelomeningocele (Fig. 14.11) [30, 31]. The reported incidence of the association of these lesions with myelomeningocele is 6% [31]. The relationship of the SCM to the neural placode can be in four different forms: above the placode, below the placode, same level with the placode and hemimyelomeningocele (Fig. 14.12). Most SCMs occur within one vertebral level of placode (mostly above). Therefore, they can be easily identified at the time of closure. In order to prevent the late occurrence of tethering, SCM should be looked for at one vertebral level above and below during the closure of myelomeningocele sac. SCM is dealt with in more detail in Chapter 38.

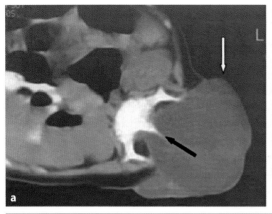
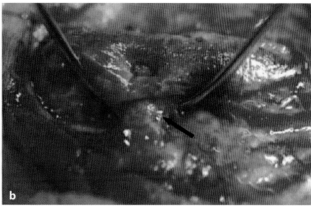

Fig. 14.11 a, b. A case of SCM associated with MMC. **a** Preoperative axial computed tomography and **b** intraoperative appearance of spur (*black arrow*) and neural placode (*white arrow*)

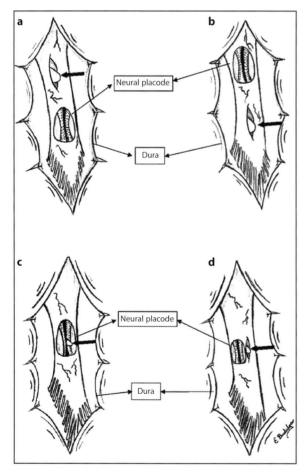

Fig. 14.12 a-d. Schematic view of the relationship between SCM and the neural placode: **a** SCM can be above the placode, **b** below the placode, **c** inside the placode and **d** hemimyelomeningocele. Bony spurs are shown with *black arrows*

Hemimyelomeningocele

First described in 1965 by Duckworth et al., hemimyelomeningocele (HMM) refers to a unique form of spinal cord dysraphism in which the myelocele or myelomeningocele is found in one hemicord of a diastematomyelia (Fig. 14.13) [11, 32-36]. Hemicords usually lie in their own dural tube and are separated in the midline by a bony septum. Few reports briefly mention this particular abnormality [11, 29, 33-37], probably because of its rare occurrence or the possible misdiagnosis as myelomeningocele [29].

The exact formation of HMM is unclear. The myelomeningocele is known to be a defect of primary neurulation with the lack of midline closure of the neural placode and contiguous structures. It takes place at 26-28 days of gestation [23, 33, 38]. On the other hand, diastematomyelia is basically known to be a defect of secondary neurulation or postneurulation [23, 38, 39]. In the detailed unified theory, Pang et al. [37] reported that SCMs and related abnormalities are results of a formation of adhesions between the ectoderm and endoderm leading to an accessory neurenteric canal around which condenses an endomesenchymal tract that bissects the notocord, thus causing formation of two hemineural plates [32]. Dias and Walker [11] explained the embryogenesis of SCMs and related malformations through a failure of midline axial integration during the process of gastrulation. The so-called disorder of gastrulation emphasizes the formation of two notochordal plates and ultimately two hemineural plates [11, 32]. The exis-

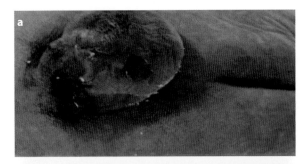

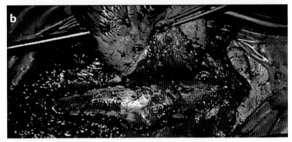

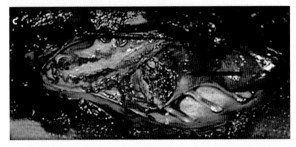

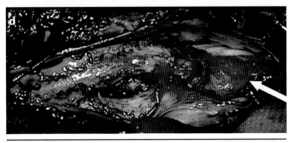

Fig. 14.13 a-d. a Preoperative and **b-d** intraoperative photographs of a hemimyelomeningocele patient. Myelomeningocele arose from the upper hemicord. The bony spur is indicated by the *black arrow*. There are asymmetries between the hemicords. Note also the concomitant fatty filum (*white arrow*)

tance of a central canal in each hemicord supports the concept that both hemicords have undergone independent neurulation after the splitting that must have occurred in the neural plate stage [36]. Describing the association of SCMs with open myelomeningocele and hemimyelomeningocele, Pang et al. [36] mentioned that in some cases of SCM, the persistence of the dorsal endomesenchymal tract interferes with normal neurulation; hence the ectodermal and mesoder-

mal structures fail to close over it to form an open myelomeningocele at the same site. This nonneurulation process is not fully understood yet.

The true incidence of HMM is therefore uncertain, but probably is much greater than was previously thought. The hemimyelomeningocele is observed in about 10% of unselected patients with myelomeningocele [33, 34]. In Duckworth's original series, it was found in 2.3% of spina bifida patients [40]. On the contrary, the association of myelomeningocele with diastematomyelia is much more frequent. Various reports have shown that between 31 and 46% of myelomeningocele patients have an associated diastematomyelia [33, 39].

The neurological deficit in children with HMM is less severe when compared to that seen in myelomeningocele patients. It has been reported that children with HMM have neurological deficits limited to the exposed hemicord and have normal function on the side of the normal hemicord [11, 29, 32, 33, 35, 40].

From a neurourological point of view, it has been reported that the urinary dysfunction arising from a neurogenic bladder and its consequences were much less pronounced in cases of HMM particularly due to the presence of the contralateral normal hemicord [11, 40]. Duckworth et al. [40] in their original paper reported that in the majority of cases HMM was associated with normal bladder function and all children with normal bladder function had one fully innervated leg. The full sacral innervation on one side enabled sphincter control to be normal.

Considered as a complication of myelomeningocele closure, McLone and Dias [29] cautioned surgeons to the possible presence of a HMM and an associated SCM. Venes and Stevens [41] mention the importace of recognition and correction of abnormalities distal or immediately proximal to the neural placode in myelomeningocele closure in order to avoid secondary tethered cord syndrome. It is well known that a second (tethering) pathology may be found in cases of spinal dysraphism. The lack of clinical diagnostic signs in some children or a simple myelomeningocele-like appearance of the defect, and the lack of preoperative radiological assessment (when the newborn undergoes urgent operation) may confuse the surgeon and lead to misdiagnosis.

Dermoid and Epidermoid Tumors

It is known that late occurrence of dermoid and epidermoid tumors is possible after myelomeningocele closure and have been reported in 16% of myelomeningocele patients [42-49]. The reason for this is the inclusion of cutaneous remnants at the time of surgical closure of the myelomeningocele repair. Hovewer, another mechanism should also be suspected because dermal elements were found within the filum terminale of a newborn with a myelomeningocele [42]. These lesions are generaly diagnosed with MRI after the occurrence of signs and symptoms of delayed retethering in myelomeningocele patients. Treatment consists of removing the tumor and detethering the spinal cord.

Teratoma

The association of teratoma and myelomeningocele in a single lesion is infrequent and there are insufficient case reports [50-54]. A teratoma is a germ cell neoplasm that contains differentiated elements derived from all three germinal layers. It is considered to be a true tumor with a neoplastic nature, which could be potentially malignant [55]. There are different hypotheses regarding the pathophysiology of teratomas [55-57]; however, the theory of dysembryogenic origin most meaningfully explains the coexistence of these lesions with myelomeningocele [50]. The most common site of concomitant teratoma and myelomeningocele is the lumbosacral area [54]. In its treatment, the entire myelomeningocele sac should be resected along with the teratomatous tissue. The prognosis of a teratoma associated with myelomeningocele is good with no recurrence of the tumor [54].

References

1. Oi S (1989) Malformations of the vertebrae. In: Raimondi ACM, Di Rocco C (eds) Principles of pediatric neurosurgery. Springer-Verlag, New York, pp 1-18
2. Tanimura T (1968) Relationship of dosage and time of administration to the teratogenic effects of thio-TEPA in mice. Okajimas Folia Anat Jpn 44:203-253
3. Egelhoff J, Prenger EC (1997) The spine. In: Ball WS (ed) Pediatric neuroradiology. Lippincott-Raven, Philadelphia
4. Moore KL, Persaud TVN (1998) Formation of germ layers and early tissue and organ differantiation. In: Moore KL, Persaud TVN (eds) Developing human. WB Saunders, Philadelphia, pp 63-80
5. Jinkins JR (2000) Atlas of neuroradiologic embryology, anatomy, and variants. Lippincott Williams & Wilkins, Philadelphia
5b. Kaplan KM, Spivak JM, Bendo JA (2005) Embryology of the spine and associated congenital abnormalities. Spine J 5:564-576
6. O'Rahilly R, Benson DR (1985) The development of vertebral column. In: Bradfort DS, Hensinger RN (eds) Pediatric spine. Thieme, New York, pp 3-17
7. Muller F, O'Rahilly R (1987) The development of the human brain, the closure of the caudal neuropore, and the beginning of secondary neurulation at stage 12. Anat Embryol (Berl) 176:413-430
8. Phillips WA (1994) Sacral agenesis. In: Weinstein SL (ed) Pediatric spine: principles and practice. Raven Press, New York, pp 259-273
9. Castillo M, Mukherji SK (1996) Imaging of the pediatric head, neck and spine. Lippincott-Raven, Philadelphia
10. Naidich TP, Harwood-Nash DC (1983) Spinal dysraphism. In: Newton TH (ed) Modern neuroradiology. Clavadel Press, San Anselmo, pp 299-353
11. Dias MS, Walker ML (1992) The embryogenesis of complex dysraphic malformations: a disorder of gastrulation? Pediatr Neurosurg 18:229-253
12. Loder RT, Hernandez MJ, Lerner AL et al (2000) The induction of congenital spinal deformities in mice by maternal carbon monoxide exposure. J Pediatr Orthop 20:662-666
13. McMaster MJ, David CV (1986) Hemivertebra as a cause of scoliosis. A study of 104 patients. J Bone Joint Surg Br 68:588-595
14. Tsou PM, Hodgson AR (1980) Embryogenesis and prenatal development of congenital vertebral anomalies and their classification. Clin Orthop Relat Res 152:211-231
15. Marin-Padilla M (1966) Study of the vertebral column in human craniorachischisis. The significance of the notochordal alterations. Acta Anat (Basel) 63:32-48
16. Barson AJ (1970) Spina bifida: the significance of the level and extent of the defect to the morphogenesis. Dev Med Child Neurol 12:129-144
17. Loder RT (2003) Congenital scoliosis and kyphosis. In: DeWald R (ed) Spinal deformities. Thieme Medical Publishers, New York, pp 684-693
18. Wynne-Davies R (1975) Congenital vertebral anomalies: aetiology and relationship to spina bifida cystica. J Med Genet 12:280-288
19. Adams MS, Niswander JD (1968) Health of the American Indian: congenital defects. Eugen Q 15:227-234
20. Carter CO, Roberts JA (1967) The risk of recurrence after two children with central-nervous-system malformations. Lancet 1:306-308
21. McMaster MJ, Ohtsuka K (1982) The natural history of congenital scoliosis. A study of two hundred and fifty-one patients. J Bone Joint Surg Am 64:1128-1147
22. Winter RB, Eilers VE (1968) Congenital scoliosis. A study of 234 patients treated and untreated. Part I: natural history. J Bone Joint Surg Am 50-A:1-15
23. Hahn YS (1995) Open myelomeningocele. Neurosurg Clin N Am 6:231-241

24. Gilbert JN, Jones KL, Rorke LB et al (1986) Central nervous system anomalies associated with meningomyelocele, hydrocephalus, and the Arnold-Chiari malformation: reappraisal of theories regarding the pathogenesis of posterior neural tube closure defects. Neurosurgery 18:559-564

25. Tortori-Donati P, Rossi A, Cama A (2000) Spinal dysraphism: a review of neuroradiological features with embryological correlations and proposal for a new classification. Neuroradiology 42:471-491

26. Warder DE (2001) Tethered cord syndrome and occult spinal dysraphism. Neurosurg Focus 10:e1

27. Tortori-Donati P, Rossi A, Biancheri R, Cama A (2005) Congenital malformations of the spine and spinal cord. In: Tortori-Donati P (ed) Pediatric neuroradiology: head, neck and spine. Springer, Berlin Heidelberg, pp 1551-1608

28. Herman JM, McLone DG, Storrs BB Dauser RC (1993) Analysis of 153 patients with myelomeningocele or spinal lipoma reoperated upon for a tethered cord. Presentation, management and outcome. Pediatr Neurosurg 19:243-249

29. McLone DG Dias MS (1991) Complications of myelomeningocele closure. Pediatr Neurosurg 17:267-273

30. Ansari S, Nejat F, Yazdani S, Dadmehr M (2007) Split cord malformation associated with myelomeningocele. J Neurosurg 107:281-285

31. Iskandar BJ, McLaughlin C, Oakes WJ (2000) Split cord malformations in myelomeningocele patients. Br J Neurosurg 14:200-203

32. Dias MS, Pang D (1995) Split cord malformations. Neurosurg Clin N Am 6:339-358

33. Barkovich AJ (1990) Congenital anomalies of the spine. In: Barkovich AJ (ed) Pediatric neuroimaging. Raven press, New York, pp 227-269

34. French BN (1990) Midline fusion defects and defects of formation. In: Youmans JR (ed) Neurological surgery. WB Saunders, Philadelphia, pp 1051-1235

35. Heffez DS, Aryanpur J, Hutchins GM, Freeman JM (1990) The paralysis associated with myelomeningocele: clinical and experimental data implicating a preventable spinal cord injury. Neurosurgery 26:987-992

36. Pang D, Dias MS, Ahab-Barmada M (1992) Split cord malformation: Part I: A unified theory of embryogenesis for double spinal cord malformations. Neurosurgery 31:451-480

37. Pang D (1992) Split cord malformation: Part II: Clinical syndrome. Neurosurgery 31:481-500

38. Lemire RJ (1988) Neural tube defects. JAMA 259:558-562

39. Shurtleff DB, Lemire RJ (1995) Epidemiology, etiologic factors, and prenatal diagnosis of open spinal dysraphism. Neurosurg Clin N Am 6:183-193

40. Duckworth T, Sharrard WJ, Lister J, Seymour N (1968) Hemimyelocele. Dev Med Child Neurol Suppl 16:69

41. Venes JL (1985) Surgical considerations in the initial repair of meningomyelocele and the introduction of a technical modification. Neurosurgery 17:111-113

42. Chadduck WM, Roloson GJ (1993) Dermoid in the filum terminale of a newborn with myelomeningocele. Pediatr Neurosurg 19:81-83

43. Bonioli E, Cama A, Bellini C et al (1983) [Importance of early diagnosis of spinal dysraphia. Dermoid cyst of the cauda equina associated with a pilonidal sinus: case report]. Minerva Pediatr 35:785-788

44. Iwasaki M, Yoshida Y, Shirane R, Yoshimoto T (2000) [Spinal dermoid cyst secondary to myelomeningocele repair: a case report]. No Shinkei Geka 28:155-160

45. Martinez-Lage JF, Masegosa J, Sola J, Poza M (1983) Epidermoid cyst occurring within a lumbosacral myelomeningocele. Case report. J Neurosurg 59:1095-1097

46. Martinez-Lage JF, Poza M, Sola J (1994) Dermoid and epidermoid tumors in myelomeningocele patients. Pediatr Neurosurg 20:274

47. Mazzola CA, Albright AL, Sutton LN et al (2002) Dermoid inclusion cysts and early spinal cord tethering after fetal surgery for myelomeningocele. N Engl J Med 347:256-259

48. Scott RM, Wolpert SM, Bartoshesky LE et al (1986) Dermoid tumors occurring at the site of previous myelomeningocele repair. J Neurosurg 65:779-783

49. Storrs BB (1994) Are dermoid and epidermoid tumors preventable complications of myelomeningocele repair? Pediatr Neurosurg 20:160-162

50. Koen JL, McLendon RE, George TM (1998) Intradural spinal teratoma: evidence for a dysembryogenic origin. Report of four cases. J Neurosurg 89:844-851

51. Ozer H, Yuceer N (1999) Myelomeningocele, dermal sinus tract, split cord malformation associated with extradural teratoma in a 30-month-old girl. Acta Neurochir (Wien) 141:1123-1124

52. Reid SA, Mickle JP (1985) Myelomeningocele occurring within a lumbosacral teratoma: case report. Neurosurgery 17:338-340

53. Semerci CN, Bebitoglu I, Kacar A et al (2001) An unusual fetus with complete absence of thoracic, lumbar and sacral vertebrae, bilateral renal agenesis, VSD, meningomyelocele, imperforate anus, and teratoma. Clin Dysmorphol 10:57-60

54. Habibi Z, Nejat F, Naeini PE, Mahjoub F (2007) Teratoma inside a myelomeningocele. J Neurosurg 106:467-471

55. Tibbs PA, James HE, Rorke LB et al (1976) Midline hamartomas masquerading as meningomyeloceles or teratomas in the newborn infant. J Pediatr 89:928-933

56. Bentley JF, Smith JR (1960) Developmental posterior enteric remnants and spinal malformations: the split notochord syndrome. Arch Dis Child 35:76-86

57. Donnellan WA, Swenson O (1968) Benign and malignant sacrococcygeal teratomas. Surgery 64:834-846

CHAPTER 15
Plastic Surgery Aspects of Large Open Myelomeningoceles

James T. Goodrich, David A. Staffenberg

The repair of large complex myelomeningoceles remains one of the most difficult challenges facing pediatric neurosurgeons. Recent collaboration with our plastic surgery colleagues has led to the joint introduction of repair techniques for these complex malformations. Our current practice is for the neurosurgical team to expose the neural elements and placode of the myelomeningocele and release them from the surrounding tissues. Once the neural reconstruction is completed the plastic surgery team completes the reconstruction with appropriate flaps and skin rotations. Our center has been using these techniques for over two decades with very gratifying results. The surgical exposures and nuances of these complex closures are discussed below.

The timing of surgical repair for complex myelomeningoceles remains controversial. Over the years we have seen a number of children with untreated myelomeningoceles that have presented with very large scarred and sclerotic sacs and have survived but with the usual lower extremity problems; fortunately these children have remained very much in the minority. In the past it has been felt that myelomeningoceles should be treated and repaired in the first 24 hours. There is now ample data confirmed by the experience from our service that it is reasonable to wait 48-72 hours, and even longer to complete the repair. This additional time allows for adequate evaluation of the child for other medical issues and also allows for the formation of a surgical team to complete whatever complex reconstruction might be needed.

There are three important concepts to keep in mind with the treatment of any form of myelomeningocele. The first and foremost is a closure of the cerebrospinal spaces to prevent leakage of cerebrospinal fluid (CSF) and potential meningitis. The surgical team must also keep in mind that the closure can, and will often accelerate the development of hydrocephalus, so they must be prepared for the treatment of hydrocephalus. The second important concept is that the neurosurgical team accomplish-

es a complete de-tethering of the spinal cord and placode at the original surgical reconstruction. Leaving dural and arachnoid adhesions in place around the neural placode will only lead to a later de-tethering operation when the child is older. Not uncommonly seen at these initial procedures are small dermoid lesions or a hypertrophied filium terminale, all of which should be dealt with at the original postnatal surgery. For the plastic surgeon the third concept – the role of cosmesis and the development of watertight, viable skin flaps – cannot be underestimated.

Surgical Considerations for the Neurosurgeon

The successful closure of a complex myelomeningocele requires an intimate understanding of its anatomy, both of the neural and the surrounding soft tissue elements. The neural placode is almost always at or near the surface of the defect. The placode is typically covered by a thin layer of leptomeninges along with skin and surrounding or bordering subcutaneous tissues; the variations seen in this theme can be enormous. The placode, typically splayed open like a fish fillet, is initially freed from the surrounding leptomeninges by following the border between the placode and the leptomeninges and skin. Once that is complete we like to tubulate the placode, sewing the pial edges together with a 6-0 prolene. Some surgeons prefer to leave the placode open and close directly over it. It has been our experience however, that if the child needs further surgery in this region, a surgically closed placode is easier to deal with anatomically than an open one due to the scarring that obscures the surgical planes. The next step in the closure is dealing with the underlying dura mater lateral to the placode. It has been our experience that the dura mater is typically opened, splayed out and attached laterally to the thoracolumbar fascia. The dura mater is freed up laterally and elevated to be brought up and over to the midline where it is closed with a running

Table 15.1. Myelomeningocele five-layer closure

1. Isolation and tubulation of the neural placode (some neurosurgeons elect to leave the placode open)
2. Lateral elevation and rotation of dura mater medially to make for a watertight dural closure
3. Elevation and closure of the lumbodorsal fascia
4. Wide subcutaneous undermining and skin closure
5. Skin closure avoiding tension and blanching of the skin. Complex plastic surgery rotations will typically be needed here

locked suture: we typically use a 6-0 prolene suture to complete the dural closure. The neurosurgeon should attempt to get a watertight closure of the dura at this point, though this is not always possible. Once the neural elements have been dealt with it is time to perform the skin closure. In complex myelomeningoceles this can be a daunting task, hence the reason we include our plastic surgery colleagues who have had more experience in complex skin closures and flap rotations (Table 15.1).

Surgical Closure of the Large Complex Myelomeningocele

In the large (typically greater than 8-10 cm) complex myelomeningocele it is not possible to just undermine the skin widely and then perform a primary skin closure. A lack of skin coverage or even worse, taunt blanching skin with poor vascularity that will dehisce and necrose, will lead to a quick and dramatic failure of this type of closure. In these children several options in the form of various flap rotations are available. With a good understanding of the anatomy and the flaps potentially available almost all myelomeningoceles can be covered with minimal morbidity to the patient. We will present three case presentations outlining potential flaps available for closure (Figs. 15.1-15.4).

Surgical Considerations for the Plastic Surgeon

A surgical plan is conceived with collaborative planning by both the neurosurgeon and plastic surgeon. General oroendotracheal intubation and intravenous access are secured well prior to turning the baby into a prone position. As these can sometimes be lengthy procedures, particular care is paid to ensure that all pressure points are appropriately padded and electrical leads are free. Antibiotic prophylaxis is started 30 minutes prior to skin incision and continued for 48 hours after the surgery. On our service we typical use oxacillin/nafcillin with a dose calculated at 25 mg/kg. The surgical area is widely prepared and draped and the surgical plan is marked out in ink. Any thinned and unhealthy skin with poor vascularity that is adjacent to the defect must be carefully debrided to allow for reliable healing. Once the neurosurgical team has the spinal cord detethered and

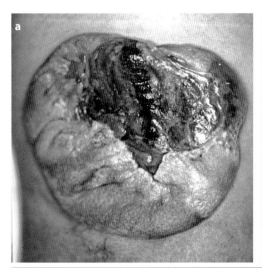 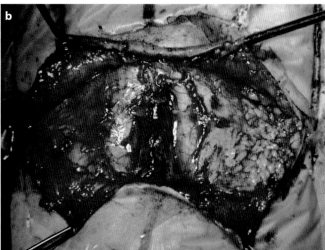

Fig. 15.1 a, b. Case 1. **a** A newborn with a large 10 x 12 cm myelomeningocele. The neural placode can be seen in the midline. **b** The placode is covered with the typical leptomeninges and surrounded by very thin remnants of skin and epidermis with the typical thin irregular margins. Once the neurosurgical repair was completed the plastic surgeon team completed the flap rotations, which are described and illustrated in Figure 15.2

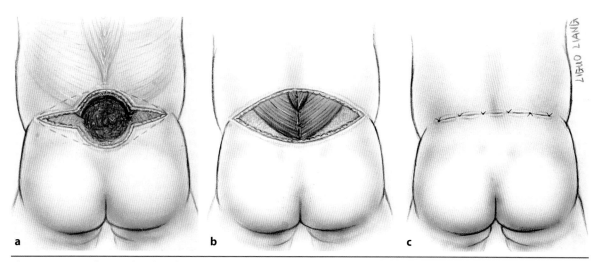

Fig. 15.2 a-c. Defects isolated to the lower back. **a** Once the defect is defined, the skin of the back is elevated deep to the latissimus dorsi muscles bilaterally. Undermining is continued cephalad and lateral until sufficient laxity is attained. While additional mobilization can be gained by dividing the latissimus dorsi distally, from deep to superficial, we avoid this so as not to weaken the arm adductors in a patient who is likely to be wheelchair-bound. **b** Closed suction drains are placed through a separate stab incision in the skin and directed as far away from the dura repair as possible. Muscle, fascia and skin are closed in layers with meticulous plastic technique. **c** Final closure leaving a suture-line across the lower back

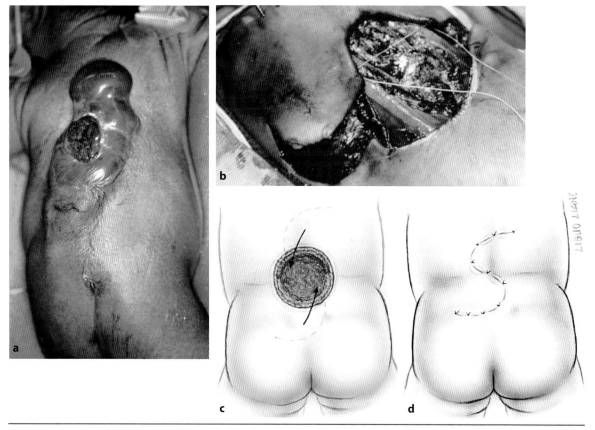

Fig. 15.3 a-d. Case 2. **a, b** A newborn child with a large extensive lumbo-sacral-thoracic myelomeningocele. Because of the extensive nature and extent of the myelomeningocele the blood supply and flap style of rotation has to be carefully considered. In this type of closure we would elect to use a "double-opposing rotation flap", the major advantage of this flap is a large lateral blood supply to the flaps, key in keeping the flaps viable. **c** A double-opposing rotation flap can be used. Large flaps must be designed with broad bases to provide adequate blood-supply. **d** Orientation of the flaps can be altered to suit the specific case needs. A meticulous plastic closure is used

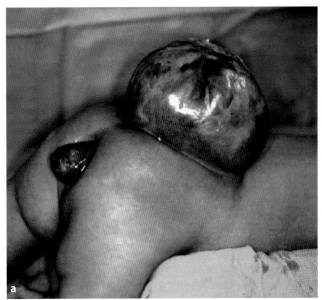

Fig. 15.4 a-d. Case 3. **a** A child that presented at age 2 with a large and unrepaired lumbo-sacral-thoracic myelomeningocele. The sac had become a large thin CSF filled myelomeningocele. The child was paraplegic and in addition had rectal prolapse. Due to the extensive nature of the myelomeningocele, a more extensive midline flap exposure was designed. Following more of a midline approach to the skin elevation the surgical team has a better opportunity to elevate large broad based flaps with preserved blood supply. **b** For defects extending up along the lumbar spine, a vertically oriented closure can be planned. Dissection is carried laterally deep to the latissimus dorsi muscle. While additional mobilization can be gained by dividing the latissimus dorsi distally, from deep to superficial, we avoid this so as not to weaken the arm adductors in a patient who is likely to be wheelchair-bound. **c** Closed suction drains are placed through a separate stab incision in the skin and directed as far away from the dura repair as possible. Muscle, fascia and skin are closed in layers with meticulous plastic technique. The wound is closed in layers. **d** Final closure leaving a suture-line along the midline

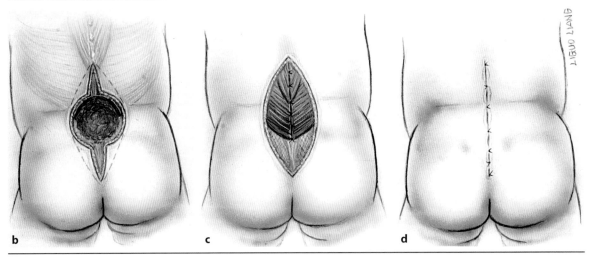

the dura repaired the defect is reassessed by the plastic surgery team.

In order to minimize tension on the repair site, wide undermining of the skin is necessary. In general, smaller defects can be closed with skin flaps dissected in the subcutaneous plane. There are many designs available for the surgeon, including opposing rotation flaps (seen in the various figures), rhomboid flaps and thoracolumbar flaps. The extent of dissection is determined by the amount of laxity gained and here prudent judgment is crucial. During dissection, care is taken to preserve the subdermal vascular plexus. When tension does not permit direct primary closure, musculocutaneous flaps may be needed. Dissection is continued laterally and cephalad deep to the thoracolumbar fascia and latissimus dorsi muscles. By dissecting deep to the fascia and muscle, additional blood

supply is recruited, often essential in good flap healing. In such cases, it is important not to dissect the plane between the skin and fascia or muscle. Throughout the surgery hemostasis is carefully maintained with bipolar cautery. We have moved away from the use of electrical bipolar currents (e.g., Malis system) to a system that uses radiofrequency current (e.g., Ellman system). With the latter system we have found better tissue healing due to less heat transmission with burning of the various tissues.

Our team normally now avoids the use of drains in general due to the concern about CSF leaks. We have completely given up the use of open drains (e.g., Penrose drains) because of the unacceptable risk of infection. In the rare cases when drains are used, closed suction drains are placed well away from the dural repair. For closure, the fascia is approximated with absorbable sutures, deep dermis is closed with inverted interrupted absorbable sutures and the skin closed with a fine running nylon. Closure of the skin must be carefully monitored to avoid excessive tension. Severe blanching of the skin edges is never a good sign. We routinely monitor the capillary refill of the skin throughout the closure. When skin tension is noted to be excessive then further mobilization of the flaps should be undertaken. An occlusive dressing is placed over the wound site. We now prefer to also place a narrow row of adhesive strips along the suture line. A clear adhesive coverlet is placed over the wound so the status of healing can be easily assessed. This dressing is left in place for five days, but removed sooner if healing is compromised. If there is a compromise in the wound healing expedient, wound revision is recommended so as to avoid any potential infection or CSF leak.

Postoperative Management of Complex Myelomeningocele Closures

The care of these complex closures does not end with the surgery. There are several themes that must be kept in mind to persevere the integrity of the surgical flaps – lack of this attention to care will lead to flap loss and necrosis. For the neurosurgeon, attention to the potential development of hydrocephalus has to be carefully monitored. Untreated hydrocephalus will lead to CSF pressure against the freshly closed wound with potential leak and possible meningitis. Hydrocephalus should therefore be treated early. Postoperative positioning of the patient is done in the prone position, typically on bolsters to reduce abdominal pressure. The wound is kept covered with an iodoform-type gauze and sterile dressing. A plastic skirt or drape is placed over the sacrum to prevent any urine or fecal material from contaminating the wound.

Additional Thoughts

Recently there has been a series of artificial materials introduced for closure of skin and dura. We personally have not had any experience with these materials in myelomeningocele repair, although there are several isolated reports of good results. To our knowledge there are no long-term (in the sense of years) reports, so we have not been able to evaluate these materials for long-term problems with respect to wound breakdown, tethered cord or other problems [1].

Reference

1. Danish SF, Samdani AF, Storm PB et al (2006) Use of allogeneic skin graft for the closure of large myelomeningoceles: Technical case report. Operative Neurosurgery 58:DNS-378

CHAPTER 16
Pathophysiology of Hydrocephalus

Giuseppe Cinalli, Pietro Spennato, Maria Consiglio Buonocore, Emilio Cianciulli,
Matthieu Vinchon, Spyros Sgouros

Incidence of Hydrocephalus in Spina Bifida Patients

The three major clinical manifestations of spina bifida (hydrocephalus, paraplegia and urinary and bowel incontinence) are easily observable and have been described since ancient times, though they were not described in relationship to spina bifida until the seventeenth century [1].

The first pathologist who came close to recognising the connection between spina bifida and hydrocephalus was Frederick Ruysch (1638-1731), whose face is familiar from Johan Van Neck's painting "Anatomy of Dr Frederick Ruysch" (1683). However, only the Italian pathologist Giovanni Battista Morgagni (1672-1771) clearly recognised the connection and that spina bifida could occur with or without hydrocephalus [2]. Gardner theorised that overdistension of the fetal neural tube caused hydrocephalomyelia and thereby explained all dysraphic states (which in his mind included the Chiari I malformation), but this interesting theory has not resisted the evidence gained from modern imaging and embryology [3].

Hydrocephalus is almost exclusively associated with the open form of spina bifida, namely myelomeningocele (MMC). Before the introduction of shunting in the early 1960s, it was the main cause of death and poor intellectual outcome in children born with myelomeningocele [4, 5].

The exact incidence of hydrocephalus in myelomeningocele is not known; however, in most surgical series the proportion of patients requiring shunting reaches 80-90% [5-7]. Correlation between the level of the spinal defect and the presence of hydrocephalus has not been shown in most series [6, 7]; however, some authors have suggested a higher incidence in thoracic level patients (97%) versus lumbar (87%) and sacral-level patients (37%) [8].

The only form of closed spinal dysraphism possibly associated with hydrocephalus is non-terminal myelocystoceles [9-11], an epithelised malformation filled with meninges and cerebrospinal fluid (CSF), which affects predominantly the cervical and upper thoracic regions [12]. The common link between open myelomeningocele and non-terminal myelocystoceles is the association with the Chiari II malformation. The presence of hydrocephalus in spina bifida patients is, in fact, almost exclusively related to the Chiari II malformation [5]. However, the incidence of such a malformation varies in the different forms of spina bifida: nearly 100% in open myelomeningocele, 44-62% in non-terminal myelocystoceles [5, 10-12]. The severity of the Chiari II malformation also differs for the two entities, with patients with open myelomeningocele being more severely affected.

Time of Onset and Prenatal Diagnosis

In immediate post-natal imaging, hydrocephalus is seen only in 15-25% of children with myelomeningocele [5, 13], often as the result of aqueductal stenosis or occlusion [14]. Thereafter hydrocephalus can be defined as congenital in only a few cases, while in a significant proportion of the remaining children it develops in the first weeks of life, usually following closure of the back lesion.

The prenatal diagnosis of hydrocephalus is possible only in the second or third trimester, because the lateral ventricles are physiologically large in the early stages of development [15, 16]. During foetal life, ventricular dilatation, with ultrasound and magnetic resonance imaging (MRI), is generally defined as an atrium larger than 10 mm. The dilatation is considered to be severe when the atrium is larger than 15 mm and mild when the atrium is between 10 and 15 mm [17].

Intrauterine ventriculomegaly is a common finding in foetuses with myelomeningocele. When performing serial sonograms Babcook et al. [18]

found that whereas only 44% of foetuses aged 24 gestational weeks or younger had ventriculomegaly, 94% of foetuses older than 24 gestational weeks had ventriculomegaly. The degree of hydrocephalus correlated with the amount of the posterior fossa deformity.

Some ultrasonographic signs in the skull, such as the lemon and banana signs (see Chapters 6, 9), characteristic of foetuses with spina bifida and the Chiari II malformation, can be demonstrated at an early stage, even in the absence of ventricular dilatation [19].

The natural history of foetal ventricular dilatation is poorly defined even in the context of spina bifida [17]. Aqueductal stenosis appears to be a factor that significantly worsens the prognosis, increasing mortality and affecting neurological development. For some authors [20], there is a significant relationship between the severity of the dilatation and future developmental delay. The prognosis is considered poor if the dilatation increases with time and, especially, if the increase in size is fast [16, 17, 21].

Late Onset Hydrocephalus

Children with a clinical picture of active hydrocephalus, with significant ventriculomegaly and, often, periventricular lucency on computed tomographic (CT) scan, require treatment early in life. Otherwise, children with mild or moderate ventriculomegaly and head circumferences within the normal range may not need treatment, but an observation policy, monitoring head circumference and neuropsychological development, repeating the ultrasound and MR imaging [5].

However, even in the absence of active hydrocephalus and progressive macrocrania, the ventricular system often remains dilated and distorted (colpocephaly). The issue of neuropsychological development in these children remains controversial [5].

It is quite common to observe older children or young adults with dilated ventricles with no clinical or radiological evidence of active hydrocephalus (headache, drowsiness, diplopia, periventricular lucency). The clinician should remember that the slow and insidious progression that characterises the evolution of this specific form of hydrocephalus might lead to a wrong diagnosis of "arrested" or "compensated" hydrocephalus, not requiring treatment: only serial IQs and psychometric testing may uncover the presence of intellectual decline [22]. In a recent study, a high incidence of intracranial hypertension has been described following intracranial pressure monitoring in patients with myelomeningocele and untreated hydrocephalus [23]. In these cases, the treatment of hydrocephalus appeared to improve IQ and overall performance (Fig. 16.1).

Therefore, these patients should be followed up with serial monitoring of intelligence and psychometric performances. Absence of clinical symptoms and stability on psychometric testing should discourage shunting. In contrast, if either subtle symptoms or evident intellectual decline is diagnosed on serial psychomotor testing, treatment or revision (in case of already implanted shunt) should be proposed. In case of doubt, invasive intracranial pressure monitoring should be employed to clarify the situation [5].

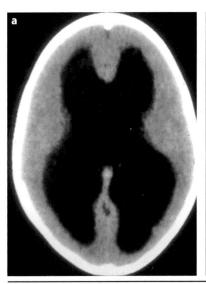
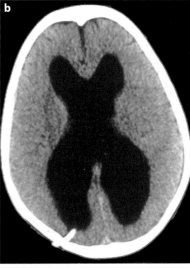

Fig. 16.1 a, b. Seven year-old girl affected by myelomeningocele and hydrocephalus. Shunted at birth, her shunt was removed at the age of 2 months because of shunt infection and never re-implanted because the hydrocephalus was considered to be "arrested". She was admitted at the age of 7 years for papilledema, macrocrania and delayed psychomotor development. **a** CT scan shows hydrocephalus. **b** Significant radiological and clinical improvement was observed after ventriculoperitoneal shunt. Reprinted from [5]

Chiari II Malformation and Hydrocephalus

Several mechanisms are implicated in the pathogenesis of hydrocephalus in patients with myelomeningoceles: aqueductal occlusion, fourth ventricular outlet obstruction, obliteration of the subarachnoid space by the crowded posterior fossa contents, obstruction at the level of the tentorial hiatus, and venous abnormalities [5, 24, 25]. These mechanisms have a common origin in the Chiari II malformation.

The Chiari II malformation is present in virtually all patients with myelomeningoceles and the majority of patients with non-terminal myelocystoceles. This malformation, first described by Hans Chiari in 1891 [26], involves the entire brain and the surrounding structures (meninges and bones), but especially the posterior fossa [25, 27]. The most characteristic finding is the hindbrain herniation; i.e., the caudal displacement of the cerebellar tonsils and vermis, together with the caudal brainstem (medulla and occasionally the pons) through an enlarged, funnel shaped foramen magnum into the cervical spinal canal (Fig. 16.2). In some instances, the brainstem becomes kinked (the medullary kink) due to the dorsal displacement of the relatively mobile medulla combined with the spinal cord being fixed by the dentate ligament (Fig. 16.3).

Often the superior vermis and cerebellar hemispheres are displaced cranially through the tentorial incisura, lying within the middle fossa, beaking the collicular plate and compressing the aqueduct (Fig. 16.4).

Associated abnormalities of the surrounding mesenchymal structures are responsible for a small posterior fossa, a low-lying tentorium with a much-enlarged tentorial incisura, a foreshortened clivus, and scalloping of the petrous bone [25]. However, the Chiari II

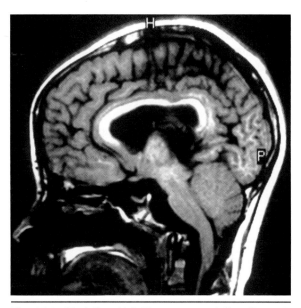

Fig. 16.3. Medullary kink. The ponto-medullary fissure is well below the level of the foramen magnum, medulla is displaced in the upper cervical canal. No CSF space is visible in the posterior fossa

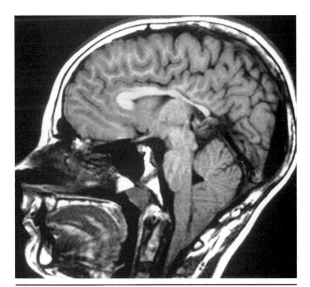

Fig. 16.2. Note the enlarged occipital foramen and the funnel-shaped upper cervical canal with the low attachment of the tentorium

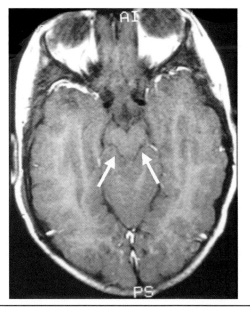

Fig. 16.4. Upward herniation of the vermis through the tentorial hiatus. Note the obliteration of the perimesencephalic cisterns, the compression and deformation of the mesencephalon (*arrows*) and the distortion and occlusion of the aqueduct

malformation also involves the supratentorial compartment: enlarged massa intermedia of the thalamus, dysgenesis of the corpus callosum, beaking of the quadrigeminal plate, polymicrogyria and cortical heterotopias are usually part of the malformation, together with characteristic deformities of the skull, such as lückenschädel or craniolacunia (characterised by irregular patches of thinning or complete erosion of the cranial vault), scalloping of the petrous pyramid, and shortening of the clivus [28]. The ventricular system appearance varies from nearly normal to severely deformed and hydrocephalic. The third ventricle is usually small, secondary to the collapse of the ventricular system during foetal life. This also results in approximation of the thalami with a large massa intermedia. The lateral ventricles, as a consequence of callosal dysgenesis, cortical heterotopias and polymicrogyria, are commonly deformed with the occipital horns disproportionately enlarged compared with the frontal horns (colpocephaly). This finding is often present even in patients with myelomeningocele who do not have hydrocephalus, and frequently persists despite shunting.

In the past it was believed that this complex malformation was part of an overall cerebrospinal dysgenesis, but there is experimental and clinical evidence that it is acquired in foetal life and progresses in severity before and after birth [18, 24].

In his initial theory, Chiari attributed the hindbrain herniation to hydrocephalus [26]. However, this theory failed to explain many of the features of the Chiari II malformation. As shown on prenatal imaging and in studies on the aborted foetal brain, hindbrain herniation is often present prior to the appearance of hydrocephalus [24]; moreover, 10-20% of children with Chiari II malformation never develop hydrocephalus [29]. In addition, the small posterior fossa, low-lying torcular herophili, and upward "herniation" of the vermis are not explained by this theory. An alternative hypothesis has been suggested by Marin-Padilla and Marin-Padilla [30], who proposed a primitive mesodermal disorder that resulted in a low-volume posterior fossa and its overcrowding as the cause of hindbrain herniation. Padget proposed a similar theory, in which chronic leaking from the open spinal defect could be the cause of an "induced" small posterior fossa [31]. However, these theories fail to explain the widespread central nervous system (CNS) abnormalities present in patients with myelomeningocele. Also the "traction" theory, in which the development of Chiari II malformation could be secondary to pulling the hindbrain caudally by the open and tethered spinal cord, resulting in the vermian and brainstem herniation [32], does not explain all the features of Chiari II malformation.

In 1989 McLone and Knepper proposed their unifying theory [33], which combined the features of the abovementioned hypotheses. According to this theory, the primum movens of the malformation is the escape of CSF from the ventricular system through the open neural tube. The absence of the CSF driving force prevents full development of the posterior fossa because both neural and calvarial development are induced by ventricular distension. At a later stage of intrauterine development, the growth of the rhombencephalon becomes more rapid; thereafter the cerebellum and the brainstem are forced into a small posterior fossa and pushed both cephalad and caudad through the tentorial incisura and foramen magnum.

The result of this disproportionate growth between the hindbrain and surrounding mesenchyme is a tightly compacted posterior fossa with little room [25]. This may also impede the development of the CSF spaces.

Several interlinked factors may impair the CSF pathway in Chiari II malformation: the vertical transhiatal translocation of the brain stem and of the cerebellum causes increased resistance to CSF flow through the tentorial incisura; crowding of the foramen magnum leads to occlusion of the foramina of Luschka and Magendie that is often not patent and the tela choroidea is dysplastic, distended and forms a sac that can extend down to the thoracic level [3, 34]. The under-developed subarachnoid space of the posterior fossa obstructs the CSF flow towards the convexity (Fig. 16.5); the small volume of the posterior fossa due to the abnormally low insertion of the tentorium may impede the egress of CSF and may also lead to venous hypertension, impeding CSF resorption [5, 25, 27]. Therefore, hydrocephalus is the result and not the cause of the Chiari II malformation.

To further support this is the observation that in the small number of children who had intrauterine repair of myelomeningocele, the incidence of hydrocephalus decreases from 91% to 59%. There is also a suggestion that this technique may prevent or reduce the severity of the Chiari II malformation [35, 36]. Tulipan et al. [37] theorise that by interrupting the continuous flow of CSF through the neural placode, the hindbrain can develop normally, and even reverse abnormal development [37]. The ascent of the hindbrain structures has been demonstrated using serial MRIs [38]. This may lead to improved flow through the aqueduct, improved compliance of CSF flow around the brain stem and the tentorial hiatus and lower venous outflow pressure in comparison with babies born with open myelomeningocele. These factors may be more important than simple ob-

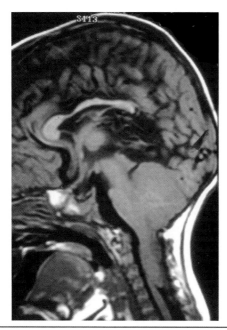

Fig. 16.5. Note the severe crowding of the posterior fossa with brainstem compression and deformation with herniation of the tonsils down to C5. Significant venous abnormalities are evident at the level of the quadrigeminal cistern

struction at the foramen magnum, considering that the incidence of hydrocephalus in patients with Chiari I malformation is much lower than in patients with Chiari II malformation [5].

The presence of Chiari II malformation in MMC often makes the clinical manifestations of hydrocephalus and of acute intracranial hypertension during shunt malfunction quite peculiar. These typically exacerbate the clinical manifestations of the Chiari II malformation, such as respiratory distress or upper extremity weakness, even in the absence of other more frequent and typical signs and symptoms of intracranial hypertension [25, 39]. The treatment of hydrocephalus usually resolves these symptoms, often avoiding the more complex (and morbid) cervical decompressive procedures [25]. For these reasons, shunt malfunction should be always suspected and ruled out when dealing with any clinical worsening of an MMC patient.

Due to anatomical anomalies of the ventricular system (enlarged massa intermedia, eccentric bulge from the head of the caudate nucleus and anteriorly pointing frontal horns) associated with the Chiari II malformation, the foramen of Monro is particularly predisposed to torsion and obstruction if overdrainage occurs, possibly resulting in isolated lateral ventricles after unilateral shunt placement [40, 41].

Role of Aqueductal Stenosis

Obstruction of the sylvian aqueduct is frequently found in MMC patients (Fig. 16.6a). It is secondary to deformation of the midbrain, which is forced both craniocaudally and ventrodorsally; the tectal plate assumes a beak like configuration, so that the aqueduct is progressively angulated to the point that, in more severe cases, it assumes a V-shape pointing dorsally (Figs. 16.4, 16.6b). This, combined with the

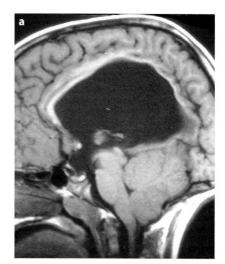

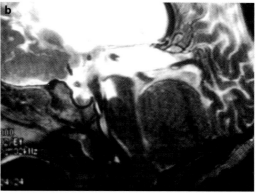

Fig. 16.6 a, b. **a** Myelomeningocele patient at the time of shunt malfunction. Note the aqueductal stenosis. Agenesis of the tentorium allows downward herniation of the lateral ventricles with obliteration of the posterior third ventricle, direct compression of the upper vermis, obliteration of the fourth ventricle and creation of a functional aqueductal obliteration. **b** Following endoscopic third ventriculostomy, significant anatomical changes are evident: the posterior third ventricle has reappeared, the aqueduct has enlarged assuming the typical V-shape pointing anteriorly, compression of the vermis has reversed with appearance of the quadrigeminal cistern, but the fourth ventricle remains compressed and obliterated. The real cause of hydrocephalus in this case was not aqueductal stenosis but fourth ventricle and posterior fossa CSF space obliteration due to the hindbrain herniation

crowding of the tentorial hiatus, creates a functional obstruction (Fig. 16.6) [28]. Histologically, agenesis, stenosis or forking of the aqueduct is a classical feature in MMC, reported in Dandy's pioneering work [42], which Gilbert found at autopsy in roughly half of MMC patients [43]. The autopsy bias may have exaggerated this figure, and this author gave no indication as to whether stenosis was malformative or secondary to infection, hemorrhage, or shunting (Fig. 16.7a, b). When live patients studied with ventriculography were considered along with autopsy data, the prevalence of aqueductal stenosis was substantially lower, around 29% [44]. In live patients studied with ventriculography at birth, the aqueduct was often stenosed but never totally occluded [34]. Forking of the aqueduct, along with beaking of the tectal plate, may be part of the deformation of the brainstem caused by hydrocephalus, rather than its *primum movens*. The contribution of obstruction of the aqueduct to the pathogenesis of hydrocephalus in patients with myelomeningocele is under debate; in fact, in contrast to typical aqueductal stenosis, the remaining CSF pathways are also abnormal and deformed [5]. Some authors have even postulated that the obstruction of the aqueduct could be the consequence of long-standing hydrocephalus, which causes axial herniation and entrapment of the midbrain with secondary compression of the ependymal surfaces of the aqueduct, leading to obstruction [45].

As a result, in patients affected by myelomeningocele and hydrocephalus, the finding of an obstructed or stenosed aqueduct is no guarantee in itself of a good outcome after endoscopic treatment.

In neuroimaging obtained early after birth in children born with severe hydrocephalus, a large third and a small fourth ventricle are usually seen, indicating the important role of aqueductal stenosis at least in congenital cases [5, 14].

While hydrocephalus in children born with myelomeningocele is always related to Chiari II malformation, in other forms of spina bifida, such as nonterminal myelocystocele, it may also occur with no evidence of hindbrain herniation. In these rare cases aqueductal stenosis has been suspected to play a determinant role in the pathogenesis of hydrocephalus [12].

Role of Venous Hypertension

The driving force for CSF resorption is the difference between CSF pressure and sagittal sinus pressure. In the presence of Chiari II malformation, the small posterior fossa volume and the abnormal anatomical disposition of the structures within it can lead to the com-

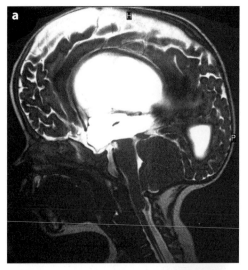

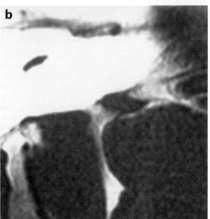

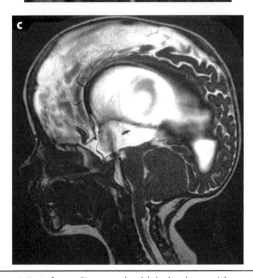

Fig. 16.7 a, b. a Six month-old baby boy with myelomeningocele, not shunted at birth, presenting with progressive macrocrania and hydrocephalus. **b** Note the deformation of the aqueduct that looks open but is filled by a web-like material. CSF spaces of the posterior fossa are well represented except at the level of the occipital foramen. **c** Hydrocephalus was successfully treated by endoscopic third ventriculostomy

pression of the sigmoid sinuses, which leads to venous hypertension [46]. Compression of the internal cerebral veins, due to deformation of the midbrain, may also contribute to venous hypertension (Fig. 16.5) [5]. Usually, collateral venous pathways, through the foramen magnum and/or through emissary veins and scalp veins, progressively develop and allow a new status quo to develop [47]. However, crowding of the foramen magnum due to cerebellar herniation may prevent the development of collateral venous pathways. If the venous obstruction is not compensated, the increasing of the sagittal sinus pressure results in a higher CSF pressure being required to maintain CSF balance. The final effect depends also on the degree of cranial and brain compliance. In children with closed sutures, intracranial pressure may rise to very high levels, overcoming the high sagittal sinus pressure; this permits absorption of CSF, with normal-sized or small ventricles, as seen in some cases of pseudotumor cerebri [47]; in infants and children with open sutures, the rise in CSF pressure may result in progressive hydrocephalus and intracranial hypertension [47].

The treatment of hydrocephalus with shunting does not necessarily improve the venous compression because the original cause is not removed. Otherwise, reduction of CSF pressure with shunting may result in accumulation of interstitial fluid and contribute to deterioration of aqueductal stenosis due to interstitial oedema [5, 46]. Intracranial hypertension can thus become a self-aggravating phenomenon, with an element of pseudotumor cerebri causing "normal volume hydrocephalus" with compression of the lateral sinuses [48]. When MMC patients grow old, obesity caused by diminished catabolism often becomes a serious concern, and raised systemic venous pressure can also interact with intracranial pressure.

Surgical procedures of internal diversion of CSF (endoscopic third ventriculostomy [ETV]), bypassing aqueductal occlusion and increasing brain compliance, may be useful in these situations [5, 49]. As the patients get older however, a higher proportion can be treated with endoscopic procedures [50]; this tends to show that with time intraventricular obstructive factors become prevalent over extraventricular ones.

Role of Closure of Myelomeningocele

The onset of hydrocephalus is often temporally related to the surgical closure of the spinal defect. It is not clear whether this is a causative relationship, or whether the operation simply precipitates an inevitable event [5]. Very rarely, the babies deteriorate dramatically following closure of the neural sac. The mechanism of this deterioration is multifactorial. Closure of the myelomeningocele may eliminate the spinal defect as a drainage pathway [38]. A significant role appears to be played by the impaction of the hindbrain herniation [5]. As already mentioned, the primary cause of hindbrain herniation is in utero escape of CSF through the open neural tube. Further loss of CSF during the first days of life and during the surgical closure of the defect may result in deterioration of the herniation of the hindbrain and the associated hydrocephalus [5], leading to acute neurological deterioration. This is secondary to intracranial hypertension related to the hydrocephalus and to brain stem dysfunction related to impaction of the hindbrain in the foramen magnum. Shunting usually reverses this neurological status [5, 13].

Role of Associated Cerebral Malformations

Spina bifida is one of the commonest congenital malformations and may be associated with several other malformations directly or indirectly related to the neural tube defect [5, 51]. Some of these may further impair CSF pathways. Severe forms of dysraphism, with the presence of bifid cranium, cervical myelomeningocele, and encephalocele are associated with a high incidence of severe hydrocephalus and a poor prognosis [5].

A non-random association between neural tube defects (anencephaly, spina bifida) and holoprosencephaly has been reported [51], indicating a possible common insult occurring early in embryological life [52]. Usually such an association is not compatible with life and had been described in about 20% of aborted embryos or foetuses with myeloschisis [53]. However, viable infants affected by both malformations have been reported [52]. In these cases, atresia of the aqueduct of Sylvius, secondary to mesencephalosynapsis and/or rhomboencephalosynapsis (fusion on the midline of the colliculi and/or cerebellar hemispheres) may be responsible for the severe congenital hydrocephalus [51].

Subependymal grey matter heterotopias are often part of Chiari II malformation. Occasionally, they may project into the ventricles, causing narrowing and, possibly, obstructing crucial areas (foramen of Monro) [54].

Arachnoid Thickening

Another factor that could explain the lower incidence of hydrocephalus following uterine reparation of

MMC is the possible resolution of subarachnoid space contamination with amniotic fluid. In fact, the arachnoid of patients with MMC is frequently thickened, especially at the level of the foramen magnum [55] and tentorial incisura [56]. In an experiment published in 1935 (and not in accordance with present ethical standards), Russell found that when India ink was injected into the ventricles of moribund MMC patients, postmortem study found that its diffusion was restricted to the spinal meninges, although in some cases, a faint supratentorial diffusion was found; she concluded that the degree of obstruction of the ventricles was variable [57]. The free communication between the arachnoid space and the amnion during intrauterine life, illustrated by spontaneous pneumocephalus diagnosed at birth [58], has raised the hypothesis that prenatal meningeal irritation by amniotic fluid could induce chronic arachnoiditis, thus adding a potential additional factor to the complex pathophysiology of hydrocephalus in MMC (Fig. 16.8).

Among 116 foetuses operated in utero for MMC and followed at least one year after birth, the shunting rate was 58%, compared to 93% in a historical cohort (MMC operated at birth in the same institution) [59, 60]. As early prenatal closing of the MMC (hence a shorter duration of exposition to amniotic fluid) appeared to be a decisive factor for the prevention of hydrocephalus in myelomeningocele (MMH), these authors considered that these data back the hypothesis that exposition to amniotic fluid plays a role in the pathogenesis of MMH [59]. However, the two groups of patients compared (before and after the introduction of intra-uterine repair) were not contemporary, the follow-up was short, and several biases restrict the reach of these figures. In particular, antenatal hydrocephalus is considered a contraindication for in utero repair; and having endured an in utero repair is also a strong motivation for the child's parents to resist shunting at birth. Furthermore, as will be discussed below, the rate of shunting in patients operated after birth may be as low as 51%, depending on the surgeon's tolerance to ventriculomegaly [61]. These data are not sufficient to ascertain the role of meningeal fibrosis as a causative factor in MMH.

Moreover, intrauterine surgery appears to increase the risk of several obstetrical complications, such as oligohydramnios, premature rupture of membranes, premature uterine contractions, premature delivery, uterine ruptures, placental abruption and maternal bowel obstruction [62, 63]. Finally, the apparent benefit may be due to selection bias; in fact, only a small number of mothers and foetuses in very good condition are considered for intrauterine repair. Only a prospective, randomised trial will be able to answer these concerns.

Communicating or Obstructive Hydrocephalus?

This issue is not without importance, due to the widespread use of ETV in the treatment of obstructive hydrocephalus in the last decade. ETV has been proposed in the management of hydrocephalus with myelomeningocele since the mid 90s, but its role remains controversial. The results, especially in the cases where ETV has been performed as first line of treatment in younger babies, are not encouraging, with a success rate rarely exceeding 30% [64-66], indicating that, in these patients, the form of hydrocephalus is mainly of the communicating type. Better results were achieved in older patients who underwent ETV as a secondary procedure at the time of shunt malfunction, in whom the reported success rate is above 70% in most series [64-66]. These data indicate a mainly obstructive hydrocephalus in older children. However, some authors failed to observe significant differences in relation to age and previous shunting [67, 68].

Recently, specific CSF biomarkers (transforming growth factor α1 [TGFα1] and aminoterminal propeptide of type 1 collagen [PC1NP]) have been found to be indicative of growth factor- and fibro-

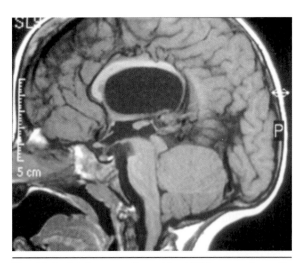

Fig. 16.8. Adolescent affected by MMC presenting with shunt malfunction. Endoscopic third ventriculostomy was attempted but resulted in a technical failure. After perforation of the third ventricular floor, dense arachnoid scarring completely filling the interpeduncular cistern was found, making communication with open subarachnoid spaces impossible. Retrospectively, dense web-like material is visible in the interpeduncular cistern on pre-operative MRI

sis-related CSF malabsorption in hydrocephalic patients [69, 70]. Thereafter, finding of such biomarkers in CSF samples could discriminate between the presence and the absence of CSF malabsorption, which should indicate communicating hydrocephalus. Heep et al. [71], assessing CSF samples during interventions performed in hydrocephalic infants, found relative low TGFα1 and PC1NP CSF concentrations in spina bifida patients and aqueductal stenosis patients, compared with high values in case of post-haemorrhagic hydrocephalus. These data indicate that, in spina bifida and non-haemorrhagic triventricular hydrocephalus, CSF obstruction, rather than malabsorption, may play a pivotal role in the pathogenesis of hydrocephalus [71].

The recent views on the pathophysiology of hydrocephalus enhance the importance of intracranial compliance that is widely dependent on the free movement of the CSF between the cranial and the spinal subarachnoid spaces. According to Greitz [49], any processes that interfere with the expansion of the arteries in the subarachnoid space and with the pulsatile CSF flow may cause communicating hydrocephalus. In Chiari I and II malformations, the impairment to the pulsatile flow at the level of the foramen magnum may be the main cause of hydrocephalus. In these cases intracranial compliance may be restored by posterior fossa decompression, which simply recreates communication with the compliant spinal canal [49]. The diversion of CSF following shunting also increases brain compliance because it causes a forced dilation of the compressed cortical veins. This increases venous compliance, decreases vascular resistance and increases cerebral blood flow [49]. Greitz also considers third ventriculostomy potentially successful in these forms of hydrocephalus [49]. The surgically created opening into the subarachnoid space ultimately should reduce the intraventricular pulse pressure, due to increased expulsion of ventricular CSF during systole. This in turn will reduce the transmantle pulsatile stress, reduce ventricular size and expand the subarachnoid spaces including the compressed cortical veins, thus again restoring intracranial compliance and cerebral blood flow.

The predominant features of hydrocephalus in children with myelomeningocele are often not clear; moreover, they may also change over time. In infants, the subarachnoid spaces' deformation and immaturity combined with the increased venous outflow resistance prevail, consequently justifying the low success rate of ETV and warranting the placement of an extrathecal CSF shunt device. However, venous hypertension would not be corrected by the procedure, subsequently leading to an accumulation of interstitial fluid which in turn would worsen the aqueductal stenosis and change the hydrocephalus from mainly communicating, to a mainly obstructive type [5, 64]. Shunting itself may be responsible for the change of the hydrocephalus from an obstructive type [72]. Placement of a ventriculo-peritoneal shunt diverts CSF to the abdominal cavity, allowing the CSF spaces to re-expand. The procedure also may induce or exacerbate an acquired aqueductal stenosis through continuous CSF diversion. This, together with re-expansion of the subarachnoid spaces, makes it more likely that a third ventriculostomy will be successful at a later date when a shunt malfunction occurs.

Conclusion

The pathophysiology of hydrocephalus in myelomeningocele is multifactorial. Aqueductal stenosis, occlusion of the foramina of Lushcka and Magendie, hindbrain herniation, obliteration of the subarachnoid spaces at the level of the posterior fossa, compression of the sigmoid sinuses with consequent venous hypertension and fibrosis of the subarachnoid spaces, are the pathophysiological factors thus far described. Each of these can induce hydrocephalus by themselves, with several if not all of them present in the same patient, and the severity of each of these factors changes over a lifetime. This leads to the pathophysiology of hydrocephalus in the same patient being completely different in the neonatal period, compared to his adolescence or his adulthood, and explains the varied response to different treatment methods according to the patient's age.

References

1. Smith GK (2001) The history of spina bifida, hydrocephalus, paraplegia and incontinence. Pediatr Surg Int 17:424-432
2. Morgagni GB (1960) The seats and causes of diseases investigated by anatomy in 5 Books, Bk 1, Letter 12. Translated from the Latin by Benjamin Alexander, vol. 1. Hafner (1760) New York, pp 244-274
3. Gardner WJ (1965) Hydrodynamic mechanism of syringomyelia: its relationship to myelocele. J Neurol Neurosurg Psychiatr 28:247-259
4. Laurence KM, Coates S (1962) The natural history of hydrocephalus. Detailed analysis of 182 unoperated cases. Arch Dis Child 37:345-362
5. Sgouros S (2004) Hydrocephalus with myelomeningo-

cele. In: Cinalli G, Maixner WJ, Sainte-Rose C (eds) Pediatric hydrocephalus. Springer-Verlag, Italia, pp 133-144

6. Mirzai H, Erşahin Y, Mutluer S, Kayahan A (1998) Outcome of patients with meningomyelocele: The Ege University experience. Childs Nerv Syst 14:120-123

7. Steinbok P, Irvine B, Cochrane DD, Irwin BJ (1992) Long-term outcome and complications of children born with meningomyelocele. Childs Nerv Syst 8:92-96

8. Rintoul NE, Sutton LN, Hubbard AM et al (2002) A new look at myelomeningoceles: functional level, vertebral level, shunting, and the implications for fetal intervention. Pediatrics 109:409-413

9. Nishino A, Shirane R, So K et al (1998) Cervical myelocystocele with Chiari II malformation: Magnetic resonance imaging and surgical treatment. Surg Neurol 49:269-273

10. Pang D, Dias MS (1993) Cervical myelomeningoceles. Neurosurgery 33:363-372

11. Rossi A, Piatelli G, Gandolfo C, Pavanello M et al (2006) Spectrum of nonterminal myelocystoceles. Neurosurgery 58:509-15

12. Salomao JF, Cavalheiro S, Matushita H et al (2006) Cystic spinal dysraphism of the cervical and upper thoracic region. Childs Nerv Syst 22:234-42

13. Dias MS, McLone DG (1993) Hydrocephalus in the child with dysraphism. Neurosurg Clin N Am 4:715-726

14. Rekate HL (1991-1992) Shunt revision: complications and their prevention. Pediatr Neurosurg 17:155-162

15. Aubry MC, Aubry JP, Dommergues M (2003) Sonographic prenatal diagnosis of central nervous system abnormalities. Childs Nerv Syst 19:391-402

16. Wilhelm C, Keck C, Hess S et al (1998) Ventriculomegaly diagnosed by prenatal ultrasound and mental development of the children. Fetal Diagn Ther 13:162-166

17. Garel C, Luton D, Oury JF, Gressens P (2003) Ventricular dilatations. Childs Nerv Syst 19:517-523

18. Babcook CJ, Goldstein RB, Barth RA (1994) Prevalence of ventriculomegaly in association with myelomeningocele. Radiology 190:703-707

19. Van der Hof MC, Nicolaides KH, Campbell J, Campbell S (1991) Evaluation of the lemon and banana signs in one hundred thirty fetuses with open spina bifida. Am J Obstet Gynecol 162:322-327

20. Bloom SL, Bloom DD, Dellanebbia C et al (1997) The developmental outcome of children with antenatal mild isolated ventriculomegaly. Obstet Gynecol 90:93-97

21. Gupta JK, Bryce FC, Lilford RJ (1994) Management of apparently isolated fetal ventriculomegaly. Obstet Gynecol Surv 49:716-721

22. Hammond MK, Milhorat TH, Baron IS (1976) Normal pressure hydrocephalus in patients with myelomeningocele. Dev Med Child Neurol Suppl 37:55-68

23. Iborra J, Pages E, Cuxart A et al (2000) Increased intracranial pressure in myelomeningocele (MMC) patients never shunted: results of a prospective preliminary study. Spinal Cord 38:495-497

24. McLone DG, Nakahara S, Knepper PA (1991) Chiari II malformation: pathogenesis and dynamics. Concepts Pediatr Neurosurg 11:1-17

25. McLone DG, Dias MS (2003) The Chiari II malformation: cause and impact. Childs Nerv Syst 19:540-550

26. Chiari H (1891) Uber Veränderungen des Kleinhirns infolge von Hydrocephaliedes Grosshirns. Dtsch Med Wschr 17:1172-1175

27. Stevenson KL (2004) Chiari Type II malformation: past, present, and future. Neurosurg Focus 16(2):Article 5

28. Naidich TP, Pudlowski RM, Naidich JB et al (1980) Computed tomographic signs of the Chiari II malformation. Part I: skull and dural partitions. Radiology 134:65-71

29. Rekate HL (1984) To shunt or not to shunt: hydrocephalus and dysraphism. Clin Neurosurg 32:593-607

30. Marin-Padilla M, Marin-Padilla TM (1981) Morphogenesis of experimentally induced Arnold-Chiari malformation. J Neurol Sci 50:29-55

31. Padget DH (1972) Development of so-called dysraphism; with embryologic evidence of clinical Arnold-Chiari and Dandy-Walker malformations. Johns Hopkins Med J 130:127-165

32. Penfield W, Coburn DF (1938) Arnold-Chiari malformation and its operative treatment. Arch Neurol Psychiatry 40:328-336

33. McLone DG, Knepper PA (1989) The cause of Chiari II malformation: a unified theory. Pediatr Neurosci 15:1-12

34. Andreussi L, Clarisse J, Jomin M et al (1977) Diagnostic value of water-soluble contrast iodoventriculography in the study of Arnold-Chiari syndrome. Mod Probl Paediatr 18:137-141

35. Tulipan N (2003) Intrauterine myelomeningocele repair. Clin Perinatol 30:521-530

36. Tulipan N, Hernanz-Schulman M, Bruner JP (1998) Reduced hindbrain herniation after intrauterine myelomeningocele repair: a report of four cases. Pediatr Neurosurg 29:274-278

37. Tulipan N, Hernanz-Schulman M, Lowe LH et al (1999) Intrauterine myelomeningocele repair reverses preexisting hindbrain herniation. Pediatr Neurosurg 31:137-142

38. Sutton L, Adzick N, Bilaniuk L et al (1999) Improvement in hindbrain herniation demonstrated by serial fetal magnetic resonance imaging following fetal surgery for myelomeningocele. JAMA 282:1826-1831

39. Holinger PC, Holinger LD, Reichert TJ et al (1978) Respiratory obstruction and apnea in infants with bilateral abductor vocal cord paralysis, meningomyelocele, hydrocephalus, and Arnold-Chiari malformation. J Pediatr 92:368-373

40. Berger MS, Sundsten J, Lemire RJ et al (1990) Pathophysiology of isolated lateral ventriculomegaly in shunt myelodysplastic children. Pediatr Neurosurg 16:301-304

41. Spennato P, Cinalli G, Carannante G et al (2004) Multiloculated hydrocephalus. In: Cinalli G, Maixner WJ, Saint-Rose C (eds) Pediatric hydrocephalus. Springer-Verlag, Milan, pp 219-244

42. Dandy WE, Blackfan KD (1914) Internal hydrocephalus: an experimental, clinical and pathological study. Am J Dis Child 8: 406-482

43. Gilbert JN, Jones KL, Rorke LB et al (1986) Central nervous system anomalies associated with meningomyelocele, hydrocephalus, and the Arnold-Chiari malformation: reappraisal of theories regarding the pathogenesis of posterior neural tube closure defects. Neurosurgery 18: 559-564

44. Shurtleff DB, Kronmal R, Foltz EL (1975) Follow-up comparison of hydrocephalus with and without myelomeningocele. J Neurosurg 42: 61-68

45. Williams B (1975) Cerebrospinal fluid pressure-gradients in spina bifida cystica, with special reference to Arnold-Chiari malformation and aqueductal stenosis. Dev Med Child Neurol Suppl 35:138-150

46. Andweg J (1989) Intracranial venous pressures, hydrocephalus and effects on cerebrospinal fluid shunts. Childs Nerv Syst 5:318-323

47. Sainte-Rose C, LaCombe J, Pierre-Khan A et al (1984) Intracranial venous sinus hypertension: cause or consequence of hydrocephalus in infants? J Neurosurg 60:727-736

48. Nadkarni TD, Rekate HL (2005) Treatment of refractory intracranial hypertension in a spina bifida patient by a concurrent ventricular and cisterna magna-to-peritoneal shunt. Childs Nerv Syst 21:579-582

49. Greitz D (2004) Radiological assessment of hydrocephalus: new theories and implications for therapy. Neurosurg Rev 27:145-165

50. Teo C, Jones R (1996) Management of hydrocephalus by endoscopic third ventriculostomy in patients with myelomeningocele. Pediatr Neurosurg 25:57-63

51. Encha-Razavi F (2003) Identification of brain malformations: neuropathological approach. Childs Nerv Syst 19:448-454

52. Rollins N, Joglar J, Perlman J (1999) Coexistent holoprosencephaly and Chiari II malformation. AJNR Am J Neuroradiol 20:1678-1681

53. Osaka J, Tanimura T, Hirayama A et al (1978) Myelomeningocele before birth. J Neurosurg 49:711-724

54. Chen CY, Zimmerman RA (2000) Congenital brain anomalies. In: Zimmerman RA, Gibby WA, Carmody RG (Eds) Neuroimaging: clinical and physical principles. Springer-Verlag, New York, pp 491-530

55. Friede RL (1989) Developmental neuropathology. Springer, Berlin Heidelberg

56. Pavez A, Salazar C, Rivera R et al (2006) Description of endoscopic ventricular anatomy in myelomeningocele. Minim Invas Neurosurg 49:161-167

57. Russell Dorothy S (1935) The mechanism of internal hydrocephalus in spina bifida. Brain 58:203-215

58. Garonzik IM, Samdani AF, Carson BS, Avellino A (2001) Pneumocephalus in a newborn with an open myelomeningocele. Pediatr Neurosurg 35:334

59. Tulipan N, Sutton LN, Bruner JP et al (2003) The effect of intrauterine myelomeningocele repair on the incidence of shunt-dependent hydrocephalus. Pediatr Neurosurg 38:27-33

60. Bruner JP, Tulipan N, Reed G et al (2004) Intrauterine repair of spina bifida: preoperative predictors of shunt-dependent hydrocephalus. Am J Obstetr Gynecol 190:1305-1312

61. Crimmins D, Hayward RD, Thompson DNP (2005) Reducing shunt placement rate in myelomeningocele patients (abstr). Childs Nerv Syst 21:828-829

62. Bruner JP, Tulipan N, Paschall RL et al (1999) Fetal surgery for myelomeningocele and the incidence of shunt dependent hydrocephalus. JAMA 282:1819-1825

63. Simpson JL (1999) Fetal surgery for myelomeningocele: promise, progress and problems. JAMA 17:1873-1874

64. Di Rocco C, Cinalli G, Massimi L et al (2006) Endoscopic third ventriculostomy in the treatment of hydrocephalus in pediatric patients. Adv Tech Stand Neurosurg 31:119-219

65. Fritsch MJ, Mehdorn HM (2003) Indication and controversies for endoscopic third ventriculostomy in children. Childs Nerv Syst 19:706-707

66. Teo C, Jones R (1996) Management of hydrocephalus by endoscopic third ventriculostomy in patients with myelomeningocele. Pediatr Neurosurg 25:57-63

67. Portillo S, Zuccaro G, Fernandez-Molina A et al (2004) Endoscopic third ventriculostomy in the treatment of pediatric hydrocephalus. A multicentric study. Childs Nerv Syst 20: 666-667

68. Tamburrini G, Caldarelli M, Massimi L et al (2004) Primary and secondary third ventriculostomy in children with hydrocephalus and myelomeningocele. Childs Nerv Syst 20:666

69. Tada T, Kanaji M, Kobayashi S (1994) Induction of communicating hydrocephalus in mice by intrathecal injection of human recombinant transforming growth factor-beta 1. J Neuroimmunol 50:153-158

70. Wyss-Coray T, Feng L, Masliah E et al (1995) Increased central nervous system production of extracellular matrix components and development of hydrocephalus in transgenic mice overexpressing transforming growth factor-beta 1. Am J Pathol 147:53-67

71. Heep A, Bartmann P, Stoffel-Wagner B et al (2006) Cerebrospinal fluid obstruction and malabsorption in human neonatal hydrocephaly. Childs Nerv Syst 22:1249-1255

72. O'Brien DF, Javadpour M, Collins DR et al (2005) Endoscopic third ventriculostomy: an outcome analysis of primary cases and procedures performed after ventriculoperitoneal shunt malfunction. J Neurosurg (5 Suppl Pediatrics) 103:393-400

CHAPTER 17
Hydrocephalus in Myelomeningocele: Shunts and Problems with Shunts

Matthieu Vinchon, Patrick Dhellemmes

Introduction

Hydrocephalus (HC) is a major problem for the majority of patients with myelomeningocele (MM). Historically, the correlation of MM with HC was suspected as early as 1769 by Morgagni [1], who hypothesized that an excess of fluid caused both the spinal cyst and the hydrocephalus. He was, however, unable to explain the relationship in more detail, and his theory had to await a better understanding of the circulation of cerebrospinal fluid (CSF) in the twentieth century, with the works of Dandy and Blackfan, to gain approval [2]. Gardner imagined that overdistension of the fetal neural tube caused hydrocephalomyelia and explained all dysraphic states (which in his mind included the Chiari I malformation), but this interesting theory has not been upheld in face of the evidence gained from modern imaging and embryology [3]. The pathophysiology of MM-related HC (MMH) is still a matter of debate, with important therapeutic implications; in particular the role of prenatal meningeal irritation caused by the amniotic fluid, and the putative effect of in utero surgery [4].

Until shunts were introduced in the late fifties, HC was generally a death sentence for patients with MM, and those who survived with "arrested" HC had a severe handicap due to brain atrophy [5]. Although shunts have dramatically improved these patients' outlooks, shunt-related morbidity and mortality, as well as long-term outcome, are poorly documented in the literature.

In the present chapter, we shall deal with hydrocephalus in myelomeningocele, and its treatment with shunts; the role of endoscopic treatment in myelomeningocele is hotly debated, and is the subject of the following chapter. We shall try to address unanswered questions by studying the data available in the literature, as well as the clinical material obtained from our database. Our department is the sole referral facility for pediatric neurosurgery in a population of 4 million people. Data have been stored since the mid-seventies, and our database now counts 452 cases of myelomeningocele, of which 363 were treated actively, and 293 were shunted. In order to compare patients with MMH to patients with other causes of hydrocephalus, we also reviewed 1,405 other children treated with permanent shunts during the same period. For statistical analysis, continuous variables were studied using Student's t-test, binary variables were studied using the Chi-square test, and survival analysis was performed with the Kaplan-Meier method using the log-rank test for statistical significance; all statistics were made using the commercially available software SPSS 11.5 for Windows.

Prevalence of Hydrocephalus in Myelomeningocele Patients

Although MM and HC are closely linked in the minds of neurosurgeons, the prevalence of shunted HC in MM varies between series published in the literature, according to the tolerance of the clinicians and to selection biases. Initially, the tenet "when in doubt, shunt" was the regular attitude in most institutions [5]; more recently, neurosurgeons have become aware of the additional burden represented by the shunt, and some have elected to avoid shunting whenever possible, with shunting rates falling from 77% in the 1980s to 58% in recent years as a result [6]. Where surgeons are particularly motivated not to insert a shunt in newborns with MM, the prevalence of hydrocephalus may be as low as 51% [7], but generally, the prevalence is no less than 80% [8, 9]. In developing countries, the prevalence of shunting can be as low as 53% for the opposite reason, because early referral is the exception rather than the rule, and HC confers a grim natural selection of patients [10].

In all series, the rate of shunting is also closely associated with the anatomical level of the myelomeningocele [10, 11]. Tulipan reported that shunts were inserted in 100% of patients with thoracic MM, versus 87% and 67% of patients with lumbar and sacral MM, respectively [4]. The mechanism linking the level of the MM to the likelihood of shunting is unclear. Greater meningeal contamination with amniotic fluid has been proposed, as well as greater loss of CSF pulsatility at the cranial level, to explain the higher prevalence of HC in high-level MM. Another explanation is that high-level and low-level MM are two different entities, resulting from defects at different stages of the closure of the neural tube [12].

Another bias influencing the prevalence of HC is antenatal diagnosis, because in many cases the attention of the obstetrician is first drawn by the dilatation of the ventricles, and the MM is identified after a closer look on the spine; as a result, MM without HC is more likely to go undetected. Pregnancies involving fetuses with MMH are more likely to be interrupted because the presence of HC has a pejorative prognostic value, and is more often associated with a higher level of the MM, another potent negative prognostic factor. In our series, in spite of these selection biases and of our reluctance to shunt unless absolutely necessary, 80.7% of the patients with MM were shunted, while MMH represented 20.8% of our shunted population.

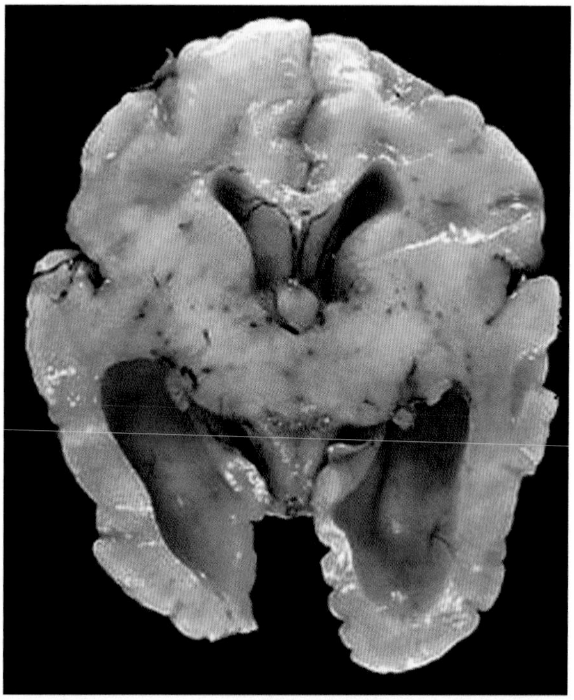

Fig. 17.1. Pathological specimen: horizontal cut of the brain of a 34-week fetus with myelomeningocele and hydrocephalus. Note the thin cerebral mantle, and the prominent massa intermedia. Courtesy of Dr. L. Devisme

Diagnosis

Prenatal Diagnosis

The diagnosis of MMH is often made during antenatal ultrasound studies, and HC is often the first clue leading to the diagnosis of MM (Fig. 17.1). However, the brain can be totally normal in fetuses with MM, especially on ultrasound studies performed during the second trimester of pregnancy [13]. MMH becomes apparent between 17 and 39 weeks [14]; the cranial image of ventricular festooning, also referred to as the "lemon deformation" (Fig. 17.2) is characteristic, as well as the "banana sign", heralding the Chiari malformation. However, antenatal diagnosis is often falsely negative: HC is diagnosed in only 30.9% of cases of MM, in contrast with the rate of postnatal MMH. Conversely, in fetuses with MMH, the myelomeningocele is missed in 24% of cases, and both HC and MM are missed in up to 57% of cases [15]. An important element of the decision to interrupt or continue the pregnancy is based on the fact that prenatal-onset MMH is associated with a poor developmental prognosis [16]. Although ultrasonography is generally enough to diagnose MMH,

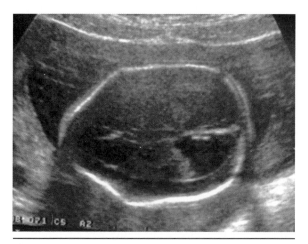

Fig. 17.2. Antenatal ultrasound showing the typical frontal festooning, the so-called lemon skull. Courtesy of Dr. A.S. Vallat

and to assess the gravity of MM [17], magnetic resonance imaging (MRI) may have an important role in studying the central nervous system in more detail, in particular, in the diagnosis of associated cerebral malformations such as microgyria or dysplasia of the corpus callosum.

Postnatal Diagnosis

Overt hydrocephalus is present at birth in 15-25% of cases of MM [18]. MMH is often associated with head deformation characteristic of the "lemon skull" (Fig. 17.3). The child may present with the classical features of intracranial hypertension (tense fontanel, poor feeding, irritability, "sun-setting" gaze), but can often be surprisingly normal. HC is then diagnosed on systematic ultrasound and due to the abnormally rapid growth of head circumference. The absence of CSF leakage in spite of a ruptured MM has been interpreted as indicative of obstructive HC [19].

In other cases, HC becomes apparent after repair of the MM, because of closure of the spinal outlet, or of loss of the cyst's absorptive capacities. MMH manifests itself by subcutaneous collection or CSF leakage through the wound, or signs and symptoms of raised intracranial pressure [18]. One of the main concerns for the surgeon is the risk of spinal wound breakdown leading to meningeal infection. Infection is the cause of both mortality and morbidity [20], precludes the insertion of a definitive shunt, and is difficult to treat by external drainage as the ventricles are not dilated when CSF leaks. MMH can also manifest itself by life-threatening signs and symptoms of brainstem compression due to the Chiari malformation, in particular, neonatal stridor [21].

In rare cases, patients with MM who have escaped shunting at birth may become shunt-dependent later due to secondary events, such as surgery for Chiari malformation or spinal cord untethering [9]. Late-onset MMH may manifest itself with the guise of spinal cord dysfunction. Hall reported a high rate of success when shunting MM patients presenting with scoliosis; he considered scoliosis as "the most common clinical manifestation of unshunted hydrocephalus in the older myelocystocele patient" [22].

Imaging

The most useful imaging tool for the diagnosis of MMH at birth is ultrasonography, because it can be easily obtained and repeated. It shows the characteristic deformation of the frontal horns ("bat wing image"); as in all newborns, the fourth ventricle is small, which may be falsely interpreted as obstructive HC [7]. Only a rounded and enlarged third ventricle contrasting with a small fourth ventricle is a reliable criterion of obstructive HC [19, 23]. MRI has few indications at birth, and is not devoid of complications, because of the risk of respiratory problems related to brainstem dysfunction [18]. MRI is useful in older patients to assess other cerebral anomalies in order to evaluate their developmental prognosis. It is also of paramount importance when the question of endoscopic treatment arises or in complicated cases for which alternative treatments need to be discussed [24].

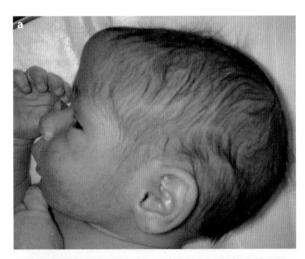
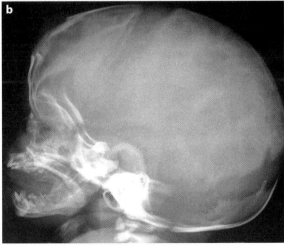

Fig. 17.3 a, b. a Newborn girl with the typically enlarged and bulging metopic suture. **b** Plain X-ray showing dysplasia of the frontal bone in the same patient; note the widening of the coronal and lambdoid sutures due to active hydrocephalus

Treatment with Shunts

Indications for Treatment or Abstention

In all cases of symptomatic HC, surgical treatment is necessary, and generally consists of shunting. Classically, abstention of shunting can be licit only when the child has no signs of brainstem dysfunction, the cortical mantle is thicker than 3.5 cm, and development is normal [5]. However, with time, our reluctance to shunt MM patients has increased, reflecting our better knowledge of shunt-related complications, of the possibility of shunt-independence in MM, and our ability to monitor patients non-invasively. Also, our tolerance toward ventricular dilatation has increased with experience gained from patients treated endoscopically for other diseases. Patients who reach the age of 5 months without a shunt can be considered as shunt-independent with a reasonable degree of confidence [5].

In cases of newborns with high-level MM, presenting with severe paraplegia and overt HC, abstention of care may be the attitude of the physician and the family. Even in such cases, shunting may be considered as part of the palliative care: in the absence of life-threatening meningitis or of symptoms relating to the Chiari malformation, the child will not die of hydrocephalus, and surgical abstention may lead to extreme macrocephaly.

The Concept of "Arrested Hydrocephalus" in Patients with Myelomeningocele

Some patients with MM may have enlarged but stable ventricles at birth, or may be diagnosed with enlarged ventricles at a later age, in which case the question of arrested HC is raised. The concept of arrested HC in MMH is hotly debated [5, 25] because of the risk of fatal complications in untreated patients on one hand [5], and of the risks associated with shunting on the other. Even in asymptomatic patients, intracranial pressure (ICP) measurements may show elevated levels and/or a B-wave pattern [26]. These patients should thus be considered as at-risk for long-term complications such as visual impairment or developmental delay, of CSF leakage in case of surgery (such as spinal cord untethering), as well as sudden deterioration [5]. As a result, primary shunt-independence in MM must be thoroughly ascertained, followed up, and the decision not to treat may need to be reversed any time. We consider that avoiding shunting at all costs may be detrimental for the patient's development, and that harboring a shunt should be considered as part of the disease for the vast majority of MM patients.

Timing of Shunt Insertion

Shunting is generally performed shortly after closure of the MM or during the same operative session. The rationale to perform MM repair and shunt insertion during the same session is that it avoids repeated anesthesia in a fragile child [27-29]. Most commonly, HC becomes overt only after closure of the MM [26], in some cases with a long delay. This delay is regarded as a guarantee that the CSF is not infected [30]. In some cases, shunting will not be necessary at all. For these reasons, most authors decide to shunt only after closure of the MM, if ever, and that simultaneous operation "should not be performed routinely, but only in clinically undoubted cases" [31]. When the child is referred several days after birth with an unclosed MM, the fear of meningitis is another reason to defer shunting: some authors prefer to delay shunting for a few days after closure of the MM in order to allow the possible infection time to declare itself [32]. In such cases, external drainage and a course of antibiotic therapy may be required before shunting, allowing closure of the wound while treating potential meningitis before inserting a shunt [30].

Surgical Technique

The endoscopic management of MMH is the subject of the next chapter, and is a hotly debated topic. In our department, as in most institutions, most patients presenting at birth with MM and HC are shunted.

As mentioned above, the decision to shunt must be taken only when there is no doubt about possible meningeal infection; since infected newborns are often afebrile and lumbar puncture is not an option, clinical (altered general status, poor suckling) and biological data (C-reactive protein and procalcitonin) are useful adjuncts. When in doubt, ventricular puncture may be necessary. As patients with MM are likely to undergo multiple surgical procedures and develop latex allergy, all surgery should be performed in a latex-free environment. The chosen type of shunt depends on the surgeon's habits and is basically not different in MMH and in hydrocephalus of other causes. We generally use a medium-pressure valve; high-pressure valves should be avoided because of the risk of lumbar wound breakdown. It is important that the shunt includes a tapping site in case monitoring of the CSF becomes necessary and because CSF can be obtained neither by lumbar puncture nor by suboccipital puncture in these patients; we use either a valve with reservoir, or a ventricular catheter with reservoir. Ventriculo-peritoneal (VP) shunts are overwhelmingly preferred over atrial shunts, which are associated with a higher risk of fatal shunt complications [33]. In the case of MMH, these patients are at special risk of pulmonary artery hypertension because of the thoracic deformity caused by scoliosis; this is an additional reason to prefer VP shunts [34]. Our general practice for the ventricular catheter is to approach the ventricle through the atrium; the posterior situation of the valve does not present any problem in case an operation for Chiari malformation becomes necessary.

Complications

Shunting is fraught with many complications, whatever the cause of hydrocephalus; however, the rate of shunt obstruction is considered higher in MMH than in other causes of HC. Tuli calculated that the hazard-ratio of shunt revision for MMH, compared with other causes of congenital HC was 1.95 [35]. The majority of these complications occur early after shunting: the rate of complications during the year following shunting for MMH is generally evaluated at 50% [30, 36]. Among these first-year complications, Caldarelli et al. [30] found that 73% were mechanical and 27% were infectious. In our experience, the one-year revision rate was 58.6% in MMH, versus 35.1% in non-MMH, the difference was highly significant (p = 0.0002). In a series of MM patients who had reached adult age, Bowman reported that 95% of the shunted patients had at least one shunt revision, and that the mean number of revisions per patient was 4.33 in this group [9]. Although the reasons for an excess morbidity in MMH in the early period are easily understood (young age, spinal wound breakdown, etc.) the reasons for persistent extra morbidity in older patients are unclear; perhaps ascribing all neurological problems in patients with MM to shunt failure may result in unnecessary shunt revisions. Also, the fear of lethal complications from shunt obstruction in MMH may lower the threshold for shunt revision in this population. Our data do not confirm these reports: in our series the mean number of past shunt revisions in adult patients with MM was 2.5, not statistically different for MMH and for HC of other causes [37].

Diagnosis of Shunt Malfunction in Spina Bifida

The clinical presentation of shunt obstruction in MMH is variable: Liptak reported that 76% of patients present with symptoms, 15% have signs of raised ICP, and 8% are diagnosed on systematic computerized tomographic (CT) scan [38]. Patients with malfunctioning shunts present with classical signs and symptoms of raised ICP: rapidly progressing headache, vomiting and drowsiness, or more subtle manifestations such as school difficulties, abulia or hyperactivity, and emotional distress [5]. In patients with MM, shunt malfunction can also manifest itself as symptomatic Chiari malformation, spinal cord malfunction with scoliosis, motor deterioration or spinal pain in case of syringomyelia [5, 18, 22]. In addition, elective shunt revision may be required for asymptomatic shunt rupture or lengthening of the peritoneal catheter. The complexity and intricacies of diseases in MM patients can make it difficult to identify new symptoms, e.g., to differentiate between shunt malfunction and bowel dysfunction or urinary infection [39]. When in doubt, surveying the patient in a neurosurgical environment is a safety measure. Figure 17.4 presents a proposed management abacus for the patients with MM and possible shunt malfunction.

The rate of shunt infection in MMH is estimated between 5 and 8% per procedure, and its cumulated rate is estimated between 17 and 24% per patient [9, 36, 40], which compares with the rates in other causes of HC. These figures are to be interpreted according to the definition of infection, and the length of follow-up in these studies [20]. In survival analysis, we found that the rate of infection associated with MMH was 22.8% at one year, compared with 12.4% in non-MMH: the difference was highly significant (p = 0.003). Early infection is clearly caused by meningeal contamination through the MM, and delayed repair of the MM is associated with a high risk of shunt infection [32]. However, delayed shunt infection is also a concern in MM: in a former study, we found that the rate of late shunt infection (more than one year after any shunt surgery) was significantly higher in MM, suggesting that risk factors for shunt infection persist throughout life [20]. Among these factors, the presence of resistant bacteria because of untimely antibiotic therapy for urinary infection, a higher risk of bowel perforation [41], and shunt contamination during abdominal surgery are to be considered.

The diagnosis of shunt infection is easy when the patient presents shortly after shunt surgery with high fever, septic shock, meningitis, or purulent discharge of the wound. It can be more difficult when the patient presents with delay, with signs and symptoms posing as aseptic shunt malfunction or intercurrent medical problems. Clinicians must therefore be wary of possible shunt infection in such unspecific con-

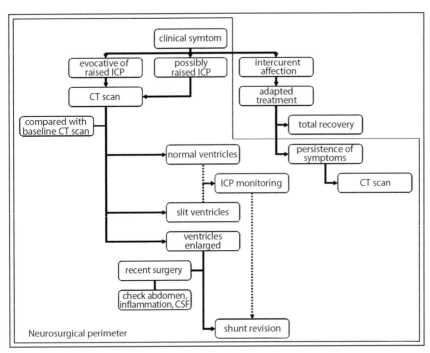

Fig. 17.4. Algorithm for the diagnosis and management of shunt malfunction in patients with myelomeningocele. Although these guidelines do not differ much from those admitted for other causes of hydrocephalus, the complexity and intricacy of diseases in MM renders the distinction between intercurrent disease and shunt malfunction more difficult, while the risk of severe complication of shunt obstruction raises the stakes. All the boxes inside the "neurosurgical perimeter" are steps and conditions for which the neurosurgeon should be involved in decision-making

ditions, especially if shunt revision or abdominal surgery has been performed recently. Blood tests can help redress the diagnosis, although mild inflammation is unspecific in that context; tapping of CSF from the shunt reservoir is a last resource in case of suspicion of shunt infection.

Abdominal problems are common in patients with MM, because of bowel disorders, surgery for cystoplasty, appendicoplasty, caecostomy, inguinal hernias, and testicular ectopia. Overall, in our experience, abdominal operations were necessary in 51 patients (14%). Remarkably, opening of the abdominal cavity, and in some cases of contaminated bowels, caused few or no cases of shunt infection; in only two instances could an operation for cystoplasty be traced as the potential source of shunt infection. This suggests that the peritoneum is an efficient anti-microbial barrier preventing contamination of the shunt material. Bowel perforation by the peritoneal catheter is a rare occurrence in patients with VP shunts, for which patients with a motor handicap such as MM appear at-risk [41]. Although MM was among the leading causes of hydrocephalus associated with bowel perforation in our experience, the trend was not statistically significant. In MM patients with severe scoliosis causing severe right heart failure, ascitis may develop, requiring the conversion of the distal catheter from peritoneal to atrial. Transitory incompetence of the peritoneum causing VP-shunt malfunction has also been reported in as-

sociation with urinary infection [39]. In the case of terminal kidney failure in a patient who has a peritoneal shunt, we consider that the use of the peritoneum for dialysis is not an option because of the risk of shunt contamination. Pregnancy is a rare occurrence in female patients with MM. In our experience, the rare cases of MM patients becoming pregnant did not present any complication due to the presence of the shunt; likewise, there was no problem during caesarean section.

Outcome

Mortality

Shunts have dramatically improved the outlook of patients with MM: survival was as low as 9.7% at 12 years of age before the introduction of shunts, and HC was the most prevalent cause of death in this population, accounting for twice as many deaths as meningitis [5]. In a more recent series, Shurtleff reported that HC was still the cause of 50% mortality at 5 years of age [25]. Actually, the incidence of mortality in MMH has been evaluated at 1% per year [42]. In addition to death indisputably caused by shunt obstruction, a number of shunted patients die suddenly, and death is therefore suspected to be shunt-related: among 13 MM patients who died during follow-up, three died of ascertained shunt obstruction, four died suddenly of unexplained causes, and two died several years after supposed shunt-independence [43]. In our series, shunt malfunction was the third cause of mortality, after infection and death from abstention of surgery at birth; shunt-related death occurred in eight out of 13 MM patients who died after 1 year of age, and in all five patients who died after their twelfth birthday.

MMH causes more shunt-related mortality than other causes of HC: among ten cases of shunt-related fatality reported by Tuli, six were MM [35]. In our series, 9.7% of patients with MM died of shunt complication, compared with 3.5% of patients with other causes of HC ($p < 0.001$). We compared shunt-related mortality in MMH and in other causes of HC in an actuarial study, and found a highly significant difference (Fig. 17.5). In MMH, the survival rates at ten years and 20 years were 88.6% and 86.6%, respectively; in HC of other causes, the survival rates at ten years and 20 years were 96.5% and 95.3%, respectively; these differences were statistically significant. Davis noted that late shunt-related mortality was almost specific to MMH: in his experience, only shunted MM patients died after 16 years of age [44]. The higher shunt-related mortal-

ity of patients with MM is most likely related to the Chiari malformation and other cerebral malformations, which cause rapidly life-threatening complications in case of intracranial hypertension, or even sudden death.

Functional Outcome

The impact of HC on the intellectual development, autonomy and achievements of patients with MM is difficult to evaluate because of the multiple neurological anomalies associated with MM, and their higher prevalence and greater severity when HC is present. Shunt-free patients generally have a higher IQ than shunted patients [31, 45]. The functional outcome of patients with MMH is considered normal in 40% of patients [18]. The better functional outcome in non-shunted patients appears mostly related to the lower anatomical level of their spina bifida. The impact of shunt infection on intellectual outcome of patients with MMH was considered important [46], but is now regarded as secondary, due to early and efficient treatment [36]. In our series, however, shunt infection was a significant predictor of intellectual delay and schooling difficulties [20]. The impact of intracranial hypertension due to HC and episodes of shunt obstruction on academic achievements has also been emphasized [40, 45, 47], but very long-term follow-up of unbiased series is necessary in order to substantiate this point.

Secondary Shunt Independence

Patients shunted for MMH can rarely, if ever, become shunt-independent. This occurs when hydrocephalus has resolved with time or because endoscopic third ventriculostomy (ETV) has been practiced successfully [40]. In other cases, a patient who has been lost to follow-up for several years shows up with a ruptured shunt but no signs of shunt malfunction: the decision to revise the shunt or declare him shunt-independent is a frequent dilemma. The rate of shunt independence in MMH has been evaluated as between 1.4% [18] and 17% [48], the difference being explained by the variability of the criteria for initial shunting, the duration of follow-up and the definition of shunt-independence. The selection of candidates and the procedure followed to ascertain that the patient is genuinely shunt independent must obey strict rules because of the seriousness of intracranial hypertension in patients with

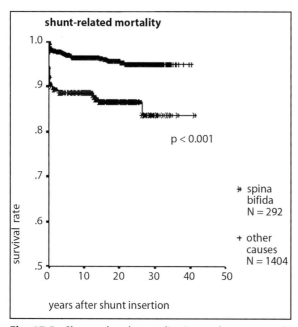

Fig. 17.5. Shunt-related mortality in myelomeningocele and in other causes of hydrocephalus. This graph shows a significantly higher shunt-related mortality in myelomeningocele. The excess mortality can be ascribed to decompensation of the Chiari malformation during intracranial hypertension

MM. For shunts in general, and in MMH in particular, we cannot accept criteria such as "shunt presumed useless because of asymptomatic rupture" or removal of the shunt at the time of elective lengthening as valid. Steinbok showed that when shunt revision was required during the first year of life, the risk of further revision during the following years was 31%, compared with only 8% if no revision was required during the first year [36]. We consider that the procedure of shunt weaning can be proposed only in patients presenting with asymptomatic shunt rupture, and having not presented before with symptomatic shunt failure. Our protocol is based on proof of shunt independence by shuntogram showing the absence of flow in the shunt, followed by catheter ligation, and finally shunt removal if the ligation has been well tolerated both clinically and radiologically for one month [49]. Following these guidelines, only eight of our patients with MMH became shunt-independent; survival analysis shows that the rate of shunt-independence can be evaluated at 7.3% after 20 years (Fig. 17.6). In the meantime, some patients who were not initially shunted became shunt-dependant, seven of these after the age of 10 years. The aim of removing shunts in MM patients should not be pursued too assiduously, because of the risk of sudden death [5], even after several years of apparent shunt-independence [43].

Conclusion

MMH is a disease in its own right, causing both morbidity and mortality in patients with MM. Shunts still

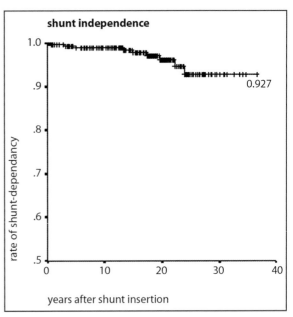

Fig. 17.6. Actuarial study of shunt-independence. Only eight patients became secondarily shunt-independent; the rate of shunt-independence in our series stabilized at 7.3% after 20 years of follow-up. In the meantime, some patients who were not initially shunted became shunt-dependant, seven of these after the age of 10 years. These figures confirm that patients with MMH should be considered as shunted for life with few exceptions

represent the sole treatment for the majority of patients with MMH. Table 17.1 summarizes some of the pathophysiology, diagnostic and therapeutic features of MMH. The frequency and severity of shunt complications justify lifelong neurosurgical follow-up of these patients.

Table 17.1. Pathophysiology, diagnostic and therapeutic features of MMH

	Data	Practical implications
Pathophysiology	Obstructive and/or communicating: varies with age	Endoscopic third ventriculostomy generally fails at birth
Incidence	Depends on the willingness to avoid shunts	Generally around 80%
Primary shunt independence	"Arrested hydrocephalus" may be associated with developmental delay	Decision to treat should be based on both clinical and radiological data
Antenatal diagnosis	Present in only 31% of fetuses; depends on the anatomical level	Poor motor and developmental prognosis
Surgical technique	Peritoneal shunt	Abdominal complications: rare
Shunt infection	Higher incidence in MM	Cause of intellectual delay
Shunt obstruction	Decompensation of Chiari malformation	Cause of mortality, both early and delayed
Secondary shunt independence	7.3% of patients after 20 years follow-up	Shunt removal is rarely an option

References

1. Russell Dorothy S (1935) The mechanism of internal hydrocephalus in spina bifida. Brain 58:203-215
2. Dandy WE, Blackfan KD (1914) Internal hydrocephalus: an experimental, clinical and pathological study. Am J Dis Child 8:406-482
3. Gardner WJ (1965) Hydrodynamic mechanism of syringomyelia: its relationship to myelocele. J Neurol Neurosurg Psychiatr 28:247-259
4. Tulipan N, Sutton LN, Bruner JP et al (2003) The effect of intrauterine myelomeningocele repair on the incidence of shunt-dependent hydrocephalus. Pediatr Neurosurg 38:27-33
5. Rekate HL (1988) Management of hydrocephalus and the erroneous concept of shunt independence in spina bifida patients. BNI Quarterly 4:17-20
6. Dirks PB, Drake JM, Lamberti-Pasculli M et al (2005) Falling ventriculo-peritoneal shunt rates in myelomeningocele (abstr). Childs Nerv Syst 19:607
7. Crimmins D, Hayward RD, Thompson DNP (2005) Reducing shunt placement rate in myelomeningocele patients (abstr). Childs Nerv Syst 21:828-829
8. De la Cruz R, Millan JM, Miralles M, Munoz MJ (1989) Cranial sonographic evaluation in children with myelomeningocele. Childs Nerv Syst 5:94-98
9. Bowman RM, McLone DG, Grant JA et al (2001) Spina bifida outcome: a 25-year prospective. Pediatr Neurosurg 34:114-120
10. Alatise OI, Adeolu AA, Komolafe EO et al (2006) Patterns and factors affecting management of spina bifida cystica in Ile-Ife, Nigeria. Pediatr Neurosurg 42:277-283
11. Rintoul N, Sutton LN, Hubbard AM et al (2002) A new look at myelomeningoceles: functional level, vertebral level, shunting, and the implications for fetal intervention. Pediatrics 109:409-413
12. Dias MS, McLone DG (1994) Spinal dysraphism. In: Weinstein SL (ed) The pediatric spine, vol 1. Raven, New York, pp 343-368
13. Aubry MC, Aubry JP, Dommergues M (2003) Sonographic prenatal diagnosis of central nervous system abnormalities. Childs Nerv Syst 19:391-402
14. Oi S, Honda Y, Hidaka M et al (1998) Intrauterine high-resolution magnetic resonance imaging in fetal hydrocephalus and prenatal estimation of postnatal outcomes with "perspective classification". J Neurosurg 88:685-694
15. Kazmi SS, Nejat F, Tajik P, Roozbeh H (2006) The prenatal ultrasonographic detection of myelomeningocele in patients referred to Children's Hospital Medical Center: a cross-sectional study. Reprod Health 3:6 doi:10.1186/1742-4755-3-6
16. Oi S (2003) Current status of prenatal management of fetal spina bifida in the world: worldwide cooperative survey on the medico-ethical issue. Childs Nerv Syst 19:596-599
17. Raybaud C, Levrier O, Brunel H et al (2003) MR imaging of fetal brain malformations. Childs Nerv Syst 19:455-450
18. Sgouros S (2004) Hydrocephalus with myelomeningocele. In: Cinalli G, Sainte-Rose C, Maixner W (eds) Pediatric hydrocephalus. Springer, Milan, pp 133-144
19. Teo C, Jones R (1996) Management of hydrocephalus by endoscopic third ventriculostomy in patients with myelomeningocele. Pediatr Neurosurg 25:57-63
20. Vinchon M, Dhellemmes P (2006) Cerebrospinal shunt infection: risk factors and long term follow-up. Childs Nerv Syst 22:692-677
21. Solan K, Glaisyer H (2006) Raised intracranial pressure in a neonate presenting as stridor. Pediatr Anesth 16:877-879
22. Hall P, Lindseth R, Campbell R et al (1979) Scoliosis and hydrocephalus in myelocele patients; the effects of shunting. J Neurosurg 50:174-178
23. Natelson SE (1981) Early third ventriculostomy in myelomeningocele infants – shunt independence? Childs Brain 8:321-325
24. Nadkarni TD, Rekate HL (2005) Treatment of refractory intracranial hypertension in a spina bifida patient by a concurrent ventricular and cisterna magna-to-peritoneal shunt. Childs Nerv Syst 21:579-582
25. Shurtleff DB, Kronmal R, Foltz EL (1975) Follow-up comparison of hydrocephalus with and without myelomeningocele. J Neurosurg 42:61-68
26. Iborra J, Pages E, Cuxart A et al (2000) Increased intracranial pressure in myelomeningocele (MMC) patients never shunted: results of a prospective preliminary study. Spinal Cord 38:495-497
27. Epstein NE, Rosenthal AD, Zito J, Osipoff M (1985) Shunt placement and myelomeningocele repair: simultaneous vs. sequential shunting. Childs Nerv Syst 1:145-147
28. Hubballah MY, Hoffmann HJ (1987) Early repair of myelomeningocele and simultaneous insertion of ventriculoperitoneal shunt: technique and results. Neurosurgery 20:21-23
29. McLone DG (1998) Care of the neonate with a myelomeningocele. Neurosurg Clin North Am 9:111-120
30. Caldarelli M, Di Rocco C, La Marca F (1996) Shunt complications in the first postoperative year in children with meningomyelocele. Childs Nerv Syst 12:748-754
31. Rolle U, Gräffe G (1999) About the rate of shunt complications in patients with hydrocephalus and myelomeningocele. Eur J Pediatr Surg 9 (suppl I): 51-52
32. Gamache FW (1995) Treatment of hydrocephalus in patients with meningomyelocele or encephalocele: a recent series. Childs Nerv Syst 11:487-488
33. Mazza C, Pasqualin A, Da Pian R (1980) Results of treatment with ventriculoatrial and ventriculoperitoneal shunt in infantile non tumoral hydrocephalus. Childs Brain 7:1-14
34. Byard RW (1996) Mechanisms of sudden death and autopsy findings in patients with Arnold-Chiari mal-

formation and ventriculoatrial catheters. Am J Forensic Med Pathol 17:260-263

35. Tuli S, Tuli J, Drake J, Spears J (2004) Predictors of death in pediatric patients requiring cerebrospinal fluid shunts. J Neurosurg (Pediatr) 100 (suppl 5):442-446

36. Steinbok P, Irvine B, Cochrane DD, Irwin BJ (1992) Long-term outcome and complications of children with myelomeningocele. Childs Nerv Syst 8:92-96

37. Vinchon M, Dhellemmes P (2007) The transition from child to adult in neurosurgery. Adv Techn Standarts Neurosurg 32:3-24

38. Liptak GS, Bolander HM, Langworthy K (2001) Screening for ventricular shunt function in children with hydrocephalus secondary to myelomeningocele. Pediatr Neurosurg 34:281-285

39. Tubbs RS, Wellons JC, Blount JP, Oakes J (2005) Transient ventriculoperitoneal shunt dysfunction in children with myelodysplasia and urinary bladder infection. J Neurosurg (Pediatr) 102 (suppl 2):221-223

40. Mirzai H, Ersahin Y, Mutluer S, Kayahan A (1998) Outcome of patients with myelomeningocele. Childs Nerv Syst 14:120-123

41. Vinchon M, Baroncini M, Thines L, Dhellemmes P (2006) Bowel perforation by peritoneal shunt catheters: diagnosis and treatment. Neurosurgery 58 (1 suppl ONS):76-82

42. Iskandar BJ, Tubbs S, Mapstone TB et al (1998) Death in shunted hydrocephalic children in the 1990s. Pediatr Neurosurg 28:173-176

43. Tomlinson P, Sugarman ID (1995) Complications with shunts in adults with spina bifida. Brit Med J 311:286-287

44. Davis BE, Daley CM, Shurtleff DB et al (2005) Long-term survival of individuals with myelomeningocele. Pediatr Neurosurg 41:186-191

45. Hunt GM, Oakeshot P, Kerry S (1999) Link between the CSF shunt and achievement in adults with spina bifida. J Neurol Neurosurg Psychiatr 67:591-595

46. McLone DG, Czyzewski D, Raimondi AJ, Sommers RC (1982) Central nervous system infection as a limiting factor in the intelligence of children with myelomeningocele. Pediatrics 70:338-342

47. Hetherington R, Dennis M, Barnes M et al (2006) Functional outcome in young adults with spina bifida and hydrocephalus. Childs Nerv Syst 22:117-124

48. Lorber J, Pucholt V (1981) When is a shunt no longer necessary? Z Kinderchir 34:327-329

49. Vinchon M, Fichten A, Delestret I, Dhellemmes P (2003) Revision for asymptomatic shunt failure: surgical and clinical results. Neurosurgery 52:347-356

CHAPTER 18
The Treatment of Hydrocephalus in Spina Bifida – Endoscopy

Benjamin Warf

Introduction

Birth rates several times those in developed countries, the lack of preventive measures, and the rarity of prenatal diagnosis all contribute to the fact that spina bifida is a very common condition among children of developing countries. At the CURE Children's Hospital of Uganda (CCHU), a center for pediatric neurosurgery established in 2001, 75-100 new infants with myelomeningocele (MMC) present for treatment annually.

In developed countries, where more than 40% of shunts fail within 2 years of placement [1] and more than 80% fail within 12 years [2], the availability of neurosurgical expertise and rapid transportation usually provide a sufficient safety net for shunt-dependent children. However, in stark contrast, those in emerging countries (representing the majority of the world's children) are without this safety net, so shunt malfunction presents a much greater threat to life. Furthermore, the risk of shunt failure and infection may even be exaggerated in infants with MMC [3, 4].

Even though the financial obstacle of shunt implantation can be overcome with the successful use of inexpensive shunts [5], the risk of shunt-dependency in developing countries is unacceptable because of the struggle for families to access urgent care in the event of shunt malfunction or infection.

This resulted in neuroendoscopic treatment being adopted as the primary management for all children coming to CCHU with hydrocephalus (HC), regardless of age or etiology of the HC, including those children with MMC [6].

General Principles for Endoscopic Treatment of Hydrocephalus in MMC Patients

Pathophysiological Basis

The endoscopic third ventriculostomy (ETV) (or ventriculcisternostomy) provides direct communication between the third ventricle and the subarachnoid spaces by way of the interpeduncular and pre-pontine cisterns. This bypasses the Sylvian aqueduct, the fourth ventricle and its outlets, and the posterior fossa subarachnoid cisterns, thus "shunting" the cerebrospinal fluid (CSF) past any obstruction to flow along these pathways. ETV should be expected to function if there is no obstruction to flow from the interpeduncular/prepontine cisterns and through the arachnoid granulations, if the dural venous sinus pressure is normal. ETV would not be expected to be a sufficient treatment if extra-ventricular CSF circulation and absorption deficiencies are significant contributors to the etiology. Among those infants for whom ETV is not sufficient to treat the HC, a likely cause for failure may be a "communicating hydrocephalus" remaining after the ETV has bypassed any obstruction at the level of the aqueduct or fourth ventricle. The hypothesis that underdeveloped extra-axial CSF circulation and absorption capacity contributed to the inferior result of ETV in young infants led to the speculation that a reduction in the rate of CSF production by choroid plexus cauterization (CPC) at the time of the ETV might be helpful. It was hoped that reducing the rate of CSF production in the face of impaired absorption would help the maturing system to accommodate the new efflux of CSF through the ventriculocisternostomy. CPC alone in the management of hydrocephalus had been reported previously, but never in combination with ETV. The largest series was that of Pople and Ettles [7], who reported a 47% success of this procedure in spina bifida infants. I thought that the conjunction of the two procedures (ETV/CPC) might be successful in those infants in whom ETV alone would fail because of a residual communicating hydrocephalus, and in those in whom CPC alone would fail because of an untreated obstructive component.

Preoperative Imaging

Magnetic resonance imaging (MRI), particularly using constructive interference in steady state (CISS), is very helpful in the preoperative assessment of anatomy [8-10]. The CISS sequences provide detailed information on the status of the aqueduct, the fourth ventricle outlets, and the status of the posterior fossa, interpeduncular, and prepontine cisterns (Fig. 18.1). We are currently investigating whether any of these features help to predict post-operative outcome for ETV/CPC.

Intraventricular Anatomy in Patients with Myelomeningocele/Chiari II Malformation

Performing endoscopic procedures in infants with hydrocephalus in association with myelomeningocele presents a singular challenge because of the abnormalities associated with the type II Chiari malformation. The intraventricular anatomy varies, but certain anomalies are especially common [6, 11]: (1) absent septum pellucidum; (2) foramen of Monro stenosis; (3) fused, thickened forniceal columns; (4) robust choroid plexus with the glomus usually loosely tethered by a pedicle of thin vascular membrane; (5) enlarged massa intermedia; (6) interhypothalamic adhesions that complicate the terrain of the third ventricular floor, which may be thick and non-translucent; (7) aqueductal narrowing (Figs. 18.2-18.5). The intracisternal anatomy is often notable for: (1) anteriorly displaced basilar artery and brainstem, often abutting the clival dura; (2) downward displacement of the basilar apex, which forms a "Y" shape; and (3) thick membrane of Liliequist that often requires separate fenestration after the floor is penetrated (Figs. 18.6 and 18.7).

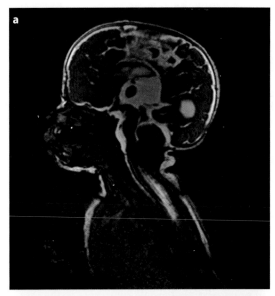

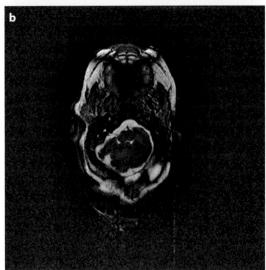

Fig. 18.1 a, b. a Sagittal CISS MRI of newborn with MM/Chiari II and hydrocephalus showing open aqueduct, but obstructed foramen of Magendie. **b** Axial CISS MRI of same patient showing obstructed foramina of Luschka

I advise against surgeons who are relatively inexperienced in neuroendoscopy undertaking the endoscopic treatment of hydrocephalus in this patient population. Competence and familiarity with the ETV should first be achieved in other patients where the anatomy is more straightforward. The variable anatomy, the thick floor of the third ventricle with its sometimes confusing topography, and the anterior displacement of the basilar apex are particularly problematic.

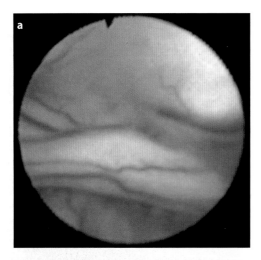

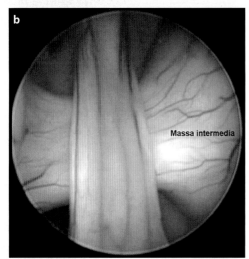

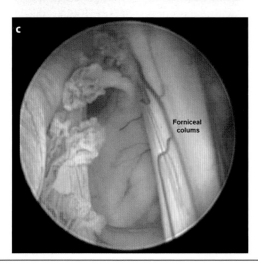

Fig. 18.2 a-c. a View from R frontal horn onto choroid plexus terminating at stenotic foramen of Monro. Note also the thick, fused forniceal columns and the absent septum pellucidum (anterior is to the *left*). **b** Thickened fused forniceal columns, and an enlarged massa intermedia. **c** The third ventricle roof is absent and choroid plexus and choroidal network in the posterior roof are seen

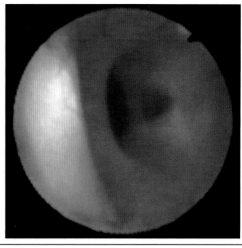

Fig. 18.3. Third ventricle with two interhypothalamic adhesions crossing posterior and inferior to the optic chiasm (anterior is to the *left*)

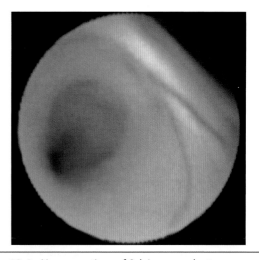

Fig. 18.4. Narrow ostium of Sylvian aqueduct

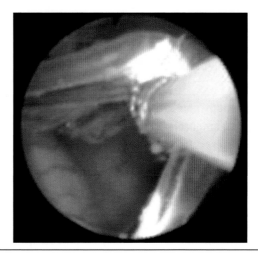

Fig. 18.5. Vascular pedicle of glomus choroidea undergoing cauterization with Bugby wire

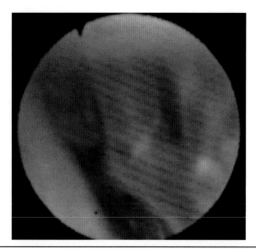

Fig. 18.6. View through ETV stoma showing "Y" shaped basilar apex and close proximity of basilar artery to the dorsum sellae and clivus (anterior is to the *left*)

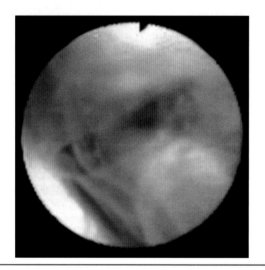

Fig. 18.7. Vertical component of Liliequist's membrane lying between the clivus (*left*) and the basilar artery (*right*) following fenestration to gain access to the pre-pontine cistern

Neuroendoscopic Techniques in Patients with Myelomeningocele

Endoscopic Third Ventriculostomy

The equipment I have used for the procedure includes the Karl Storz 3.7 mm flexible steerable neuroendoscope (11282 BN) with a standard xenon light source and video system (Karl Storz Company, Tuttlingen, Germany). Rigid endoscopes have the advantage of superior optics and

that they can be autoclaved. However, they do not allow sufficient maneuverability to perform the bilateral CPC procedure. The flexibility of the fiberoptic endoscope with the additional feature of its steerable tip provides many degrees of freedom to allow safe maneuvering of the scope throughout both lateral ventricles as well as within the interpeduncular and prepontine cisterns. The fiberscope filter setting options for the camera aid in enhancing the image quality. All images presented here (except Fig. 18.1) were obtained with the fiberoptic endoscope.

The endoscope and camera are both sterilized and placed directly on the operative field, or can be supported with a holder rigidly affixed to the operating table. The camera and light cables exit the field toward the video cart (which houses the monitor, video box, light source, and image capture system) at the foot of the table. The patient is positioned supine as for a right frontal ventriculo-peritoneal shunt placement, with the head turned to the left. I prep and drape the patient for a shunt placement in case of technical failure of the ETV/CPC. After the set up and white balancing of the endoscope and video system, a gently curved 90-degree angle incision is made in the lateral corner of the anterior fontanel with the flap centered in the mid-pupillary line. The small scalp flap is reflected to expose the dura of the fontanel and is tacked back with a suture. The dura is incised sharply, allowing for its primary closure to avoid CSF leak. After opening the dura, the pia and cortical surface are coagulated, then penetrated with the obturator of a peel-away sheath or a ventricular cannula. The endoscope is then inserted into the frontal horn of the right lateral ventricle just as one would pass a ventricular catheter, and the camera orientation is adjusted appropriately such that anterior is at 9 o'clock and posterior at 3 o'clock on the video image. The bulk of the endoscope rests on the operative field, or is supported by the holder, and the surgeon's right hand rests on the patient's head while the tip of the scope is inserted and subsequently manipulated. I control the endoscope with my right hand, which I stabilize by resting my fourth and fifth fingers lightly on the patient's head, and manipulate the scope between my right thumb and index finger (for depth, gross angulation, and torque). I control the steering mechanism with my left hand (to flex the tip in either of two directions while simultaneously twisting the scope with my right thumb and forefinger to point the tip in any direction through 360-degrees). The depth of the Bugby wire is also controlled with my left hand.

The flexible neuroendoscope has one working channel with two access ports – each with a stopcock. I do not use continuous irrigation, but rather intermittent manual irrigation with a 10 cc syringe as needed. If irrigation is required while the Bugby wire is occupying the working channel via port A, the syringe can be connected to port B and irrigation performed after the stopcock on port A is clamped down on the wire to prevent egress of the irrigant.

The variations in ventriculoscopic anatomy among these patients have been described above. The foramen of Monro is identified and the scope is passed into the third ventricle. The typically enlarged massa intermedia only rarely precludes access to the floor, which is almost always thickened with no evidence of the basilar artery (BA) position below. Inter-hypothalamic adhesions are common, but are usually preserved as the floor is approached around them en passant. The floor is gently and bluntly penetrated using the Bugby wire (but without the use of electrocautery) posterior to the infundibular recess and anterior to the mammillary bodies, taking advantage – if possible – of a small segment of the floor that is often thinned out. There is commonly a prominent inter-hypothalamic adhesion crossing the floor in this vicinity. It is best to perforate the floor just over the dorsum sellae to avoid entering over the basilar apex or brainstem, which are typically anteriorly displaced and close against the clivus (Fig. 18.8). As the floor is gradually penetrated, the dorsum sellae, pituitary, and brainstem come into view. The ETV stoma is widened by gentle traction in different directions on

its edges with the Bugby wire. Flexing the tip and rotating the scope (by applying torque with the right thumb and forefinger) accomplish this, and the stoma is widened to a diameter of 5-7 mm. This requires virtually no gross translation of the proximal portion of the endoscope. The flexible fiberoptic neuroendoscope is then gently threaded over the wire into the interpeduncular and prepontine cisternal spaces (after fenestration of Liliequist's membrane if needed), which are typically very crowded from the anterior displacement of the brainstem and BA complex. Blunt dissection of arachnoid adhesions using the tip of the Bugby wire and the tip flexion control of the flexible endoscope is sometimes required to open up the cistern. If penetration through the floor is made anterior to the vertical portion (mesencephalic leaf) of Liliequist's membrane, which obscures the basilar artery, blunt dissection is accomplished with the tip of the wire to fenestrate the membrane (Fig. 18.7). The goal of the dissection below the floor is to visualize a "naked" basilar artery complex. I find that the flexible endoscope allows this dissection to be accomplished delicately and safely. I do not recommend such maneuvers with a rigid endoscope because the required movements are too gross. The scope is withdrawn from the ventriculostomy, and evidence for flow across the stoma is noted.

Lamina Terminalis (LT) Fenestration

If an ETV in the floor is not technically feasible, then fenestration of the lamina terminalis can be attempted [6]. The technique is similar to that for the floor. I often perform a partial thickness cauterization of the LT with the Bugby wire followed by a blunt penetration without cautery and subsequent stretching of the stoma as described for the floor. The endoscope often needs to be rotated between the right thumb and index finger while simultaneously flexing the tip with the steering mechanism in order to achieve a more perpendicular angle of attack for the Bugby wire upon the LT.

Choroid Plexus (CP) Cauterization

Following the ETV, attention is turned to cauterization of the choroid plexus. Beginning at the right foramen of Monro and gradually moving posteriorly, the CP of the lateral ventricle is thoroughly cauterized using the Bugby wire and monopolar coagulating current adjusted to the lowest setting that can be efficiently used (Fig. 18.9a). Care is taken to avoid

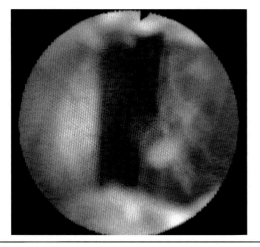

Fig. 18.8. View through ETV stoma placed over dorsum sellae (at *left*) with basilar apex positioned immediately posterior (at *right*)

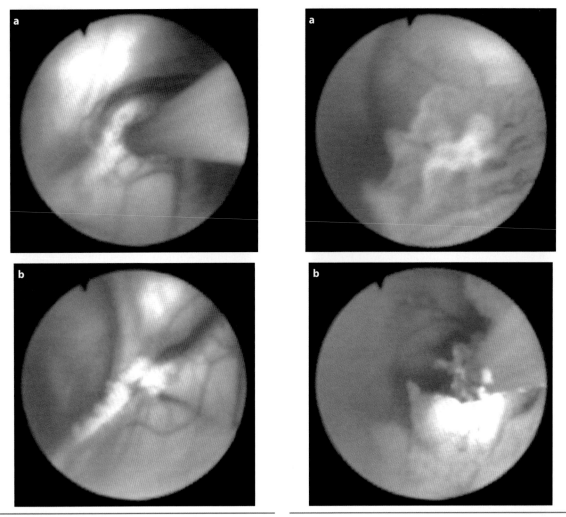

Fig. 18.9 a, b. a Cauterization of CP with Bugby wire beginning at foramen of Monro. Note superior choroidal vein. **b** Result of cauterization showing distinction between cauterized and uncauterized CP and superior choroidal vein

Fig. 18.10 a, b. a Anterior extent of CP in temporal horn. Note contour of hippocampus in ventricular wall behind CP. **b** Cauterization of temporal horn CP with Bugby wire

injury to the thalamostriate and internal cerebral veins or ependymal surfaces. Special attention is paid to the complete coagulation of all vessels within the plexus, including the superior choroidal vein along its entire length. At the level of the atrium the glomus portion of the CP is thoroughly cauterized. In MMC patients there is typically redundant, robust CP loosely tethered by a thin vascular sheet-like membrane in addition to a carpet of CP adherent to the ependymal surface along the curve of the thalamus. With the patient's head turned to the left, the right glomus choroideum often drops across the midline, dangling into the left lateral ventricle (when the septum pellucidum is absent) by this elongated vascular pedicle, which I thoroughly cauterize in addition to the glomus (Fig. 18.5). Then, passing the scope

posterior to the thalamus, its tip is flexed and turned to direct the procedure along the CP of the temporal horn, which is then cauterized in a similar fashion beginning from its anterior extreme and advancing the wire posteriorly along its length (Fig. 18.10). Cautery is continued until all visible CP has been coagulated and shriveled. For cases in which the septum pellucidum is intact, a septostomy is performed superior to the posterior edge of the foramen of Monro to gain access to the contralateral CP, where the same procedure is carried out in the left lateral ventricle. Uncommonly, bleeding (usually venous) from the CP may be encountered. In such cases, I have found it most efficiently controlled by tamponading it with the Bugby wire while gently irrigating for a couple of minutes until it stops.

Results

Treatment with Endoscopic Third Ventriculostomy Alone

The pathophysiology of HC in infants with MM can include intra-axial obstructive components such as aqueductal stenosis or fourth ventricle outlet obstruction, as discussed in Chapter 17. Therefore, primary treatment by ETV to bypass these sites of obstruction would seem a rational approach. Successful outcomes for ETV have been reported in 64-80% of older patients and those previously shunted; however, results in the limited published experience with ETV as the primary treatment in infants with MMC and HC have been less successful, ranging from 12 to 53% success, depending upon the age under consideration (< 6 months or < 24 months, respectively) [12-14]. My own experience with ETV in MMC infants less than 12 months old is similar, with success in 7 of 20 infants (35%) [15]. Therefore, ETV alone is not effective as the primary treatment for HC in most MM infants.

ETV in MMC Patients with Shunt Malfunction

In contrast to the success of ETV alone in MMC infants as the primary treatment for hydrocephalus, previously shunted MMC patients presenting with shunt malfunction can be freed from shunt-dependency in the majority of cases by performing an ETV instead of a shunt revision. Teo and Jones [13] reported success in 46 of 55 such patients (83%). My current routine for MMC patients with shunt malfunction is to offer ETV as an option whenever possible, and we have had similar success. We have even found ETV to be a successful alternative to shunt revision in a patient presenting with symptomatic hydromyelia resulting from shunt malfunction, which resolved dramatically following ETV [16]. This provides a good illustration of ETV bypassing obstruction to CSF flow at the level of the posterior fossa.

My experience in these previously shunted patients has been similar to that reported by Cinalli and co-authors [17], in that a temporary period of elevated ICP postoperatively may occur, presumably as the extra-axial CSF circulation and absorption pathways are accommodating the new efflux of CSF. Allowing sufficient time for this to run its course in the postoperative period is necessary in order to avoid a premature erroneous conclusion that the ETV will not be successful.

Treatment with Combined Endoscopic Third Ventriculostomy and Choroid Plexus Cauterization (ETV/CPC)

In a consecutive series of 65 children affected by MMC and HC treated at the CURE Children's Hospital of Uganda (CCHU), CPC was added non-selectively to ETV as the primary treatment in 45 cases, and the result was compared to those obtained in 20 children treated with ETV alone in this homogenous patient group [15]. As illustrated in Table 18.1, 34 of 45 (76%) patients were successfully treated in this way, compared to the 35% success rate described above for ETV alone. This difference was statistically significant ($p = 0.0045$). Thus, the addition of CPC significantly enhanced the effectiveness of ETV in MMC infants. Since the initial publication, this population continues to be studied. Currently, 80 MMC infants (mean age 2.8 months) with primary treatment of HC by ETV/CPC have been followed up to 41 months, with a mean follow up of 15.7 months. Successful long-term treatment of the HC has been accomplished in 72.5% of patients. The mean time to failure is 2.1 months, with more than 80% of failures occurring by 3 months postoperatively, and no failures manifest after 6 months at the time of this writing.

In conclusion, ETV alone has been shown to be an effective treatment for hydrocephalus associated with myelomeningocele in older patients, but it has not been successful as the primary treatment for hydrocephalus in newborns. However, the combined ETV/CPC technique can avoid the creation of shunt-dependency from the beginning of life in 70-75% of MMC infants. In environments where shunt-dependency is particularly undesirable, ETV/CPC provides an excellent alternative treatment.

ETV/CPC Versus Shunting

In the developed world, shunts can better be maintained and thus high failure rates and repeat operations can be tolerated, despite the inconvenience and potential morbidity and mortality for the patient. Whether ETV/CPC should supplant shunt-dependency

Table 18.1. Difference in outcome for ETV vs. ETV/CPC in MM infants < 1 year old, p = 0.0045

Procedure	Success/total
ETV only	7/20 (35%)
ETV/CPV	34/45 (76%)

as the standard of care for MMC infants with HC is unknown, and revolves around two unresolved questions.

ETV/CPC Longevity

First is the question of ETV/CPC longevity. Thus far, it is clear that most ETV/CPC failures are apparent very soon after the operation, and there have been no failures recognized among MMC infants treated in this way beyond 6 months. However, the results of truly long-term follow up to the order of 5 or 10 years are not yet available.

"Late rapid deterioration" among patients of all sorts treated with ETV alone has recently been highlighted [18]. Sixteen cases, accumulated from a review of the world's literature plus an international survey, included seven patients who died within a year of surgery, five within 6 months, and two within 2 months. This would suggest that, although failures can occur at intervals distant from the procedure, this is a rare occurrence. In my own ongoing follow up of those MMC infants initially treated with ETV alone in the first year of life [6, 15], success appears to be long-lasting. The mean follow up for successful cases has now been more than 32 months (range 14-49 months). The mean time to failure was 3.4 months, with 10 of 13 (77%) failing by 2 months postoperatively, and no failures after 6 months. Teo and Jones [13], in their large series of MMC patients undergoing ETV (mostly as an alternative to shunt revision) reported the majority of failures were evident within 6 weeks of surgery; but they did have individual failures at 1, 3, 4, and 5 years postoperatively. On balance, it would seem that successful results for ETV are durable in this patient population in contrast to the continued attrition over time that is seen with shunt function.

At this time, in the absence of a prospective randomized trial, only general comparisons can be made between ETV/CPC and shunting in MMC patients as regards failure in the short-term. In one study, 64% of MMC patients had a first shunt failure with a median time to failure of about 10 months, 32% had a second shunt failure, 20% had a third, and 19% had four or more shunt failures during a follow up period of 1-10 years [3]. In another study with follow up of 9-19 years [4], 54% of patients required between one and three shunt revisions, and 32% had more than three shunt revisions. Fifty-one percent of children required a shunt revision in the first year of life and only 14% did not have a shunt revision. It was determined that there was a 10% per year risk

of shunt failure after 2 years. ETV/CPC, then, appears to be a superior treatment modality in terms of shorter-term success. Whereas around one-half of shunted MMC infants will fail within one year of surgery, only around one-quarter of those treated by ETV/CPC will fail (the majority within 3 months). If a 10 year result similar to this were sustained, i.e., no – or even a few – additional patients requiring a second operation for shunt placement (or repeat endoscopy), this would represent a significant improvement in morbidity, infection, cost, and quality of life for the patient and the family, given the known continuing risk of shunt failure. Only time will tell.

It is also worth calling attention to a recent study that demonstrated a decreased life expectancy in shunt-dependent spina bifida patients compared to those without a shunt. These authors suggested that shunting should be avoided by delaying the decision to shunt during infancy until "absolutely necessary" and by "making more frequent use of a third ventriculostomy" to avoid the hazards of shunting [19]. On the other hand, it has been suggested that the presence of a shunt allows easier diagnosis of treatment failure in these patients, and that this may be an argument against using ETV in spina bifida patients [20].

Neurocognitive Outcome

The second unresolved question is whether either procedure offers any advantage in the ultimate neurocognitive and developmental outcome. It is recognized that, following ETV, ventricular size is not typically reduced to the degree that has come to be the expectation with shunting [21]. The long-term consequences of persistently enlarged ventricles are not known. There is, however, no evidence that normal-sized ventricles are essential to normal neurocognitive development. In fact, evidence suggests that psychomotor development and the progress of myelination correlate well with one another and (negatively) with elevated intracranial pressure, but do not correlate with ventricular volume [22-25]. In another study, the postoperative change in ventricular volume did not correlate with neurodevelopmental outcome in infants treated for hydrocephalus [26].

It should not be ignored that shunt infections have a deleterious effect on IQ in spina bifida children [27, 28]. A per procedure shunt infection risk of 5-15% can be expected in spina bifida infants [3, 4], compared to an infection risk of less than 1% for the ETV/CPC procedure [15]. Therefore, preventing shunt-dependency avoids the negative impact of these infections on cognitive development. Furthermore, the chronic and difficult problems of children with slit-like ventricles from shunting are far from insignificant, and this problem is avoided when the hydrocephalus is treated without a shunt [29]. Interestingly, one study found that spina bifida children with shunted hydrocephalus performed worse on neuropsychological evaluations than either those with arrested (unshunted) hydrocephalus or those without hydrocephalus [30].

There is currently no data to suggest that either shunt-dependence or endoscopic treatment is superior in regard to developmental outcome. Only long-term prospective studies that compare neurocognitive outcomes can answer this question definitively. This is one of the goals of the International Infant Hydrocephalus Study [31] that proposes to address this question in infants with isolated congenital aqueductal stenosis. It is reasonable to suggest that the result of this study will help illuminate the issue also in regard to infants with spina bifida.

Conclusion

ETV/CPC represents the novel combination of two older techniques using new technology. The procedure addresses both "communicating" and "non-communicating" mechanisms (extraventricular and intraventricular obstruction) of hydrocephalus that may co-exist in infants with MMC, and treats it successfully without introducing shunt dependency in 70-75% of these infants. This appears to be holding true in the first 2-3 years of follow up available thus far. As regards failure rate, infection rate, and the need for repeat operations over this time period, ETV/CPC appears superior to shunting in this population. Thus, from what is known, this would appear to be the preferred initial treatment.

Two important things are yet to be determined: (1) whether ETV/CPC longevity beyond 2 or 3 years is superior to that for shunts (of which only around 20% survive in the first decade); and (2) whether there is any difference between the two treatments as regards neurocognitive development, given any as yet unknown effect of the differences in ventricular volume reduction balanced with the different rates of infection and reoperation between the two procedures. Given what is well known regarding the performance of shunts, any perceived advantage of shunt-dependency would necessarily be predicated on the existence of a sufficient "safety net" that efficiently supports their urgent maintenance. However, the majority of the world's children with spina bifida and hydrocephalus are not born into such a supportive environment, and the data in hand for ETV/CPC at present argue strongly, in my opinion, for its application in that context.

References

1. Drake JM, Kestle JR, Milner R et al (1998) Randomized trial of cerebrospinal fluid shunt valve design in pediatric hydrocephalus. Neurosurgery 43:294-305
2. Sainte-Rose C, Piatt JH, Renier D et al (1991) Mechanical complications in shunts. Pediatr Neurosurg 17:2-9
3. Tuli S, Drake J, Lamberti-Pasculli M (2003) Long-term outcome of hydrocephalus management in myelomeningoceles. Childs Nerv Syst 19:286-291
4. Steinbok P, Irvine B, Cochrane DD et al (1992) Long-term outcome and complications of children born with meningomyelocele. Childs Nerv Syst 8:92-96
5. Warf BC (2005) Comparison of one - year outcomes for the Chhabra™ and Codman Hakim Micro Precision™ shunt systems in Uganda: A Prospective Study in 195 Children. J Neurosurg (Pediatrics 4) 102:358-362
6. Warf BC (2005) Hydrocephalus in Uganda: predominance of infectious origin and primary management with endoscopic third ventriculostomy. J Neurosurg (Pediatrics 1) 102:1-15
7. Pople IK, Ettles D (1995) The role of endoscopic choroid plexus coagulation in the management of hydrocephalus. Neurosurgery 36:698-702
8. Laitt RD, Mallucci CL, Jaspan T et al (1999) Constructive interference in steady-state 3D Fourier-transform MRI in the management of hydrocephalus and third ventriculostomy. Neuroradiology 41(2):117-123
9. Kurihara N, Takahashi S, Tamura H et al (2000) Investigation of hydrocephalus with three-dimensional constructive interference in steady state MRI. Neuroradiology 42(9):634-638
10. Aleman J, Jokura H, Higano S et al (2001) Value of constructive interference in steady-state three-dimensional, Fourier transformation magnetic resonance imaging for the neuroendoscopic treatment of hydrocephalus and intracranial cysts. Neurosurgery 48(6):1291-1295
11. Kadri H, Mawla AA (2004) Variations of endoscopic ventricular anatomy in children suffering from hydrocephalus associated with myelomeningocele. Minim Invas Neurosurg 47:339-341
12. Jones RF, Kwok BC, Stening WA et al (1994) The current status of endoscopic third ventriculostomy in the management of non-communicating hydrocephalus. Minim Invas Neurosurg 37:28-36
13. Teo C, Jones R (1996) Management of hydrocephalus by endoscopic third ventriculostomy in patients with myelomeningocele. Pediatr Neurosurg 25:57-63

14. Kadrian D, van Gelder J, Florida D et al (2005) Long-term reliability of endoscopioc third ventriculostomy. Neurosurgery 56:1271-1278

15. Warf BC (2005) Comparison of endoscopic third ventriculostomy alone and combined with choroid plexus cauterization in infants younger than 1 year of age: a prospective study in 550 African children. J Neurosurg (6 Suppl Pediatrics) 103:475-481

16. Warf BC, Campbell JW. Case report in preparation

17. Cinalli G, Spennato P, Ruggiero C et al (2006) Intracranial pressure monitoring and lumbar puncture after endoscopic third ventriculostomy in children. Neurosurgery 58:126-136

18. Drake J, Chumas P, Kestle J et al (2006) Late rapid deterioration after endoscopic third ventriculostomy: additional cases and review of the literature. J Neurosurg (2 Suppl Pediatrics) 105:118-126

19. Dillon CM, Davis BE, Duguay S et al (2000) Longevity of patients born with myelomeningocele. Eur J Pediatr Surg 10(suppl 1):33-34

20. Marlin AE (2004) Management of hydrocephalus in the patient with myelomeningocele: an argument against third ventriculostomy. Neurosurg Focus 16(2):E4

21. St George E, Natarajan K, Sgouros S (2004) Changes in ventricular volume in hydrocephalic children following successful endoscopic third ventriculostomy. Childs Nerv Syst 20:834-838

22. van der Knaap MS, Valk J, Bakker CJ et al (1991) Myelination as an expression of the functional maturity of the brain. Dev Med Child Neurol 33:849-857

23. Hanlo PW (1995) Noninvasive intracranial pressure monitoring in infantile hydrocephalus and the relationship with transcranial Doppler, myelination and outcome. Thesis, Utrecht, The Netherlands

24. Hanlo PW, Gooskens RJ, van Schooneveld M et al (1997) The effect of intracranial pressure on myelination and the relationship with neurodevelopment in infantile hydrocephalus. Dev Med Child Neurol 39 (5):286-291

25. Hanlo PW, Gooskens RH, Vandertop PW (2004) Hydrocephalus: intracranial pressure, Myelination, and neurodevelopment. In: Cinalli G, Maixner WJ, and Sainte-Rose C (eds) Pediatric hydrocephalus. Springer-Verlag Italia, Milan, pp 113-119

26. Horner E, Marchand S, Kaiser GL (2001) Ventricular and parenchymal surface before and after shunting--do they have prognostic value for outcome? Eur J Pediatr Surg 11(supp 1):S28-31

27. Brown J, McLone D (1980) The effect of complications on intellectual function in 167 children with myelomeningocele. Z Kinderchir 34:17

28. McLone DG, Czyzewski D, Raimondi AJ et al (1982) Central nervous system infections as a limiting factor in the intelligence of children with myelomeningocele. Pediatrics 70:338-342

29. Di Rocco C, Massimi L, Tamburrini G (2006) Shunts vs. endoscopic third ventriculostomy in infants: are there different types and/or rates of complications?: A review. Childs Nerv Syst 22(12):1573-1589

30. Casari EF, Fantino AG (1998) A longitudinal study of cognitive abilities and achievement status of children with myelomeningocele and their relationship with clinical types. Eur J Pediatr Surg 8(suppl 1):52-54

31. Sgouros S, Kulkharni AV, Constantini S (2006) The international infant hydrocephalus study: concept and rationale. Childs Nerv Syst 22:338-345

Section IV
SECONDARY MANAGEMENT NEUROLOGY AND NEUROSURGERY

CHAPTER 19
Chiari II Malformation and Syringomyelia

Spyros Sgouros

Introduction

The Chiari II malformation was described at the end of the nineteenth century (1891-1896) by Hans Chiari, a German pathologist, as a congenital malformation in a post-mortem examination of a child who died from a constellation of malformations including prolapse of the cerebellum, part of the brain stem and part of the hindbrain, involving the upper part of the cervical spine, with hydrocephalus and myelomeningocele. Around the same time (1894) similar observations were made by Arnold, hence the malformation is often called the Arnold-Chiari malformation. Cleland made similar observations in 1883 and 1913. Subsequently, the term Chiari malformation has been used to describe all forms of hindbrain herniation, of which three subtypes have been described. Chiari type I malformation refers to the prolapse of the cerebellar tonsils more than 5 mm below the foramen magnum, with no spina bifida malformation. In severe forms of Chiari I malformation there may be some brain stem descent, and occasionally this is incorrectly called a Chiari II malformation. The term Chiari II should only be used for patients born with spina bifida aperta (myelomeningocele) and hindbrain herniation. Equally incorrect is the labeling of a mild hindbrain herniation in children with spina bifida aperta as a Chiari I malformation.

Chiari type III malformation is a severe type II form that includes severe hindbrain herniation with cervical myelomeningocele. A fourth type, Chiari type IV malformation, has been described and includes brain stem descent with severe cerebellar hypoplasia, but is not universally accepted as part of the Chiari spectrum of malformations.

General Characteristics of Chiari II Malformation

Anatomy – Radiology

The Chiari II malformation includes a constellation of complex malformations of the skull, brain, spine and spinal cord, the severity of which can vary between patients. There have been many anatomical, cadaveric descriptive studies, but from the clinical perspective, appreciation of the anatomical features of Chiari II malformation in vivo is well achieved with magnetic resonance (MR) scanning, hence study of the anatomy is effectively through radiological study of the malformation. Computerized tomography (CT) scanning shows the anatomy of the ventricular system well, but does not offer the anatomical detail necessary to visualize all other complex malformations. In the last decade it has been possible to obtain a MR scan antenatally, allowing early accurate diagnosis of the malformation in utero. The most notable abnormalities are outlined below (Figs. 19.1-19.3).

Posterior Fossa Malformations

The features of posterior fossa malformations are as follows:
- The brain stem has abnormal disposition and angulation with respect to the midbrain and the tentorial hiatus.
- The posterior fossa has a smaller capacity than normal [1].
- The fourth ventricle is caudally displaced and elongated.

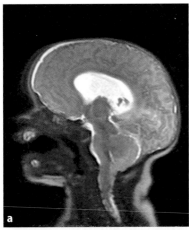
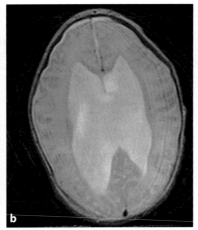
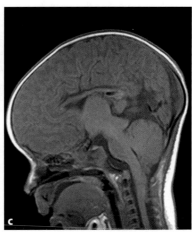

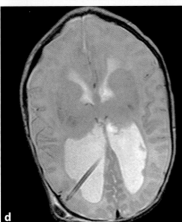

Fig. 19.1 a-d. MR scans of a boy born with myelomeningocele, Chiari II malformation and hydrocephalus. **a** Sagittal T2-weighted head scan obtained the first day of life. The movement artifact is obvious and is degrading image definition. There is a Chiari II malformation with most of the characteristic features: small posterior fossa, cerebellar ectopia down to possibly C4 (it is difficult to count the exact level), the fourth ventricle is at the level of the foramen magnum, there is a dilated third ventricle, abnormal disposition/angulation of the midbrain, and the aqueduct of Sylvius is not clearly shown. **b** Axial T2-weighted head scan obtained the first day of life showing characteristic appearance of the lateral ventricles in the presence of acute hydrocephalus; their long axes are almost parallel. The movement artifact is obvious. The child had closure of myelomeningocele and insertion of ventriculo-peritoneal shunt. **c** Sagittal T1-weighted head scan was performed at the age of 24 days, because the patient continued to have episodes of respiratory distress, stridor and cyanosis. The scan was obtained with the patient intubated, in order to exclude shunt malfunction prior to performing cranio-vertebral decompression. The Chiari II malformation is clearly shown, the tonsillar ectopia is extending down to the inferior border of C3. The fourth ventricle is at the level of the foramen magnum. The third ventricle is small in comparison to the scan of Fig. 19.1a. Anomalous deep venous drainage can be seen at the region of the quadrigeminal plate, which is deformed. **d** Axial T2-weighted scan showing the ventricular catheter in the right lateral ventricle. The characteristic dilatation of the occipital horns is seen. The ventricles are smaller than the scan of Figure 19.1b. The gyration pattern is abnormal for his age. The child had cranio-vertebral decompression, but despite some improvement he required long-term tracheostomy and feeding gastrostomy

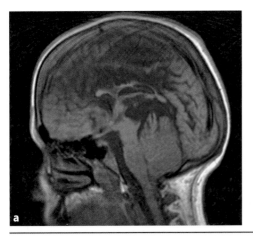
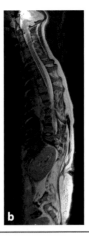
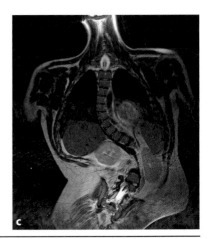

Fig. 19.2 a-c. MR scan of a 6-year-old girl who had closure of lumbar myelomeningocele and insertion of ventriculo-peritoneal shunt at birth. She had been stable for many years with no new symptoms. The scan was performed as a baseline because she had just migrated to the area and it was thought necessary to have baseline radiological appearances for future reference. **a** Sagittal T1-weighted head scan showing the Chiari II malformation with cerebellar ectopia down to C2. **b** Sagittal T2-weighted spine scan showing a thin syringomyelia in the thoracic cord. **c** Coronal T2-weighted body scan showing significant scoliosis. She required no treatment for the syringomyelia and remained stable for several years

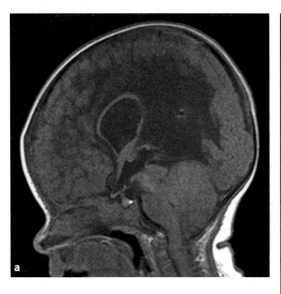

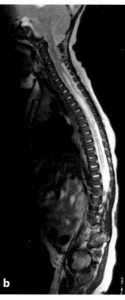

Fig. 19.3 a, b. MR scan of a 13-month-old boy who had closure of lumbar myelomeningocele and insertion of ventriculo-peritoneal shunt at birth. After the repair he had good thigh movements but poor movements below the knee. For 4 weeks prior to the scan he had deteriorating proximal leg movement and stiffness, increased tone and pronounced knee reflexes. **a** Sagittal T1-weighted head scan showing the Chiari II malformation. The shunt tube can be seen in the parietal region. **b** Sagittal T2-weighted spine scan showing a significant syringomyelia occupying most of the thoracic cord. In the upper and middle part of the cord the cavity is very wide, occupying more than half the width of the cord. In the lower thoracic region the cavity is thin. The patient underwent shunt revision, following which his symptoms rapidly improved, to the previous state

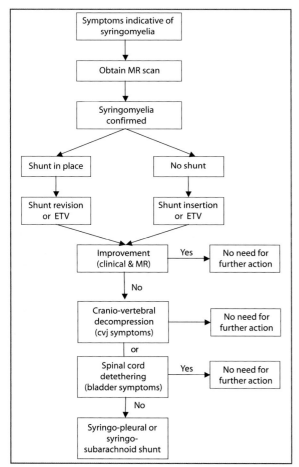

Fig. 19.4. Management scheme for patients with Chiari II malformation and syringomyelia

- There is significant prolapse of the cerebellar vermis through the foramen magnum [2], causing crowding of the foramen magnum.
- As a result of the caudal migration of the medulla the lower cranial nerves are elongated and stretched. There is also defective myelination and hypoplasia of the brain stem nuclei.
- Up to 50% of the patients have skull base and upper cervical spine abnormalities such as Klippel-Feil syndrome and atlanto-axial assimilation.

Midbrain Malformations

The features of midbrain malformations are as follows:

- There is aqueduct stenosis of variable degree in patients with myelomeningocele and Chiari II. In neuro-imaging obtained early after birth in severe cases, a large third and a small fourth ventricle are often seen, indicating aqueduct stenosis.
- The midbrain is deformed in the majority of patients [3].
- The tectal plate is deformed cranio-caudally and ventro-dorsally, in a beak-like configuration, so that the aqueduct is progressively angulated to the point that in severe cases it assumes a V-shape, pointing dorsally ("beaking" of the aqueduct) [3-5].

Brain and Ventricular System Malformations

The features of brain and ventricular system malformations are as follows:
- There is dysgenesis or absence of septum pellucidum in a high proportion of patients [6].
- The long axes of the lateral ventricles are almost parallel.
- In the lateral ventricles the atria and the occipital horns are disproportionately larger than the frontal horns, a condition known also as colpocephaly. This in association with cortical heterotopia and polymicrogyria, which are often present and create a very characteristic appearance of the ventricular system [7, 8].
- There is partial or complete absence of the falx in almost all patients.
- There is often an enlarged massa intermedia, associated with closer approximation of the two thalami.
- The floor of the third ventricle is commonly malformed [6].
- It has been postulated that the defects are part of a wider neurodevelopmental defect affecting the cerebrum, as the shape of the ventricular system resembles the fetal configuration more closely than that of normal newborns [8, 9].

Epidemiology

The incidence of myelomenigocele ranges between 0.2 to 2 per 1000 live births, with regional and racial variations [10]. The incidence of Chiari II malformation in newborns with myelomeningocele is very high, of the order of 90-100% [10, 11], but in recent years there has been the perception that the severity of the anatomical malformations seen is considerably milder in comparison to those seen a decade ago. This may reflect improved standard of living and antenatal care.

Clinical Manifestations

Clinical manifestations of the Chiari II malformation can be classified as follows:
- Problems related to the open myelomeningocele, seen at birth (discussed in another chapter of this book).
- Problems related to hydrocephalus, seen commonly at birth or developing in the first few weeks of life. Active hydrocephalus can develop later on in life as well, in childhood or adulthood.

Shunted patients can develop problems of shunt malfunction at any time in their life.
- Problems related to brain stem compression from the Chiari II malformation, usually seen in the first few weeks of life, but can be seen in the first year of life.
- Problems related to the hindbrain hernia seen later in life, in childhood or adulthood.
- Problems related to syringomyelia, seen usually in childhood and adulthood.
- Problems related to scoliosis, seen usually in childhood and adulthood.
- Problems related to spinal cord tethering, seen usually in childhood and adulthood.
- Problems related to bladder and bowel function, affecting most patients with myelomeningocele, even those who ambulate unaided: these are established in the first few years of life and require life-long treatment.
- Neuro-orthopedic problems of the lower limbs affecting most patients, but paraplegics more severely, from the first few months of life, and requiring life-long treatment.

Problems in the Neonatal Period due to Chiari II Malformation

Symptoms of brain stem dysfunction due to brain stem compression from the hindbrain hernia are not always easy to appreciate in neonates. Poor feeding due to dysphagia, recurrent vomiting, poor sucking, depressed or absent gag reflex, generally subdued behavior with poor crying, high pitched cry or stridor due to vocal cord paralysis, episodes of apnea, nystagmus, episodes of bradycardia, and recurrent aspiration often manifesting with recurrent pneumonia, can all be manifestations of brain stem and lower cranial nerve dysfunction. Other symptoms are torticollis, opisthotonus, unilateral facial paresis and long tract signs in the form of limb weakness. Inexperienced observers can easily overlook these symptoms in neonates. The incidence of these symptoms in children with Chiari II malformation and myelomeningocele is estimated at 5-10%. Such symptoms can be present at birth and deteriorate after closure of the myelomeningocele, and may coincide with the development of ventriculomegaly.

Whenever such symptoms are present the ventricular system ideally should be imaged with MR or with a CT scan, to establish the presence of hydrocephalus. If there is ventriculomegaly, a ventriculoperitoneal shunt should be inserted as soon as possible. If there is no ventriculomegaly, or the insertion of a ventricular shunt has not improved the symptoms, then a cranio-vertebral decompression should be considered early. The indications for cranio-vertebral decompression have been regarded as controversial in this clinical situation, but it has been shown that early decompression is associated with better clinical results [12, 13]. Clinical studies have demonstrated that when decompression is performed in the first two months of life it is associated with worse clinical outcomes, probably because such severe brain stem dysfunction is due to the intrinsic malformation rather than compression (Fig. 19.1). In the first 2 months of life vocal cord paresis is a sign of irreversible damage, and an indirect sign that cranio-vertebral decompression is unlikely to achieve clinical improvement. In contrast, when decompression is performed in children over the age of 2 months before the establishment of vocal cord paralysis there is a better outcome, with most symptoms improving dramatically [12, 13]. In cases where surgical treatment has not resulted in clinical improvement, often tracheostomy is required to overcome the severe respiratory problems, and a feeding gastrostomy is performed to overcome dysphagia and improve the nutritional status of the neonate (Fig. 19.1).

Problems in Childhood and Adulthood due to Chiari II Malformation

Brain stem compression, manifested with lower cranial nerve paresis, can be seen later in life in patients with Chiari II malformation, although this is uncommon. Patients with Chiari II malformation may have symptoms similar to those of patients with Chiari I malformation at any time throughout life, but these tend to be uncommon. Such symptoms include occipital headaches, worse with cough or other straining, nystagmus, syncopal episodes, recurrent episodes of aspiration pneumonia, limb weakness or clumsiness, delayed deterioration of ambulation in patients who walk, delayed deterioration of scoliosis and delayed deterioration of bladder function. Clinical signs can include new long tract signs, increased tendon reflexes and spasticity, or deterioration of long standing neurological deficits in the arms and legs. When such symptoms are present with a ventricular shunt, shunt malfunction should be excluded first. Imaging of the head ideally with MR scan, or at least with a CT scan, should be performed in order to exclude shunt obstruction. Even if the head scan is inconclusive, shunt tap or even explo-

ration should be contemplated, before it is decided that the symptoms are due to the hindbrain hernia. If the shunt has been verified to be working, or it has been revised and the symptoms and signs still persist or deteriorate, then cranio-vertebral decompression should be performed.

Cranio-vertebral Decompression in Chiari II Malformation

Cranio-vertebral decompression in children with Chiari II malformation includes occipital craniectomy in the region of the foramen magnum (usually more limited than needed in Chiari I malformation), upper cervical laminectomy that extends according to the level of the cerebellar prolapse, as low as C5 in severe cases, and dural decompression. Cranio-vertebral decompression in patients with Chiari II malformation is considerably more difficult than in patients with Chiari I. The torcular is commonly low-lying and dural opening should be performed with care to avoid opening the low-lying venous sinuses, which would be fatal for a neonate. The hindbrain hernia may contain not only cerebellum but also lower medulla. It is not uncommon for the fourth ventricle to be at the level of the foramen magnum or even lower (Fig. 19.1). When the dura is opened, care should be taken as dissection may result in unexpected exposure of the floor of the fourth ventricle. Inadvertent damage to that area can have severe neurological side effects and bulbar palsy.

In contrast to Chiari I, where intradural dissection requires exploration of the exit foramina of the fourth ventricle, in Chiari II there are significant adhesions and commonly the procedure is limited to decompression without fourth ventricle exploration. At the end of the procedure, closure is performed either with a duraplasty using pericranium or artificial materials, or by leaving the dura open in the pseudo-meningocele technique. Controversy still exists as to which of these two techniques is better. Duraplasty is favored in North America, while pseudo-meningocele is favored in parts of Europe and elsewhere in the world. Cranio-vertebral decompression in patients with Chiari II has mixed results [13, 14]. Severe bulbar symptoms tend not to improve and long tract signs show moderate improvement. As stated already, bilateral vocal cord paresis and very young age are poor prognostic factors [13]. Despite the extensive laminectomy performed in the cervical region, late spinal deformities or subluxations are uncommon following cranio-vertebral decompression, but radiological follow up should be continued for several years to monitor the evolution of spinal deformities.

Hydrocephalus in Chiari II Malformation

Epidemiology of Hydrocephalus in Myelomeningocele

In a significant proportion of patients, hydrocephalus is absent at birth but develops in the first few weeks or months of life, indicating that there is a spectrum of manifestations [10]. Hydrocephalus is seen in 15-25% of children with myelomeningocele who are imaged post-natally prior to closure of the defect [7, 10]. Many patients develop hydrocephalus in the first few weeks of life. In most surgical series the proportion of patients with myelomenigocele who required shunting reaches 80-90%, although inevitably there must be some sample bias of such series [15, 16]. No obvious correlation between the level of the lesion and the presence of hydrocephalus has been shown [15, 16].

Clinical Manifestations of Hydrocephalus in Chiari II Malformation

As in other forms of infantile hydrocephalus, children with myelomeningocele can develop an enlarging head with a bulging fontanelle, enlarged scalp veins, macrocrania, suture diastasis, and positive 'crack-pot' signs. If left untreated they develop 'sunset' eyes, recurrent vomiting and later respiratory arrest. The particular consideration of children with Chiari II malformation is the presence of hindbrain herniation, which can cause clinical symptoms of bulbar palsy early, and can remain unnoticed by inexperienced observers. Manifestations of brain stem dysfunction due to hindbrain herniation can be aggravated by ventricular dilatation. Persistent cerebrospinal fluid (CSF) leak from the repaired spinal wound almost invariably indicates active hydrocephalus, even if the ventricular size is only modestly enlarged and the anterior fontanelle is not bulging.

Radiological Considerations of Hydrocephalus in Chiari II Malformation

Most children born with myelomeningocele will have had in utero ultrasound scans, which provide information on the state of the ventricular system. Even if these scans are available, it is important to obtain neuro-imaging soon after birth, to assess the state of the ventricular system and of the hindbrain. Postnatal MR shows the ventricles, the aqueduct and the hindbrain in good detail. However, there are often significant movement artifacts degrading the image definition (Fig. 19.1a), as the newborn baby moves and sedation is avoided due to possible respiratory complications from intracranial hypertension and bulbar dysfunction. Whenever MRI cannot be obtained CT scan provides enough information on the state of the ventricular system, and assists in deciding on the need for ventricular shunt. In up to 15-20% of cases there is marked hydrocephalus with periventricular lucency indicating raised CSF pressure, and in a further 20% there is moderate ventriculomegaly [8, 17]. The features of the ventricular system in Chiari II malformation have been described already. The third ventricle is moderately dilated in most cases [6]. The lateral ventricles have a characteristic appearance. The dilatation of the occipital horns seen in children with Chiari II malformation should not be mistaken for hydrocephalus (Fig. 19.1d).

Management of Hydrocephalus

Indications for Surgery

Children with a clinical picture of active hydrocephalus and with significant ventriculomegaly will need surgical treatment early in life [7, 18-21]. While shunting has a higher infection risk in the first few weeks of life, Acetazolamide (Diamox®), ventricular tapping or lumbar puncture serve no purpose as they cannot delay shunting for 6 months and are therefore not recommended.

Children with mild or moderate ventriculomegaly and head circumference within the normal centiles may not need shunting at first, and an observation policy can be adopted for the first few months of life. Monitoring of the head circumference and repeat ultrasound or MR scanning will help decide whether they will finally require shunting.

Patients who have been shunted already and present with symptoms of possible shunt malfunction or symptoms thought to be related to the Chiari II malformation should have shunt malfunction excluded with shunt tap or even shunt revision.

Patients with shunts who have established shunt obstruction can be considered for a third ventriculostomy to have the shunt removed.

An important consideration is the relationship between hydrocephalus and scoliosis, which develops in a very high proportion of these patients in early childhood. It has been observed that scoliosis deteriorates in the presence of untreated hydrocephalus, and improves following successful shunting [22, 23]. The underlying mechanism is not fully understood, but it is postulated that active hydrocephalus exacerbates the compressive effect of the hindbrain hernia on the descending pathways at the cranio-vertebral junction, inducing neuromuscular balance on the already compromised spine from the bifid deformity.

Syringomyelia in Chiari II Malformation

Pathophysiological Aspects

Syringomyelia is the cavitation of the spinal cord for more than two spinal segments [24]. It is commonly associated with subarachnoid obstruction to CSF flow. The commonest cause of CSF obstruction is hindbrain herniation, which leads to protrusion of the inferior part of the cerebellum through the foramen magnum on to the upper cervical spine. The commonest form of hindbrain hernia is the Chiari I malformation. All the theories of formation and propagation of syringomyelia have been formulated on the basis of Chiari I malformation. Several theories have been proposed, such as the hydrodynamic 'water hammer' theory [24] and the 'suck and slosh' theory [25]. The latest theory on the formation of syringomyelia, the 'piston' theory, stems from intraoperative CSF pressure measurements and CSF velocity measurements on phase contrast cine magnetic resonance (PC Cine MR) scans of patients with Chiari I, where it has been observed that the cerebellar tonsils act like a piston in the foramen magnum during the cardiac cycle, obstructing the free flow of CSF and creating a raised CSF pressure wave in the subarachnoid space below the foramen magnum, forcing CSF into the spinal cord [26, 27].

Syringomyelia is seen in association with Chiari II malformation (Figs. 19.2 and 19.3) as indeed is seen in other forms of spinal dysraphism such as spinal lipoma or diastematomyelia. There are many anatomical and physiological differences between the two types of Chiari malformations and the theoretical models that explain syringomyelia creation and propagation in Chiari I malformation do not easily apply to patients with Chiari II malformation. To date, there is no detailed investigative work in the literature that attempts to explain the formation of syringomyelia in Chiari II patients. All evidence is based on clinical retrospective observations.

Some of the main differences between the two malformations are:

- In Chiari II malformation most of the prolapsed cerebellar tissue is part of the vermis and not the tonsils, as the malformation is created in utero before formation of the cerebellar tonsils. Often, the lower medulla and part of the fourth ventricle is also below the foramen magnum. While in Chiari I the mobile tonsillar tissue can move with every cardiac cycle and 'plug' the foramen magnum, in Chiari II the hindbrain hernia contains less 'mobile' structures such as the vermis and the lower medulla, so the analogy may not be appropriate.

- In support of the previous point, during craniovertebral decompression, in patients with Chiari II malformation there are always significant and dense arachnoid adhesions in the region of the foramen magnum and foramens of Magendie and Luschka, more than seen in patients with Chiari I malformation. This is evident at operation, even in children who are only a few weeks old.

- The majority of patients with Chiari I malformation are symptomatic, whereas the majority of patients with Chiari II malformation do not experience symptoms directly caused by the malformation [20, 28].

- In contrast to Chiari I malformation where syringomyelia is found in a high proportion of patients, over 60% in most clinical series [25, 29, 30], in Chiari II malformation the co-existence of syringomyelia is considerably less frequent, varying from 25 to 45% in different reports [14, 31-36] and a third of them require treatment [14]. Overall, patients with Chiari II malformation account for approximately 4% of all patients with syringomyelia of all causes and types [25]. This reflects not only the low incidence of syringomyelia in Chiari II, but also the low incidence of the Chiari II malformation itself.

- In the context of the Chiari I malformation, although the phenomenon of progressive development of syringomyelia has been well described, in most patients syringomyelia is present from the beginning, at the first clinical presentation [37], and very often is responsible for the symptoms. In the context of Chiari II malformation, syringomyelia is rarely present at birth, and commonly develops many years later. The average age of children with Chiari II who have syringomyelia is between 4 and 7 years [14, 33-36], although it can be seen at an earlier age as well.

- In patients with Chiari I malformation and syringomyelia commonly there is no clinically significant hydrocephalus, whereas in most patients (80-90%) with Chiari II and syringomyelia there is almost always long standing hydrocephalus that has been treated in the first few weeks of life with ventriculo-peritoneal shunt [7, 20]. There is indirect evidence that development of syringomyelia in patients with Chiari II malformation is associated with insufficient shunt function because in most patients shunt revision leads to radiological improvement of the syrinx [14, 31-36]. In contrast, in most patients with Chiari I malformation, syringomyelia improves with establishment of free flow of CSF in the foramen magnum [25, 29, 30]. On the other hand, similar to Chiari II, in the few patients who have Chiari I, syringomyelia and hydrocephalus, when there is shunt malfunction the syringomyelia cavity increases and when the shunt is revised the syringomyelia cavity decreases.

There has been no study demonstrating a correlation between the extent of herniation of the hindbrain and the incidence of syringomyelia. In recent years antenatal repair of myelomeningocele has been performed, and this has been shown to lead to reduced incidence of hindbrain herniation at birth [38]. Nevertheless, as this treatment has been performed only for about 15 years and only in two centers worldwide, it is too early to know if it also leads to reduced syringomyelia incidence in these patients.

This complex association between hindbrain hernia, hydrocephalus and syringomyelia in Chiari II malformation creates significant problems in the clinical management of such patients. It is not always easy to distinguish whether symptoms are due to the syringomyelia, the hindbrain herniation, the hydrocephalus or the spinal cord tethering that is commonly present radiologically in patients who have had primary closure of myelomeningocele at birth.

Clinical Presentation of Syringomyelia in Chiari II Malformation

It is common for patients who have had closure of myelomeningocele at birth and have Chiari II malformation, hydrocephalus and syringomyelia and have been stable for many years, to present with gradual progressively deteriorating neurological symptoms and signs related to bulbar, long tract or bladder function [14, 33-35]. Bulbar symptoms include respiratory distress, stridor or sleep apnea, vocal cord

paresis, difficulty in swallowing, episodes of aspiration, impaired gag reflex and ocular motor paresis with squint or diplopia and nystagmus. Motor symptoms and signs include deterioration of leg function in ambulatory patients with progressive difficulty in walking and clumsiness or even spasticity and, if the cervical spinal cord is affected, new problems in the upper limbs with clumsiness in fine hand movements and dexterity (e.g., deterioration of writing pattern). Sensory symptoms include new pain or an increase in previously existing pain in trunk and lower limbs, altered sweating pattern especially below the level of the paraplegia and patchy altered sensation in a non-dermatomal distribution. Patients who have intact bladder function can develop deterioration of the micturition pattern. Many paraplegic patients with spina bifida have scoliosis and the development of syringomyelia can coincide with deterioration of the scoliotic curve [39].

While most of these symptoms are seen also in relation to syringomyelia in the context of the Chiari I malformation, in patients with Chiari II malformation the causative link of such symptoms with syringomyelia is not always obvious or firm. Patients with Chiari II, hydrocephalus and a shunt often develop many of the symptoms outlined above, even in the absence of syringomyelia, when their shunt is malfunctioning, and they improve after successful shunt revision. Even scoliosis deterioration has been reported in association with shunt malfunction [21]. Moreover, most patients who had myelomeningocele repaired at birth have a radiological appearance of tethered cord at the repair site in MR scans. Regardless of how successful and anatomically correct the repair has been, the spinal cord never ascends to its correct level and always appears attached to the area of the repaired defect. This situation is established in the first few weeks after the repair and remains unchanged even when the patient is clinically very well and stable.

Radiology of Syringomyelia in Chiari II Malformation

In the pre-MR era it was very difficult to diagnose syringomyelia in patients with spina bifida aperta. CT scan shows cavitation in the spinal cord but cannot be used easily to image the entire spinal cord, especially in children, as it would give the patient a significant dose of radiation. Myelography was used but this was not an easy procedure to perform as many patients have a degree of scoliosis and in general they do not tolerate invasive procedures well.

MR scans improved the ability to diagnose syringomyelia, and offered a better appreciation of the magnitude of the problem for patients with myelomeningocele. The presence of syringomyelia is easily diagnosed in the sagittal spinal T1- and T2-weighted MR scans in patients with Chiari II. In contrast to Chiari I-related syringomyelia, which is most often cervical in location, in Chiari II the center of gravity of the cavity is usually located in the thoracic cord. It can be either 'segmental', occupying a few segments of the spinal cord, or 'holocord', occupying the entire spinal cord (Figs. 19.2 and 19.3). Although in Chiari II the syringomyelia cavity is commonly longer than in Chiari I, its transverse diameter is usually less than that seen in cavities associated with Chiari I malformation. Rarely, the syringomyelia cavity is in the cervical cord and threatens to become syringobulbia. Large cavities can have septations, as in patients with Chiari I malformation. In patients with scoliosis, the estimation of the length of syringomyelia can be difficult, as the whole length of the spine may not be seen in one sagittal view.

While most of the patients with Chiari II and syringomyelia have had treatment for hydrocephalus, in a small proportion the ventricles have been either normal or borderline enlarged at birth and these patients have not had surgical ventricular drainage procedures [7]. An even smaller proportion of patients have moderate ventriculomegaly without symptoms of raised pressure, which represents a state of arrested hydrocephalus and is not treated surgically in most cases.

Surgical Management of Syringomyelia in Chiari II Malformation

With modern imaging the challenge with these patients is no longer how to establish the diagnosis, but to decide which patients need surgical treatment for the syringomyelia. In departments where routine MR scanning of patients with Chiari II malformation is performed every 2-3 years, occasionally the presence of syringomyelia is discovered incidentally, in the course of such a routine MR scan [14]. These patients tend to have mild to moderate syringomyelia (Fig. 19.2). In the absence of symptoms, and if the cavity's transverse diameter is less than half the width of the spinal cord, most often we would elect to avoid surgery and instead observe first and repeat the scan in a few months, before we decide to consider surgical treatment. Clinically 'silent' syringomyelia cav-

ities often remain radiologically stable and do not require treatment for years. However, in most units routine MR scans of patients with Chiari II malformation are not performed, reserving that examination for when new clinical problems arise.

In most cases, the presence of new neurological symptoms prompts an MR scan, which can demonstrate syringomyelia. The difficulty in distinguishing whether the clinical symptoms are due to the syringomyelia, the hydrocephalus or the tethered cord has created inconsistencies in the management of patients with Chiari II and syringomyelia. There are no agreed protocols or robust evidence originating from randomized studies on how these patients should be managed [40, 41], and different schemes and algorithms have been suggested based on clinical series, often reflecting prevailing tendencies at the time, and differences in experience, training and attitude. While there have been many attempts to classify and group different neurological symptoms, the situation is even more confusing with scoliosis, as there is no clear evidence if deterioration is directly related to syringomyelia [39].

If the syringomyelia is extensive, with a transverse diameter more than half of the width of the spinal cord, and appears threatening, in association with the onset of new symptoms, then surgical action is required.

A proposed algorithm for the management of these patients is shown in Fig. 19.4. This algorithm is a variation of other similar schemas proposed in the past [34] and should be used as a guideline rather than a rigid protocol. It is universally accepted that in a patient who has had treatment for hydrocephalus with a ventriculo-peritoneal shunt and who presents with clear neurological deterioration and significant syringomyelia, the shunt must be investigated first, and even in the absence of ventriculomegaly or symptoms of raised intracranial pressure, shunt revision should be performed to exclude shunt malfunction and establish that the shunt is functioning [14, 31-36, 41]. In most patients, shunt revision leads to improvement of the clinical symptoms and radiological improvement of the syringomyelia or at worst stabilization, thus not requiring any further surgical measures (Fig. 19.3). Recently, endoscopic third ventriculostomy (ETV) has been tried with some success when a patient presents with a blocked shunt, in order to remove the shunt completely [42].

In the presence of moderate ventriculomegaly, patients who have not had shunts before should be considered for surgical drainage of the ventricles. Most surgeons would insert a ventricular shunt, although in the last few years there have been reports of successful treatment and resolution of the syringomyelia cavity with ETV [42].

After surgical treatment of hydrocephalus, in the presence of clinical improvement, even if the syringomyelia cavity has not reduced in size it is best to avoid immediate surgical action, and to observe and repeat the MR scan in 6 months to verify that the syringomyelia cavity is remaining stable. The remaining treatment options are more difficult and complex and risk significant complications, thus careful consideration should be given before further surgical action is taken.

If hydrocephalus treatment (shunt revision/insertion or ETV) has not resulted in clinical and/or radiological improvement, cranio-vertebral decompression should be performed to establish CSF circulation in the cranio-cervical junction if the predominant symptoms are those of cranio-vertebral junction compression, and tethered cord release should be undertaken if the predominant symptoms are those of bladder dysfunction [34, 36]. Both surgical options pose significant difficulties.

Cranio-vertebral decompression in patients with Chiari II malformation is considerably more difficult than in Chiari I, as already described. When it is performed for syringomyelia, especially in the absence of bulbar symptoms, results are better, with a good chance of clinical and radiological improvement in over 60% of patients [13, 14].

The decision to perform tethered cord release should not be taken hastily, as repeat exploration of the spina bifida site is fraught with problems. The quality of the skin is usually poor, as the dermis is mostly scar tissue, without substantial subcutaneous layers. Even if the repair after birth manages to recreate satisfactory layers, a few years later the area is mostly scar tissue and has no normal anatomical planes. This makes dissection difficult, with high risk of operative damage of the remaining rootlets, and difficulty in closing the wound at the end, with high risk of CSF leak, and all the associated problems. Due to the poor skin quality, wound healing is often difficult. For this reason, if the repeat exploration is unavoidable, we often take the opportunity to employ plastic surgical techniques to mobilize normal skin from nearby and improve on the skin closure.

If despite all these measures the clinical symptoms and the radiological appearances of syringomyelia persist, insertion of a syringo-pleural or syringo-subarachnoid shunt can be considered [14, 32, 33, 43]. The use of syrinx shunts is controversial. Many authors have suggested them as an early surgical option, before cranio-vertebral decompression [31, 34]. There is no conclusive evidence on the best time to use these options. There have been reports of good results in spina bifida patients [43]. Nevertheless, in the analogy of Chiari I malformation, if a syrinx shunt is inserted before addressing the block at the foramen magnum, the beneficial effect tends to be short lived [44]. Insertion of a syringo-pleural or syringo-subarachnoid shunt requires laminotomy in the site of the widest diameter of the syrinx and intradural exposure of the spinal cord. A midline myelotomy is performed. A fine ultrasound probe is recommended prior to performing the myelotomy, to confirm the presence of a cavity. After a small myelotomy is performed, a T-shaped catheter is inserted in the syrinx cavity and secured with pial fine sutures. The other end is placed in the subarachnoid space or threaded towards the chest wall in the midaxillary line and in the pleural cavity. As for all shunts, syrinx shunts have mechanical and infective complications.

For paraplegic wheelchair bound patients with severe bladder and bowel disorders and with relentlessly deteriorating syringomyelia, the option of cordotomy and terminal ventriculostomy exists. This was practiced infrequently in the 70s and 80s but has fallen out of favor in the last decade due to its amputating nature, and is no longer performed.

Outcome of Syringomyelia in Chiari II Malformation

Syringomyelia is seen in 25-40% of patients with myelomeningocele and Chiari II malformation, but only a small proportion of these patients require surgical treatment [14]. When a new syringomyelia cavity is seen and is associated with new neurological symptoms, in most cases shunt revision results in good clinical and radiological resolution. If the patient has had no treatment for hydrocephalus and there is mild ventriculomegaly, surgical drainage of the ventricles with a shunt or endoscopic third ventriculostomy is usually sufficient to control the syringomyelia. This is fortunate and obviates the need for other surgical maneuvers, which have a significant risk of complication. A small proportion of patients develop relentlessly deteriorating syringomyelia and may require multiple operations in the form of cranio-vertebral decompression, cord detethering or syrinx shunts. In clinical practice though, it is rare for syringomyelia to be a difficult problem in patients with repaired myelomeningocele and Chiari II malformation.

References

1. Naidich TP, Pudlowski RM, Naidich JB et al (1980) Computed tomographic signs of the Chiari II malformation part I: skull and dura partitions. Radiology 134:65-71
2. Naidich TP, McLone DG, Fulling KH (1983) The Chiari II malformation: Part IV. The hindbrain deformity. Neuroradiology 25:179-197
3. Naidich TP, Pudlowski RM, Naidich JB (1980b) Computed tomographic signs of Chiari II malformation II: Midbrain and cerebellum. Radiology 134:391-398
4. Parent AD, McMillan T (1995) Contemporaneous shunting with repair of myelomeningocele. Pediatr Neurosurg 22:132-135; discussion 136
5. Vogl D, Ring-Mrozik E, Baierl P et al (1987) Magnetic resonance imaging in children suffering spina bifida. Z Kinderchir 42 (Suppl I):60-64
6. Naidich TP, Pudlowski RM, Naidich JB (1980) Computed tomographic signs of the Chiari II malformation III: Ventricles and cisterns. Radiology 134:657-663
7. Dias MS, McLone DG (1993) Hydrocephalus in the child with dysraphism. Neurosurg Clin N Am 4:715-726
8. Van Roost D, Solymosi L, Funke K (1995) A characteristic ventricular shape in myelomeningocele-associated hydrocephalus? A CT stereology study. Neuroradiology 37:412-417
9. Bannister CM, Russell SA, Rimmer S (1998) Pre-natal brain development of fetuses with a myelomeningocele. Eur J Pediatr Surg 8 Suppl 1:15-17
10. Dias MS (1999) Myelomeningocele. In: Choux M, Di Rocco C, Hockley A, Walker M (eds) Pediatric neurosurgery. Churchill Livingstone, pp 33-59
11. McLone DG (1998) Care of the neonate with a myelomeningocele. Neurosurg Clin N Am 9:111-120
12. Pollack IF, Kinnunen D, Leland Albright A (1996) The effect of early craniocervical decompression on functional outcome in neonates and young infants with myelodysplasia and symptomatic Chiari II malformations: results from a prospective series. Neurosurgery 38:703-710
13. Pollack IF, Pang D, Albright AL et al (1992) Outcome following hindbrain decompression of symptomatic Chiari malformations in children previously treated with myelomeningocele closure and shunts. J Neurosurg 77:881-888
14. Caldarelli M, Di Rocco C, La Marca F (1998) Treatment of hydromyelia in spina bifida. Surg Neurol 50:411-420
15. Mirzai H, Ersahin Y, Mutluer S et al (1998) Outcome of patients with meningomyelocele: the Ege University experience. Childs Nerv Syst 14:120-123
16. Steinbok P, Irvine B, Cochrane DD et al (1992) Long-term outcome and complications of children born with meningomyelocele. Childs Nerv Syst 8:92-96
17. Babcock CJ, Goldstein RB, Barth RA et al (1994) Prevalence of ventriculomegaly in association with myelomeningocele: correlation with gestational age and severity of posterior fossa deformity. Radiology 190:703-707
18. Gamache FW (1995) Treatment of hydrocephalus in patients with meningomyelocele or encephalocele: a recent series. Childs Nerv Syst 11:487-488
19. Hubballah MY, Hoffman HJ (1987) Early repair of myelomenigocele and simultaneous insertion of ventriculoperitobeal shunt: technique and result. Neurosurgery 20:21-23
20. McLone DG (1992) Continuing concepts in the management of spina bifida. Pediatr Neurosurg 18:254-256
21. Sgouros S (2004) Hydrocephalus with myelomeningocele. In: Cinalli G, Maixner WJ, Sainte-Rose C (eds) Pediatric hydrocephalus. Spinger-Verlag, Milano, pp 133-144
22. Geiger F, Parsch D, Carstens C (1999) Complications of scoliosis surgery in children with myelomeningocele. Eur Spine J 8:22-26
23. Hall P, Lindseth R, Campbell R et al (1979) Scoliosis and hydrocephalus in myelocele patients. The effect of ventricular shunting. J Neurosurg 50:174-178
24. Gardner JW (1965) Hydrodynamic mechanism of syringomyelia: its relationship to myelocele. J Neurol Neurosurg Psychiatry 28:247-259
25. Williams B (1990) Syringomyelia. Neurosurg Clin North Am 1:653-685
26. Heiss JD, Patronas N, DeVroom HL et al (1999) Elucidating the pathophysiology of syringomyelia. J Neurosurg 91:553-562
27. Oldfield EH, Muraszko K, Shawker TH, Patronas NJ (1994) Pathophysiology of syringomyelia associated with Chiari I malformation of the cerebellar tonsils. Implications for diagnosis and treatment. J Neurosurgery 80:3-15
28. Haines SJ, Berger MD (1991) Current treatment of Chiari malformations type I and II: a survey of the Pediatric Section of the American Association of Neurological surgeons. Neurosurgery 28:353-357
29. Dyste GN, Menezes AH, Van Gilder JC (1989) Symptomatic Chiari malformations. An analysis of presentation, management, and long-term outcome. J Neurosurg 71:159-168
30. Milhorat TH, Johnson WD, Miller JI et al (1992) Surgical treatment of syringomyelia based on magnetic resonance imaging criteria. Neurosurgery 31:231-245
31. Caldarelli M, Di Rocco C, Colosimo C Jr et al (1995) Surgical treatment of late neurological deterioration in children with myelodysplasia. Acta Neurochir (Wien) 137:199-206
32. Craig JJ, Gray WJ, McCann JP (1999) The Chiari/hydrosyringomyelia complex presenting in adults with myelomeningocele: an indication for early intervention. Spinal Cord 37:275-278
33. Koyanagi I, Iwasaki Y, Hida K et al (1997) Surgical treatment of syringomyelia associated with spinal dysraphism. Childs Nerv Syst 13:194-200

34. La Marca F, Herman M, Grant JA, McLone DG (1997) Presentation and management of hydromyelia in children with Chiari type-II malformation. Pediatr Neurosurg 26:57-67
35. Rauzzino M, Oakes WJ (1995) Chiari II malformation and syringomyelia. Neurosurg Clin N Am 6:293-309
36. Zerah M (1999) Syringomyélie de l'enfant (Syringomyelia in childhood) Neurochirurgie 45 Suppl 1:37-57 (article in French)
37. Milhorat TH, Miller JI, Johnson WD et al (1993) Anatomical basis of syringomyelia occurring with hindbrain lesions. Neurosurgery 32:748-754
38. Tulipan N, Hernanz-Schulman M, Bruner JP (1998) Reduced hindbrain herniation after intrauterine myelomeningocele repair: A report of four cases. Pediatr Neurosurg 29:274-278
39. Dias MS (2005) Neurosurgical causes of scoliosis in patients with myelomeningocele: an evidence-based literature review. J Neurosurg 103(1 Suppl):24-35
40. Piatt JH Jr (2004) Syringomyelia complicating myelomeningocele: review of the evidence J Neurosurg 100(2 Suppl Pediatrics):101-109
41. Tubbs RS, Oakes WJ (2004) Treatment and management of the Chiari II malformation: an evidence-based review of the literature. Childs Nerv Syst 20:375-381
42. Buxton N, Jaspan T, Punt J (2002) Treatment of Chiari malformation, syringomyelia and hydrocephalus by neuroendoscopic third ventriculostomy. Minim Invasive Neurosurg 45:231-234
43. Vernet O, Farmer JP, Montes JL (1996) Comparison of syringopleural and syringosubarachnoid shunting in the treatment of syringomyelia in children. J Neurosurg 84:624-628
44. Sgouros S, Williams B (1995) A critical appraisal of drainage in syringomyelia. J Neurosurg 82:1-10

CHAPTER 20
Challenging Problems of Shunt Management in Spina Bifida

Harold L. Rekate

Introduction

Hydrocephalus in the context of spina bifida may represent the most complicated and confusing form of congenital hydrocephalus. Essentially all patients with spina bifida aperta have an associated Chiari II malformation. In some, especially those with very low lesion levels, this malformation may be very mild. Experimental evidence suggests that the Chiari II malformation results from in utero loss of cerebrospinal fluid (CSF) into the amniotic fluid and subsequent failure of distension of the fetal head leading to a very small posterior fossa and severe herniation of the hindbrain [1]. One of the major indications for prenatal repair of the myelomeningocele is to minimize this descent of the cerebellum and brainstem and therefore maximize the chance that the patient may be able to thrive without a shunt [2-4].

The complexity of the hydrocephalus relates to the anatomy of the Chiari II malformation and the sites of obstruction within the CSF pathways leading to the hydrocephalus. Figure 20.1 shows an artist's representation of the Chiari II malformation documenting the potential sites of obstruction to the flow of CSF resulting in hydrocephalus [5, 6]. In an individual patient with spina bifida, obstruction can be documented in any of these sites and many will have multiple sites of obstruction.

In the Chiari II malformation, the tentorium tends to be oriented vertically and to be incompetent at the incisura. This leads to upward migration or herniation of the superior cerebellar vermis. This herniation can lead to distortion of the aqueduct of Sylvius and therefore to secondary aqueductal stenosis. It is this subset of spina bifida patients with hydrocephalus overt at birth that often require early delivery secondary to rapidly increasing head circumference and rapidly evolving hydrocephalus with loss of brain volume. In the context of the Chiari II malformation, the degree of herniation can be so severe

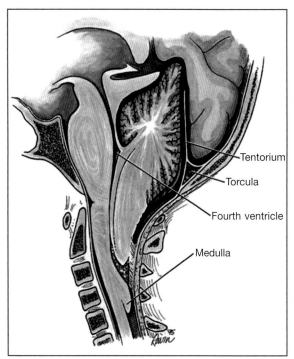

Fig. 20.1. Artist's concept of the Chiari II malformation demonstrating the four potential sources of obstruction of the flow of cerebrospinal fluid causing hydrocephalus in patients with spina bifida. Reprinted with permission from Barrow Neurological Institute

that the foramina of Luschka can reside within the cervical canal. The foramen of Magendie is almost uniformly closed due to scarring and extrusion of the choroid plexus of the fourth ventricle into the subarachnoid space of the cervical spine. The chronic arachnoiditis that occurs as a result of the mixing of the CSF with amniotic fluid in utero also contributes to the failure of the foramina of Luschka to serve as pathways for the egress of CSF from the fourth ventricle into the spinal subarachnoid space. The pathophysiology of this form of hydrocephalus will be discussed in greater detail in the case examples below.

Relatively often, the degree of hindbrain herniation is such that there is occlusion of the pathway between the spinal and cortical subarachnoid spaces. Since there is flow of CSF between the ventricle and the spinal subarachnoid space, this form of hydrocephalus is viewed as "communicating" hydrocephalus despite the fact that there is a complete, or nearly complete, obstruction of the flow of CSF from the spinal to the cortical subarachnoid space. This form of hydrocephalus may lead to insidious deterioration over a long period of time. Insidious deterioration is very unlikely except in the context of spina bifida and there is no evidence to support routine asymptomatic scanning in this condition except in spina bifida patients. The diagnosis of shunt independent arrest of hydrocephalus is most dangerous in this context and sudden death and near miss cardiac and respiratory arrests are well reported [7].

Finally, venous abnormalities are frequent in the Chiari II malformation and it is not unusual to find the torcula at or even below the level of the foramen magnum (Fig. 20.2). Venous hypertension does not lead to hydrocephalus in older children or adults who have fixed skull volumes. It leads to pseudotumor cerebri. In infants, however, the fontanel is open and the sutures are not fused. In the context of increased pressure in the superior sagittal sinus the intracranial pressure does not rise high enough for CSF to be absorbed. Following shunting the fontanels and sutures

close. The skull is no longer distensible and CSF can be absorbed because the intracranial pressure (ICP) can rise sufficiently. The cost, however, is marked increases in ICP. In this situation the ventricles do not expand at the time of shunt failure, a condition referred to by Engel and colleagues as normal volume hydrocephalus (NVH) [8, 9]. These patients are frequently misdiagnosed as drug seeking or malingerers due to the radiology report indicating "good shunt function" or "no evidence of hydrocephalus". In patients with hydrocephalus and spina bifida, clinical evidence of increased ICP must be taken seriously and an assessment of ICP needs to be made even in the context of ventricles that have not increased in size.

Obstruction of the Outlet Foramina of the Fourth Ventricle

Prior to the introduction of magnetic resonance imaging (MRI) the diagnosis of syringomyelia was very challenging. Imaging studies with myelography or air myelography required a high index of suspicion and were often difficult to interpret. In 1973 Hall and Lindseth [10] recognized that scoliosis in the context of spina bifida could result from severe syringomyelia at the time of shunt failure. These authors recommended that if a patient with spina bifida presents with rapidly progressive scoliosis without an anatomic basis such as one or more hemivertebrae, one should assume that the cause of the scoliosis is a failed shunt resulting in syringomyelia. Shunt repair is usually all that is needed to treat the syringomyelia. This and other observations led Dr. David McLone, who proposed that when anything goes wrong with a patient with spina bifida it should first be determined whether or not the shunt is working, to repeat famous words: "it's the shunt stupid" [11].

Case Example 1

This 15-year-old male born with an L5 level myelomeningocele presented to another center with severe headaches, neck pain and rapid progression of scoliosis. MRI of his spine showed the expected Chiari II malformation and syringomyelia (Fig. 20.3). He initially underwent a Chiari II malformation decompression with C1 to C4 decompression, with no improvement in the symptoms or change in the MRI. Over this time he began to complain of severe pain in his hands and decrease in hand strength so that he

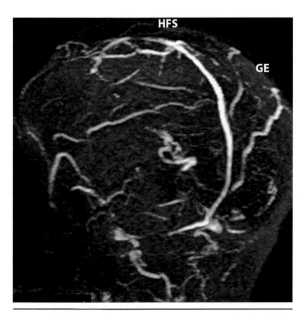

Fig. 20.2. MR venogram in a patient with Chiari II malformation demonstrating low placement of torcula and abnormal venous drainage leading to hydrocephalus in infants with the Chiari II malformation

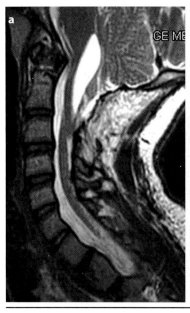
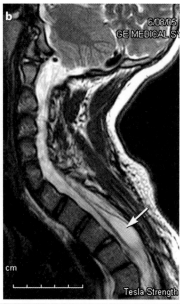

Fig. 20.3 a, b. Sagittal MRI of patient in example 1 demonstrating the expected Chiari II malformation and syringomyelia. Severe scoliosis required two images. **a** Cephalad sagittal image showing Chiari II and fourth ventricular dilatation and **b** showing the syrinx identified by *white arrow*

needed help with dressing and personal hygiene. With progression of symptoms and lack of radiographic response the patient underwent a syrinx-to-pleural shunt. This procedure resulted in radiographic improvement of the syrinx and stabilization of the weakness in his hands but with minimal improvement. He developed weakness in his neck musculature and had difficulty holding his head up. He was placed in a rigid cervical collar. At this point he was unable to remain upright for more than 30 minutes at a time and had to leave school and undergo home-schooling.

On presentation, the patient was in significant pain and on narcotic medication. He remained recumbent most of the day and was required to lie down frequently due to severe headaches that could only be ameliorated with recumbency. His hands were very weak and showed early atrophy of both the thenar and hypothenar eminences. Reflexes were absent in his upper extremities and brisk at his knees. He did not have ankle reflexes and had never had them.

MRI of the brain showed mild ventricular enlargement but the presence of significant extracerebral CSF collections (Fig. 20.4). MRI of the cervical spine showed a syrinx at the C6 and C7 level (Fig. 20.5).

The syrinx-to-pleural shunt that had been implanted was a straight tube with only a distal slit valve. On hearing the overall history and analysis of his current condition, we suspected that the underlying cause of his problems from the beginning was an insidious failure of his ventriculoperitoneal shunt. The initial cause of his hydrocephalus had been complete obstruction of the outlet foramina of the fourth

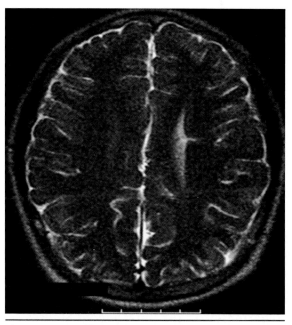

Fig. 20.4. MRI of brain showing mild ventricular dilatation but marked prominence of extracerebral fluid

ventricle and the failure of the shunt resulted in an acute development of syringomyelia. The valveless shunt that was employed for the treatment of the syringomyelia had also drained the ventricles at a very low ICP, leading to severe intracranial hypotension.

With this in mind he underwent removal of the distal end of the syrinx shunt and connection to a drainage system. At the same time the shunt was ex-

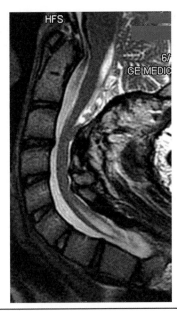

Fig. 20.5. MRI of cervical spine following shunt revision and removal of syringopleural shunt

plored and complete proximal obstruction was demonstrated. This was repaired. On the day following surgery the shunt was injected with indigo carmine and within two hours the dye was seen to pass into the syrinx drainage system. After MRI revealed no increase in the size of the syrinx, this tube was removed. All symptoms have improved. He no longer has headaches, no longer needs his collar, has had improvement in the scoliosis and improvement in the strength of the hand. The message here, which has been often repeated, is that when there is evidence of neurological deterioration in a patient with spina bifida, first make absolutely certain that the shunt is working. Also a new syrinx in patients with spina bifida is most likely to be caused by failure of the ventricular shunt.

Hypertension in the Dural Venous Sinuses

As stated above, venous abnormalities are common in patients with the Chiari II malformation. In most cases this is due to the low position of the insertion of the falx and therefore the presence of the torcula at the level of the foramen magnum or within the cervical spine. Between one-quarter to one-third of patients with hydrocephalus in the context of spina bifida will have little or no change in ventricular size at the time of shunt failure, so-called normal volume hydrocephalus [8]. In most cases this enigmatic condition can be managed with a ventricular shunt with

a device to retard siphoning with an opening pressure that is higher than the pressure in the venous sinuses. In severe cases in which the venous pressures are very high this strategy is not successful. This then requires new strategies for management. In patients without spina bifida but with this severe form of the slit ventricle syndrome, it is best to manage this condition using a lumboperitoneal shunt, which can access both the intraventricular CSF and the CSF within the cortical subarachnoid space. This is not practical because of the spinal anatomy in spina bifida and an alternative strategy to drain both the ventricles and the cortical subarachnoid space is needed [12, 13].

Case Example 2

The present case illustration deals with a 20-year-old woman who was born with hydrocephalus and a high lumbar myelomeningocele. She underwent staged repair of the myelomeningocele perinatally, and ventriculoperitoneal shunt was placed before discharge from the hospital. About 6 weeks prior to this admission she began to experience severe intermittent headaches and pain along the shunt track. The shunt was explored and completely replaced with a Codman Hakim programmable valve with siphonguard™ (Codman Corp, a Johnson and Johnson Company, Raynham, MA) initially set at an opening pressure of 100 mm H_2O. Postoperatively she was unimproved. The ventricular catheter was found on computed tomography (CT) scan to be in the appropriate position and the ventricles were not enlarged. A shunt tap was performed with poor proximal flow. ICP monitoring utilizing a parenchymal pressure transducer was undertaken and the ICP was found to be 60 mm Hg with a good waveform. By this time she was found to have a pulse that intermittently dropped below 40 beats/minute. Figure 20.6 is an MRI demonstrating the size of the ventricles at the time of the documented high ICP. Figure 20.6a is an axial T2 image demonstrating small lateral and third ventricles. Figure 20.6b is a sagittal image at the same time revealing small ventricles, Chiari II malformation and significant CSF in the cortical subarachnoid space. MR venography revealed severe abnormalities of venous drainage with absence or high grade stenosis of the transverse sinuses bilaterally.

Reestablishing a functioning ventriculoperitoneal shunt in this situation was felt to be futile. It was felt that we would need to do something that would effectively drain both the ventricles and the cortical subarachnoid spaces. As stated above, our usu-

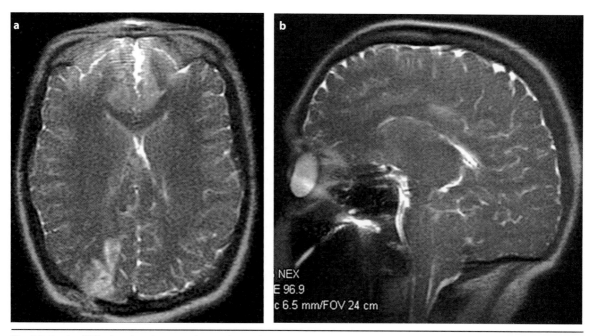

Fig. 20.6 a, b. MRI of patient in example number 2 showing small ventricles at the time of shunt failure and documented life threatening intracranial pressure. **a** Axial T2 image showing small ventricles and the presence of fluid in cortical sub-arachnoid space. **b** Sagittal MRI showing expected Chiari II malformation with small ventricles and the presence of ex-tracerebral CSF

al strategy in this situation would be to perform a lumboperitoneal shunt but due to the spina bifida and a previous spinal fusion we felt that this would not be possible [13]. Johnston and colleagues [14] had recommended direct shunting of the cisterna magna as an appropriate treatment for patients with pseudo-tumor cerebri. Our previous experiences with direct shunting to the cisterna magna had been problem-atic, with the tendency of the shunt to break with movements of the neck. Patients with the Chiari II malformation also lack a cisterna magna, making the performance of such a shunt very difficult, if not im-possible.

In order to access the cortical subarachnoid space we decided to create a new cisterna magna by doing a standard Chiari II decompression of C1 to C3 with a generous dural patch to create this new cisterna magna. A piece of lumboperitoneal shunt tubing was then placed into this newly created cis-terna magna and affixed to the patch by suturing a stepdown connector and splicing a standard piece of peritoneal shunt tubing and bringing it to the site of insertion of the ventricular catheter where it was spliced into the existing shunt system with a "Y" or "T" connector. This system allows mixing of the various compartments of the CSF and balances the inward and outward stresses that tend to distort the ventricular system [15, 16]. Following the proce-

dure, ICP was monitored and was found to be com-pletely normalized with recumbent pressures of 5-15 mm Hg and the upright pressures -5 to +5 sitting up. She has done well in the subsequent 4 years.

The cisterna magna-to-ventricle-to-peritoneal shunt has been shown to be useful in patients with severe difficulties with intracranial hypertension and non-responding ventricles, and not only in patients with this problem and the Chiari II malformation, but also in patients with Chiari I malformation and in the specific case of hydrocephalus and achondroplasia where the lumbar theca cannot be shunted due to the severe spinal stenosis. We have now performed the procedure in 22 subsequent patients with success [16]. As the procedure has developed we now uti-lize a titanium plate over the exposed dural patch to tent up the patch and assure the continued filling of the newly created cisterna magna (Fig. 20.7). It is very complex. We have had to reposition catheters on six occasions. Troubleshooting the system is rel-atively simple. In these patients imaging studies with CT scanning or MR do not reveal changes in ven-tricular volume. In order to know whether or not the shunt is working it is necessary to perform a shunt tap with a very small needle, measure the pressure with a manometer and inject about 5 cc of myelo-gram dye into the system and perform a CT scan of

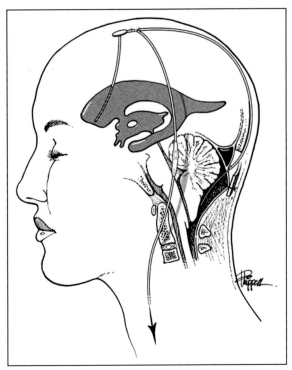

Fig. 20.7. Artist's representation of the cisterna magna-to-ventricle-to-peritoneal shunt as it has been developed. Reprinted with permission from Barrow Neurological Institute

the brain and spinal subarachnoid space to reveal that both limbs of the shunt system are patent and the pressure is normal.

Endoscopic Third Ventriculostomy in the Chiari II Malformation

As described in another chapter in this work, endoscopic third ventriculostomy in the context of the Chiari II malformation is problematic. There are several reasons for this. The most widely held reason is correct, in that the anatomy of the third ventricle is very different than the ventricle in other forms of hydrocephalus. The massa intermedia is very large and the width of the third ventricle is frequently not enlarged despite rather massive enlargement of the lateral ventricles. The floor of the third ventricle is usually vertical, being parallel to the trajectory of the endoscope when performing the procedure, thus making the perforation of the floor very difficult. The visual clues, especially the infundibular recess, are distorted and the point of perforation difficult to dis-

cern without the assistance of frameless stereotaxis. Even so, the procedure is technically difficult. It is possible to find the perforation into the sella or actually into the brainstem rather than in the very small interpeduncular cistern.

Our previous work on programmed shunt removal has shown that an increase in ventricular size is the most important predictor of the success of ETV [17]. This is true in all conditions except spina bifida and we no longer employ this program for such patients. Based on cisternography we have shown that all patients with an enlarged ventricular volume at the time of the shunt occlusion have an obstruction between the ventricles and the cortical subarachnoid space. If there is communication between the ventricle and cortical subarachnoid space the ventricles cannot expand at the time of the failure in older children or adults because the pressure in the cortical subarachnoid space and ventricles is balanced. Spina bifida is unique in that the ventricles can be isolated from the cortical subarachnoid space and therefore dilate at the time of shunt failure. However, as discussed in the introductory portion of this chapter, frequently there are multiple sites of obstruction in this complex abnormality. We have found that while ETV can result in free flow of CSF, the ICP remains very high because of the increased pressure in the dural venous sinuses.

Conclusion

Hydrocephalus is subject to the laws of physics and can be described using mathematical models based on hydrodynamics [18]. All hydrocephalus is obstructive in nature but relates to various points of obstruction [18-21]. While there are complicated problems, most hydrocephalus is due to a single site of obstruction to flow of CSF, from its point of production within the ventricles to its absorption in the dural venous sinuses. Hydrocephalus in spina bifida is particularly difficult because it has four different potential points of obstruction and one or more, or all four of them, may be part of the problem. It is difficult to predict in these situations what syndrome will occur at the time of shunt failure. Internal shunting such as ETV may not function because of the possible downstream source of obstruction. This discussion has attempted to demystify this situation and provide a thought process to help choose among treatment options in individual patients with hydrocephalus and spina bifida.

References

1. McLone DG, Knepper PA (1989) The cause of Chiari II malformation: a unified theory. Pediatr Neurosci 15:1-12
2. Bruner JP, Tulipan N, Reed G et al (2004) Intrauterine repair of spina bifida: preoperative predictors of shunt-dependent hydrocephalus. Am J Obstet Gynecol 190:1305-1312
3. Johnson MP, Gerdes M, Rintoul N et al (2006) Maternal-fetal surgery for myelomeningocele: neurodevelopmental outcomes at 2 years of age. Am J Obstet Gynecol 194:1145-1150
4. Sutton LN, Adzick NS (2004) Fetal surgery for myelomeningocele. Clin Neurosurg 51:155-162
5. Rekate HL (1988) Management of hydrocephalus and the erroneus concept of shunt independence in spina bifida. BNI Quarterly 4:17-20
6. Rekate HL (1991) Neurosurgical management of the child with spina bifida. CRC Press, Boca Raton
7. Rekate HL, Nulsen FE, Mack H et al (1982) Establishing the diagnosis of shunt independence. Monogr Neural Sci 8:223-226
8. Engel M, Carmel PW, Chutorian AM (1979) Increased intraventricular pressure without ventriculomegaly in children with shunts: "normal volume" hydrocephalus. Neurosurgery 5:549-552
9. Rekate HL (1993) Classification of slit-ventricle syndromes using intracranial pressure monitoring. Pediatr Neurosurg 19:15-20
10. Hall P, Lindseth R, Campbell R et al (1979) Scoliosis and hydrocephalus in myelocele patients. The effects of ventricular shunting. J Neurosurg 50:174-178
11. Dias MS, McLone DG (1993) Hydrocephalus in the child with dysraphism. Neurosurg Clin N Am 4:715-726
12. Le H, Yamini B, Frim DM (2002) Lumboperitoneal shunting as a treatment for slit ventricle syndrome. Pediatr Neurosurg 36:178-182
13. Rekate HL, Wallace D (2003) Lumboperitoneal shunts in children. Pediatr Neurosurg 38:41-46
14. Johnston IH, Sheridan MM (1993) CSF shunting from the cisterna magna: a report of 16 cases. Br J Neurosurg 7:39-43
15. Nadkarni TD, Rekate HL (2005) Treatment of refractory intracranial hypertension in a spina bifida patient by a concurrent ventricular and cisterna magna-to-peritoneal shunt. Childs Nerv Syst 21:579-582
16. Rekate HL, Nadkarni T, Wallace D (2006) Severe intracranial hypertension in slit ventricle syndrome managed using a cisterna magna-ventricle-peritoneum shunt. J Neurosurg 104:240-244
17. Baskin JJ, Manwaring KH, Rekate HL (1998) Ventricular shunt removal: the ultimate treatment of the slit ventricle syndrome. J Neurosurg 88:478-484
18. Rekate HL, Brodkey JA, Chizeck HJ et al (1988) Ventricular volume regulation: a mathematical model and computer simulation. Pediatr Neurosci 14:77-84
19. Ransohoff J, Shulman K, Fishman RA (1960) Hydrocephalus: a review of etiology and treatment. J Pediatr 56:399-411
20. Rekate HL (1989) Circuit diagram of the circulation of cerebrospinal fluid. In: Marlin AE (ed) Concepts in Pediatric Neurosurgery. Karger, Zurich, pp 46-56
21. Rekate HL (1989) Resistance elements within the cerebrospinal fluid circulation. In: Gjerris F, Borgesen SE, Solberg-Sorensen P (eds) Alfred Benzon symposium. Munksgaard, Copenhagen, pp 45-52

CHAPTER 21
Supratentorial Cerebral Malformations in Spina Bifida

Pietro Spennato, Luciano Savarese, Maria Consiglio Buonocore, Emilio Cianciulli, Giuseppe Cinalli

Introduction

In 1957, Cameron [1] first noted the association of spina bifida with several supratentorial abnormalities such as polymicrogyria, cortical heterotopia, corpus callosum dysgenesis, thickening of the massa intermedia, hypoplasia of the falx and aqueductal stenosis and forking. All of Cameron's patients also suffered from the Chiari II malformation [2].

Even if reliable epidemiological data are not available, these malformations appear to occur with a high frequency in spina bifida patients. In the postmortem evaluation of 25 children with myelomeningocele Gilbert et al. [3] found 23 cases of supratentorial malformations, including cortical heterotopias in 11 cases, polymicrogyria in 14 and cortical dysplasia ranging from disordered lamination to profound primitive development in 12 children. True agenesis of the corpus callosum was demonstrated in three cases. Aqueductal stenosis or forking was present in almost all 23 cases. This study was based on patients who had died at an early age, and therefore were presumably the most severely affected. However, the incidence of supratentorial malformations in spina bifida patients is also high in the neuroradiological literature. In a recent paper in which a population of 24 patients affected by different forms of spina bifida was evaluated with MR imaging [4], all patients with myeloschisis (9/9) and the majority of patients with meningo(myelo)cele (8/10) presented magnetic resonance imaging (MRI) supratentorial abnormalities, with partial agenesis of the corpus callosum and polymicrogyria being the most frequent. Only a minority of patients with spina bifida occulta (2/5) demonstrated cerebral abnormalities, consisting of cervicomedullary deformity and elevation of the hypothalamus. Also in the series of Yoshida et al. [5], the entire population of patients with cerebral abnormalities belonged to the group with myeloschisis/myelomeningocele, in

which these abnormalities (above all polymicrogyria and hypogenesis of corpus callosum) were diagnosed with very high frequency (50/51 patients).

Usually, multiple supratentorial malformations are described in the same patient, generally together with caudal displacement of the cerebellar tonsils and vermis, a condition known as Chiari II malformation, which is almost invariably associated with all the open forms of spina bifida and often with hydrocephalus.

Correlation between the level of the spinal defect and the presence of supratentorial anomalies has been recently emphasized by Fletcher and co-workers [6], who highlighted a more anomalous brain development in the cerebrum, midbrain and corpus callosum of children with upper-level lesions than those with lower-level lesions. The spinal lesion level and the degree of anomalous brain development also appeared to correlate with neurobehavioral outcomes, with upper-level lesions having a poorer outcome. The authors concluded that the differences between lesion-level groups represented the effects of hydrocephalus, shunt revisions or other perinatal variables potentially related to outcome.

In 1989, McLone and Knepper [7, 8] proposed a unified pathogenetic theory to explain the occurrence of anomalies of both supra- and infratentorial neuroectoderm and also of the surrounding mesoderm. According to their theory, the continued cerebrospinal (CSF) leak from an open myelomeningocele (MMC) defect results in reduced ventricular distension. As both the neural and calvarial development are induced by ventricular distension, the absence of a CSF driving force prevents the posterior fossa and the supratentorial neural elements from fully developing. As a result, transcranial disorganization occurs involving both the neuroectoderm and the surrounding mesoderm. As the third ventricle does not distend, the thalami remain approximated and contact to form a large massa intermedia. The lack of support for the developing telencephalic hemispheres results in ectopia, disorganization of future cerebral gyri, and dysgenesis of the corpus callosum. McLone and Knepper's hypothesis is based on previous studies concerning the role of mechanical factors, including cerebrospinal fluid pressure, in brain morphogenesis [9, 10]. In experimental animals, the developing cerebral cortex became disorganized, following drainage of CSF from the telencephalic ventricles.

McLone and Knepper [7] identified, in their experimental model, a metabolic defect in the glycosylation of neuroepithelial proteins as the primary cause of deficient closure of the neural tube, possibly related to genetic factors or nutritional deficiencies (e.g., folic acid). The concomitant cerebral and cranial malformations may also arise from this enzymatic defect, which is presumably not limited to the site of defective neurulation and tube closure, but can influence, at a later stage, cell surface interaction, cell activity, adhesion and distension of the primitive ventricular system.

Another possible reason for the abnormal cortical development in these patients has been suggested by Mashayekhi [11], who underlined the role of growth factors in the developing cortex. The CSF contains growth factors, inhibitors and other signaling molecules that are required for the normal activity of the stem and progenitor cells of the germinal matrix. Escape of CSF from the ventricular system or its accumulation in case of intrauterine hydrocephalus may alter the equilibrium between the inhibitory and stimulating factors in CSF, leading to secondary effects on germinal matrix activity.

Heterotopias

Epidemiology

Cameron et al. [1] noted cerebral heterotopias in 38% of patients with myelomeningocele and Chiari type II malformations, and Gilbert et al. [3] reported a frequency of 44%; in contrast, this malformation was described in only one of 26 patients (4%) in a study by Gross et al. [12].

Both types of heterotopias (subependymal and subcortical) have been found in patients with neural tube closure defects [3].

Embryology

Gray matter heterotopias are collections of normal neurons in abnormal locations that result from the arrest of radial migration of neurons. Currently, the most accepted theory of heterotopias in the context of spina bifida has been described by McLone et al. [8], who postulated that abnormality of cortical development may be the result of reduced ventricular distension secondary to continued CSF leak from an open MMC defect.

Normally the neurons that constitute the mammalian brain are generated in proliferative zones situated along the ventricular surface of the developing brain. At the end of the second gestational month, the neurons migrate from their site of origin along radially aligned glial cells to relatively distant final positions. At this point they further differentiate, grow axons and dendrites, and develop synaptic contacts with other neurons. Any insult to the brain during this period results in a migration anomaly, leading to cortical heterotopias [13]. Distension of the ventricular system appears to be an important factor to guide neuronal migration from the ventricular germinal zone to the cortical layers. Collapse of the ventricles may disorganize the migrational process, leading to accumulation of neurons in subependymal or subcortical locations.

Radiology

Heterotopias may be divided into three types on the basis of the MRI appearance: subependymal, focal subcortical and diffuse heterotopias (Band type) [14]. The most common is the subependymal nodular type. This appears to be the most benign form, causing little or no distortion of the remaining brain [14]: usually the surrounding white matter is normal in signal intensity and volume, the deep gray matter nuclei have normal configuration and the cerebral cortex has a normal thickness and gyral pattern. On the contrary, the less frequent focal subcortical heterotopias may cause marked distortion of the ventricles and deep gray matter nuclei, reduction of hemisphere size and apparent herniation of the hemisphere across the interhemispheric fissure. The surrounding white matter may be altered, and the cerebral cortex thinned [15, 16].

Clinical Features

Together with polymicrogyria, the presence of cortical heterotopias appears associated with seizure disorders and developmental delay. However in such patients, usually also afflicted with the Chiari II malformation and hydrocephalus, the real role of heterotopias in the genesis of symptoms and neurocognitive development is very difficult to ascertain. Subependymal heterotopias are generally thought to have the fewest clinical manifestations [17].

Barkovich et al. [14] reported that seizures are relatively uncommon and are of late onset in patients with subependymal heterotopias, regardless of the primary etiology. He also reported that intellectual and motor development is normal or only mildly impaired in almost 100% of patients. On the other hand, patients with focal subcortical heterotopias had a 50% prevalence of developmental delay and contralateral hemiplegia.

Polymicrogyria

Neuropathology

Polymicrogyria is the presence of an excess number of abnormally small gyri separated by shallow sulci that produce an irregular cortical surface [18]. It is often superimposed on areas of apparently broad gyri that represent fusion of superficial cortical cellular layers (particularly the molecular one). Polymicrogyria usually results from insults to the developing brain in the late migrational period or after neuronal migration has stopped. Histologically, the six-layered lamination of the normal cerebral cortex is deranged [19]. Two broad histological types have been described: four layered polymicrogyria and unlayered polymicrogyria; however, various intermediate gradations exist. Brain injury occurring during the early second trimester of pregnancy has been associated with unlayered polymicrogyria; injury occurring later (before the 24th week of gestation) may result in layered polymicrogyria [20]. In an unlayered cortex, only a molecular layer is present with a single band of unlayered neurons or poorly laminated cortex [21]; on the contrary, in layered polymicrogyria four individual layers are distinctly evident; a molecular layer, and a second layer of unlaminated neurons arranged in a sinuous band with two underlying layers of horizontal, unlaminated neurons. In "parallel four-layered cortex", the four layers described above are horizontal and parallel to each other [21]. The basic cytoarchitectonic abnormality of layered polymicrogyria is that of ischemic laminar necrosis predominating in layer 5, resulting in a cell-sparse layer. Superficial to this, layers 4, 3, and 2 are normal. However the appearance of each case of polymicrigyria is unique and may vary within the brain even in the same patient [21].

According to some authors [3, 22], the gyration disorder occurring in spina bifida patients should not be considered as a true polymicrogyria: the cortex is histologically normal, even if it is thrown into innumerable small closely spaced folds, and has no derangement of the normal six layered lamination [19]. To underline this difference Muller [22] used the term "stenogyria" to describe the abnormal convolutional pattern associated with the normal cortical layering of the cortex in spina bifida/Chiari II malformation. However, subsequent studies have not provided histological confirmation of this difference, thereafter the term polymicrogyria as well as stenogyria has been used to describe all patterns of gyration disorder, regardless of cortical organization and the presence of the Chiari II malformation.

Epidemiology

An abnormal convolutional pattern has been described in about 50% of patients with Chiari II malformation: MacFarlane and Maloney [23] observed it in 65% of patients with myelomeningocele and Chiari type II malformation, and Peach et al. [24] in 55% of his series. Kawamura et al. [4] found an anomalous pattern of gyration in six of nine patients with myeloschisis and in three of the ten patients with myelomeningocele, but in no patients with lumbar lipoma.

Radiology

The combination of three features on MRI has been used to identify polymicrogyria: abnormal gyral pattern, increased thickness, and irregularity of the cortical-white matter junction due to packing of microgyri [25, 26].

Polymicrogyria associated with spinal neural tube closure defects is usually localized bilaterally in the parieto-occipital region (Fig. 21.1) [5]. The location and topological extent of the polymicrogyria are often best determined from the sagittal images than from the axial or coronal images (Fig. 21.2). Barkovich et al. and Takanashi et al. [25, 26] have described two different cortical patterns on T2-weighted images; the first was a small, fine, undulating appearance with normal thickness (3-4 mm), and the other thick and bumpy in appearance (5-8 mm). The first pattern was observed on T2-weighted images of neonates and infants, whereas the latter was recognized later in childhood: the first seeming to evolve into the second as the brain underwent myelination.

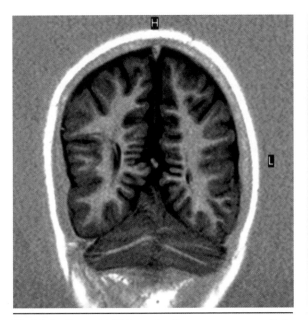

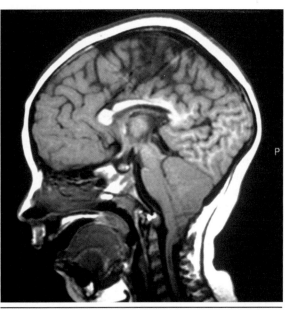

Fig. 21.1. Coronal MRI, Inversion-Recovery sequence: Note the abnormal gyration pattern of the parieto-occipital cortex, more evident in the interhemispheric fissure

Fig. 21.2. Sagittal T2W MRI sequence. Polymicrogyria of the occipito-parietal lobe. Note the difference in gyration pattern compared with the medial surface of the frontal lobe

Clinical Features

The clinical presentation of patients with polymicrogyria is variable and depends on the severity of involvement and its location. The outcome is worse in those with a smaller head size and more extensive polymicrogyria (especially in case of involvement of the fronto-temporal regions). Most patients without spina bifida/Chiari II malformation but with polymicrocryria present with seizures, usually focal motor, and developmental delay [19]. Dysplasia of the motor strip causes hemiparesis of varying severity. Speech delay may result from malformation of primary speech and language areas. Diffuse polymicrogyria results in microcephaly, hypotonicity, and infantile seizures with marked developmental delay. These manifestations, however, may also be related to the intrauterine brain insult that was the origin of the polymicrogyria, such as congenital cytomegalovirus infection. The high incidence of seizures (more than 80%) in non-spina bifida polymicrogyria is probably attributable to the presence of lesions in cortical layer 5 (which is a source of epilepsy) and in layer 4, which normally inhibits input into layer 5 [20].

In patients with spina bifida/Chiari II malformation, polymicrogyria is generally limited to parieto-occipital regions; moreover, the cortex is often histologically normal, with the six layered lamination preserved. Thereafter the real role of such a malformation in the pathogenesis of symptoms such as seizures and mental retardation in children also affected by Chiari II malformation and hydrocephalus (who usually undergo several shunt procedures) is not clear.

Bourgeois et al. [27], studying a population of 802 children with hydrocephalus of various etiologies, observed that children with myelomeningocele experienced a significantly lower overall prevalence of epilepsy (7%), compared with those born prematurely (30%) and those with prenatal hydrocephalus (38%). They also noted that the presence of supratentorial anomalies, such as agenesis of the corpus callosum and focal migration abnormalities was statistically associated with a higher incidence of epilepsy. Most studies that investigated seizures in spina bifida patients found that the presence of a shunt, number of shunt procedures, history of shunt infection or ventriculitis and shunt location (frontal versus parieto-occipital) significantly increased the potential for developing seizures [28, 29]. Different conclusions were reached by Yoshida et al. [5] in a recent paper. They evaluated 75 spina bifida patients and observed cerebral abnormalities such as polymicrogyria or hypogenesis of the corpus callosum in all epileptic cases. Locations of cerebral abnormalities topographically correlated with areas of interictal electroencephalography (EEG) abnormalities.

Although all epileptic cases had a ventriculoperi-toneal shunt inserted for hydrocephalus before the onset of epilepsy, interictal EEG abnormalities could not be explained by the location of the ventriculoperitoneal (VP) shunt. These data are in agreement with those of Talwar et al. [29], who found a prevalence of epilepsy of 17% in their population of 81 spina bifida patients, with most patients harboring other CNS pathology to account for their seizures. Recent magnetoencephalographic studies have revealed that interictal irritative zones were localized within the lesion in polymicrogyria comparable to other malformations that have intrinsic epileptogenicity [5].

However, all these findings indicate that epileptogenesis in spina bifida is multifactorial, since not all patients with spina bifida and cerebral abnormalities have epilepsy, and not all patients with epilepsy have cerebral abnormalities [5]. In addition, the role of severe apneic episodes and cardiac arrest secondary to Chiari malformation, with developing of areas of encephalomalacia and/or stroke, cannot be discounted.

Dysgenesis of the Corpus Callosum

Epidemiology

Although agenesis of the corpus callosum is occasionally found in combination with multiple malformation syndromes, it was not considered a component of the central nervous system pathology in infants with spinal dysraphism until Gross et al. [12] described partial agenesis in two of 27 cases (7%). Gilbert et al. [3] also described three cases of complete or nearly complete agenesis of the corpus callosum in a series of 25 autopsies of children with Chiari type II malformations.

Kawamura et al. [30] examined images of the brain in patients with spinal dysraphic lesions to characterize abnormalities of the corpus callosum and found that 14 of 23 patients with spinal dysraphic lesions (61%) had a dysgenetic corpus callosum. Corpus callosum dysgenesis was found in seven of eight patients with myeloschisis, and seven of ten with myelomeningocele. None of five patients with lumbosacral lipoma had a callosal anomaly. No isolated callosal anomaly was found, but all patients had associated hemispheric abnormalities. Yoshida et al. [5] showed dysgenesis of the corpus callosum in the nine epileptic patients with spinal tube closure defects.

Embryology

As well as other disorders of migration and maturation of the telencephalon, dysgenesis of the corpus callosum may be considered the result of the disorganization of the cerebral hemispheres, a frequent finding of Chiari II malformation [8]. Development of the corpus callosum begins at 8-12 weeks of gestation with formation of the massa commissuralis between the laminae reuniens in the dorsal aspect of the primitive lamina terminalis. The massa commissuralis acts as an induction bed for the decussation of callosal commissural fibers. As early as 11-12 weeks of gestation, fibers from the developing hemispheres extend across the massa commissuralis, forming a thin corpus callosum [30]. The corpus callosum develops from a rostral to caudal direction. The posterior genu and anterior body appear first, followed by the posterior body, inferior genu, splenium, and finally the rostrum.

Since the normal development of the corpus callosum depends on the uncomplicated closure of the neural tube, as well as proper formation of the massa commissuralis and appropriate development of the cerebral hemispheres, an insult to the massa commissuralis or to the developing cerebral hemispheres at any time during the embryonic period can cause callosal dysgenesis [30].

On the basis of embryology, Dobyns [31] described two types of true callosal abnormalities. They include: (1) defects in which axons develop but are unable to cross the midline because of absence of the massa commissuralis and leave large aberrant longitudinal fiber bundles (the Probst bundles) along the medial hemisphere walls; and (2) defects in which the commissural axons or their parent cell bodies fail to form in the cerebral cortex. Probst bundles are absent in this type of agenesis of the corpus callosum [32]. Dysgenesis of the corpus callosum among patients with spinal dysraphism was not associated with Probst bundles [30]. This pattern suggests a disturbed developmental relationship between the corpus callosum and the cerebral hemispheres rather than primary callosal dysgenesis after agenesis of the massa commissuralis. A reduced number of commissural fibers projecting from the dysgenetic cerebral hemispheres would be likely, considering the abnormal configurations observed. Since dysgenesis of cerebral hemispheres often appears somewhat random, incomplete and asymmetric, the corpus callosum may correspondingly demonstrate varying degrees of unifocal, multifocal, or generalized hypoplasia [30]. McLone et al. [8] attributed primary dysgenesis of cerebral hemispheres to the disorder of neuronal histogenesis, secondary to collapse of the ventricular system.

Radiology

Morphologically, callosal anomalies in patients with spinal dysraphism were categorized into three types according to the overall configurations and the abnormal regions of the corpus callosum [30]. Kawamura et al. [30] classified the abnormal callosal configurations of this group of patients with spinal dysraphism as hypoplasia of the corpus callosum, hypoplasia with partial agenesis or partial agenesis.

In the first type, all parts (rostrum, genu, body, and splenium) can be identified, but the corpus callosum is hypoplastic, with diminished width and total cross sectional area (Fig. 21.3). In the second group the corpus callosum is both small overall and also partially agenetic (Fig. 21.4). In the third group, the posterior third of the corpus callosum is partially absent or hypoplastic while the anterior two-thirds have a nearly normal appearance.

Clinical features

Recently, Huber-Okrainec et al. [33] related the presence of neuropsychologic problems, particularly involving language, to the grade of dysgenesis of the corpus callosum in patients with spina bifida. Corpus callosum agenesis, causing interhemispheric transfer deficits, disrupts figurative language comprehension in children with myelomeningocele. The language processing limitation of such children may be related to their pattern of idiom comprehension. Idioms are non-literal phrases whose figurative meanings cannot be derived from the literal meanings of their individual words. Children with myelomeningocele have impaired idiom comprehension, a difficulty that appears to be related not only to features intrinsic to the idioms, but also to differences in the extent of corpus callosum dysmorphology [33]. As a result, when context is not provided, their ability to understand isolated idioms is poor.

Holoprosencephaly

Holoprosencephaly refers to a spectrum of forebrain malformations characterized by the failure of the

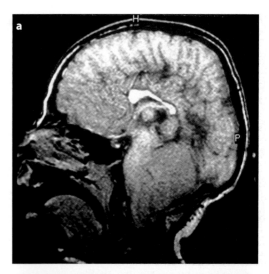

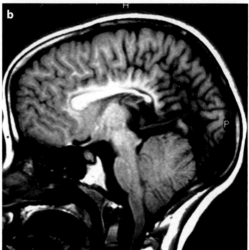

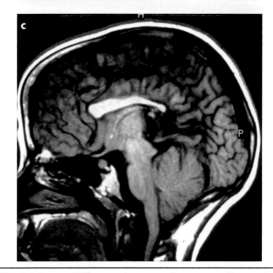

Fig. 21.3 a-c. Different degrees of corpus callosum hypoplasia. All parts of the corpus callosum are visible but **a** severely or **b**, **c** less significantly reduced in length and thickness. Corpus callosum hypoplasia in some cases can be associated with polymicrogyric patterns of gyration diffuse to the whole medial cortex (**a**, **b**)

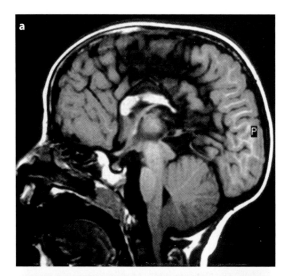

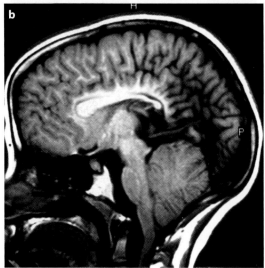

Fig. 21.4 a, b. Different degrees of corpus callosum hypoplasia with partial agenesis. The posterior third of the corpus callosum can be **a** completely absent or **b** reduced to a very thin layer, without the typical thickening of the splenium

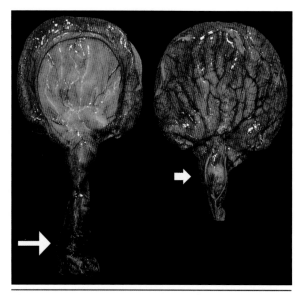

Fig. 21.5. Anatomical specimen of a fetus affected by myelomeningocele and holoprosencephaly. Courtesy of Prof. Aydın Sav, Marmara University, Istanbul

Rollins et al. [36] reported the only case of association of holoprosencephaly with myelomeningocele in a viable infant, who had been followed for thirteen months after surgical closure of myelomeningocele, shunting of hydrocephalus and suboccipital decompression for life threatening apnoic episodes, secondary to severe Chiari II malformation. At the time of the last follow up, the baby had microcephaly, seizures, global developmental delay and intermittent apnea.

An alteration in the primitive mesenchyme may be considered a common link in both malformations, explaining their association. It can probably be related to defective glycosylation of proteins, which influences the interaction of cells. Barkovich and Quint [37] suggested that the paucity of mesenchyme that normally invests the deepening interhemispheric groove separating the developing cerebral hemispheres is the pivotal anomaly in holoprosencephaly.

The importance of the supportive role of mesenchyme in the initial phase of neurulation in the rat has been stressed by embryologists who note that mesenchymal deficiency may prevent further neurulation [36].

prosencephalon to form two lateral telencephalic vesicles [34]. Its association with spinal dysraphism is known mainly from autopsy series. Osaka et al. [35] observed holoprosencephaly in 18 of 92 aborted embryos or fetuses with myeloschisis, embryos showing a higher incidence than fetuses, suggesting that the malformations were incompatible with later fetal development (Fig. 21.5).

References

1. Cameron AH (1957) The Arnold-Chiari and other neuroanatomical malformations associated with spina bifida. J Pathol Bacteriol 73:195-211

2. Cameron AH (1957) Malformations of the neurospinal axis, urogenital tract and foregut in spina bifida attributable to disturbances of the blastopore. J Pathol Bacteriol 73:213-221

3. Gilbert JN, Jones KL, Rorke LB et al (1986) Central nervous system anomalies associated with meningomyelocele, hydrocephalus, and the Arnold-Chiari malformation: Reappraisal of theories regarding the pathogenesis of posterior neural tube closure defects. Neurosurgery 18(5):559-564

4. Kawamura T, Morioka T, Nishio S et al (2001) Cerebral abnormalities in lumbosacral neural tube closure defect: MR imaging evaluation. Childs Nerv Syst 17:405-410

5. Yoshida F, Morioka T, Hashiguchi K et al (2006) Epilepsy in patients with spina bifida in the lumbosacral region. Neurosurg Rev 29:327-332

6. Fletcher JM, Copeland K, Frederick JA et al (2005) Spinal lesion level in spina bifida: a source of neural and cognitive heterogeneity. J Neurosurg (Pediatrics 3) 102:268-279

7. McLone DG, Knepper PA (1989) The cause of Chiari II malformation: a unified theory. Pediatr Neurosci 15:1-12

8. McLone DG, Dias MS (2003) The Chiari II malformation: cause and impact. Childs Nerv Syst 19:540-550

9. Coulombre AG, Coulombre JL (1958) The role of mechanical factors in brain morphogenesis (abstract). Anat Rec 130:289-290

10. Desmond ME, Jacobson AG (1977) Embryonic brain enlargement requires cerebrospinal fluid pressure. Dev Biol 57:188-198

11. Mashayekhi F, Draper CE, Bannister CM et al (2002) Deficient cortical development in the hydrocephalic Texas (H-Tx) rat: a role for CSF. Brain 125:1859-1874

12. Gross H, Jellinger K, Kaltenbac E (1974) Progressive hydrocephalus associated with spina bifida caused by a peculiar cerebellum-brain stem syndrome. Presented at the VIIth International Congress of Neuropathology, Budapest, Hungary

13. Barkovich AJ, Chuang SH, Norman D (1988) MR of neuronal migration anomalies. AJR 150:179-187

14. Barkovich AJ, Kjos BO (1992) Gray matter heterotopias: MR characteristics and correlation with developmental and neurologic manifestations. Radiology 182:493-499

15. Barkovich AJ (1996) Subcortical heterotopias: a distinct clinicoradiologic entity. AJNR Am J Neuroradiol 17:1315-1322

16. Barkovich AJ, Jackson DE, Boyer R (1989) Band heterotopias: a newly recognized neuronal migration anomaly. Radiology 171:455-458

17. Cho WH, Seidenwurm D, Barkovich AJ (1999) Adult-onset neurologic dysfunction associated with cortical malformations. AJNR Am J Neuroradiol 20:1037-1043

18. Sisodiya S M (2004) Malformations of cortical development: burdens and insights from important causes of human epilepsy. Lancet Neurol 3:29-38

19. Thompson JE, Castillo M, Thomas D et al (1997) Radiologic-pathologic correlation polymicrogyria. AJNR Am J Neuroradiol 18:307-312

20. Barkovich AJ, Gressens P, Evard P et al (1992) Formation, maturation, and disorders of brain neocortex. AJNR Am J Neuroradiol 13:423-446

21. Norman MG, McGillivray BC, Kalousek DK et al (1995) Neuronal migration diseases and cortical dysplasia. In: Norman MG, McGillivray BC, Kalousek DK et al (eds) Congenital malformations of the brain. Oxford University Press, New York, pp 223-279

22. Muller J (1983) Congenital malformations of the brain. In: Rosenberg RN (ed) The clinical neurosciences, vol 3. Churchill, New York, pp 1-33

23. MacFarlane A, Maloney AFJ (1957) The appearance of the aqueduct and its relationship to hydrocephalus in the Arnold-Chiari malformation. Brain 80:479-493

24. Peach B (1965) Arnold-Chiari malformation. Anatomic features of 20 cases. Arch Neurol 12:613-621

25. Takanashi J, Barkovich J (2003) The changing MR imaging appearance of polymicrogyria: a consequence of myelination. AJNR Am J Neuroradiol 24:788-793

26. Barkovich AJ, Hevner R, Guerrini R (1999) Syndrome of bilateral polymicrogyria. AJNR Am J Neuroradiol 20:1814-1821

27. Bourgeois M, Sainte-Rose C, Cinalli G et al (1999) Epilepsy in children with shunted hydrocephalus. J Neurosurg 90:274-281

28. Chadduck W, Adametz J (1988) Incidence of seizures in patients with myelomeningocele: A multifactorial analysis. Surg Neurol 30:281-285

29. Talwar D, Baldwin MA, Horbatt CI (1995) Epilepsy in children with meningomyelocele. Pediatr Neurol 13:29-32

30. Kawamura T, Nishio S, Morioka T, Fukui K (2002) Callosal anomalies in patients with spinal dysraphism: correlation of clinical and neuroimaging features with hemispheric abnormalities. Neurol Res 24:463-467

31. Dobyns WB (1996) Absence makes the search grow longer. Am J Hum genet 58:7-16

32. Sztriha L (2005) Spectrum of corpus callosum agenesis. Pediatr Neurol 32:94-101

33. Huber-Okrainec J, Blaser SE, Dennis M (2005) Idiom comprehension deficits in relation to corpus callosum agenesis and hypoplasia in children with spina bifida meningomyelocele. Brain Lang 93:349-368

34. Razavi FE (2003) Identification of brain malformations: neuropathological approach. Childs Nerv Syst 19:448-454

35. Osaka K, Tanimura T, Hirayama A, Matsumoto S (1978) Myelomeningocele before birth. J Neurosurg 49:711-724

30. Rollins N, Joglar J, Perlman J (1999) Coexistent holoprosencephaly and Chiari II malformation. AJNR Am J Neuroradiol 20:1678-1681

36. Barkovich AJ, Quint DJ (1993) Middle interhemispheric fusion: an unusual variant of holoprosencephaly. AJNR Am J Neuroradiol 14:431-440

CHAPTER 22
Tethered Cord in Children with Spina Bifida

Robin M. Bowman, David G. McLone

Introduction

Any process that attaches and fixes the spinal cord, inhibiting movement of the cord in the spinal canal, has the potential to cause tethered cord syndrome. Motion of the head and trunk changes the length of the spinal canal and the cord must move cranially to accommodate increases in length. If the cord is unable to move, it must lengthen to accommodate increased distance. The epipial layer of the spinal cord contains abundant collagen and extension narrows the cord and causes this layer to squeeze the interior of the cord, elevating intramedullary pressure. This is much like the children's toy, the "finger trap". The harder you pull the tighter the squeeze. When intramedullary pressure exceeds perfusion pressure, the cord becomes ischemic and metabolism ceases. Repetitive or prolonged stretching of the spinal cord leads to infarction and a deficit. As would be expected, the deterioration is usually subtle, progressive, may be reversible and only rarely catastrophic. Hoffman, Hendrick, and Humphreys described this problem in children in 1976 [1]. Yamada demonstrated the physiology in the laboratory in 1981 [2].

All children born with an open neural tube defect have a low-lying cord on magnetic resonance imaging (MRI), even after initial repair and untethering; consistent with tethering, or scarring, in the area of the prior exposed neural placode (Fig. 22.1). It is likely that almost all children are anatomically tethered within months of their initial repair. Fortunately, only approximately one-third or less of these children will develop neurological, orthopedic, or urologic decline related to spinal cord tethering [3, 4].

Spina Bifida is a birth defect, not a degenerative disease. Deterioration almost always has a treatable cause. Early detection of deterioration offers the best chance for recovery and limits the deficit. Recognition of deterioration requires the collection of reliable objective data of the child's functional state.

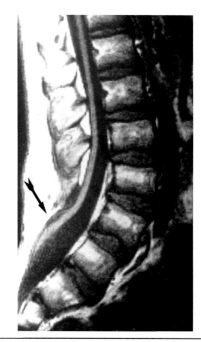

Fig. 22.1. A T1 sagittal lumbar MRI demonstrating tethering at the area of the prior exposed neural placode (*arrow*)

Mom's opinion that the child is worse is usually not an adequate reason for surgery. More often the parents are unaware that their child has lost function. Therefore, throughout childhood, children born with a myelomeningocele are closely monitored in our multi-disciplinary Spina Bifida Clinic at Children's Memorial Hospital (CMH). Our team consists of: Neurosurgery, Orthopedic Surgery, Urology, Neurology, Physical/Occupational Therapy, Physical Medicine and Rehabilitation, Nursing, and Social Work. Although all children born with a myelomeningocele usually have neurologic, orthopedic and/or urologic deficits, it is our goal that the children remain neurologically stable or improve throughout their childhood. It is possible that congenital deficits are the result of intrauterine tethered cord. This requires diligence both from the medical team and family. The children are evaluated in the clinic at least every 3 months during the first year of life and then every 4-6 months until school age. Subsequently, they are examined on a yearly basis. The family is instructed to contact us should they note a neurologic, orthopedic or urologic change in their child between office visits.

We have found, as have others, that a shunt malfunction is often the cause of neurological change in a child with a myelomeningocele [5]. The second most common cause of neurologic decline is symptomatic tethering of the spinal cord at the initial site of the placode closure [4].

We have reported the outcome of children who had their original back closure at CMH and subsequently required a tethered cord release (TCR). This study has the advantage of a population followed from birth into adult life and treated at a single institution. We have analyzed the clinical presentation and subsequent neurologic outcome as well as the surgical procedure and complications. A majority of these surgical procedures were performed by the senior author (DGM) and all were undertaken at CMH.

Management

The multidisciplinary Spina Bifida Clinic at CMH was originally established in 1975. Since that time, we have aggressively managed all children born with a myelomeningocele in a prospective manner with the goal of maintaining or improving their long-term neurologic outcome.

Since 1975, 502 newborns with an open neural tube defect have had their back closure at CMH. In this cohort, 114 children (23%) have undergone a tethered cord release at CMH. Eighty-one patients (71%) have had one untethering, 20 patients (17%) have had two untetherings, ten patients (9%) have had three untetherings and three patients (3%) have had four untetherings. Therefore, there were 163 tethered cord release procedures in 114 patients.

In this group of 114 patients, one patient (1%) has an asymmetrical motor exam, 14 patients (12%) have an upper lumbar or thoracic motor level, six patients (5%) have an L3 motor level, 25 patients (22%) have an L4 motor level, 33 patients (29%) have an L5 motor level and 35 patients (31%) have a sacral motor level. Obviously, the lower the lesion the more the child has to lose. Fifty-eight patients are female and 56 are male. In this cohort, 108 patients (95%) have shunted hydrocephalus.

The average age at the time of the first untethering is 7 years, with a range of 7 months-21.8 years. The average length of follow-up after the initial untethering is 12 years, with a range of 1 month-23.3 years.

All newborns undergo a baseline motor evaluation by the physical therapist, who administers a standardized manual motor test exam (MMT). The MMT has been tested by our therapist and found to be highly reliable as an indicator of deterioration. The MMT is then repeated on a yearly basis and following any surgical intervention. Baseline evaluations are obtained by Neurosurgery, Orthopedic Surgery and Urology. The child is subsequently followed with intermittent team examinations, which may include renal ultrasound, cystometrogram (CMG), voiding cystourethrogram (VCUG), brain and spine MRI/computerized tomography (CT), plain radiographs and/or a gait study. When a child is suspected of having a neurologic decline, he/she undergoes at least a MMT, CMG and brain/spine MRI with an evaluation by the full team.

Prior to diagnosing a child with a symptomatic tethered spinal cord, shunt function is always confirmed. The child is examined clinically and brain imaging is obtained. If concern arises regarding possible shunt malfunction, the shunt is either tapped and/or surgically explored prior to any untethering procedure.

The clinical signs or symptoms we utilize as indicative of spinal cord tethering are: progressive scoliosis, decline in lower extremity motor strength, lower extremity contractures, lower extremity spasticity, change in gait, in urologic function, and/or back pain.

One child has undergone a tethered cord release with resection of a recurrent teratoma at the site of the neural placode. A second child has undergone both a posterior cervical decompression and tethered cord release simultaneously for progressive upper extremity weakness.

Surgery

After confirming adequate shunt function, the child is positioned in the prone position on chest gel rolls to avoid pressure sores. Prior to positioning, a urinary catheter is placed. A prophylactic antibiotic is administered.

The pre-operative MRI will assist in determining the location and extent of the surgical incision. Most of the time, the entire prior myelomeningocele scar will need to be reopened. If the child was originally closed in a transverse incision, we create a longitudinal incision dorsal to the placode. The incision is started superiorly, dorsal to the last intact lamina, and carried deep to the fascial layer. The paraspinal musculature is dissected laterally, exposing the last intact lamina. The ligamentum flavum is released from the undersurface of the intact lamina utilizing periosteal elevators, thereby exposing the superior epidural plane. If adequate normal dura is not present, then a small inferior laminectomy is completed with bone-biting rongeurs. The carbon dioxide laser is a useful tool for dissection, removing fat, and controlling blood loss.

Prior to dural opening, the child is tipped into a gentle Trendelenburg position to limit the amount of spinal fluid loss. Subsequently, the dura is opened superiorly and retracted laterally. If the placode is imbricated at the time of back closure, the tether is usually along the dorsal pial suture line and significantly easier to release (Fig. 22.2). If the placode was not closed at the time of the original repair, the area of adhesion is much larger and more difficult to dissect free from the dura.

With dissection, one continually works distally on either side of the cord, taking care to preserve all dorsal nerve roots. It is often useful to begin the

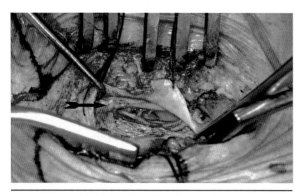

Fig. 22.2. Tether along dorsal pial suture line (*arrow*)

dissection in the subdural space that allows the dorsal roots to be safely swept medially. All intradural dissection is completed with operating loupes and a head light. If the spinal cord is densely adherent to the dorsal dura, dissection is carried out laterally on either side of the adherent zone, eventually circumferentially untethering the cord, except for the dorsally adherent dura. At this point, usually by working gently in all directions, the small, adherent dorsal dura can be removed. At the conclusion of the untethering, the spinal cord relaxes into the anterior spinal canal. The spinal canal of the newborn is very shallow, but fortunately with growth of the pedicles it deepens in older children and allows the cord to rest some distance from the dural closure.

Once the spinal cord is completely untethered, the spinal column should be inspected for other pathologies such as dermoid tumor in the distal spinal cord, fatty or thickened filum, or split cord malformation. If another pathology is confirmed, it is resected or released. After confirming that no other pathology is present, the dura is then closed in a watertight fashion, with a dural patch if necessary. We attempt to create a capacious dural closure. The deep layers are closed and the skin is closed with non-absorbable suture. If a dural patch is used and the integrity of the dural closure is in doubt, an intrathecal drain can be placed superior to the closure suture line. Fortunately, this is not normally necessary. Post-operatively, the child is maintained at flat bedrest for 4 days and then slowly mobilized.

Outcome

In this cohort of 114 patients, there are 163 tethered cord release procedures. The data from each procedure is analyzed separately. Table 22.1 summarizes the outcome data for each clinical indicator.

Table 22.1. A summary of the outcome data for each clinical indicator for a tethered cord release

Clinical indicators	Pre-op symptom	Improved	Stable	Worse	Progression
Scoliosis	46 (28%)	7 (15%)	4 (9%)		25 (54%) (21 spinal fusion)
Muscle Test change	47 (29%)	33 (70%)	13 (28%)	1 (2%)	
Contracture	34 (21%)	7 (21%)	27 (79%)		
Spasticity	54 (33%)	34 (63%)	20 (37%)		
Gait change	29	23 (79%)	5 (17%)	1 (3%)	
Back/leg pain	19	19 (100%)			
Urinary changes	30 (18%)	20 (67%)	9 (30%)		

Scoliosis

Forty-six patients (40%) were untethered secondary to progressive scoliosis with 13 patients (11%) having only this symptom. Sixty-seven tethered cord releases (41%) were performed secondary to progressive scoliosis.

Ten children have had severe scoliosis and have undergone an untethering immediately prior to their spinal fusion to prevent neurologic decline secondary to possible spinal column lengthening. If the orthopedic surgeon feels the column will not be lengthened, it is reasonable to do only a fusion. Of the remaining 36 patients, seven patients (19%) have improvement in their scoliosis, with four patients (11%) demonstrating no further progression. Four patients (11%) have developed more than ten degrees of progression in their scoliosis post-operatively, but have been managed conservatively and have not required a spinal fusion. Twenty-one patients (58%) have had continual progression in their scoliosis and subsequently have required a spinal fusion.

Of the 13 children in whom scoliosis was their only presenting symptom, four patients have undergone an immediate spinal fusion. Of the remaining nine children, five patients eventually have required a spinal fusion and four either have stabilized or improved.

Decline in MMT

Forty-seven children (41%) were diagnosed with a symptomatic tethered cord after developing a decline in their lower extremity strength. Fifty-four tethered cord releases (33%) were performed on these 47 children. In six procedures (11%), a change in the MMT was the only indication of neurologic worsening.

In these 54 releases, there was a 70% improvement in motor functioning post-operatively with 28% remaining stable. One child (2%) had a further decline in lower extremity motor strength post-operatively.

Contractures

Thirty-seven tethered cord releases (23%) were undertaken in 34 patients (30%) secondary to development of lower extremity contractures. In one procedure, the development of contractures was the only indicator of tethering. Post-operatively, 22% of the contractures have improved, with 78% remaining stable.

Spasticity

Spasticity is one of the indications of tethering in 75 procedures (46%) completed on 54 patients (47%), being the only indication in 11 cases. Spasticity was improved in 63% and remains stable in 37%.

Gait Change

A worsening in the child's gait was one of the clinical signs of symptomatic tethering in 29 patients (25%) who have undergone 32 procedures (20%). Two releases were performed for a change in gait only. Post-operatively, there was a 78% improvement in this symptom and 19% stability. One child (3%), the same one who had a worsening MMT post-operatively, has a worse gait due to increased weakness in her quadriceps.

Urinary Changes

In 30 children (26%), a worsening in urologic functioning was a clinical sign of tethering. Thirty-seven procedures (23%) were performed for deteriorating urologic functioning. In ten cases, this was the sole indication for intervention. One child is currently in the early post-operative period and hence has not yet had post-operative studies. In the remaining 36 cases, there is a 64% improvement with a 36% stabilization in urologic symptoms. Post-operatively, no child is worse urologically.

Interestingly, nine children have undergone an untethering for reasons other than urologic decline, but experienced an improvement in their urologic functioning post-operatively. One child, however, developed a decrease in his bladder capacity that has gradually improved back to baseline.

Pain

Nineteen patients (17%) complained of low back pain pre-operatively and have undergone 24 untetherings (15%). Post-operatively, all patients have had improvement in their pain. In only one patient, back pain was the sole indicator for tethering. Another patient with back pain was diagnosed with an anterior meningocele and pelvic dermoid. After closure of the meningocele and resection of the tumor, her pain has resolved. At 1 year of age, one infant has undergone an untethering for back fullness and irritability (questionable back pain). The symptoms have resolved post-operatively.

Unique Indicators

As a newborn, one child was diagnosed with a teratoma at the site of the placode. This tumor was resected at the time of the myelomeningocele closure. The infant was followed closely for possible tumor recurrence with frequent MRIs and alpha-fetoprotein (AFP) levels. At 7 months of age, he was noted to have a regrowth of the tumor and an increase in his AFP level. He underwent an untethering with subsequent gross total resection of the tumor. He is now 2 years post-operative and has had no further recurrence. He functions at a thoracic motor level and has had no neurologic change since birth.

Two children have developed upper extremity weakness. One child has improved after a simultaneous tethered cord release and posterior cervical decompression. The other patient is paraplegic and has undergone a lower thoracic spinal cord transection. Post-operatively, her upper extremity strength has improved.

Additional Pathology

Nineteen children (17%) had at least one other form of spinal pathology, some of which are tethering in nature. Seven children (6%) had distal spinal cord dermoids and seven patients (6%) had a thickened, fatty filum. Four patients (4%) had a split cord malformation. One child had a distal lipoma and a second child had an associated subcutaneous fibroma. One of the children with dermoids had an associated anterior meningocele. Lastly, one newborn had a teratoma ventral to his placode.

Complications

Overall, only four children of the 114 (3.5%) are neurologically worse following an untethering. All patients declined by at least one motor level on their MMT. For three patients, their weakness was after the first untethering, and for one patient it was after the second surgery. In two patients, there has been associated pathology consisting of a large, distal dermoid tumor in one child and a diastematomyelia with a thickened, fatty filum in another. Other complications have consisted of a cerebrospinal fluid leak following seven releases (4%) and wound dehiscence after 11 cases (7%).

Discussion

As previously stated, we are strong advocates of aggressive management of children born with a myelomeningocele to prevent neurologic decline. The most common cause of neurologic change in this group of patients is a shunt malfunction [5]. Most children will require 2-3 shunt revisions throughout childhood [3, 4]. A shunt malfunction can mimic signs of a tethered cord and consequently, shunt function must always be confirmed prior to any surgical untethering. Opening of the central nervous system inferior to the foramen magnum in a child with a Chiari II malformation and an unrecognized shunt malfunction may have life-threatening consequences [6]. The second most common cause of deterioration in a child born with an open neural tube defect is tethering of the distal spinal cord. As reported by Phuong et al. [7], without surgical release of a symptomatic tethered cord, 60% of children will have further orthopedic and urologic deterioration within 5 years.

Dr. Yamada and colleagues [2] have supplied the physiologic data that support the concept of stretch-induced trauma to the distal spinal cord when it is held under tension. Consequently, it is not surprising that symptoms of a spinal cord held taut by a scar are referable to the thoracic and lumbosacral spinal cord. The most common presenting symptoms of spinal cord tethering are: spasticity of the lower extremities (47% patients, 46% TCRs), decline in lower extremity strength (41% patients, 33% TCRs), and scoliosis (40% patients, 41% TCRs) (Figs. 22.3 and 22.4). Approximately 25% of the cohort present with either urinary changes or a worsening, crouched gait. The least common presentation is pain in 17% of the children.

Outcome is best assessed by reviewing each individual presenting symptom given that 73% of cases presented with more than one clinical indicator of tethering. Fortunately, of all of the neurologic problems exacerbated by a tethered spinal cord, pain has the best response to an untethering in children. Unfortunately this is not true in adults. In our children, 100% of the patients have improvement in their pain post-operatively. Rinaldi et al. [8] and Cochrane et al. [9] have also found that pain responds well to an untethering in children with spinal dysraphism. The pain is usually vague and difficult for the child to localize. The pain often radiates into the anterior thigh or even up the spine. Flexion of the neck can exacerbate the pain and lordotic posture with bent knees, the "crouched gait", seems to reduce the pain.

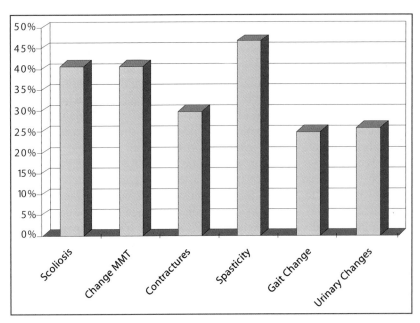

Fig. 22.3. Clinical indicators of tethering in 114 patients. Clinical indicators are plotted on the x-axis and percentage of patients affected on the y-axis. MMT: manual motor test

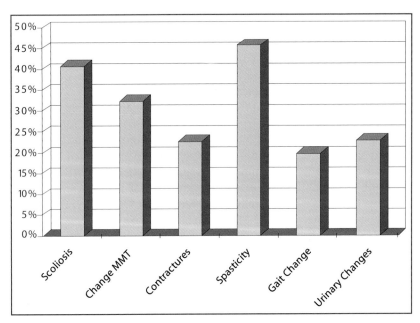

Fig. 22.4. Clinical indicators of tethering in 163 procedures. Clinical indicators are plotted on the x-axis and percentage of patients affected on the y-axis. MMT: manual motor test

Gait and lower extremity motor strength are significantly improved with release of a symptomatic tethered cord. Seventy-eight percent of children experience an improvement in their gait, with 70% improvement in lower extremity motor strength as tested by physical therapy. These findings are in contrast to those of Schoenmaker et al. [10], who note that a majority of their patients (82%) remain stable post-operatively with only 7% improving. Although only one paraplegic patient in this cohort has undergone a cord transection for upper extremity weak-

ness, she has experienced significant improvement in her hand strength post-operatively. Blount et al. [11] have reported similar findings in several patients.

In a long-term outcome study from the Netherlands on children with different types of spinal dysraphism, five of 44 patients (11%) have deteriorated in their motor exam post-operatively [10]. Our overall risk of lower extremity motor strength decline is 3.5%. One child has weaker quadriceps post-operatively that affected her gait initially. Although she gradually has had some improvement in strength, weight gain has prevented ambulation. Three other children have lost motor strength post-operatively, although weakness was not a presenting symptom. Two of these children have associated pathology, with one child having a very large distal dermoid. In an attempt to close the dura in a water-tight fashion, the last child had a very snug primary dural closure. In the immediate post-operative period, he was noted to have increased weakness in his lower extremities. He promptly underwent re-exploration with dural patching with some long-term improvement in his lower extremity strength.

As expected, a majority of children with contractures (78%) are stable post-operatively and require subsequent orthopedic procedures. This finding is supported by the work completed by Archibeck et al. [12] who found a significant increase in orthopedic procedures per year following an initial untethering. These results mirror our clinical practice. When a child develops a contracture, we initially recommend an untethering prior to corrective orthopedic procedures. A corrective orthopedic procedure without a release of the tether will not prevent further orthopedic, or urologic, decline [7].

In children with urologic decline as an indictor of tethering, 64% of patients experience improvement and 36% remain stable on post-operative testing. This result is in contrast to the study by Abrahamsson et al. [13], who found that all six patients with deterioration prior to untethering had improved urodynamics post-operatively. In this study, we note improvement in the urodynamic testing and function of nine children following an untethering for reasons other than urologic decline. Interestingly, the one child who had an initial decrease in bladder capacity, but stable pressures, on his 3 month post-operative CMG also experienced a very impressive increase post-operatively in strength in all muscle groups of his lower extremities. It is possible that the untethering of his spinal cord improved his oxidative metabolism [2] and thereby increased the sacral reflex arch to his bladder. Fortunately, gradually over 15 months, his bladder capacity has improved and returned to baseline.

Scoliosis is an indicator of tethering in this series of patients. In prior studies, untethering is felt to be beneficial for stabilization or improvement of the spinal curvature [1, 14, 15]. Indeed, this is shown to be true within the first year post-operatively. In a prior study of 30 children with scoliosis who underwent an untethering, 96% have either an improvement or stabilization in their curves at one year follow-up [16]. In the Sarwark et al. [15] study of children with an L3 level and below, 75% are either stable or improved at one year, but more than 41% are noted to have developed progression at long-term follow-up (range of 3-7 years). In two separate studies by McLone's team, scoliosis progresses to approximately 38% of the cohort at long-term follow-up (2-7 years) [14, 16].

Our results are comparable to the findings of Pierz et al. [17] who note a 57% progression, 48% undergoing spinal fusion, at a 5 year follow-up period. The unique difference between this study and the other reports is the extended length of follow-up (average 12 years, range 1 month-23.3 years). In our long-term study, 58% of the cohort has undergone spinal fusion. Thirty percent of the cohort have improved or stabilized. In the four children with some progression, but no fusion, three children are at skeletal maturity and will most likely never require a fusion.

Further extensive evaluation of this cohort is needed to determine if an early untethering is beneficial in stabilizing a child's spinal curvature long enough to allow for skeletal maturity. Untethering of the distal spinal cord, however, does not appear to prevent the need for eventual spinal fusion in a majority of children born with an open neural tube defect.

Conclusion

Symptomatic tethering of the closed neural placode occurs in approximately 23% of the children cared for at CMH since 1975. Release of the tethered spinal cord is beneficial in a majority of patients in maintaining or improving their neurologic disabilities at relatively low risk (3.5%).

References

1. Hoffman HJ, Hendrick EB, Humphreys RP (1976) The tethered spinal cord. Its protean manifestations, diagnosis, and surgical correction. Childs Brain 2:145-155
2. Yamada S, Won DJ, Yamada SM (2004) Pathophysiology of tethered cord syndrome: correlation with symptomatology. Neurosurg Focus 16(2):E6
3. Bowman RM, Seibly JM, McLone DG (in press) Tethered cord release: A long-term study of 114 patients
4. Bowman RM, McLone DG, Grant JA et al (2001) Spina bifida outcome: a 25-year prospective. Pediatric Neurosurgery 34:114-120

5. Dias MS, McLone DG (1993) Hydrocephalus in the child with dysraphism. Neurosurg Clin N Am 4(4):715-726

6. Tomita T, McLone DG (1983) Acute respiratory arrest. Am J Dis Child 137:142-144

7. Phuong LK, Schoeberl KA, Raffel C (2002) Natural history of tethered cord in patients with meningomyelocele. Neurosurgery 50(5):989-993

8. Rinaldi F, Cioffi FA, Columbano L et al (2005) Tethered cord syndrome. J Neurosurg Sci 49(4):131-135

9. Cochrane DD, Rassekh SR, Thiessen PN (1998) Functional deterioration following placode untethering in myelomeningocele. Pediatric Neurosurgery 28(2):57-62

10. Schoenmakers MA, Gooskens RH, Gulmans VA et al (2003) Long-term outcome of neurosurgical untethering on neurosegmental motor and ambulation levels. Dev Med Child Neurol 45(8):551-555

11. Blount JP, Tubbs RS, Okor M et al (2005) Supra-placode spinal cord transection in paraplegic patients with myelodysplasia and repetitive symptomatic tethered spinal cord. J Neurosurg 103(1 Suppl):36-39

12. Archibeck MJ, Smith JT, Carroll KL et al (1997) Surgical release of tethered spinal cord: survivorship analysis and orthopedic outcome. J Pediatr Orthop 17(6):773-776

13. Abrahamsson K, Olsson I, Sillen U (2007) Urodynamic findings in children with myelomeningocele after untethering of the spinal cord. J Urol 177(1):331-334

14. Herman JM, McLone DG, Storrs BB, Dauser RC (1993) Analysis of 153 patients with myelomeningocele or spinal lipoma reoperated upon for a tethered spinal cord. Pediatr Neurosurg 19:243-249

15. Sarwark JF, Weber DT, Gabrieli AP et al (1996) Tethered cord syndrome in low motor level children with myelomeningocele. Pediatr Neurosurg 25(6):295-301

16. McLone DG, Herman JM, Gabrieli AP, Dias L (1990-91) Tethered cord as a cause of scoliosis in children with a myelomeningocele. Pediatr Neurosurg 16:8-13

17. Pierz K, Banta J, Thomson J et al (2000) The effect of tethered cord release on scoliosis in myelomeningocele. J Pediatr Orthop 20(3):362-365

CHAPTER 23
Pathophysiology and Clinical Features of Tethered Cord Syndrome

Joon-Ki Kang

Pathophysiology

The proposed normal function of the terminal filum of the spinal cord is to fixate, stabilize and buffer the distal cord from normal and abnormal cephalic and caudal traction. The filum is a viseoelastic band that usually allows the conus medullaris to move slightly during flexion and extension of the spine. It is theorized that if the viscoelasticity of the filum is lost or compromised by fatty infiltration [1] or abnormal thickening, then caudal tension and traction may cause stress upon the conus, resulting in a tethered spinal cord (TSC).

The abnormal inelastic filum is thought to interfere with normal cord ascension resulting in a low-lying conus medullaris (a conus below the L1-2 interspace). Clasically believed to be the hallmark of TCS, other authors have demonstrated that TCS can exist when the conus is positioned normally [2-7]. In dorsal and transitional lipomas, the conus is often tautly pulled toward the site of insertion of the fibrofatty stalk. The nerve roots arising from a low-lying conus frequently course laterally or even cephalad and appear more relaxed than usual because their points of origin are brought closer to their exit foramina. Clinical and intraoperative evidence suggests that the neurological lesion in the TCS is within the spinal cord and not in the lumbosacral nerve roots.

Underlying the pathogenesis of TCS is the theory probably best termed the "ischemic hypothesis", which has been proposed by several authors [8-12]. The natural history begins with the dysraphic abnormality causing increased tension on the conus. Chronic or intermittent tension then leads to deformation of the conus, impaired local spinal cord blood flow and finally, local spinal cord ischemia. It is this local ischemia that causes neurological dysfunction and is presumably improved by the detethering procedure.

There are several corollaries to this theory. The first is that the mechanical properties of the terminal filum are important so that a thicker terminal filum or one with more fibrous tissue causes higher tension [13]. Second, such mechanical properties prevent normal spinal cord migration, which exacerbates this tension. Finally, asymmetrical growth of the vertebrae vis a vis the spinal cord is particularly evident during periods of rapid growth, which explains the occurrence of neurological deterioration during these times [14].

Based on experimental tethering in growing cats, Kang et al. [9] reported a reduction in spinal cord blood flow (SCBF) in the distal spinal cord, adjacent to the site of tethering, of 32% of the normal flow in 2 weeks. Detethering of the cord 2 weeks after tethering resulted in an increase in SCBF, returning to normal levels (Fig. 23.1). This study supports the hypothesis that spinal cord dysfunction in the early stage of tethering results from mechanical and vascular damage to a spinal cord segment, which results in widespread ischemic involvement of the

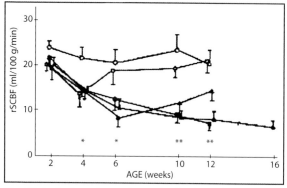

Fig. 23.1. Tethered growing animals showed progressive reduction of regional spinal cord blood flow (rSCBF): similar findings were made in growing animals detethered after 8 weeks. However, growing animals detethered after 2 weeks showed progressive increase of rSCBF (L3) to normal control level. *Open circles* - normal control growing animals; *closed circles* - tethered growing animals; *open squares* - 2 week old detethered growing animals; *open triangles* - 4 week old detethered growing animals; *closed triangles* - 8 week old detethered growing animals. *$p < 0.05$; **$p < 0.01$. Reproduced from [12], with permission

cord with prolonged tethering during growth. There are several reported cases of adult presentation of a tethered conus, and it is unclear why these patients were symptom-free and the diagnosis overlooked for so long. Sostrin et al. [15] described three patients with acquired spinal stenosis and a tethered conus, and suggested that the stenosis induced the primary tethered conus to become symptomatic. Pool [16] theorized that a tethered conus eventually became symptomatic in one patient due to local stretching and ischemia occurring from the repetitive and insidious low back trauma associated with the patient's occupation. The description of spinal vasculature in patients with scoliosis given by Hilal and Keim [17] supports this hypothesis. They demonstrated that tension on the conus caused arterial stretching and ischemia with resultant cord damage.

Yamada et al. [12] defined TCS as "a stretch-induced functional disorder of the lumbosacral spinal cord due to excessive tension" between the lowest pair of dentate ligaments and the caudal end of the spinal cord anchored to an inelastic terminal filum. However, in an anatomical study of the dentate ligament we observed no evidence that this structure significantly interferes with either cranial or caudal traction on the spinal cord [18]. Nevertheless, Yamada et al. showed that caudal traction on the distal cord resulted in impairment of oxidative metabolism and that the degree of impairment correlated with the severity of the neurological deficits. Using animal models, they also showed that the dysfunction seen in TCS involves the gray matter of the distal cord (below L1) and occurs due to derangement of oxidative metabolism. This metabolic dysfunction is at the mitochondrial level with a significant reduction shift of cytochrome A and A_3 (similar to that seen in hypoxic and ischemic brain/spinal cord models). This reduction is proportional to the amount of caudal traction applied to the distal cord. These authors also demonstrated a corresponding reduction in spinal cord blood flow in proportion to the traction force. They then postulated that such cord traction caused "traction induced hypoxia" and neuronal membrane stretch with "loss of transmembrane ion homeostasis and electrical activity depression" [19, 20].

Clinical Features

Symptoms and Signs in Children and Adolescents

Pain

Unlike adults with TCS, who universally suffer from excruciating and unrelenting pain [21], children with TCS seldom complain of severe pain (Table 23.1). The quality of the pain in children is also different from that of adults. The dysesthetic, poorly localized diffuse pain in the legs, groin and perineum, or the electric shock pain along the spine so commonly seen in adults is rarely encountered in children. The pain in children is more often confined to the lower back, with only occasional radiation to the legs. Occasionally, the back pain is aggravated by prolonged bed rest presumably from thickening of the intervertebral discs due to absorption of water and from straightening of the cervical and lumbar curvature on recumbency, which increase the total length of the spine and place additional tension on the conus [23].

Table 23.1. Comparison between childhood and adolescent tethered cord syndrome. Reproduced from [22], with permission

Parameter	Childhood (0-6 years)	Adolescence (7-25 years)
Pain	Uncommon	Common: localized anorectal, diffuse, bilateral
Sensorimotor deficits	Common early signs: walking difficulty, abnormal gait	Common: frank leg weakness
Sphincter disturbance	Common: incontinence, dribbling delayed toilet training	Common: urinary frequency urgency, incontinence
Trophic ulcerations of the legs, foot	Relatively common Common early signs: neuromuscular deformities	Uncommon
Back lesions	Common	Uncommon
Spine deformity	Common: worsening scoliosis	Uncommon
Aggravating factors	Growth spurts	Precipitating factors: trauma, stretching of conus, lumbar spondylosis, disc herniation

However, the suffering of pain in young children does sometimes manifest in unusual ways and is expressed with unfamiliar vocabulary.

Sensorimotor Deficits

Motor deficits manifest themselves in different ways, depending on the age of the child. In infants, the loss of motor neuron function is most often seen as atrophy of the buttocks and calves although abundant baby-fat makes this difficult to detect. The affected foot may also be smaller, with exaggerated pedal arches and/or hammer toes. Muscle weakness may be very subtle and difficult to elicit; unilateral weakness is best detected by observing spontaneous kicking and flexion of the leg and the infant's attempts to right itself when alternatively placed in the prone and supine positions. The deep tendon reflexes are often absent on the affected side: signs of corticospinal tract involvement are extremely uncommon in infants. Insensitivity to pinprick may be confined to the genital region or noted as an absent anal wink reflex. In toddlers, lower extremity weakness presents as delayed motor milestones in the legs, regression in gait training or a wide-based divergent, wobbly gait, depending on the age of onset of symptoms. Parents notice their child having a clumsier leg, an in- or out-turned foot, dragging of the foot or neglect of the affected side. Sometimes matching the left and right shoes for the child becomes a problem as the disparity of growth between the feet becomes more apparent. Characteristically, the weakness is bilateral and involves several cord segments. With increasing age, corticospinal tract deficits become superimposed on signs of anterior horn cell injury with spasticity and upper motor neuron signs accompanying a rapidly progressive atrophy. Long tract signs are seen in 80% of adults with TCS [24], but are rarely encountered in young children.

Cutaneous Signs

The correlation between cutaneous and intradural lesions is such that the presence of cutaneous signs is a sufficient indication for neuroimaging studies.

Almost all children with TCS have some cutaneous stimata of underlying dysraphism, which affects less than 50% of adults. Several helpful points may be made about the cutaneous lesions. Midline hairy patches are highly correlated with split cord malformations [25]. Over 80% of intradural lipomas are associated with cutaneous signs; about two-thirds of these signs are subcutaneous lipomas, and one-third are capillary hemangiomas, dermal pits, or hypertrichosis without a subcutaneous lipoma [26]. If the subcutaneous lipoma is low, the gluteal cleft sometimes veers eccentrically so that one buttock appears larger, or the cleft bifurcates into two deep furrows cradling the fat lump. Dermal dimples can lead into a dermal sinus tract but are just as likely to be associated with other tethering lesions. Features that distinguish a "dysraphic" dimple from an innocuous "terminal" dimple (remnants of the posterior neuropore) are overhanging skin edges around the opening, a high location (above the lowest sacral vertebra), and the presence of hair tuffs. Capillary hemangiomas can be midline but frequently extend far laterally. Proboscis-like skin and subcutaneous protrusions akin to residual human tails are almost always associated with cord tethering.

Bladder and Bowel Dysfunction

Bladder and bowel dysfunction are difficult to detect in infants. The examiner should specifically ask whether there are any dry periods between diaper changes, which gives some idea about the retentive capacity of the bladder neck, and whether the infant ever urinates in a forceful arc, which is a rough measure of detrusor power. Complete absence of detrusor contraction is uncommon in infancy, since even a denervated bladder, as long as its muscular wall is sufficiently contractile and not totally fibrotic, has the ability to expel urine on a reflexive level at the right filling threshold [27].

In toddlers, the most common bladder symptom is delayed or unsuccessful toilet training. The normal age for full toilet training varies between individuals and cultures, but if control is still unsatisfactory by the age of 4 or 5 years, a neuropathic bladder should be suspected. Usually incontinence occurs during both day and night: enuresis with perfect daytime control points more to a psychogenic etiology, but exceptions have been reported. The symptoms of urgency, frequency, urge or stress incontinence, poor voluntary control, and post-void dribbling are mainly seen in older children and adults. Frequent urinary tract infections are seen at any age and more in girls than boys. Tethering of the conus rarely causes a pure lesion in any single neural pathway, but rather mixed abnormalities of the parasympathetic, sympathetic, and somatic pathways. Blaivas [28] found that sympathetic innervation was often the first to be impaired in TCS. The nonfunctioning internal urethral sphincter causes sagging of the proximal urethra and effacement of the bladder neck on the voiding cystourethrogram, which characteristically leads to postvoid dribbling and stress incontinence, both of which are early symptoms of neuropathic bladder. When the parasympathetic pathways are primarily injured, the detrusor mechanism is weakened and the bladder becomes hypotonic and areflexic [29]. Poor bladder emptying leads to the subjective feeling of incomplete voiding, and when the parasympathetic and sympathetic pathways are injured together, patients have both an inability to empty the bladder and incontinence due to sphincteric incompetence. A hypotonic bladder poses little threat to the upper urinary tract, but parasympathetic denervation sometimes results in an areflexic hypertonic bladder, which maintains high intravesicular pressure and promotes ureterovesicular reflux.

The most severe reflux is encountered with detrusor-sphincter dyssynergia. Normally, efferent discharges from the pudendal nucleus (supplying the external sphincter) and pelvic nucleus (supplying the detrusors) are mutually inhibitory via cross-linked collateral fibers, so that the two target muscles are never simultaneously activated. This delicate and polysynaptic connection is also tightly coordinated by descending inputs from the pontine micturition center. Dyssynergia is seen both with diseases involving the descending pathways and with diseases of the sacral cord itself, although more commonly with the latter. The detrusor contracts involuntarily against uncontrolled spasm or contractions of the external sphincter [30], causing huge rises in bladder pressure. These patients are partially obstructed by the closed sphincter (pseudocontinent), yet are intermittently incontinent owing to overriding contractions of the detrusor. They have a 50% chance of developing hydronephrosis.

Foot and Spine Deformities

Progressive talipes is one of the most common presenting features in children with TCS [14]. The mildest form of talipes is hammer toes, that is, fixed flexion at the interphalangeal and extension at the metatarsophalangeal joints. Sometimes the entire forefoot shows a valgus or varus drift at the tarsometatarsal articulations. More profound and higher denervation causes exaggeration of the horizontal and vertical arches, hollowing of the instep and neuromuscular imbalance at the ankle, giving rise to the various combined forms of equinus, calcaneal, varus, and valgus deformities of the foot.

Foot deformities most likely result from neuromuscular imbalance at a time when the tarsal, metatarsal, and phalangeal bones are actively growing and aligning with each other along closely set joint surfaces; that is, during childhood. The formation and orientation of these joint surfaces are affected by forces acting on their respective levers (participating bones). Confusion in this network of forces will cause malalignment to occur. If normal growth and alignment of these joints are undisturbed during the formative years, permanent deformities are unlikely to occur in later life. Adults with a tethered cord who did not have a pre-existing talipes never develop foot deformities with the onset of other symptoms [21].

Progressive scoliosis or kyphosis is seen in approximately one-quarter of children with TCS [26]. As with foot deformities, adults with a tethered cord do not develop new scoliosis with the onset of other neurological symptoms. However, once preexisting scoliosis has progressed beyond a certain angle (about 40-degrees), gravity itself will worsen the curvature regardless of age, whether or not the cord has been adequately detethered. When scoliosis secondary to cord tethering requires surgical correction, the tight conus must first be released before the spine is distracted to avoid catastrophic neurological deterioration.

Progressive Neurological Deterioration and Aggravating Factors due to Tethering

Occasionally, children with a lipoma or tight filum terminale deteriorate or become symptomatic for the first time during a period of rapid growth. Presumably, the disproportionate lengthening of the vertebral column in relation to the cord accentuates the tension in the conus and precipitates neurological dysfunction. Catastrophic leg weakness and bladder dysfunction have also been reported in adolescents after specific activities that have acutely stretched the spine [24]. These activities include ballet high-kicks; gymnastics, especially cart-wheel jumps; and exercises focusing on knee-chest bends. Medical examination and obstetric procedures in the lithotomy position, and automobile accidents in which the body is thrown into the jack-knife position, have also been implicated [24]. Breig showed that full flexion of the head on the chin is associated with a sudden upward movement of the spinal cord by as much as 2 cm [31]. When full neck flexion is combined with flexion of the lower spine, an already taut conus would be momentarily stretched beyond its physiologic limit and past the tissue's ability to maintain normal function. Finally, direct blunt trauma to the subcutaneous component of a lipoma can occasionally precipitate severe pain and unbearable dysesthesia down the legs, followed by accelerated neurological deterioration and a cascade of recurrent symptoms. The sudden deterioration in the tight conus is probably brought about by the shock-wave stresses directed through the subcutaneous connection [23, 32].

Both indirect and direct evidence suggests that the likelihood of neurological deterioration in TCS increases with age and ultimately becomes very high. For example, Hoffman divided the neurological status of 73 children with lipomeningocele into five grades, ranging from grade 0 for children who were neurologically normal to grade 5 for children unable to ambulate [29]. He found that most of the infants had either grade 0 or grade 1 status, whereas the pro-

portions of children with higher grades increased progressively with age. Almost all the teenagers were grade 3 or 4. This close correlation between the severity of disability and the age at diagnosis indirectly supports the argument that TCS is a progressive disease. Hoffman further reviewed 24 individuals who had undergone inadequate childhood operations for TCS and found that most of them had unequivocally deteriorated over a period of 1-18 years [33]. Certainly, many adult TCS patients who enjoy years of perfect health deteriorate precipitously after a minor automobile accident, a fall, or even a bout of vigorous exercise. In these instances, successful detethering "after the fact" does not guarantee full neurological recovery. It is therefore advisable to treat most cases of TCS as soon as diagnosis is made.

References

1. Dubowitz V, Lober J, Zachary RB (1965) Lipoma of the cauda equine. Arch Dis Child 40:207-213
2. Hogg ID (1941) Sensory nerves and associated structures in the skin of human fetuses of 8 to 14 weeks of menstrual age correlated with functional capability. J comp Neurol 75:371-410
3. Hendrick EB, Hoffman HJ, Humphreys RP (1983) The tethered spinal cord. Clin Neurosurg 30:457-463
4. Metcalfe PD, Luerssen TG, King SJ et al (2006) Treatment of the occult tethered spinal cord for neuropathic bladder: results of sectioning the filum terminale. J Urol 176:1826-1829; discussion 1830
5. Drake JM (2006) Occult tethered cord syndrome: not an indication for surgery. J Neurosurg 104:305-308
6. Selden NR (2006) Occult tethered cord syndrome: the case for surgery. J Neurosurg 104:302-304
7. Wehby MC, O'Hollaren PS, Abtin K et al (2004) Occult tight filum terminale syndrome: results of surgical untethering. Pediatr Neurosurg 40:51-57
8. Huse T, Patrickson JW, Yamada S (1989) Axonal transport of horse-radish peroxidase in the experimental tethered spinal cord. Pediatr Neurosci 15:196-301
9. Kang JK, Kim MC, Kim DS, Song JU (1987) Effects of tethering on regional spinal cord blood flow and sensory – evoked potentials in growing cats. Childs Nerv Syst 3:35-39
10. Koca KA, Kilie A, Nurlu G et al (1997) A new model for tethered cord syndrome: a biochemical electrophysiological and electron microscopic study. Pediatric Neurosurg 26:120-126
11. Tani S, Yamada S, Knighton RS (1987) Extensibility of the lumbar and sacral cord. Pathophysiology of the tethered spinal cord in cats. J Neurosurg 66:116-123
12. Yamada S, Iacono RP, Androde T et al (1995) Pathophysiology of tethered cord syndrome. Neurosurg Clin N Hm 6:311-323
13. Selcuki M, Vatansever S, Inan S et al (2003) Is a filum terminale with a normal appearance really normal? Childs Nerv Syst 19:3-10
14. Hoffman HJ, Hendrick EB, Humphreys RP (1976) The tethered spinal cord: its protean manifestations, diagnosis and surgical correction. Childs Brain 2:145-155
15. Sostrin RD, Thompson JR, Rouhe SA (1977) Occult spinal dysraphism in the geriatric patient. Radiology 125:165-169
16. Pool JL (1952) Spinal cord and local signs secondary to occult sacral meningoceles in adults. Bull NY Acad Ned 28:655-663
17. Hilal SK, Keim HA (1972) Selective spinal angiography in adolescent scoliosis Radiology 102:349-359
18. Tubbs RS, Oakes WJ (2004) Can the conus medullaris in normal position be tethered? Neurol Res 26:727-731
19. Yamada S, Sanders D, Maeda G (1981) Oxidative metabolism during and following ischemia of cat spinal cord. Neurol Res 3:1-16
20. Yamada S, Knerium DS, Mandybur GM et al (2004) Pathophysiology of tethered cord syndrome and other complex factors. Neurol Res 26:722-726
21. Pang D (1985) Tethered cord syndrome in adults. In: Holtzman RNN, Stein BM (eds) The tethered spinal cord. Thieme-Stratton, New York, pp 99-115
22. Kang J-K (2000) In: Matsumoto S, Sato H (eds) Spina Bifida. Springer-Verlag Tokyo, pp 131-137
23. Joned PH, Love JG (1956) Tight filum terminale. Arch Surg 73:556-566
24. Pang D, Wilberger JE Jr (1982) Tethered cord syndrome in adults. J Neurosurg 57:32-47
25. Pang D (1992) Split cord malformation: Part II: clinical syndrome. Neurosurgery 31:481-500
26. Pang DC (1995) Spinal cord syndrome. In: Pang D (ed) Disorders of the pediatric spine. Raven Press, New York, pp 175-201

27. Pang D (1991) Tethered cord syndrome: newer concepts. In: Wilkins RH, Rengachary SS (eds) Neurosurgery update II. McGraw-Hill, New York, pp 336-344

28. Blaivas JG (1985) Urological abnormalities in the tethered spinal cord. In: Holtzman RNN, Stein BM (eds) The tethered spinal cord. Thieme-Stratton, New York, pp 59-73

29. McGuire, EJ, Woodside JR, Borden TA (1981) Prognostic value of urodynamic testing in myelodysplastic patients. J Urol 126:205-209

30. Blaivas JG, Sinha HP, Zayed AA, Labib KB (1981) Detrusor-external sphincter dyssynergia. J Urol 125:542-544

31. Breig A (1970) Overstretching of and circumscribed pathological tension in the spinal cord: a basic cause of symptoms in cord disorders. J Biomech 3:7-9

32. Pang D (1986) Tethered cord syndrome. In: Hoffman HG (ed) Advances in pediatric neurosurgery (Neurosurgery: State of the art reviews. Vol 1, no 1) Hanley's Beefus, Philadelphia, pp 45-79

33. Hoffman HJ (1985) The tethered spinal cord. In: Holtzman RNN, Stein BM (eds) The tethered spinal cord. Thieme-Stratton, New York, pp 91-98

CHAPTER 24
Spasticity in Spina Bifida

David Douglas Cochrane, Richard Beauchamp, Carol King, Andrew MacNeily

Introduction

Progressive deterioration in function due to neurological, musculoskeletal and urological complications in patients with spina bifida is not uncommon.

Dynamic factors invoked by progressive hydrocephalus, hindbrain compression, syringohydromyelia, diastematomyelia, cord tethering and the effects of gravity, growth and existing congenital deformity conspire to result in gait deterioration, motor weakness, urinary incontinence, scoliosis, or progressive joint deformity and contractures [1-11]. Developmental maturation, growth and existing musculoskeletal deformity play an important role in this deterioration, but the final common pathway for central nervous system (CNS) causes is often a progressive and relentless increase in muscular tone: spasticity.

Fundamental to current management of patients with spina bifida is multidisciplinary monitoring [12] that focuses on early clinical recognition of functional deterioration in at risk patients, investigation to define etiological factors, and timely intervention, directed to the presumed etiological cause(s), with the goal of maintaining or recovering function.

This chapter describes the clinical consequences of increased muscle tone in patients with spina bifida, describes the CNS anomalies that play a role in generating spasticity, and outlines an approach to treatment that can be used to modulate tone or its consequences in these patients.

Definition

Spasticity is a motor disorder and is recognized physiologically by the finding of a velocity dependent increase in the tonic stretch reflex evident on passive movement of a joint. It is due to hyperexcitability of the stretch reflex and is one component of the upper motor neuron syndrome [13-15]. The underlying pathogenesis is the loss of central inhibition of the spinal reflex arcs, resulting in hyperexcitability of primary motor neurons that are activated by inputs which otherwise would not provoke a response and consequent inappropriate co-activation of muscles.

The National Institutes of Health [16] built on this definition, defining spasticity as hypertonia in which one or both of the following signs are present: 1) resistance to externally imposed movement that increases with increasing speed of stretch and varies with the direction of joint movement; and/or 2) resistance to externally imposed movement which rises rapidly above a threshold speed or joint angle. Hypertonia is defined as increased resistance to externally imposed movement about a joint and is seen in rigidity and dystonia and as part of the constellation of motor symptoms in spasticity [16].

Pathogenesis of Hypertonicity in Spasticity

There continues to be debate as to the nature of the neurological lesion in the spina bifida placode. It has been thought to be a lower motor neuron lesion resulting in flaccid paraparesis [17, 18]. Stark and Drummond [19] believed that the lesion was frequently an upper motor neuron lesion, based on electrical stimulation studies of the neural plaque. Geerlink et al. [20] have described the results of cranial and lumbar magnetic stimulation in children with spinal dysraphism. In the study population, no infant responded to cranial stimulation, as is the case in the normal newborn, however lumbar stimulation resulted in responses in the majority of subjects even if their lower limbs were clinically paralyzed, inferring the integrity of the lower motor neuron.

Menelaus recognized on clinical grounds that a spastic and/or a flaccid paralysis could be present [21]. Sival et al. [22, 23] postulate that neuronal lesions can affect both the lower motor neuron in the placode and the upper motor neurons as they traverse the placode and that these lesions can be progressive.

Many authors have observed that the neurological deficit seen at birth can change over time. Sival and colleagues [22-24] have reaffirmed that progression of both lower and upper motor dysfunction can occur, with loss of motor functions in the early postnatal period and subsequently more slowly, spasticity can increase. The etiology of these changes is not well understood. Leg movements served by motor functions within the placode disappeared in some patients during the first postnatal week and appear to be due to the loss of lower motor neuron function, while upper motor neurons traversing the placode remain intact. Loss of motor movements and reflexes can occur prior to closure as well as after. Whether this is due to the care provided to the placode pre- or intraoperatively is not known.

Preservation of the upper motor neurons in the placode, relieved of normal suprasegmental modulation, provides the neuroanatomical substrate for spasticity affecting musculoskeletal and urinary systems.

Placode tethering is often considered in the assessment of the spina bifida patient with evolving spasticity and consequent deformity. The surgical pathology consistently reveals dense adhesions between the placode or conus and the overlying dura. Arachnoiditis in the subarachnoid space ventral to the dural-placode scar was also always seen, enveloping the nerve roots and radicular vessels. The pathogenesis of symptomatic retethering in myelomeningocele patients is postulated to be multifactorial and includes mechanical compression, arachnoiditis, mechanical distortion and stretching of neural and vascular elements at and above the placode [3, 7-11, 25].

Processes rostral to the neuroplacode can also affect the functioning of the upper motor neuron, causing spasticity to worsen. Hydrocephalus due to shunt dysfunction is the most common cause of worsening spasticity. This can be due to lateral ventricular dilatation, central transtentorial or foramen magnum herniation or syringohydromyelia. The Chiari II malformation with its associated cerebral and brain stem malformations, its hind brain herniation and secondary deformational brainstem dysfunction, with or without adhesive arachnoiditis, can result in increasing spasticity over time. Syringomyelia in patients with myelomeningocele is commonly associated with shunt dysfunction and/or the Chiari malformation. While this can result in lower motor neuron lesion at the level of the maximal syrinx, upper motor neuron signs are traditional accompani-

ments more caudally. Moreover, the degree of neurological impairment can change, usually worsening with time [3, 8, 9, 11, 26, 27]. Extensive spasticity discordant with the level of the spina bifida, upper extremity dysfunction and cognitive impairment are suggestive of other cerebral malformations or concomitant cerebral palsy [28, 29].

Systematic factors including acute and chronic urinary tract infections, perianal fissures and abscess formation, decubiti and contractures, and immobility in bed or chair can alter reflex sensitivity and muscle tone, increasing spasticity.

Spasticity as the Cause of Deterioration in Spina Bifida

In spasticity, resting muscle tone is increased and is associated with hyperreflexia, clonus, involuntary movements (spasms), enlarged receptive fields for cutaneous reflex responses, exaggerated withdrawal responses and the absence of voluntary movement and central perception of stimulation [30]. The consequence of increasing muscle tone in patients with spina bifida is abnormal static posturing of a limb, despite the presence of a full range of movement at the involved joint(s) and muscle weakness [30-32]. Abnormal static posturing results in contractures by limiting the range of joint movement and by altering the mechanical advantage of muscles acting across the joint. These features, in addition to increasing weakness, result in loss of range, coordination and postural integrity that support standing and ambulation [30]. Increasing muscle tone in the detrusor and the sphincter produces a small capacity, high pressure, irritable bladder that results in incontinence, and enuresis. This effectively increases the resistance to bladder emptying, aggravating any tendency to reflux and threatening the upper tracts.

There are other causes for deterioration in patients with spina bifida that are not the subject of this chapter but that need to be considered in the assessment of functional loss in these patients. Scoliosis, in particular in patients with thoracic or thoracolumbar myelomeningocele, is commonly due to structural congenital anomalies of the vertebrae that predispose to the development and progression of the spinal curvature. Congenital dysplasias of the hip, ankle and hind foot are evident at birth, due in part to the muscular imbalance present during intrauterine life. With ambulation and sitting, the effects of gravity are borne by the skeletal deformities, resulting in further progression. In addition, muscles weakened as a result of partial innervation can further lose function as limbs lengthen and the lever arm over which muscles act are lengthened, placing the muscles at greater mechanical disadvantage. Confinement to a wheelchair or bed for any reason, with the resultant inactivity, also facilitates muscular atrophy and weakening. Recognizing the roles of neurological and nonneurological factors, the most important final effecter of progressive functional loss is spasticity [33-36].

Functional Expectations and the Evolution Due to Spasticity

With the exception of the infant or child whose neuroplacode is excised at closure or detethering, who undergoes rhizotomy or has the most caudal sacral lesion, the majority of children and adults with spina bifida will develop spasticity and its consequences [30, 35]. The reported incidence appears to be less in patients with lipomyelomeningocele than in myelomeningocele, however the differences are likely to be a reflection of the duration of follow-up and the methods used to detect neuromotor and urinary changes in these populations.

Spasticity in myelomeningocele does not always present in a symmetrical or predictive pattern. Tonal changes may be isolated to one muscle group and may be unilateral. Occasionally there is a reflexive flexor synergy pattern present. Increased tone in the proximal muscle groups is usually associated with the higher level lesions and distal tone in the lower level lesions. Higher level lesions may also exhibit ankle clonus or a lower extremity reflexive flexor patterning. Bladder involvement can be present in patients with any pathological form of spina bifida, high or low. The functional status of the bladder cannot be predicted based upon the level of the neurological lesion. The following outlines the functional expectations based on the level of the dysraphic spinal lesion and the impact of spasticity on these functions [18, 30].

Myelomeningocele

Thoracic and Upper Lumbar Level Lesions

Infants who present with a thoracic level lesion have no voluntary muscle activity and often no fixed deformity in the legs. Patients with partial or complete innervation at the L1 and 2 levels have unopposed hip flexion due to sartorius and iliop-

soas muscle activity and they may have weak hip adductors. The legs lie in hip external rotation, abduction and slight flexion, with slight flexion at the knees and equinus at the ankles. They acquire postural deformities as a consequence of the effect of gravity. Hip dislocation and scoliosis are often present but not as a consequence of spasticity. Paralysis limits these patients to wheelchair mobilization, standing devices, catheterization and bowel management protocols.

In patients with higher level lesions, spasticity may not aggravate motor disability. There may be reflexive spasticity present, such as ankle clonus impacting ankle foot orthotic wear. In patients with innervation of L1 and L2 musculature, spasticity may interfere with the maintenance of hip-pelvic articulation resulting in the inability to stand because of hip flexion contractures. The upper renal tracts are protected by the low pressure high compliance bladder due to lower motor neuron lesion; however, if the placode reflex arcs are intact, a contracted, high pressure bladder is more common, putting the upper urinary tracts at risk from reflux.

Mid Lumbar Level Lesion

With preservation of hip flexors and adductors and the quadriceps and the lack of hip extension and abduction power, hip subluxation progressing to dislocation commonly occurs. When the fourth lumbar levels are functional, the quadriceps muscles, the medial hamstring muscles, tibialis anterior and posterior muscles are present in decreasing order of power. The knee is often in extension or hyperextension and there is a high incidence of calcaneal foot deformities due to unopposed tibialis anterior activity and absent gastrosoleus and other variables such as intrauterine position.

Due to the development of increasing tone in hip and knee flexors, with the consequent flexion contractures, ambulation with orthotics becomes increasingly inefficient. In addition to spasticity, gravity, increasing weakness of the quadriceps and the increasing mechanical disadvantage of short muscles and growing bones, aggravate the problem.

Spasticity may cause hip dislocation or subluxation, especially if there is over-pull of hip adductors. A pelvic X-ray evaluating the acetabular index and migration percentage are objective measures of change in hip pathology. However, one study noted that in myelomeningocele patients with an L3-4 lesion, two thirds of hips become dislocated or subluxed at the end of the first year (86% of patients with an L3 level lesion and 45% of those with an L4 level) [33]. A posterior pelvic tilt may result in sacral sitting predisposing a non-ambulatory child with myelomeningocele to pressure sores. If the hamstring pull is asymmetrical, pelvic obliquity may result, predisposing the individual to a secondary scoliosis and pressure sores. Hip flexor spasticity can also increase the lumbar lordosis.

These patients, like others with lower lesions, commonly exhibit incontinence despite anticholinergic medication and clean intermittent catheterization. Typically there is a variable degree of increased detrusor tone (hyperreflexia and hypocompliance) leading to poor bladder storage function. The external urinary sphincter tends to be set at a fixed resistance, independent of detrusor function. This combination of bladder and outlet dysfunction results in unpredictable ultimate continence.

Lumbosacral and Sacral Level Lesions

With the fifth lumbar root, innervation is present in the tensor fasciae latae, gluteus medius, and gluteus minimus. Hip abduction of sufficient power is usually present to provide hip stability, while the anterior and posterior tibial muscles are sufficiently strong to become deforming forces about the foot and ankle. These unopposed muscles often cause a calcaneus ankle or a cavus deformity. The first sacral root provides antigravity power in the hip extensors, allowing for a more normal gait with gastrosoleus providing, and toe flexors supplementing, plantar flexion. Foot posture may be relatively normal. Minimal motor loss in the feet occurs with paralysis below the second sacral root, resulting in clawing of the toes due to weakness in the intrinsic muscles of the foot.

Patients with lumbosacral and sacral lesions declare the development of spasticity with clawing of toes and pes cavus or cavovarus deformity or with bladder dysfunction, specifically incontinence and infection. Spasticity limited to the ankle joint muscles influences the gait pattern, standing position and balance [32].

Spasticity may cause an asymmetrical pull on the paraspinal or lower extremity muscles, resulting in scoliosis and pelvic obliquity. Trivedi [37] reviewed the association between scoliosis and the clinical motor level, the ambulatory status, spasticity, motor asymmetry and hip instability. The clinical motor level, ambulatory status and the last intact laminar arch were all found to be predictive factors for the development of scoliosis [37, 38].

Upper Limb Spasticity in Myelomeningocele

A significant proportion of patients with myelomeningocele exhibit spasticity in their upper limbs due to associated CNS anomalies such as the Chiari malformation and its various components, hydrocephalus, syringomyelia, and space occupying lesions [35]. Upper extremity tonal changes will usually be flexor in myelomeningocele, involving the forearm pronators and wrist flexors, with occasion resistance to full shoulder elevation. Upper limb spasticity was found in 22% of Mazur's patient population [35]. Those with spastic upper limbs and flaccid lower limbs most commonly had thoracic level lesions, but lumbar level patients exhibiting this combination were also seen. No patients with a sacral level myelomeningocele exhibited upper limb spasticity. In the patients with upper limb spasticity, the degree of spasticity correlated with the control of hydrocephalus as reflected by the number of shunt revisions and episodes of shunt infection.

Spasticity in the upper and lower limbs is particularly disabling. Upper limb spasticity results in the limb weakness and dyscoordination, making the use of wheelchair and aids of daily living more difficult. Spasticity in the lower limbs results in persistent contractures and deformity, making orthotic fitting difficult, limiting mobility and therefore rendering community and household mobility less likely.

Spina Bifida Occulta

There is no characteristic set of neurological symptoms, signs, or both that occur in a patient with closed spinal dysraphism. The presentations range from the presence of a cutaneous marker, back or leg pain, subtle bladder disturbance detected with urodynamics, a mild sensory disturbance in one foot, to a severe motor deficit and resultant muscular atrophy. The one common factor that the neurological deficits share is that they are typically asymmetrical, regardless of the type or location of the spinal lesion [39, 40]. Prior to the onset of walking, it is often difficult to detect muscular weakness. Often, the deficit is only evidenced by a slight asymmetry of the feet (possibly indicating long-standing motor weakness) or a predisposition to painless foot ulcers due to unnoticed absence of pain sensation. The difficulty with diagnosis is especially true in the newborn population, in whom a thorough neurological examination is particularly challenging. The abundant subcutaneous fat and decreased spontaneous movements may hide unilateral atrophy of the leg muscles in the infant, or an unusual posture of one extremity may be an indication of subtle motor weakness. Delayed or asymmetrical ambulation in an infant may be the initial complaint.

With the onset of weight bearing, inversion and forefoot adduction occur and with time, cavovarus movement becomes fixed and noticeable at rest. Paralysis of the evertors of the foot may be present initially in more severely affected children or may appear subsequently with a progressive neurological deficit. Because of underlying malformed bone and joint, the foot deformity may worsen after repair of the spinal anomaly [40, 41].

Urological Consequences of Spasticity in the Spina Bifida Patient

Although patients with spina bifida can have primary deformity of the upper and lower urinary tract and renal dysplasia, the fundamental threat to renal function in the longer term is detrusor sphincter dyssynergia, creating functional bladder outlet obstruction and causing obstructive neuropathy [42]. The pelvic floor activity and detrusor activity can be abnormal, overactive or inactive and may be completely independent from each other. Knoll and others have described the patterns of sphincter activity with in the range of 45% of these children showing sphincter over-activity, 34% combined with detrusor over-activity, and 11% exhibiting detrusor under-activity [42]. Chronic renal failure remains an important case of morbidity and mortality in patients with myelomeningocele [43].

Urologic problems are a common accompaniment of spina bifida occulta, in particular lipomyelomeningocele, and are easily overlooked in infancy and early childhood. In older children and adults, the most common presenting urologic complaints are frequent urinary tract infections and incontinence; other symptoms include frequency and urgency of urination and enuresis that is refractory to conservative medical management. Because it is less socially acceptable in older patients, incontinence is a symptom that usually compels patients to seek medical care. Encopresis, when it is of neurological origin, is almost never seen without concomitant bladder involvement.

Evaluation of Spasticity

Neuromotor Evaluation

The multidisciplinary team and in particular physical therapists play an integral role in obtaining an ac-

curate baseline assessment of the neuromotor status in patients with spina bifida. The assessment needs to be reproducible over time and with various examiners, in order to detect changes in motor function.

A motor level must be determined shortly after birth by evaluating the muscle strength of all muscle groups in each lower extremity and the trunk. Standardized manual muscle strength testing [44] and myometers can be used in older children. The motor level should not change over time unless there are complicating factors.

Tonal changes impacting range of motion must be differentiated from loss of range secondary to changing bony pathology and muscle contractures. Assessment tools for measuring spasticity in spina bifida can help differentiate between muscles that have contractures and those that are spastic. The Ashworth Scale, Modified Ashworth Scale (MAS) and the Tardieu, and modified Tardieu scales have been utilized [45-50].

The Ashworth scale has been shown to measure resistance to passive stretch adequately but does not differentiate between resistances due to muscle shortening and muscle stiffness. The Tardieu Scale differentiates contracture from spasticity and is the preferable scale for detecting discriminatory changes in tone as a result of interventions [51]. The Tardieu Scale compares the occurrence of a catch at low and high speeds. The modified Tardieu scale uses standardized conditions and measures the quality of the muscle reaction as well as the angle at which it occurs for the hip adductors, hamstrings and gastrosoleus muscles [46]. The point of resistance to maximum velocity stretch is synonymous with the 'over-active stretch reflex' defined by Boyd as 'R1'. This is compared to the amount of muscle contracture or muscle length 'R2' obtained when a standardized velocity and force is applied [45]. The catch point can be measured using a goniometry. A large measure between 'R1' and 'R2' characterizes a large reflexive component, whereas a small difference means that there is predominantly a fixed muscle contracture present [45, 46].

Spasticity may alter gait patterns and detailed computerized gait analysis is a valuable tool for objectively assessing changes that may result from spasticity. If this is not available, a standardized approach to the use of a two-dimensional (2D) video should be obtained. Biomechanical functional activities such as the ability to rise up to sitting from lying, rising to stand from a chair, rising to stand from the floor, rising to stand from squatting, floor mobility, toe walking, heel walking and stair climbing ability should be recorded. Balance agility in one legged standing and hopping should be assessed. Sitting balance, bed mobility, floor mobility, transfer ability and wheelchair skills should be evaluated in those patients who are non-ambulatory. The time taken to complete these tasks can be used to monitor their efficiency. Spasticity may increase fatigue levels and therefore energy expenditure should also be looked at in gait and during other functional tasks. Fine motor dexterity skills need to be reviewed to screen for upper extremity neurological dysfunction.

Various tools for standardizing and assessing motor function are being utilized in spina bifida patients. The timed 'Up & Go' (TUG) is a quick and easy measure of functional mobility. It assesses the individual's ability to maneuver his or her body capably and independently to accomplish every day tasks [52, 53].

The Functional Motor Scale (FMS) [54] designed for children with cerebral palsy is now being applied to the children with spina bifida. It has been constructed to classify functional mobility in children, taking into consideration the mobility aides they might use. The FMS rates walking ability at three specific distances: 5, 50, and 500 meters. This represents the child's mobility in the home, at school and in the community. Its sensitivity in documenting change in the same child or to evaluate change with interventions has not yet been determined in patients with spina bifida.

Urological Evaluation

The assessment and follow-up for patients with neurogenic bladder requires a complete urodynamic study, renal ultrasound, urine analysis and culture. Monitoring should include clinical assessment, renal ultrasound and urine and biochemical surveillance, at least on an annual basis. The performance of, and interpretation of urodynamic studies in young children is difficult and subjective. This has led many urologists to apply them selectively (e.g., onset of new hydronephrosis, refractory incontinence, contemplation of urinary tract reconstructive surgery) [55, 56]. Considering these challenges, Tarcan et al. [57] have reported their experience in spinal bifida infants with apparently normal urinary function. Twenty-five newborns with normal neurourological evaluation after surgical repair of the spinal defect were reevaluated every three months until the age of three years, semiannually until the age of six years and thereafter yearly, with the longest follow up at 18.6 years. During a mean follow up of 9.1 years, urodynamics subsequently showed neurourological deterioration in eight children. No change in urodynamics was observed in any patients after the age of six years [57]. The findings in this small subset of patients with normal bladder function should not at this time be generalized to the entire myelodysplasia population as it is well known that the risks of spinal cord tethering with consequent urological impairment exist into the pubertal years [58].

An Approach to the Treatment of Spasticity in Spina Bifida

The consequence of progressive and persistent spasticity is the formation of joint contractures leading to the development of joint subluxations and dislocations, progressive weakness in voluntary movement, resulting in muscle imbalance, and impaired ambulation and seating for patients with higher lesions. Spasticity aggravated by intermittent and/or chronic infection is the prime contributor to the development of detrusor hypertonicity and high urinary storage pressures, sphincter spasticity with secondary reflux, hydronephrosis and the risk of renal deterioration.

Spasticity requires treatment when it results in functional interference with seating, standing or moving, or when it leads to the development of a deformity. Spasticity may also need to be modified for comfort, fitting of orthoses, to promote ambulation and to facilitate intermittent bladder catheterization in order to deal with bladder neck obstruction and detrusor hypertonicity that would threaten the upper urinary tract. The decision to treat spasticity should be arrived at only after careful multidisciplinary input.

Prior to embarking on any treatment to relieve spasticity that is directed to the neuroplacode, the ventral or dorsal roots or joints, a thorough review of other CNS anomalies must be undertaken. The clinical worsening may be related simply to a malfunctioning shunt, with an expanded cerebral ventricular system and the ultimate channeling of cerebrospinal fluid (CSF) into a progressively enlarging syringohydromyelia [59]. A straightforward shunt revision may reverse the problem. A second rostral dysraphic lesion may have been hidden from view at the time of the first operation and may be uncovered by magnetic resonance imaging (MRI) of the spinal cord. These lesions include diastematomyelia, inclusion dermoid tumor, and hindbrain herniation with or without syringohydromyelia. Surgery on these lesions usually has a favorable outcome [3, 7, 11].

In the situation of progressive functional deterioration in a child with spina bifida, the treating team is faced with task of differentiating the role of concurrent congenital anomalies and spasticity as causes for the deterioration. In the case of musculoskeletal deterioration, accurate physical evaluation will confirm progression of the dysfunction and will aid in the differentiation of contracture and spasticity [45, 46]. In the case of contracture, releases will be necessary along with ancillary bracing and physiotherapy. Where spasticity is deemed the primary etiology or is of major importance, a trial of intramuscular botulinum toxin is useful to evaluate the correctness of the diagnosis and to determine in a reversible fashion, the extent to which spasticity is interfering with function and is being used by the patient for support.

When spasticity relief is deemed beneficial, and a long-term permanent solution is required, the decision-making then focuses on tendon lengthening, transfer or joint capsule releases. When the joints are mobile and spasticity is the primary cause, cord detethering and targeted rhizotomies are recommended.

When progressive bladder dysfunction is the primary indication for treatment and where the response to nonoperative methods is not adequate, intradetrusor injection of Botulinum toxin (Botox®, Allergan) or intravesical antimuscarinic therapy have been trialed to determine the clinical and urodynamic response. When the clinical response to these time limited agents is as expected and a permanent solution is required, cord detethering and targeted rhizotomy is pursued.

In the clinical situation when cord detethering has failed to provide long term spasticity relief, whether in the musculoskeletal or urinary systems, and other causes have one again been excluded, repeat detethering and rhizotomy is recommended using preoperative clinical evaluation and intraoperative electromyography and nerve root stimulation to define root bundles to be sectioned. Treatments are detailed in the next section.

Treatment Methods, Goals and Techniques – Prophylactic Interventions

Physiotherapy

The goal of physiotherapy is to create purposeful movements that can be incorporated into activities of daily living, and to prevent postural abnormalities that limit function. Specifically, physiotherapy is designed to maintain or increase range of joint movement, maintain muscle length and prevent contractures, to

prevent or minimize bone deformities, improve orthotic fit, improve mobility, decrease pain, decrease spasms, improve positioning and seating, and decrease energy expenditure with the result that function and activities of daily living are improved [60].

The treatment of spasticity begins preemptively with passive range of movement exercises in infancy. To optimize the range of joints which support weakened muscles and to delay the development of permanent contractures, splinting/orthotics, exercises and medications may be required. The aggressive and complete treatment of urinary tract infections prevents aggravation of spasticity and minimizes the effects of infection of the lower urinary tract.

Treatment Methods, Goals and Techniques – Therapeutic Interventions

Physiotherapy

Although spasticity cannot be altered directly by physical therapy, the therapist plays a role in the management of secondary changes caused by spasticity. However, not all spasticity is detrimental to motor function, as sometimes children with myelomeningocele use the hypertonicity for standing transfers or weight bearing.

Stretching has often been used as a tool to reduce the secondary effects of spasticity. A slow stretch is applied to the spastic muscle and maintained for a prolonged period of time to dampen the reflex activity response. The effectiveness of stretching in the management of spasticity and the duration that the stretch needs to be maintained remains controversial. Evidence for the efficacy of passive stretching on individuals with spasticity is limited [61, 62].

Stretching may need to be augmented with bracing, splinting, orthotics and serial casting to optimize joint alignment, reduce joint stress and optimize function. The physical therapist plays a role in the selection and evaluation of appropriate bracing. The type of bracing and orthotics needed are dependent on the level of lesion and on which muscles are impacted by the spasticity. Night-time splints and braces are sometimes utilized. If spasticity results in overactivation of an unopposed muscle group, such as the strong over-pull of tibialis posterior in the equinovarus foot deformity in children with lipomyelomeningocele, strapping changes in the orthotics may be needed. A lateral to medial pull from an ankle strap may contain a varus hind foot more effectively in equinovarus foot deformities. Orthotic/brace intolerance or asymmetrical wear may indicate a change in neurological status.

Serial casting has been used to stretch out tight spastic muscles such as heel cords. Once the desired range of motion (ROM) has been obtained by serial casting, splints and orthotics are utilized to maintain the alignment [47]. Serial casting has recently been utilized in conjunction with Botulinum toxin (Botox®, Allergan) to improve joint alignment and muscle elongation. Botox is felt to be most effective when there is a large difference between the 'R1' and the 'R2' values as noted on modified Tardieu testing [46]. Botulinum toxin has been utilized in spina bifida patients to reduce ankle clonus, thereby reducing the pressure sore predisposition and brace wear intolerance, and to improve muscle imbalance secondary to increased spasticity.

Seating and positioning may be impacted if there are tonal changes in the hip adductors and hamstrings, resulting in lower extremity asymmetry, pelvic obliquity or scoliosis. This may impair upper extremity function, sitting balance and increase pain. Wheelchair set up and seating systems need to be reviewed for optimal self wheeling, improving upper extremity function, optimizing comfort and to prevent pressure sores [63].

Spastic muscles are also weak. They may be slow to reach their maximum contractility power and slow to relax. Strength training may improve function and overall well being, but their benefit requires further study [64].

Pharmacotherapy

Oral Anticholinergic Agents

Anticholinergic medication plays an important role in the conservative management of children with neurogenic detrusor hyperreflexia [65]. In a study of 41 children with myelomeningocele and detrusor hyperreflexia who were evaluated urodynamically before and within three months after the initiation of combined therapy, oxybutynin significantly increased the maximal bladder capacity, and decreased the detrusor pressure at maximal capacity. Continence was improved also in 70% of patients over six years of age who were incontinent before therapy [66].

Tolterodine tartrate is a newer oral muscarinic antagonist that is currently being used in children. It is thought to possess a better side effect profile than oxybutynin based upon pharmacokinetic data, indicating

a more selective affinity for muscarinic receptors of the bladder compared to those in the salivary gland [67, 68]. The main drawbacks are high cost and that the only available oral formulation is as a pill.

Intravesical Therapy

Intravesically administered agents are better tolerated that their oral counterparts from the perspective of anticholinergic effects, although side effects including oxybutynin associated cognitive impairment, can occur [69].

Intravesical resiniferatoxin, acting to block the afferent C fibers in the reflex arc, has been used in patients who have been unresponsive to oral and intravesical oxybutynin [70], but currently this remains investigational.

Injection Therapies - Botulinum Toxin

Botox® (Allergan) is the most popular botulinum toxin in clinical practice. There are a total of seven botulinum toxins potentially available for clinical use. Of these toxins, 'A' is the most potent and is the one most frequently used for spasticity management [71-73]. Botulinum toxin A is a drug that blocks the release of acetylcholine at the neuromuscular junction in the muscle. To be effective, it has to be injected directly into that muscle. Ophthalmologists have used botulinum toxin A for 30 years for management of strabismus and other conditions. It has also been used for many years in the management of cervical dystonia. More recently, it has been shown to be very effective in reducing spasticity in selected muscles in children with spasticity from cerebral palsy. Botox® has been used in our center in over 1500 children, with various diagnoses, and is a useful spasticity controller in most situations, especially in younger children and smaller muscles. It is most useful in gastrocnemius muscles to control equinus in children under 30 kilograms in weight. Its efficacy is augmented by a three to six week period of intensive splinting or casting combined with stretching. The clinical effect usually lasts from four to six months. Repeated injections can be scheduled at six monthly intervals.

Intradetrusor injection of botulinum toxin has been used to control detrusor spasticity in patients with myelomeningocele [74-77]. Significant improvement in maximal bladder capacity and decrease in maximal detrusor have been regularly reported. Overall improvement in continence was seen in 73% of treated patients [75]. The effect would seem to last in the order of six months and subsequent injections retained efficacy without a decrease in bladder compliance [75-77]. The main impediment to the universal adoption of intradetrusor botulinum therapy is the cost, and need for repeated procedures.

Functional Neurostimulation

Biofeedback and functional electrical stimulation have limited application in the spina bifida population for muscle strengthening [78]. Some patients with myelomeningocele who have an intact sacral reflex arc may be candidates for sacral root stimulation. While this is not a treatment for spasticity, it has been used in selected patients to achieve continence following posterior sacral rhizotomy to increase compliance and decrease spontaneous reflex contractions [75, 79].

Orthopedic Procedures

Releases

Spasticity eventually results in inhibition of a muscle's growth in the face of continued skeletal growth. Control of spasticity does not address this relative muscle shortening. In this situation, surgical lengthening of the musculo-tendinous unit is required. This involves either an open tendon lengthening or a closed, per-cutaneous tenotomy. Surgical lengthening of contracted (e.g., dislocated hip, crouch gait) [31] or dynamically overactive muscles and tendons is done when development of the child's function is thought to be in jeopardy or when serious complications would occur if the muscles were allowed to remain contracted. Tendon lengthening does not change the spasticity 'cause', but it does weaken the muscular pull on the tendon or joint, making range of movement as well as voluntary control easier for the child. Because the underlying tone in the muscle is usually not changed following tendon lengthening, recurrence of contractures can be seen when the surgical lengthening is done in the very young child [80].

Hip Adductor Releases

Indications include limitation of abduction of less than 30 degrees of each hip and/or subluxation of the hip of greater than 25% on radiograph. Methods include open release of adductor longus, gracilis and usually a portion of adductor brevis. Post-operative management often requires six weeks in an abduction (Petrie) cast followed by resting night splint for three to six months. Occasionally a Standing, Walking and Sitting Hip orthosis (SWASH®) is useful [81-84].

Hamstring Releases

There are no absolute indications for release of the hamstrings unless it can be shown that the spasticity is interfering either with sitting or ambulation. Occasionally a detailed gait analysis will show the presence of a posterior pelvic tilt and reduced knee extension in stance and swing phases (crouch gait), which may require surgery [85, 86]. The surgical technique usually releases the medial insertion of the hamstrings behind the knee. This is a transection of the semi-tendinosis and gracilis tendons and a fractional lengthening of the tendonus portion of the semimembranosis. Following operation, the leg is immobilized in a long-leg cast for four weeks, and then the child uses an anti-crouch ankle-foot orthosis (AFO) or a knee-ankle foot orthosis (KAFO).

Equinus Releases

Equinus releases are considered when the foot cannot be placed in an AFO, when a midfoot break is imminent or has occurred, or when knee hyperextension is excessive [87, 88]. The typical cause of this deformity is combined gastrocnemius and soleus spasticity requiring a tendo-achilles tenotomy to release both muscles. Following operation, the foot is immobilized in a below-knee cast for four weeks then placed in an AFO.

Tendon Transfers

A joint may become unbalanced when a single muscle such as an antagonist muscle is much stronger than its agonist. Before a contracture occurs, however, there may be sufficient mobility and movement to allow a tendon's insertion to be moved surgically to produce a different, more balanced result when that motor unit fires and the muscle-tendon unit contracts.

The basic requirements for any tendon transfer apply to the myelomeningocele patient. These include an expendable tendon that can be transferred, with the muscle strength at least grade 4 (MRC Scale). The transfer should be 'in synchrony' and the direction of pull should follow a straight course to optimize the mechanical advantage of the transfer [89, 90]. Some examples of common tendon transfers include:

1. Anterior tibial tendon transfer from the dorsum of the foot to the calcaneus, done for a calcaneus deformity [91].
2. Posterior tibial (or split posterior tibial) tendon transfer for varus or inverted foot or a drop foot [92].

The patient who develops an increasing foot deformity, most commonly a unilateral, progressive cavovarus foot, most likely has a symptomatic tethered cord. Such deformities eventually become rigid, leading to disability and pressure sores. Surgical correction includes maintaining as much mobility as possible and avoiding sub-talar or triple arthrodeses [93]. This involves a combination of cord detethering, in addition to plantar fasciectomy, metatarsal osteotomy, tendon transfers and capsular releases.

Urological Procedures

Vesicostomy

As discussed above, at risk children are monitored for evidence of hydronephrosis, urinary infection and urodynamic deterioration. If attempts at medical management with oral and/or intravesical agents in conjunction with clean intermittent catheterization fail to prevent or correct these adverse outcomes, then vesicostomy is often recommended. Failure is typically the result of a combination of anatomic and social factors. Vesicostomy involves exteriorization of the dome of the bladder at the cutaneous level below the umbilicus. The result is conversion of the hostile bladder from a high pressure storage chamber, to a conduit with little or no pressure. The upper tracts are thus preserved. The incontinent stoma drains directly into the diaper, but is usually socially acceptable only up until approximately school age, when further reconstructive options to reverse the procedure are entertained [94].

Augmentation Cystoplasty

The concept of enlarging the bladder and lowering storage pressures by the incorporation of a segment of the gastrointestinal tract into the urinary system has been present for decades [95]. All segments of the intestine from stomach to sigmoid colon, alone or in combination, have been employed, but the ileum is most commonly employed today [96]. If conservative management of the hostile bladder fails, then augmentation cystoplasty is recommended. This procedure involves isolating a segment of intestine from the fecal stream, detubularizing it, with subsequent anastomosis to the opened bladder. The resultant storage chamber is then part bowel, part detrusor, of lower pressure, and greater capacity. Complications relate to mucous production by the intestinal epithelium, which must be cleared by regular catheterization and irrigation to prevent stone formation and infections. Metabolic acidosis secondary to reabsorption of urinary ammonium can occur, but is rare in the presence of adequate renal function [97]. Augment rupture, an abdominal catastrophe, can occur, and, in our experience, is most often related to noncompliance with an intermittent catheterization regimen [98].

Placode Detethering, Rhizotomy and Cordectomy

Detethering is the most commonly performed procedure on the neuroplacode to address spasticity. Placode detethering is a challenging operation because of the difficulty in defining and protecting normal and functional structures in the face of scarring and arachnoiditis. Some authors suggest that the neural-dural cicatrix is minimized by intubulation of the neuroplacode, and the creation of a generous subarachnoid space at the time of the original repair. This is not always possible [3].

Electrophysiological monitoring (free running electromyography (EMG) and bipolar stimulation) is used by some to improve recognition of functional structures and to thereby minimize the risk of operative injury. Care in the induction and maintenance of anesthesia is required to optimize the recordings. Our monitoring technique is based on our experience using multi-muscle and perianal sphincter EMG monitoring and bipolar stimulation for selective dorsal rhizotomy in spastic cerebral palsy.

When monitoring is to be used, the active and ground needle electrodes are placed in the tibialis anterior, gastrocnemius, vastus medialis, lateral hamstrings, adductor magnums, iliopsoas and the perianal sphincter bilaterally, following the induction of analgesia. The previous skin incision is prepared with chlorhexidine and the surgical site is draped. The incision is opened and the dissection carried down to the last intact lamina rostral to the spina bifida defect. The lamina is exposed by reflecting the multifidus and interspinales muscles. Following laminectomy of the exposed lamina, the area of the extradural cicatrix overlying the dura can be explored, using the exposed normal dural as a guide. Nonabsorbable sutures, if used at the primary closure, may serve as a guide to the dura. With the dorsal dura exposed, and depending on the relationship of the placode to the midline, an incision is made in the dura directly over the placode in the midline or laterally into the subarachnoid space. The dura is elevated from the dorsal surface of the placode using sharp dissection or a contact laser. Dural retention sutures are placed to facilitate access to the placode and subarachnoid space. Stimulation with the bipolar electrode and observation of the EMG and clinical responses guide the aggressiveness of dissection.

Once the placode is defined, it can be rotated to expose the roots if rhizotomy is being considered. Reconstitution of the dural tube is usually straightforward. It is rare that a dural graft is necessary. The paraspinal muscular scar and skin are closed in layers. Postoperatively, patients are nursed prone to minimize the risk of CSF leak and adhesion of the placode to the dural repair.

Detethering alone provides good immediate and short term results [11, 99], however in our experience, spasticity returns in many patients between 6-12 months postoperatively, despite continued aggressive physiotherapy. Others have reported similar findings [8, 9]. To address this, rhizotomy or excision of the placode in whole or in part has been recommended [9, 100].

If rhizotomy or cordectomy is being considered, pre-operative planning must begin with a detailed clinical examination to define the muscle groups that are responsible for the spasticity. Critical to this evaluation is the forecasting of muscle power, joint postures and mobility that will occur following rhizotomy. A trial of intramuscular botulinum toxin can greatly assist the determination. Intraoperative stimulation is designed to define the innervation to the spastic muscles.

In contrast to the clear delineation of the ventral and dorsal roots when rhizotomy is undertaken in cerebral palsy, the definition of ventral and dorsal roots, even at the intervertebral foramen, is often difficult because of the arachnoid scar in patients with spina bifida. As a result, the root bundles are often combinations of anterior and posterior roots. Teasing these into smaller bundles ('rootlets') allows them to be individually stimulated. Typically responses occur at higher thresholds than seen in anterior roots in patients with cerebral palsy; rootlets

responding at greater than 0.2-0.4 mA and sensory roots greater that 1 mA. More important than the threshold to response is the pattern of muscles activated by the stimulation. If stimulation provokes an EMG response in the problematic spastic muscles as defined preoperatively, the rootlet is sectioned. In general, it is more effective to section more rootlets than less and to include rootlets, even those with lower thresholds that replicate the activity of the spastic muscles. The final determination of what rootlets and the extent of rhizotomy relies on matching the intraoperative stimulatory response with the clinical assessment of the spasticity.

Complete rhizotomy involving all ventral and dorsal roots with or without placode excision is performed in paraplegic patients with problematic spasticity that interferes with sitting, and who have threatened upper urinary tracts. This can be done at the time of spinal fusion [100].

Intrathecal Baclofen

Continuous intrathecal baclofen has not been used extensively in the treatment of refractory spasticity in spina bifida. Bergenheim [101] has reported its successful use in a single shunted paraplegic patient with a high lumbar myelomeningocele. Spasticity developed in early childhood, followed by scoliosis at age three years. Placode detethering was performed twice and a hindbrain decompression failed to control painful spasticity and the scoliosis. A trial injection was performed through a catheter placed in the thoracic subarachnoid space prior to pump implantation. No complications were seen due to the drug's subarachnoid.

Conclusion

Spasticity is commonly seen in patients with spina bifida and when present, threatens functional abilities by restricting range of movement, underpinning contractures, and weakening muscles and renal function through the development of bladder outlet obstruction and detrusor hypertonicity, with subsequent upper track failure and hydronephrosis. The management of spasticity should be aggressive and requires a team, which should include a physiotherapist, occupational therapist, neurologist, orthopedic surgeon, neurosurgeon, nurse, and social worker [12]. Accurate and consistent assessment and functional evaluation are critical to the timely recognition of deterioration due to spasticity and the application of appropriate investigations to diagnose causation. Specific pathologies that exacerbate spasticity must be treated directly. In their absence, interventions must focus on the reflex arcs of the neuroplacode, the muscular-tendon unit or the muscle itself. Pharmaco-logical treatments often provide temporary and reversible relief and are helpful in defining the involved muscles. Placode detethering combined with rhizotomy or placode excision may be necessary to provide sustained relief of spasticity.

References

1. Alexander E, Garvey FK, Boyce W (1954) Congenital lumbosacral myelomeningocele with incontinence. J Neurosurg 11:183-191
2. Asher M, Olson J (1983) Factors affecting the ambulatory status of patients with spina bifida cystica. J Bone Joint Surg Am 65:350-356
3. Cochrane DD, Rassekh SR, Thiessen PN (1998) Functional deterioration following placode untethering in myelomeningocele. Pediatr Neurosurg 28:57-62
4. Koyanagi I, Iwasaki Y, Hida K et al (1997) Surgical treatment of syringomyelia associated with spinal dysraphism. Childs Nerv Syst 13:194-200
5. La Marca F, Herman M, Grant JA et al (1997) Presentation and management of hydromyelia in children with Chiari type-II malformation. Pediatr Neurosurg 26:57-67
6. Rauzzino M, Oakes WJ (1995) Chiari II malformation and syringomyelia. Neurosurg Clin N Am 6:293-309
7. Reigel DH, Tchernoukha K, Bazmi B et al (1994) Change in spinal curvature following release of tethered spinal cord associated with spina bifida. Pediatr Neurosurg 20:30-42
8. Sarwark JF, Weber DT, Gabrieli AP et al (1996) Tethered cord syndrome in low motor level children with myelomeningocele. Pediatr Neurosurg 25:295-301
9. Storrs BB (1987) Selective posterior rhizotomy for treatment of progressive spasticity in patients with myelomeningocele. Preliminary report. Pediatr Neurosci 13:135-137
10. Tamaki N, Shirataki K, Kojima N et al (1988) Tethered cord syndrome of delayed onset following repair of myelomeningocele. J Neurosurg 69:393-398
11. Venes JL, Stevens EA (1983) Surgical pathology in tethered cord secondary to myelomeningocele repair. Concepts Pediat Neurosurg 4:165-185
12. Chambers GK, Cochrane DD, Irwin B et al (1996) Assessment of the appropriateness of services provided by a multidisciplinary meningomyelocele clinic. Pediatr Neurosurg 24:92-97
13. Lance JW (1990) What is spasticity? Lancet 335:606
14. Lance JW, Burke D (1974) Mechanisms of spasticity. Arch Phys Med Rehabil 55:332-337
15. Lance JW (1980) Symposium Synopsis In: Feldman RG, Young RR, Koella WP (eds) Spasticity: disordered motor control. Yearbook Medical, Chicago, pp 485-494
16. Sanger TD, Delgado MR, Gaebler-Spira D et al (2003) Task Force on Childhood Motor D: Classification and definition of disorders causing hypertonia in childhood. Pediatrics 111:e89-97
17. Sharrard WJW (1963) Spina bifida. Paraplegia 1:190-199
18. Sharrard WJW (1964) The segmental innervation of the lower limb muscles in man. Ann R Coll Surg Engl 35:106-122
19. Stark GD, Drummond M (1971) The spinal cord lesion in myelomeningocele. Dev Med Child Neurol 13 suppl 25:1-15
20. Geerdink N, Pasman JW, Roeleveld N et al (2006) Responses to lumbar magnetic stimulation in newborns with spina bifida. Pediatr Neurol 34:101-105
21. Menelaus MB (1980) The orthopaedic management of spina bifida cystica. Churchill Livingstone, Edinburgh
22. Sival DA, Brouwer OF, Bruggink JL et al (2006) Movement analysis in neonates with spina bifida aperta. Early Hum Dev 82:227-234
23. Sival DA, Brouwer OF, Sauer PJ et al (2003) Transiently present leg movements in neonates with spina bifida aperta are generated by motor neurons located cranially from the spinal defect. Eur J Pediatr Surg 13 Suppl 1:S31-32
24. Sival DA, van Weerden TW, Vles JS et al (2004) Neonatal loss of motor function in human spina bifida aperta. Pediatrics 114:427-434
25. Caldarelli M, Di Rocco C, Colosimo C et al (1995) Surgical treatment of late neurological deterioration in children with myelodysplasia. Acta Neurochir (Wien) 137:199-206
26. McLone DG, Herman JM, Gabrieli AP et al (1990) Tethered cord as a cause of scoliosis in children with a myelomeningocele. Pediatr Neurosurg 16:8-13
27. McLone DG, La Marca F (1997) The tethered spinal cord: diagnosis, significance, and management. Semin Pediatr Neurol 4:192-208
28. Ozaras N, Yalcin S, Ofluoglu D et al (2005) Are some cases of spina bifida combined with cerebral palsy? A study of 28 cases. Eura Medicophys 41:239-242
29. Sival DA, Brouwer OF, Meiners LC et al (2003) The influence of cerebral malformations on the quality of general movements in spina bifida aperta. Eur J Pediatr Surg 13 Suppl 1:S29-30
30. Mazur JM, Menelaus MB (1991) Neurologic status of spina bifida patients and the orthopedic surgeon. Clin Orthop Relat Res 264:54-64
31. Bartonek A, Gutierrez EM, Haglund-Akerlind Y et al (2005) The influence of spasticity in the lower limb muscles on gait pattern in children with sacral to mid-

lumbar myelomeningocele: a gait analysis study. Gait Posture 22:10-25

32. Bartonek A, Saraste H (2001) Factors influencing ambulation in myelomeningocele: a cross-sectional study. Dev Med Child Neurol 43:253-260

33. Fraser RK, Hoffman EB, Sparks LT et al (1992) The unstable hip and mid-lumbar myelomeningocele. J Bone Joint Surg Br 74:143-146

34. Frawley PA, Broughton NS, Menelaus MB (1998) Incidence and type of hindfoot deformities in patients with low-level spina bifida. J Pediatr Orthop 18:312-313

35. Mazur JM, Stillwell A, Menelaus M (1986) The significance of spasticity in the upper and lower limbs in myelomeningocele. J Bone Joint Surg Br 68:213-217

36. Wright JG, Menelaus MB, Broughton NS et al (1991) Natural history of knee contractures in myelomeningocele. J Pediatr Orthop 11:725-730

37. Trivedi J, Thomson JD, Slakey JB et al (2002) Clinical and radiographic predictors of scoliosis in patients with myelomeningocele. J Bone Joint Surg Am 84-A:1389-1394

38. Isu T, Chono Y, Iwasaki Y et al (1992) Scoliosis associated with syringomyelia presenting in children. Childs Nerv Syst 8:97-100

39. Cochrane DD, Finley C, Kestle J et al (2000) The patterns of late deterioration in patients with transitional lipomyelomeningocele. Eur J Pediatr Surg 10 Suppl 1:13-17

40. James C, Lassman L (1981) Spina bifida occulta. Orthopedic, radiological and neurosurgical aspects. Academic Press, London

41. Carroll N (1987) Assessment and management of the lower extremity in myelodysplasia. Orthop Clin North Am 18:709–724

42. van Gool JD, Dik P, de Jong TP (2001) Bladder-sphincter dysfunction in myelomeningocele. Eur J Pediatr 160:414-420

43. McDonnell GV, McCann JP (2000) Why do adults with spina bifida and hydrocephalus die? A clinic-based study. Eur J Pediatr Surg 10 Suppl 1:31-32

44. Kendall FP, Rodgers MM, McCreary EK et al (2005) Muscle testing and function with posture and pain. Lippincott Williams and Wilkins, Baltimore

45. Boyd NR, Ada L, Barnes MP et al (2001) Physiotherapy management of spasticity. In: Upper motor neurone syndrome and spasticity. Clinical management and neurophysiology. Cambridge University Press, Cambridge, pp 96-121

46. Boyd RN, Barwood SA, Ballieu C et al (1998) Validity of a clinical measure of spasticity in children with cerebral palsy in a randomized clinical trial. Dev Med Chid Neurol 40:7

47. Boyd RN, Graham HK (1999) Objective measurement of clinical findings in the use of botulinium toxin A in the management of children with cerebral palsy. Eur J Neurol 69 Suppl 4:S23-S35

48. Haugh AB, Pandyan AD, Johnson GR (2006) A systematic review of the Tardieu Scale for the measurement of spasticity. Disabil Rehabil 28:899-907

49. Johnson GR, Barnes MP, Johnson GR (2001) Measurement of spasticity. In: Upper motor neurone syndrome and spasticity. Clinical management and neurophysiology. Cambridge University Press, Cambridge, pp 79-95

50. Scholtes VA, Becher JG, Beelen A et al (2006) Clinical assessment of spasticity in children with cerebral palsy: a critical review of available instruments. Dev Med Child Neurol 48:64-73

51. Patrick E, Ada L (2006) The Tardieu Scale differentiates contracture from spasticity whereas the Ashworth Scale is confounded by it. Clin Rehabil 20:173-182

52. Hoffer MM, Feiwell E, Perry R et al (1973) Functional ambulation in patients with myelomeningocele. J Bone Joint Surg Am 55:137-148

53. Williams EN, Carroll SG, Reddihough DS et al (2005) Investigation of the timed 'up & go' test in children. Dev Med Child Neurol 47:518-524

54. Graham HK, Harvey A, Rodda J et al (2004) The Functional Mobility Scale (FMS). JPO 24:514-520

55. Kaefer M, Pabby A, Kelly M et al (1999) Improved bladder function after prophylactic treatment of the high risk neurogenic bladder in newborns with myelomentingocele. J Urol 162:1068-1071

56. Wu HY, Baskin LS, Kogan BA (1997) Neurogenic bladder dysfunction due to myelomeningocele: neonatal versus childhood treatment. J Urol 157:2295-2297

57. Tarcan T, Bauer S, Olmedo E et al (2001) Long-term follow up of newborns with myelodysplasia and normal urodynamic findings: Is follow up necessary? J Urol 165:564-567

58. Kaplan WE, McLone DG, Richards I (1988) The urological manifestations of the tethered spinal cord. J Urol 140:1285-1288

59. Hall PV, Campbell RL, Kalsbeck JE (1975) Meningomyelocele and progressive hydromyelia. Progressive paresis in myelodysplasia. J Neurosurg 43:457-463

60. Gage J, Gormley M, Krach L et al (2004) Managing spasticity in children with cerebral palsy requires a team approach. In: A pediatric perspective, Gillette Children's Specialty Healthcare, pp 1-6

61. DeJong S (2006) Contracture management of children with neuromuscular disabilities. In: APTA CSM Meeting, San Diego

62. Pin T, Duyke P, Chan M (2006) The effectiveness of passive stretching in children with cerebral palsy. Dev Med Child Neurol 48:855-862

63. Kirwood CA, Bardsley GI, Barnes MP et al (2001) Seating and positioning in spasticity. In: Upper motor neurone syndrome and spasticity. Clinical management and neurophysiology. Cambridge University Press, Cambridge, pp 122-139

64. Sharp SA, Brouwer BJ (1997) Isokinetic strength training of the hemiparetic knee: effects on function and spasticity. Arch Phys Med Rehabil 78:1231-1236

65. Aslan AR, Kogan BA (2002) Conservative management in neurogenic bladder dysfunction. Curr Opin Urol 12:473-477

66. Goessl C, Knispel HH, Fiedler U et al (1998) Urodynamic effects of oral oxybutynin chloride in children with myelomeningocele and detrusor hyperreflexia. Urology 51:94-98

67. Goessl C, Sauter T, Michael T et al (2000) Efficacy and tolerability of tolterodine in children with detrusor hyperreflexia. Urology 55:414-418

68. Nilvebrant L, Andersson KE, Gillberg PG et al (1997) Tolterodine--a new bladder-selective antimuscarinic agent. Eur J Pharmacol 327:195-207

69. Madersbacher H (2002) Neurogenic bladder dysfunction in patients with myelomeningocele. Curr Opin Urol 12:469-472

70. Seki N, Ikawa S, Takano N et al (2001) Intravesical instillation of resiniferatoxin for neurogenic bladder dysfunction in a patient with myelodysplasia. J Urol 166:2368-2369

71. Jankovic J, Brin MF (1997) Botulinum toxin: historical perspective and potential new indications. Muscle Nerve Suppl 6:S129-145

72. Pierson SH, Katz DI, Tarsy D et al (1996) Botulinum toxin A in the treatment of spasticity: functional implications and patient selection. Arch Phys Med Rehabil 77:717-721

73. Skeil D, Barnes M (1994) The local treatment of spasticity. Clin Rehabil 8:240-246

74. Altaweel W, Jednack R, Bilodeau C et al (2006) Repeated intradetrusor botulinum toxin type A in children with neurogenic bladder due to myelomeningocele. J Urol 175:1102-1105

75. Kajbafzadeh AM, Moosavi S, Tajik P et al (2006) Intravesical injection of botulinum toxin type A: management of neuropathic bladder and bowel dysfunction in children with myelomeningocele. Urology 68:1091-1096

76. Patel AK, Patterson JM, Chapple CR (2006) Botulinum toxin injections for neurogenic and idiopathic detrusor overactivity: A critical analysis of results. Eur Urol 50:684-709; discussion 709-610

77. Schulte-Baukloh H, Michael T, Sturzebecher B et al (2003) Botulinum-a toxin detrusor injection as a novel approach in the treatment of bladder spasticity in children with neurogenic bladder. Eur Urol 44:139-143

78. Karmel-Ross K, Cooperman DR, Van Doren CL (1992) The effect of electrical stimulation on quadriceps femoris muscle torque in children with spina bifida. Phys Ther 72:723-730

79. Madersbacher H, Fischer J (1993) Sacral anterior root stimulation: prerequisites and indications. Neurourol Urodyn 12:489-494

80. Schmale GA, Eilert RE, Chang F et al (2006) High reoperation rates after early treatment of the subluxating hip in children with spastic cerebral palsy. J Pediatr Orthop 26:617-623

81. Abel MF, Blanco JS, Pavlovich L et al (1999) Asymmetric hip deformity and subluxation in cerebral palsy: an analysis of surgical treatment. J Pediatr Orthop 19:479-485

82. Miller F, Cardoso Dias R, Dabney KW et al (1997) Soft-tissue release for spastic hip subluxation in cerebral palsy. J Pediatr Orthop 17:571-584

83. Noonan KJ, Walker TL, Kayes KJ et al (2001) Varus derotation osteotomy for the treatment of hip subluxation and dislocation in cerebral palsy: statistical analysis in 73 hips. J Pediatr Orthop B 10:279-286

84. Turker RJ, Lee R (2000) Adductor tenotomies in children with quadriplegic cerebral palsy: longer term follow-up. J Pediatr Orthop 20:370-374

85. Moen T, Gryfakis N, Dias L et al (2005) Crouched gait in myelomeningocele: a comparison between the degree of knee flexion contracture in the clinical examination and during gait. J Pediatr Orthop 25:657-660

86. Westberry DE, Davids JR, Jacobs JM et al (2006) Effectiveness of serial stretch casting for resistant or recurrent knee flexion contractures following hamstring lengthening in children with cerebral palsy. J Pediatr Orthop 26:109-114

87. Greene WB (2000) Cerebral palsy. Evaluation and management of equinus and equinovarus deformities. Foot Ankle Clin 5:265-280

88. Park ES, Kim HW, Park CI et al (2006) Dynamic foot pressure measurements for assessing foot deformity in persons with spastic cerebral palsy. Arch Phys Med Rehabil 87:703-709

89. Kling Jr TF, Kaufer H, Hensinger RN (1985) Split posterior tibial-tendon transfers in children with cerebral spastic paralysis and equinovarus deformity. J Bone Joint Surg Am 67:186-194

90. Mulier T, Moens P, Molenaers G et al (1995) Split posterior tibial tendon transfer through the interosseus membrane in spastic equinovarus deformity. Foot Ankle Int 16:754-759

91. Piazza SJ, Adamson RL, Sanders JO et al (2001) Changes in muscle moment arms following split tendon transfer of tibialis anterior and tibialis posterior. Gait Posture 14:271-278

92. Kagaya H, Yamada S, Nagasawa T et al (1996) Split posterior tibial tendon transfer for varus deformity of hindfoot. Clin Orthop Relat Res:254-260

93. Romanini L, Carfagni A, Amorese V (1983) Grice's operation for spastic flat foot. Ital J Orthop Traumatol 9:439-449

94. Morrisroe SN, O'Connor RC, Nanigian DK et al (2005) Vesicostomy revisited: the best treatment for the hostile bladder in myelodysplastic children? BJU Int 96:397-400

95. Duckett JW, Gazak JM (1983) Complications of ureterosigmoidostomy. Urol Clin North Am 10:473-481

96. Metcalfe PD, Cain MP, Kaefer M et al (2006) What is the need for additional bladder surgery after bladder augmentation in childhood? J Urol 176:1801-1805

97. Gilbert SM, Hensle TW (2005) Metabolic consequences and long-term complications of enterocystoplasty in children: a review. J Urol 173:1080-1086

98. Metcalfe PD, Casale AJ, Kaefer MA et al (2006) Spontaneous bladder perforations: a report of 500 augmentations in children and analysis of risk. J Urol 175:1466-1470

99. Tarcan T, Onol FF, Ilker Y et al (2006) Does surgical release of secondary spinal cord tethering improve the prognosis of neurogenic bladder in children with myelomeningocele? J Urol 176:1601-1606; discussion 1606

100. McLaughlin TP, Banta JV, Gahm NH et al (1986) Intraspinal rhizotomy and distal cordectomy in patients with myelomeningocele. J Bone Joint Surg Am 68:88-94

101. Bergenheim AT, Wendelius M, Shahidi S et al (2003) Spasticity in a child with myelomeningocele treated with continuous intrathecal baclofen. Pediatr Neurosurg 39:218-221

CHAPTER 25
Seizures in Children with Myelomeningocele

Uğur Işik

Seizures in Children with Myelomeningocele

Seizures are reported to occur frequently in children born with myelomeningocele. For patients with hydrocephalus, the reported incidence of seizures ranges from 14.7-29% [1-7] whereas a much lower incidence, roughly 2-8%, has been reported for children with myelomeningocele but without shunts [4, 8]. Not every study in the literature specifies seizures versus epilepsy (recurrent unprovoked seizures) in these children. According to Bourgeois et al. [9], patients with myelomeningocele experienced a significantly low incidence of epilepsy (7%) compared to other etiologies. Those with prenatal hydrocephalus demonstrated a prevalence of 38% and, in the same study, those with meningitis and postinfective hydrocephalus carried a high risk of epilepsy, in the order of 50%. In a different study, the incidence of seizures was 21%, whereas the incidence of epilepsy was 17.3% in children with myelomeningocele [10].

According to Bowman et al. [11], out of 71 patients, 16 patients had seizures, all with shunted hydrocephalus. In a different series, 17 of 89 children (21%) with myelomeningocele had seizures, all with shunted hydrocephalus, however seizures were not observed in the 15 children without hydrocephalus [10]. Chadduck reported the overall incidence of seizures in patients with shunts as 22%, whereas it was only 2% in a nonshunted group [8]. In a study of a group of patients with hydrocephalus, including patients with myelomeningocele, 28.6% of patients with seizures experienced their first seizure before shunt insertion, while seizures developed after insertion in the remaining 71.4%, suggesting a strong influence of the shunting procedure on the development of epilepsy [9]. There are, however, some reports that do not show a difference in epileptic incidence between myelomeningocele patients with and without hydrocephalus, stressing the role played by possible underlying pathology, such as migration disorders or other malformations [4, 7]. The incidence of seizures and/or epilepsy in myelomeningocele patients in the presence and absence of hydrocephalus according to major reports is summarized in Table 25.1.

The increased incidence of seizures in patients with myelomeningocele and hydrocephalus may result from minor cortical injury at the time of shunt insertion, shunt complications such as infection or malfunction, and the pathology underlying or asso-

Table 25.1. Seizure and/or epilepsy incidence in patients with myelomeningocele in the presence or absence of hydrocephalus

	N. of patients	Seizure incidence	Epilepsy incidence	N. or percent of hydrocephalic children with seizures	N. or percent of non-hydrocephalic children with seizures
Talwar et al.	81	17 (21%)	14 (17.3%)	17	0
Bowman et al.	71	16 (23%)	Not mentioned	16	0
Chadduck et al.	190	24%	Not mentioned	22%	2%
Noetzel et al.	140	24 (17.1%)	Not mentioned	18	6
Bourgeois et al.	160	Not mentioned	7%	7% or all	Not mentioned
Bartoshesky et al.	111	25	Not mentioned	24	1

ciated with the development of hydrocephalus [8]. In addition, the role of severe apneic episodes and cardiac arrest secondary to Chiari malformation contributing to the later development of epilepsy cannot be discounted [10].

The incidence of seizures in patients requiring shunt modification was 22%, whereas patients who never required a modification had an incidence of seizures of only 9% [8]. In children with hydrocephalus with different etiologies, the incidence of epilepsy was 20% without revision, while it was 52% in the patients in whom more than three revisions were needed [9]. There is strong evidence to suggest a significant correlation between the frequency of revisions and the occurrence of seizures, as only 5.9% of those who did not have a catheter revision developed epilepsy, compared with 24.2% of those with two or more proximal site revisions [12]. Seizures associated with shunt malfunction have been reported in other studies [6, 7, 13].

Even low-grade infections of the central nervous system (CNS) with bacteria such as *Staphylococcus epidermidis* cause inflammation, arteritis, changes in the glucose concentration in the cerebrospinal fluid (CSF) and diffuse cerebral injury. In a study performed on children with myelomeningocele, the incidence of seizures in the group free of infection was 15%, whereas it was 47% in patients with a history of infection [8]. According to Blaauw et al. [3], infection appeared to be closely connected with late epilepsy. The increased incidence of postshunt epilepsy was 46% when complicated with infection, compared with 20% in patients without infection [14].

In children with myelomeningocele, age at the time of shunt insertion was not predictive of seizures and none of these children had recurrent seizures in follow-up periods up ranging from 10-16 years [7]. Most other studies suggest no correlation between the age at shunt insertion and seizure risk [12, 15].

There was no difference in the incidence of seizures according to ventricular catheter entry points [8]. Only a single study stated a higher incidence of seizures associated with frontal entry points (54.5%), as opposed to a lower incidence associated with posterior parietal entry points (6.6%) [12].

Other anomalies of the CNS have been described with myelomeningocele, the most important of which are cortical malformations. 92% of the brains with myelomeningocele showed cerebral cortical dysplasias and 40% had overt polymicrogyria [16]. The occurrence of seizures in about 20-25% of children with myelomeningocele might be accounted for in part by cortical dysgenesis [4, 7, 10]. According to Talwar et al. [10], 50% of the children with epilepsy had areas of encephalomalacia and/or stroke, in contrast to only 5% of the patients who had hydrocephalus and no seizures. In shunted patients, seizures may precede placement of the shunt [9, 17]. Mental retardation is an important factor that aggravates the risk of having or developing seizures and furthermore, in children with meningomyelocele, mental retardation was statistically more common when associated with seizures, regardless of the presence or absence of hydrocephalus [7, 15]. The presence of seizures before shunting and the increased risk of seizures in patients with intellectual impairment indicate that underlying brain abnormalities, particularly of the cerebral cortex, are of importance in the development of seizures.

Electroencephalogram (EEG) and Hydrocephalus

In an uncontrolled study, 40 children who had shunts for hydrocephalus underwent EEG testing following the onset of clinical seizures. Specific abnormalities (spikes, sharp waves and spike and wave discharges) and nonspecific abnormalities (monomorphic and polymorphic slow wave activity) both occurred more frequently over the shunted hemisphere [18]. Ines and Markand [19] compared the EEGs of 81 shunted hydrocephalic children with those of 11 children with nonshunted hydrocephalus. Shunted patients had a significantly higher prevalence of abnormal EEGs and seizures. All types of focal abnormalities and especially slow wave foci were more frequently lateralized over the shunted hemisphere [19]. Hydrocephalus in children, regardless of the cause, may be associated with generalized or focal EEG abnormalities [20]. Graebner and Celesia [21] compared 21 nonshunted children with hydrocephalus with 26 of their shunted counterparts. The shunted group showed a higher prevalence of abnormal EEGs, focal paroxysmal discharges and clinical seizures. In the shunted group, focal discharges were seen most frequently over the shunted hemisphere. An example of lateralized epileptiform abnormalities in patient with shunted hydrocephalus is shown in Figure 25.1.

It is difficult to know whether EEG abnormalities are due to brain injury related to the shunt or previous lesions on the same side. To explore this issue, Bourgeois defined a small group of patients in which there were no abnormal findings on computed tomography (CT) scan or magnetic resonance imaging (MRI), and a right posterior parietal ven-

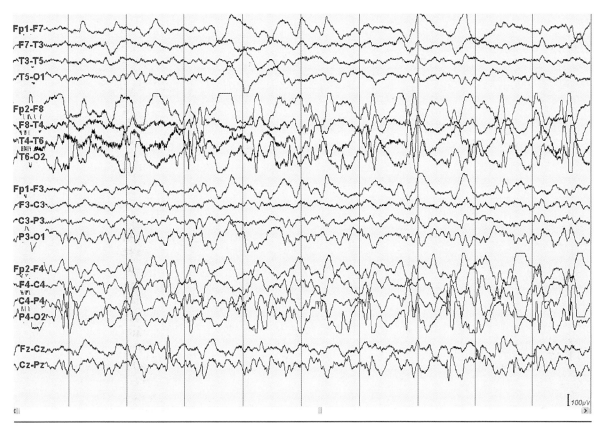

Fig. 25.1. Multifocal high amplitude spike and wave epileptiform discharges over the shunted hemisphere (R) in a 2-year-old boy with hydrocephalus

tricular catheter remained in place even after shunt revision [9]. In this selected group, bilateral abnormalities were found in 76% before shunt insertion, but spike-and-wave activity was recognized in only 8% before shunting, whereas an epileptic focus appeared in 30% in the right hemisphere after a shunt tube was placed. In children without cerebral parenchymal lesions on CT scan, the focal side of the interictal EEG abnormalities was identical to the area of shunt insertion [9].

The spectrum of epileptic abnormalities in children with hydrocephalus changes from mild focal interictal abnormalities to generalized or bilaterally synchronous spike waves to continuous spike waves during slow wave sleep (CSWS) [22]. CSWS has recently been described in two children with shunted hydrocephalus due to myelomeningocele [23]. In the report, the presence of thalamic injury in addition to hydrocephalus in one of the patients is discussed in the pathogenesis. An example of CSWS in a patient with multicompartmental hydrocephalus and shunt is shown in Figure 25.2.

Prognosis of Seizures

Noetzel found that 75% of patients with myelomeningocele and seizures were successfully taken off antiepileptic drugs, without recurrence of seizures over a mean follow-up period of 9.3 years, while 20.8% had well-controlled seizure disorders while being maintained on medication [7]. The single most useful predictor of outcome was normal intellectual development. In a different study, out of 14 children with epilepsy with myelomeningocele, 12 were taking antiepileptic drugs, and seizures were controlled on medication in five children and, in the other seven, seizures were relatively infrequent (1-6/year) [10]. At the time of initial CSF shunt surgery, 12% of patients had already been treated with antiepileptic drugs (AEDs), and the hazard rate for initiation of AEDs was a constant 2% a year; in consequence, the estimated prevalence of AED treatment had risen to 33% by ten years after initial shunt insertion [24]. The debate continues on prophylactic use of AEDs after shunt surgery.

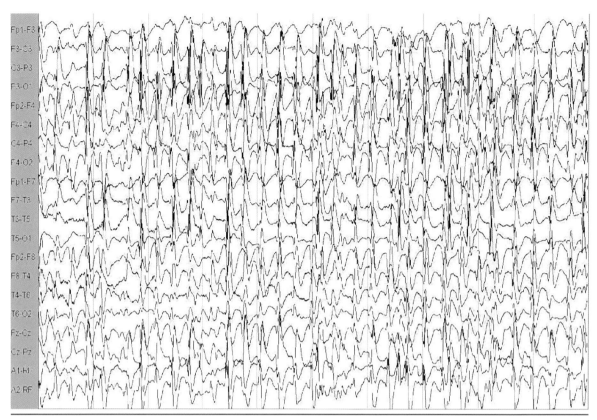

Fig. 25.2. Continuous spike and wave pattern in a patient with multicompartmental hydrocephalus and a shunt

Conclusion

Myelomeningocele is associated with seizures and epilepsy, although this association is not as strong as the other causes of hydrocephalus. The presence of other cerebral malformations and mental retardation are related to the development of epilepsy in these children. In addition, shunt dysfunction and infection further predispose a child to seizures. The prognosis is better compared to other causes of hydrocephalus.

References

1. Hosking GP (1974) Fits in hydrocephalic children. Arch Dis Child 49:633-635
2. Varfis G, Berney J, Beaumanoir A (1977) Electroclinical follow-up of shunted hydrocephalic children. Child's Brain 3:129-139
3. Blaauw G (1978) Hydrocephalus and epilepsy. Z Kinderchir 25:341-345
4. Bartoshesky LE, Haller J, Scott RM et al (1985) Seizures in children with meningomyelocele. Am J Dis Child 139:400-402
5. Stellman GR, Bannister CM, Hillier V (1986) The incidence of seizure disorder in children with acquired and congenital hydrocephalus. Z Kinderchir 41 (suppl 1):38-41
6. Hack CH, Enrile BG, Donat JF et al (1990) Seizures in relation to shunt dysfunction in children with meningomyelocele. J Pediatr 116:57-60
7. Noetzel MJ, Blake JN (1991) Prognosis for seizure control and remission in children with myelomeningocele. Dev Med Child Neurology 33:803-810
8. Chadduck W, Adametz J (1988) Incidence of seizures in patients with myelomeningocele: a multifactorial analysis.Surg Neurol 30:281-285
9. Bourgeois M, Sainte-Rose C, Cinalli G et al (1990) Epilepsy in children with shunted hydrocephalus. J Neurosurg 90:274-281
10. Talwar D, Baldwin M, Horbatt CI (1995) Epilepsy in children with myelomeningocele. Pediatr Neurol 13:29-32

11. Bowman RM, McLone DG, Grant JA et al (2001) Spina bifida outcome: a 25-year prospective. Pediatr Neurosurg 34:114-120

12. Dan NG, Wade MJ (1986) The incidence of epilepsy after ventricular shunting procedures. J Neurosurg 65:19-21

13. Fallace WJ, Canady AI (1990) Cerebrospinal fluid shunt malfunction signaled by new or recurrent seizures. Childs Nerv Syst 6:37-40

14. Copeland GP, Foy PM, Shaw MDM (1982) The incidence of epilepsy after ventricular shunting operations. Surg Neurol 17:279-281

15. Noetzel MJ, Blake JN (1992) Seizures in children with congenital hydrocephalus: long-term outcome. Neurology 42:1277-1281

16. Gilbert JN, Jones KL, Rorke LB et al (1986) Central nervous system anomalies associated with meningomyelocele, hydrocephalus and the Arnold-Chiari malformation: reappraisal of theories regarding the pathogenesis of posterior neural tube closure defects. Neurosurgery 18:559-564

17. Saukkonen AL, Serlo W, von Wendt L (1990) Epilepsy in hydrocephalic children. Acta Paediatr Scand 79:212-218

18. Ligouri G, Abate M, Buono S et al (1986) EEG findings in shunted hydrocephalic patients with epileptic seizures. Ital J Neurol Sci 7:243-247

19. Ines DF, Markand ON (1977) Epileptic seizures and abnormal electroencephalographic findings in hydrocephalus and their relation to the shunting procedures. Electroencephalogr Clin Neurophysiol 42:761-768

20. Al-Sulaiman AA, Ismail HM (1998) Pattern of electrographic abnormalities in children with hydrocephalus: A study of 68 patients. Childs Nerv Syst 14:124-126

21. Graebner RW, Celesia GG (1973) EEG findings in hydrocephalus and their relation to shunting procedures. Electroencephalogr Clin Neurphysiol 35:517-521

22. Veggiotti P, Beccaria F, Papalia G et al (1998) Continuous spikes and waves during sleep in children with shunted hydrocephalus. Childs Nerv Syst 14:188-194

23. Battaglia D, Acquafondata C, Lettori D et al (2004) Observation of continuous spike-waves during slow sleep in children with myelomeningocele. Child Nerv Syst 20:462-467

24. Piatt JH, Carlson CV (1995) Hydrocephalus and epilepsy: an actuarial analysis. Neurosurgery 39:722-728

Section V
ORTHOPEDIC PROBLEMS

CHAPTER 26
Management of Vertebral Problems and Deformities

M. Memet Özek, Bülent Erol, Junichi Tamai

Introduction

Children with myelomeningocele have a high incidence of scoliosis, kyphosis and lordosis [1]. These spinal deformities are usually progressive and may cause severe disability, interfere with rehabilitation, and negate previous treatments aimed at maintaining ambulation. Spinal deformities may be congenital or acquired, specific to myelomeningocele or similar to deformities seen in other conditions. Although the majority of these deformities are paralytic and occur in childhood, as many as 15% may be congenital [2]. The most obvious and consistent congenital abnormality is the incomplete posterior arch in the lumbosacral spine (Fig. 26.1). This abnormality affects many aspects of scoliosis and kyphosis treatment. Other congenital malformations may also be present, including hemivertebrae, butterfly vertebrae, diastematomyelia, and unsegmented bars. Acquired deformities include idiopathic-like scoliosis, pelvic obliquity-related scoliosis, and neuromuscular curves secondary to spinal muscle asymmetry, or closed spinal dysraphism. Deformities occur with any level of paralysis and without regard to ambulation ability or history.

In myelomeningocele the spinal curvature often appears at a younger age than typical for most developmental abnormalities. It may be present by 2-3 years of age, becoming severe by 7 years of age [1-3]. Due to the early onset of the deformity, treatment strategies that anticipate the growth of the spine are needed. However, the projections for growth in children with myelomeningocele are different from those for children with normal growth potential. Children with myelomeningocele may have slow growth due to growth hormone deficiency, and mature earlier than usual, often by 9-10 years of age in girls and 11-12 years in boys [3].

Patients with myelomeningocele who undergo spinal surgery are particularly likely to sustain peri-and postoperative complications. Even under the care of an experienced team, pressure sores, wound breakdown, deep infections, pseudoarthrosis, and progression of the deformity are much more frequent than in most other patient populations. These patients are subject to frequent septicemias due to urinary tract infections. The treating surgeon must ensure preoperatively that the patient's shunt function is stable, that the weight-bearing skin of the

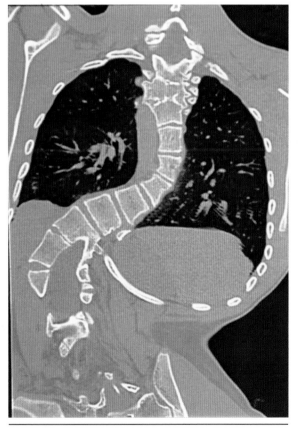

Fig. 26.1. Spinal computed tomography scan of a child with myelomeningocele demonstrates congenital incomplete posterior arch defects in the lumbosacral spine

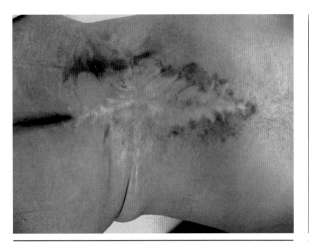

Fig. 26.2. The skin in the area of the meningocele repair is often of poor quality

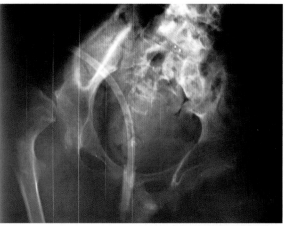

Fig. 26.3. Pelvic obliquity and hip deformities frequently cause spinal deformities in children with myelomeningocele

pelvis and upper thighs is free of pressure sores, and that the skin over the portion of the spine to be operated upon is healthy. The skin in the area of the myelomeningocele repair is often of poor quality, and gives minimal coverage for instrumentation (Fig. 26.2). Postoperatively, the wound must be monitored carefully for evidence of infection, and promptly debrided if there is evidence of either superficial or deep infection or tissue necrosis. In those patients with potential closure problems, tissue expanders are implanted 2-3 months prior to the primary surgery.

Children with myelomeningocele frequently have pelvic obliquity and hip deformities that affect spinal balance (Fig. 26.3). For example, asymmetric hip contractures may cause lumbar scoliosis, pelvic obliquity, and abnormal lordosis in the standing or sitting position. Similarly, correction of the spine in the treatment of scoliosis may position the legs in a way that prevents functional sitting or standing. When the patient performs independent transfers with flail or nearly flail extremities, the surgeon must observe these transfers preoperatively to determine whether fixation of the pelvis will enable these movements postoperatively.

The goals of treatment of spinal curvatures in children with myelomeningocele are the prevention of further deformity and the creation of a stable, balanced spine. These children require more precise correction of their spinal deformities than other children, as residual deformity may prevent them from sitting, standing, or walking. Pressure sores are likely to develop if pelvic obliquity remains, and their sagittal plane alignment must allow them to perform intermittent self-catheterization.

Scolisosis and Lordosis

The review by Trivedi and colleagues [4] has provided useful definitions and information on the incidence and prevalence of scoliosis in children with myelomeningocele. Scoliosis in this population has been defined as curves with a Cobb angle greater than 20 degrees, because smaller curves have typically improved. Most curves develop early in life, but approximately 40% of curves develop after 9 years of age, with some not appearing until the age of 15.

Scoliosis in patients with myelomeningocele may be congenital, idiopathic-like, or related directly or indirectly to the spinal dysraphism and associated paralysis (associated spinal cord anomalies such as thick and tight filum terminale, diastematomyelia, lipoma, hydromyelia or paralytic pelvic obliquity, asymmetric paralysis). Children with a thoracic neurological level or a thoracic level for their last intact laminar arch have a 90% incidence of scoliosis [1, 3, 4]. Eighty-five percent of these curves are greater than 45 degrees (Fig. 26.4a). As the paralysis level lowers, so does the incidence of scoliosis. At the fourth lumbar level of paraplegia the incidence of curvature decreases to about 60%, with only 40% requiring surgical intervention. Those children with a level below L4 have an incidence closer to 10% [4, 5]. Ambulatory status of these children also has a strong correlation with the development of scoliosis. Community ambulators have half the incidence of scoliosis of noncommunity ambulators [3, 4].

Noncongenital scoliosis in young myelomeningocele patients is highly likely to progress. In a study

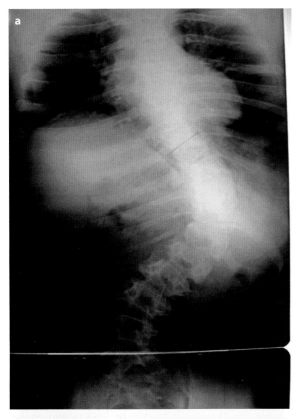

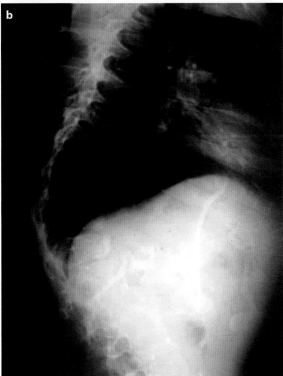

Fig. 26.4 a, b. A C-shaped scoliosis associated with high level paraplegia. **a** Children with high level paraplegia frequently have severe scolisosis which requires surgical correction. **b** These C-shaped curves are frequently associated with kyphosis

by Muller and colleagues [6], noncongenital scoliosis increased by an average of 5 degrees per year. The severity of the curve and the age of the patient were risk factors for progression: curves of more than 40 degrees were much more likely to progress, and curves progressed only slightly after the age of 15.

Several causes for the scoliosis have been identified in patients with myelomeningocele. A C-shaped scoliosis is usually caused by muscle weakness due to high level paraplegia. It also may be associated with asymmetric levels of paralysis or a spastic hemiplegia due to hydrocephalus. This type of scoliosis may be associated with kyphosis rather than lordosis (Fig. 26.4b). Typically, this curve pattern occurs at a young age, often in infancy, and is usually progressive. A surgical procedure may be necessary to relieve severe spasticity, if present [7].

Another cause of scoliosis in this population is hydromyelia or hydrosyringomyelia associated with uncompensated hydrocephalus. Typically, an S-shaped scoliosis is observed in the thoracic or thoracolumbar spine. Shunt dysfunction or progressive hydromyelia may present with scoliosis at any age, even early in childhood. Typical clinical symptoms of hydromyelia may be absent. It has been shown that reinserting a functional shunt may decrease the scoliosis if it is less than 50 degrees [1].

Secondary tethered cord syndrome is caused by attachment of the spinal cord to the area of primary surgery, preventing its upward migration with growth. This syndrome may be associated with other intraspinal pathologies, such as dermoid cysts, lipomas, and diastematomyelia and can cause scoliosis, usually in the thoracolumbar or lumbar region. Releasing the tethered cord may prevent progression of the spinal deformity in the majority of the patients, although variable results have been reported. If the curve is more than 50 degrees, the scoliosis should be corrected and stabilized with a spinal fusion [1, 3].

Congenital vertebral malformations, including formation and segmentation defects, may be another cause of scoliosis in children with myelomeningocele (See Chapter 14). These malformations may exist in combination with hydromyelia, tethered cord, or muscle paralysis, so that the treating physician must consider each component of the scoliosis in the treatment program. An increasing scoliosis should be an indication for a referral to a pediatric neurosurgeon. A shuntogram and computed tomography (CT) are necessary to evaluate potential mechanical or dynamic shunt failure. In case of shunt dysfunction, an immediate shunt replacement is recommended. As a second step a spinal magnetic resonance imaging

(MRI) should be performed to rule out the existence of additional spinal cord malformations or a secondary tethering of the cord.

Each child with myelomeningocele should have a regular clinical and radiological follow-up of their spinal deformity. At each visit a thorough neurological examination of muscle strength, levels of sensation, and reflex activity of the upper and lower extremities should be carefully documented. If there is a progressive deformity, the changes in neurological function may have diagnostic importance with respect to etiology. Radiographic evaluation should be carried out annually from the age of 1 year. If possible, the radiographs of the spine should be taken while the child is sitting; this eliminates the problems related to hip flexion contracture and asymmetric abduction and adduction. Spinal dysraphism and congenital vertebral anomalies are often best appreciated on infant films. In all infants with myelomeningocele, radiographs of the entire spine should be obtained and studied for evidence of these anomalies.

Rapidly progressive curves or curves associated with deteriorating neurological level should be imaged with MRI [8]. The head and the entire spinal canal should be scanned. While the MRI of the head and cervical spine can show the hydrocephalus, additional cranial malformations and the degree of Chiari Type II malformation, the appearance of a syrinx is best evaluated by a cervical and thoracic MRI. The scan of the lumbar spine provides information on the posterior displacement, and the presence of a low lying conus and spinal malformations. The MRI studies must be interpreted in association with the clinical findings to determine the cause of scoliosis.

Even mild scoliosis can affect balance and impair the walking and sitting ability of children with myelomeningocele. Balance problems can force a child to stabilize the body with the hands, which can then not be used for other tasks. As the curve progresses, pelvic obliquity may develop followed by pressure sores, typically over the ischial tuberosities. Large curves can cause pain, make positioning in a chair nearly impossible, and even affect cardiopulmonary function [9, 10]. In severe cases, deformity of the thorax can lead to a restrictive pulmonary insufficiency that could improve with surgery.

Treatment

If the scoliosis continues to progress after neurological problems have been corrected, orthopedic treatment is indicated. Curves with a Cobb angle of 30 degrees or less can generally be observed, but progressive curves require treatment. If the curve is unbalanced or greater than 30 degrees the center of gravity falls outside of the pelvic base of support, the spine will become unstable, and progression of the deformity is almost assured. A trial of bracing is indicated in children younger than 7 years of age if the curve is supple and can be corrected easily. A Swedish study has shown brace treatment to be moderately effective with relatively few complications [11]. However, paralytic curves are notoriously resistant to brace therapy, and children with myelomeningocele can experience skin problems as a result of curves, including pressure ulcers, which are challenging to heal. In infants special care is needed to avoid abdominal compression, which may make it difficult for the child to breathe and eat. Therefore, the use of a spinal brace is only a temporary measure, which may delay the necessity of surgery until the child is 8 or 9 years old [1, 3, 12].

Spinal orthotics such as the Boston brace may be difficult to incorporate into the overall management of the child with myelomeningocele, especially an ambulatory child, because a spinal orthosis may be hot, uncomfortable, and cumbersome. The most effective spinal orthosis for a child with myelomeningocele is a two-piece, polypropylene, bivalved, molded body jacket [1, 3]. This design allows the brace to be expanded or contracted throughout the day, to allow for eating, and allows some adjustability for growth. Meticulous care is required because pressure sores are frequent, and once they develop it is almost impossible to continue using the brace for control of the curve. The skin of the child should be inspected frequently by the family or caregivers, particularly at the beginning of brace treatment. If any redness does not disappear within 4 hours, the orthosis must be modified. The time in the brace should be increased gradually over 2-3 weeks until the child is wearing it throughout the day except for naps and nighttime.

Spinal fusion with correction of scoliotic deformity can have a positive effect on pulmonary function in myelomeningocele patients. Several studies have reported improvements in vital capacity and forced expiratory volume of patients, probably secondary to improved thoracic mechanics after spinal stabilization [9, 10].

Curves of greater than 30 degrees that are documented to progress are generally considered candidates for posterior fusion and instrumentation. Levels of fusion depend on the age of the child, the location of the curve, the level of paralysis, and the ambulatory status. Surgical treatment should provide a precise correction of the spinal deformity in children with myelomeningocele: because of their paralysis these children are unable to compensate for any residual deformity, which may prevent them from sitting or from standing and walking. Generally, the same guidelines for instrumentation and fusion in idiopathic scoliosis are applicable to the myelomeningocele spine. The fusion should extend from neutral vertebrae to neutral vertebrae, and the end vertebrae should be located within the stable zone. However, in double curves, uncompensated curves, and primary lumbar curves, these guidelines may differ from those for idiopathic scoliosis. In general, it is a mistake to fuse short; if there is a question, fuse long. A compensatory thoracic curve should be fused for its entire length, and the fusion should not end in the middle of a sagittal curve or at a junctional kyphosis [3].

Several aspects of myelomeningocele make considerations regarding surgery for scoliosis unique in this condition. Foremost among these is the presence of a posteriorly deficient spinal column, presenting challenges to both fixation and fusion. An open vertebral arch prevents attachment of the instrumentation to the end vertebra. Second, because the curves are neuromuscular, the treatment of many curves will entail fusion to the pelvis, a condition which may negatively impact upon mobility and self-care [13, 14]. There will invariably be significant scarring around the neural elements, and distraction correction must be done carefully in patients with useful lower extremity function to avoid the potential loss of neurological function. Finally, these challenges, combined with scarring of the posterior soft tissues, make for a much higher than average incidence of wound breakdown and deep infections.

The indications for extending the fusion mass to the sacrum are not well established. The lack of a posterior vertebral arch makes lumbosacral arthrodesis very difficult to obtain in children with myelomeningocele. Besides, pseudoarthroses and instrumentation failures are commonly seen. If a successful fusion to the sacrum is obtained it may deprive ambulatory patients of the ability to walk. A lumbosacral fusion may also increase the incidence of pressure sores in wheelchair-bound patients. On the other hand, if the lumbosacral joint is not fused, the scoliosis tends to increase, unless the lumbar scoliosis can be corrected to less than 20 degrees and pelvic obliquity to less than 15 degrees [3, 15-18]. Therefore, it is important to treat the scoliosis while the curve is small, whether fusion to the sacrum is planned or not. The delay of surgical correction of the scoliosis to allow the spine to grow may lead to an unsatisfactory correction. If a significant amount of residual pelvic obliquity remains after surgical treatment, then a bilateral iliac osteotomy, with transfer of a wedge of bone from the long side to the short side, can be performed in order to prevent the development of ischial ulcers [19].

In general, children with a thoracic or upper lumbar level of paraplegia should be fused to the sacrum. In children with low lumbar and sacral levels of paraplegia, the lumbosacral joint should be spared if they are walkers, and the spine can be aligned satisfactorily.

The sagittal deformity also must be evaluated because increased lumbar lordosis is a common deformity. Assessment of sitting, supine and standing posture must be made before correcting the lumbar lordosis. These children often require a greater degree of lordosis than normal. Restoring the lumbar lordosis to the normal range may uncover a hip flexion contracture and prevent the child from standing or walking. The degree of lordosis left in the spine after fusion needs to be tailored to each patient. It is best to treat the hip contractures before correcting the spine. If the deformity is not corrected first, positioning of the spine on the operating table will be difficult and torque the spine postoperatively, leading to instrument failure and pseudoarthrosis.

Extensive spinal fusion, which is necessary to treat progressive noncongenital scoliosis in myelomeningocele, has potential negative impacts on the child's overall mobility. Mazur and colleagues [14] found that whereas sitting balance improved in 70% of 27 patients treated by anterior and posterior fusion for paralytic scoliosis, ambulatory ability was adversely affected in 67%, unchanged in 33%, and improved in none. Muller and colleagues [20] also reported a decrease in overall mobility level in the majority of 14 patients who had undergone spinal fusion for scoliosis. Thus, the decision to perform anterior and posterior fusion, especially to the pelvis, must be carefully weighed against the potential impact on the child's mobility and independence. Activities of daily living, including self-catheterization, may also be adversely affected by extensive spinal fusion [13, 20]. Finally, the incidence of pressure sores in sitting weight-bearing areas may actually be increased by spinal fusion to the pelvis, irrespective of whether there is residual pelvic obliquity. Presumably, the loss of flexibility of the lumbar spine and the lumbosacral junction, combined with altered locations of weight-bearing in the sitting position are the causes of this increased incidence of pressure sores.

Deep wound infections are of particular concern, and achieving wound healing is enormously challenging for most patients with spinal deformity in myelomeningocele. An infection rate as high as 33% has been described [14], although later studies have cited a rate closer to 8% [21]. The frequency of wound problems, which include superficial infection and wound breakdown, has led many surgeons to recruit plastic surgeons to assist with mobilizing local flaps for closure in children with myelomeningocele (Fig. 26.5).

In a child with a progressive curve that cannot be controlled by a brace and who is younger than 8 years old, the preferred treatment is extraperiosteal segmental Luque instrumentation without spinal fusion. Distal fixation of the rods in the area of the open spine is difficult. The ilium can be used, although loosening of the rod in the ilium with loss of fixation and erosion of the rod through the skin has been reported [3]. The use of the first sacral foramen as the anchor point or the use of an 'S' rod attached to the ala are the other possibilities. Postoperative brace treatment is still indicated, and complications from this approach include rod breakage, wire breakage, and spontaneous fusion. To provide a definitive solution, reoperation is often necessary when the child reaches maturity.

In many children, the combination of posterior element deficiency and relative skeletal immaturity mandates anterior or combined anterior and posterior spinal fusion [22-26]. Posterior fusion or anterior fusion alone appears to be inadequate for most patients with paralytic scoliosis in myelomeningocele. If the child has not yet reached adolescence, there is an almost 100% assurance that the curve will continue to progress despite posterior fusion, unless the anterior spine is fused to the same level.

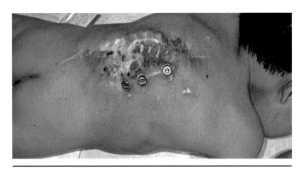

Fig. 26.5. Wound breakdown. This boy had a spine fusion for severe scoliosis and had skin breakdown over his hardware. Obtaining adequate skin coverage in children with myelomeningocele for surgical procedures can be a major challenge, especially in the spine

Several authors reported that the combination of anterior and posterior fusions with a variety of instrumentation has significantly lowered the pseudoarthrosis rate when compared to isolated anterior or posterior fusion with or without instrumentation [23, 25, 27]. The role of the instrumentation is to improve spinal alignment and the fusion rate, and reduce the need for postoperative immobilization. It is important to carry out an early fusion when the deformity is manageable. The amount of correction that is possible is probably limited to about 60 degrees, so it is better to correct a 60 degree curve than to correct a 120 degree curve to 60 degrees.

The best results of spinal fusion for paralytic scoliosis in myelomeningocele occur in patients treated by combined anterior and posterior fusion with stable segmental fixation achieved by a combination of sublaminar wires, pedicular remnant wires, and/or pedicular screws. Banta and colleagues [22] reported the results of combined anterior and posterior fusion with Luque rods and sublaminar and pedicular remnant wires in 50 patients with scoliosis or kyphosis. The authors concluded that the addition of anterior fusion to posterior fusion and instrumentation provided greater correction of spinal deformity and pelvic obliquity and improved the fusion mass over that achieved with posterior fusion alone.

The current preferred surgical treatment for scoliosis in patients with myelomeningocele is a single-stage, combined anterior spinal release and fusion and posterior spinal fusion with Luque instrumentation to the pelvis (Fig. 26.6) [1, 3]. Sublaminar wires are used under the intact lamina; however, in the area of posterior element insufficiency, pedicular wires or screws should be used. Fixation to the pelvis can be achieved either by Luque-Galveston instrumentation to the iliac crests or Dunn-McCarthy modification of Luque instrumentation to the sacrum [1, 15, 28]. Luque instrumentation provides segmental fixation to each vertebra and achieves a better control over the spine [3, 29-31]. Postoperative immobilization is not required in most patients. However, this technique does not fix the length of the spine as well as a rod with hooks does; therefore, the spine may settle or collapse along the rod, with loss of some correction in the immediate postoperative period. Fixation to the open posterior spine in the lumbar area by wires around the pedicle is weak, and extension of the instrumentation to the ilium is usually necessary. Even this distal attachment of the Luque rods is weak, because there may be significant osteoporosis of the pelvis. Loosening of the instrumentation and pseudo-

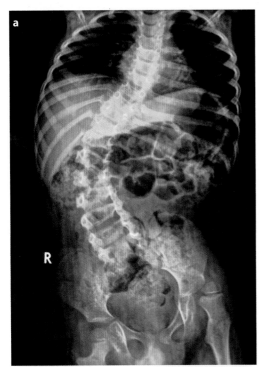

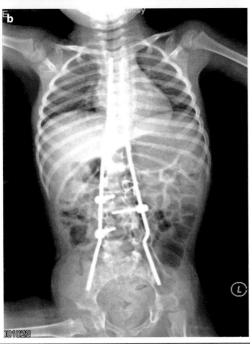

Fig. 26.6 a, b. A 10-year-old girl with high level paraplegia. She has a progressive thoracolumbar scoliosis and pelvic obliquity. Also note the unilateral hip dislocation. A tethered spinal cord previously was released. **a** Posterior-anterior radiograph demonstrates a 70 degree uncompensated thoracolumbar curve. **b** Postoperative radiograph shows almost complete correction of the deformity. This patient had a single-stage, combined anterior spinal release and fusion and posterior spinal fusion with Luque instrumentation. Fixation to the pelvis was achieved by Luque-Galveston instrumentation to the ilium. Pedicle screws were used to secure the segmental instrumentation in the lumbar spine

arthrosis of the lumbosacral joint is frequent. The use of pedicle screws may solve this instrumentation problem in the lumbar area; the pedicle screws allow the end vertebra to be positioned in three planes, and provide stable segmental instrumentation (Fig. 26.6b) [3, 32]. The use of pedicle screws in combination with Luque instrumentation may also lessen the need for anterior instrumentation. Long-term studies have not yet been performed, but early experience indicates that satisfactory results can be obtained.

Whatever the instrumentation used posteriorly, it should be low-profile in design. In the area of the myelomeningocele sac there is poor skin and soft tissue coverage. Prominence of hardware invariably leads to ulceration over the hardware, eventual infection, and the need to remove the instrumentation.

Congenital Scoliosis

As previously mentioned, about 15% of children with myelomeningocele also have congenital abnormalities of the vertebrae separate from the posterior element defects [2]. The defect is one of formation, whereby the vertebra is incompletely developed and often wedge-shaped, or one of segmentation, in which a bony bridge connects two or more consecutive vertebrae (Fig. 26.7). A combination of formation and segmentation defects may also be seen. Certain patterns of these abnormalities predictably lead to scoliosis and often require surgery for correction. Nonoperative methods of treatment do not correct congenital scoliosis, nor prevent it from worsening. Children with myelomeningocele, because of their neurological abnormalities, are unable to tolerate an unbalanced spine. Therefore, it is important that treatment be carried out in infancy when the deformity is small, rather than waiting until the child is older and complex measures are needed to obtain satisfactory alignment [3]. Several factors may be in effect simultaneously in these children, all of which must be explored before a course of treatment is chosen. Although a progressive curve must be arrested, it is essential to protect intact spinal levels to avoid worsening these patients' neurological and functional status.

Posterior spinal fusion is rarely successful in preventing the progression of congenital curves. Anterior and posterior fusion is the procedure of choice, and it should be performed when a diagnosis of progressive scoliosis is made, usually at 1 year of age. The spine may be approached in staged or separate

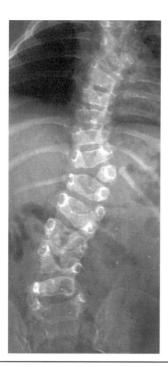

Fig. 26.7. Congenital abnormalities of the spine associated with myelomeningocele. Posterior-anterior view of the spine demonstrates multiple congenital vertebral anomalies, including hemivertebrae of the thoracic and lumbar spine and block vertebrae of the lumbar spine. Combination of these formation and segmentation defects frequently leads to severe scoliosis which requires surgical treatment

anterior and posterior procedures, or anterior and posterior interbody fusions may be performed through a posterior approach, using the pedicle as the access conduit to the anterior spine [3]. If the lumbar curve is already so severe that the pelvic obliquity is greater than 15 degrees, an osteotomy of the spine to correct the deformity should be considered.

Hyperlordosis

A less common but potentially difficult to treat spinal deformity in patients with myelomeningocele is hyperlordosis, with or without associated scoliosis [33, 34]. Hyperlordosis can lead to difficulty in sitting, intertriginous skin breakdown, and difficulty with self-catheterization in females because of the posterior rotation of the perineum. In the past, this deformity was associated with lumboperitoneal shunting [34], but this method of shunting is rarely used today. Treatment, when required, is by a combination of anterior and posterior spinal release and posterior instrumentation [1, 3].

Kyphosis

Kyphosis of the lumbar spine is a very common deformity in spina bifida patients. The incidence has been reported from 10% to as high as 46% in this population [20, 35-37]. Carstens and colleagues [37] found that 20% of over 700 myelomeningocele patients had lumbar kyphosis on lateral radiographs. Kyphotic deformity is particularly common in thoracic and upper lumbar level paraplegics. In Carstens's series, the most common level of paralysis was lower thoracic (ranging from upper thoracic to L5). Shurtleff and colleagues [36] reported that although one in ten children with a thoracic lesion had kyphosis at birth, one in three demonstrated kyphosis by adolescence. Kyphosis often measures 80 degrees or more at birth, and usually progresses with growth.

The kyphosis deformity has been described as paralytic and congenital. The paralytic kyphosis is seen much more commonly and can be divided into two types: collapsing kyphosis and rigid, sharp-angled kyphosis. In the review of Carstens and colleagues [37], collapsing kyphosis was the most common (44%), followed by rigid, sharp-angled kyphosis (38%). True congenital kyphosis was the least common. The collapsing kyphosis is often C-shaped and supple, at least during the initial stages. The apex may occur anywhere from the lower thoracic spine to the lumbosacral joint (Fig. 26.8). Rigid, sharp-angled kyphosis is usually S-shaped with a proximal thoracic lordosis. The kyphosis is usually centered at L2 and the proximal rigid lordosis at about T10. This is the most common variety in the older child because the C-shaped curve often progresses to the S-shaped curve with time.

The natural history of both kinds of paralytic curves is one of constant progression, making them difficult to treat. Long, gentle C-shaped curves tend to progress by about 3 degrees per year, whereas short, sharp curves are more malignant, progressing by 8 degrees per year. It is not unusual to see a 2 or 3 year old child with a kyphosis greater than 100 degrees. The progression of true congenital kyphosis is variable during growth.

Lumbar kyphosis can be problematic from birth, causing difficulty in closing the skin and meningeal defects. Untreated, progressive kyphosis leads to loss of truncal height, difficulty with sitting, and, in advanced cases, skin ulceration over the kyphos posteriorly and impingement of the ribs on the iliac crest (Fig. 26.8c, d). Chronic skin breakdown can leave the neural elements and the spinal column exposed

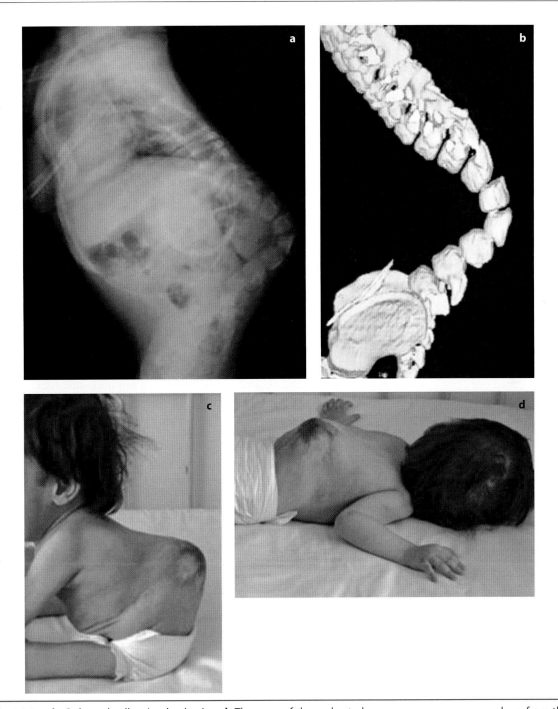

Fig. 26.8 a-d. C-shaped collapsing kyphosis. **a, b** The apex of these short, sharp curves may occur anywhere from the lower thoracic spine to the lumbosacral joint. **c, d** Untreated kyphotic curves progress rapidly in children with myelomeningocele and may lead to loss of truncal height, difficulty in sitting, and skin ulceration over the kyphos

and at risk of infection. Progression of the kyphosis may lead to breathing difficulty because the abdominal contents are crowded into the chest cavity by increasing upward pressure on the diaphragm. These children also have difficulty eating because of loss of abdominal size, which results in a failure to thrive. They also have difficulty using their hands as they need them to support their body in the sitting position. They are underweight and short in stature. The increased flexion of the trunk may also interfere with drainage of urine if the child has an urethrostomy, a vesicotomy, or an ileostomy.

Treatment

Kyphosis is almost always progressive, and attempts to delay definitive treatment until the child is older leads to a more severe deformity [1, 3]. The treatment should be carried out early, even though it may be only a temporizing procedure. A more definitive procedure can be performed later. The goals of treatment are to increase abdominal height, to allow more room for abdominal contents, and relieve pressure on the diaphragm and the lungs. In addition, the kyphosis must be minimized to lessen the incidence of pressure sores and move the center of gravity posteriorly to center it over the ischium. This provides the child with a better truncal balance that improves the child's ability to interact with the environment by freeing the arms, improving brace fitting, and enhancing seating.

The treatment of myelomeningocele-related kyphosis is never easy. The curve usually progresses rapidly. In those few instances in which the collapsing curve does not progress rapidly and is less than 20-30 degrees, an initial period of observation may be worthwhile. If the curve is supple and the skin is in excellent condition, a brace can be tried. However, braces frequently fail to control the deformity and can actually cause problems, including skin ulceration and compression of the thoracic cage and abdominal wall. Therefore, despite the high complication rate, surgical correction is the treatment of choice in the vast majority of these children.

Patients with skin breakdown over a stable kyphosis that does not itself need treatment should first have their wheelchair support and activities carefully evaluated and any irritants found to be causing the breakdown removed. If these efforts are unsuccessful, rotational or free flaps may be used to cover the kyphotic area with thicker, more stable skin. Soft tissue expanders have been used for this purpose both independently and in conjunction with spinal deformity correction (Fig. 26.9).

Collapsing Kyphosis

Collapsing kyphosis in the skeletally immature child is difficult to treat surgically. Posterior spinal fusion without instrumentation usually fails because of tension forces in the fusion mass. Instrument failure is common when instrumentation is used [1, 21, 29]. Attempts to provide stability by anterior strut fusion with a strut graft also tend to fail in young patients. The fusion creates an anterior unsegmented bar, with growth potential remaining posteriorly. As the child grows, the kyphosis increases. If the surgeon waits until the child is older to carry out anteroposterior fusion with instrumentation along the thoracolumbar spine, the curve is often so severe that satisfactory correction is difficult, if not impossible, to obtain.

Spinal fusion may not be advisable in infancy, because without spinal growth there will be inadequate room for the abdominal and thoracic organs, resulting in pulmonary insufficiency. Instrumentation without fusion can buy time until the child is large enough for a definitive fusion. In very small children, apical tension-band wiring of the posterior elements may be adequate. An extraperiosteal Luque wiring technique is required for segmental instrumentation in most children older than 1 or 2 years [3]. At least three sublaminar wires on each rod superior to the kyphosis are needed to provide sufficient support. In older children and adolescents, fusion (to the pelvis) is usually possible at the time of the definitive procedure.

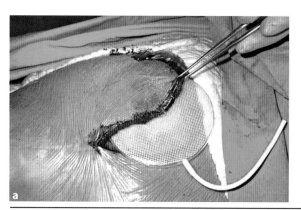 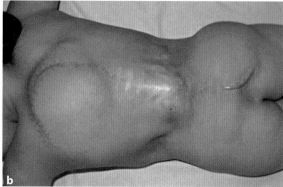

Fig. 26.9 a, b. Soft tissue expanders can be used independently and in conjunction with spinal deformity correction to cover the kyphotic area, with thicker and more stable skin, in order to prevent skin breakdown

Spinal shortening may be required in severe deformities because the anterior structures, including the abdominal wall, the aorta, and the vena cava tether the kyphosis anteriorly [38-40]. Many different procedures have been described to shorten the posterior spine and allow the spine to be straightened and put into a more normal sagittal alignment [26, 41, 42]. To shorten the spine in skeletally immature patients, partial excision of the periapical vertebrae with creation of a posterior tension band creates both imme-

diate correction and the potential for gradual, long-term correction when the anterior column grows against the surgically tethered posterior elements [38]. The definitive management of kyphosis in older children or adolescents consists of kyphectomy and posterior spinal fusion and instrumentation [43-45]. Fixation to pelvis is frequently required and this can be achieved either by Luque-Galveston instrumentation to the iliac crests or Dunn-McCarthy modification of Luque instrumentation to the sacrum (Fig. 26.10).

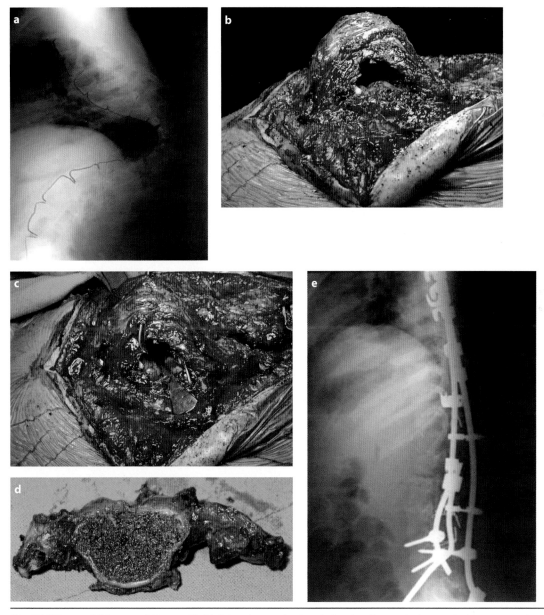

Fig. 26.10 a-e. A 14-year-old boy with high level paraplegia. **a** Lateral radiograph demonstrates a severe kyphotic deformity. **b-e** In older children and adolescents the treatment of this deformity consists of kyphectomy and posterior fusion and instrumentation. Fixation to pelvis is usually required

Rigid S-shaped Kyphosis

Treatment of the rigid form of kyphosis is difficult and controversial. Conservative nonoperative treatment invariably leads to an increased deformity and difficulty in later correction. Sharrard was the first to describe the technique of apical vertebral body resection for the treatment of kyphosis [41]; since then, most authors have recommended vertebral excision as a part of the operative treatment [43-46]. Most of these reports also showed that excision of the apical vertebra may lead to initial correction of the deformity. However, the deformity has a tendency to recur, often to a worse degree than the initial kyphosis [42].

Treatment of the rigid form of kyphosis requires a different approach. In patients with no function below the level of resection, the nerve roots and cauda equina remnants may be resected by ligating the roots, elevating the distal cord, and transecting it. The spinal cord should not be tied, as acute hydrocephalus may result, which in turn can cause sudden death [1]. After resection of the cord, the lumbar spine is dissected extraperiosteally from the posterior approach to the anterior aspect of the vertebral bodies. Both the kyphosis and the proximal lordosis are rigid, so it is necessary to correct both deformities at the same time. This can be accomplished by excising the vertebra(e) (usually two) between the kyphosis and lordosis and fusing the apical vertebra to the distal end of the thoracic spine at the level of the resection [42, 47]. In a young child, this is the only area fused, and the osteotomy is held in position by tension-band wiring around the pedicle above and below the resected vertebrae [48]. The correction can also be held by use of rods anchored in the first sacral foramen distally and sublaminar wires proximally, similar to the fixation used in the collapsing kyphosis. If the child is Risser sign I or above, the spine may be fused along the length of the instrumentation.

It should be kept in mind that kyphectomy and instrumentation is a major surgical procedure: intraoperative blood loss is usually well in excess of 1,000 mL, perioperative deaths have occurred, and postoperative complications, including skin breakdown, infection, loss of fixation, and recurrence of deformity, are more frequent than after most other orthopedic procedures [3, 21].

Summary

Scoliotic, kyphotic, or lordotic deformities are seen frequently in patients with myelomeningocele. The deformity is either congenital or the result of paralysis. Since it is always progressive, spinal deformity in combination with trophic skin and soft-tissue disturbances can lead to secondary problems such as decubital sores and contractures. Bracing is usually ineffective, allowing significant progression. Surgical correction is therefore an acceptable treatment of choice when the benefits of surgery outweigh the risks. With the new types of instrumentation, together with changes in postoperative management, there has been considerable improvement in the final outcome of scoliosis surgery in children with myelomeningocele. The surgical management of kyphosis is more complex. Kyphectomy is a challenging procedure with high complication rates. However, new techniques, longer fusion, and early intervention have also resulted in remarkable improvements in the final outcome.

References

1. Herring JA (2002) Tachdjian's pediatric orthopaedics. WB Saunders, Philadelphia, pp 1249-1302
2. Samuelsson L, Eklof O (1988) Scoliosis in myelomeningocele. Acta Orthop Scand 59:122-127
3. Lindseth RE (2001) Myelomeningocele. In: Morrissy RT, Weinstein SL (eds) Lovell and Winter's pediatric orthopaedics. Lippincott Williams & Wilkins, Philadelphia, pp 601-632
4. Trivedi J, Thomson JD, Slakey JB et al (2002) Clinical and radiographic predictors of scoliosis in patients with myelomeningocele. J Bone Joint Surg 84A:1389-1394
5. Mackel JL, Lindseth RE (1975) Scoliosis in myelodysplasia. J Bone Joint Surg 57A:1031
6. Muller EB, Nordwall A, Oden A (1994) Progression of scoliosis in children with myelomeningocele. Spine 19:147-150
7. McLaughlin TP, Banta JV, Gahm NH et al (1986) Intraspinal rhizotomy and distal cordectomy in patients with a myelomeningocele. Pediatr Neurosurg 68:88-94
8. Breningstall GN, Marker SM, Tubman DE et al (1992) Hydrosyringomyelia and diastematomyelia detected by MRI in myelomeningocele. Pediatr Neurol 8:267-271
9. Carstens C, Paul K, Niethard FU et al (1991) Effect of scoliosis surgery on pulmonary function in patients with myelomeningocele. J Pediatr Orthop 11:459-464
10. Banta JV, Park SM (1983) Improvement in pulmonary function in patients having combined anterior and posterior spine fusion for myelomeningocele scoliosis. Spine 8:765-770
11. Muller EB, Nordwall A (1994) Brace treatment of scoliosis in children with myelomeningocele. Spine 19:151-155
12. Bunch WH (1975) The Milwaukee brace in paralytic scoliosis. Clin Orthop 110:63-68

13. Boemers TM, Soorani-Lunsing IJ, de Jong TP et al (1996) Urological problems after surgical treatment of scoliosis in children with myelomeningocele. J Urol 155:1066-1069

14. Mazur J, Menelaus MB, Dickens DR et al (1986) Efficacy of surgical management for scoliosis in myelomeningocele: correction of deformity and alteration of functional status. J Pediatr Orthop 6:568-575

15. Allen Jr BL, Ferguson RL (1984) The Galveston technique of pelvic fixation with L-rod instrumentation of the spine. Spine 9:388-394

16. Neustadt JB, Shufflebarger HL, Cammisa FP (1992) Spinal fusions to the pelvis augmented by Cotrel-Dubousset instrumentation for neuromuscular scoliosis. J Pediatr Orthop 12:465-469

17. Perra JH (1994) Techniques of instrumentation in long fusions to the sacrum. Orthop Clin North Am 25:287-299

18. Widmann RF, Hresko T, Hall JE (1999) Lumbosacral fusion in children and adolescents using the modified sacral bar technique. Clin Orthop 364:85-91

19. Lindseth RE (1978) Posterior iliac osteotomy for fixed pelvic obliquity. J Bone Joint Surg 60A:17-22

20. Muller EB, Nordwall A, von Wendt L (1992) Influence of surgical treatment of scoliosis in children with spina bifida on ambulation and motoric skills. Acta Paediatr 81:173-176

21. Todore I, Dickens D (1998) The spine. In: Broughton N, Menelaus M (eds) Menelaus' orthopaedic management of spina bifida cystica. WB Saunders, Philadelphia, pp 145-167

22. Banta JV (1990) Combined anterior and posterior fusion for spinal deformity in myelomeningocele. Spine 15:946-952

23. Osebold WR, Mayfield JK, Winter RB et al (1982) Surgical treatment of paralytic scoliosis associated with myelomeningocele. J Bone Joint Surg 64A:841-856

24. Stark A, Saraste H (1993) Anterior fusion insufficient for scoliosis in myelomeningocele, 8 children 2-6 years after the Zielke operation. Acta Orthop Scand 64:22-24

25. Ward WT, Wenger DR, Roach JW (1989) Surgical correction of myelomeningocele scoliosis: a critical appraisal of various spinal instrumentation systems. J Pediatr Orthop 9:262-268

26. Warner WC Jr, Fackler CD (1993) Comparison of two instrumentation techniques in treatment of lumbar kyphosis in myelodysplasia. J Pediatr Orthop 13:704-708

27. McMaster MJ (1988) The long-term results of kyphectomy and spinal stabilization in children with myelomeningocele. Spine 13:417-424

28. Odent T, Vincent A, Ouellet J et al (2004) Kyphectomy in myelomeningocele with a modified Dunn-McCarthy technique followed by an anterior inlayed strut graft. Eur Spine 13:206-212

29. Allen BL Jr (1979) The operative treatment of myelomeningocele spinal deformity. Orthop Clin North Am 10:845-862

30. Boachie-Adjei O, Lonstein JE, Winter RB et al (1989) Management of neuromuscular spinal deformities with Luque segmental instrumentation. J Bone Joint Surg 71A:548-562

31. Broom MJ, Banta JV, Renshaw TS (1989) Spinal fusion augmented by Luque-rod segmental instrumentation for neuromuscular scoliosis. J Bone Joint Surg 71A:32-44

32. Farcy JP, Rawlins BA, Glassman SD (1992) Technique and results of fixation to the sacrum with iliosacral screws. Spine 17(Suppl):S190-195

33. Baker RH, Sharrard WJ (1973) Correction of lordoscoliosis in spina bifida by multiple spinal osteotomy and fusion Dwyer fixation: a preliminary report. Dev Med Child Neurol Suppl 29:12-23

34. Steel HH, Adams DJ (1972) Hyperlordosis caused by the lumboperitoneal shunt procedure for hydrocephalus. J Bone Joint Surg 54A:1537-1542

35. Hoppenfeld S (1967). Congenital kyphosis in myelomeningocele. J Bone Joint Surg 49B:276-280

36. Shurtleff DB, Goiney R, Gordon LH et al (1976). Myelodysplasia: The natural history of kyphosis and scoliosis: A preliminary report. Dev Med Child Neurol Suppl 37:126-133

37. Carstens C, Koch H, Brocai DR et al (1996). Development of pathological lumbar kyphosis in myelomeningocele. J Bone Joint Surg 78B:945-950

38. Roye BD (2005) Neuromuscular disorders. Myelomeningocele. In: Dormans JP (ed) Pediatric orthopaedics. Core knowledge in orthopaedics. Elsevier Mosby, Philadelphia, pp 483-504

39. Fromm B, Carstens C, Niethard FU et al (1992) Aortography in children with myelomeningocele and lumbar kyphosis. J Bone Joint Surg 74A:691-694

40. Lintner SA, Lindseth RE (1994) Kyphotic deformity in patients who have a myelomeningocele. Operative treatment and long-term follow-up. J Bone Joint Surg 76A:1301-1307

41. Sharrard WJ, Drennan JC (1972) Osteotomy-excision of the spine for lumbar kyphosis in older children with myelomeningocele. J Bone Joint Surg 54B:50-60

42. Lindseth RE, Stelzer L (1979) Vertebral excision for kyphosis in children with myelomeningocele. J Bone Joint Surg 61A:699-704

43. McCall RE (1998) Modified Luque instrumentation after myelomeningocele kyphectomy. Spine 23:1406-1411

44. Nolden MT, Sarwark JF, Vora A et al (2002) A kyphectomy technique with reduced perioperative morbidity for myelomeningocele kyphosis. Spine 27:1807-1813

45. Niall DM, Dowling FE, Fogarty EE et al (2004) Kyphectomy in children with myelomeningocele. A long-term outcome study. J Pediatr Orthop 24:37-44

46. Heydermann JS, Gillespie R (1987) Management of myelomeningocelekyphosis in the older child by kyphectomy and segmental spinal instrumentation. Spine 12:37-41

47. Hall JE, Poitra B (1977) The management of kyphosis in patients with myelomeningocele. Clin Orthop 128:33-40

48. Eyring EJ, Wanken JJ, Sayers MP (1972) Spinal osteotomy for kyphosis in myelomeningocele. Clin Orthop 88:24-30

Chapter 27
Spina Bifida: The Management of Extremity Deformities in Myelomeningocele

Bülent Erol, Junichi Tamai

The spectrum of congenital neural tube defects, referred to as myelomeningocele (spina bifida), produces a wide variety of disabilities, ranging from benign defects in the skin of the back to devastating paralysis and deformity of the lower extremities, urinary and fecal incontinence, hydrocephalus, spasticity, and mental retardation. The care of children with myelomeningocele usually requires a multidisciplinary approach. Early intervention by a team of trained caregivers can significantly improve the disabilities and permit many children to be integrated into normal social environments with high levels of independence. This chapter describes the overall management of myelomeningocele with special emphasis on the orthopedic management.

Orthopedic Treatment

In children with myelomeningocele, orthopedic treatment is intertwined with the neurosurgical treatment. It is also tied in with urologic treatment. Almost all children with myelomeningocele have urologic abnormalities that require bladder drainage by conduits or intermittent catheterization. Frequent infection may spread to orthopedic surgical areas, and the orthopedic treatment of spine deformity influences the ability of the patient to self-catheterize.

The goal of the orthopedic surgeon participating in the care of children with myelomeningocele should be to serve as a partner in the health care team seeking to maximize function and minimize disability and illness. Over time, the specifics of the requirements for achieving that goal will change, based on the child's needs and abilities and changes in neurologic health. Orthopedic treatment of myelomeningocele has three major goals. The first goal is to provide for maximal use of residual ability to maintain range of motion and stability of the spine and extremities. The second is to provide for mobility by means of a wheelchair and other wheeled devices, or by ambulation. The third goal is to prevent deterioration of neurologic function.

Nearly all patients with myelomeningocele will need orthoses to replace muscle strength and joint stability so that they can stand and walk. Similarly, most children, irrespective of the extent of deformity and paralysis, can be enabled to walk at a young age with a combination of deformity correction, bracing, an upper extremity aid, and instruction. Thus, one of the primary functions of the orthopedic surgeon is to correct foot and hip deformities that prevent the patient from using orthotics to ambulate in childhood. Although it is possible for most paraplegic children to walk to some degree during preschool and school age, many adults (especially those with thoracic or upper lumbar level paralysis) are not able to continue walking, since the extent of bracing and the energy consumption required for community ambulation is too great or onerous for the adult. There are four necessary requirements for walking: alignment of trunk and legs; range of motion; control of the hip, knee, and ankle joints; and power to provide forward motion [1].

The alignment of the spine and the legs must be such that the center of gravity passes through the joints of the pelvis, the hip, the knee, and the foot. There is a very high incidence of both congenital and neurologically related scoliosis and kyphosis in children with myelomeningocele, and these conditions can jeopardize posture or sitting comfort by preventing the center of gravity from passing through the center of the hip joint. Contractures of the hip or knee will also prevent stable weight-bearing.

Motion of the lumbosacral spine and the hip are essential for functional walking. Motion of the knee is less important, and is useful only in clearing the swing leg. Mobility of the spine must allow the center of gravity to be shifted from side to side over the stance leg. Motion of the hip is the most important part of walking; thirty degrees of motion is necessary for forward progression. If there is less motion than this, then pelvic motion must help compensate for this decreased motion.

The child must be able to control the position of the trunk and hip, knee, and ankle joints during the gait cycle. If this cannot be performed by muscle activity then it must be provided by an orthotic device. The determination of available muscles to control the joints is dependent on the level of paralysis.

Patients with thoracic level paraplegia essentially have flail lower extremities and, based solely on the total lower extremity flaccid paralysis, would be expected not to develop muscle imbalance-induced lower extremity deformities. These children have no active muscle contraction across the hip joint, and no feeling below the groin or in the hip. In these children, the hips are unstable and stability for walking can only be provided by an orthosis that crosses the hip joint.

Patients with upper lumbar level paraplegia have hip flexor power and some adductor power, but no motor control of the knees or feet. These children have some sensation crossing the hip joint. Their ambulation potential and needs parallel those of patients with thoracic level function. There is no way of surgically providing stability to the hip in upper lumbar paraplegia, the stability must be provided by an orthosis.

Patients with middle or lower lumbar level paraplegia have greater hip adductor strength and, more importantly, quadriceps power to provide active knee extension. Although theoretically these patients could walk with ankle-foot orthoses (AFOs) only, in practice this is not commonly the case, since strength around the knee is not completely normal, and the weakness of the foot, ankle, and hip abductors and extensors leads to the lurching gait, which imposes a great deal of stress on the unbraced knee [2, 3]. The force imbalance around the hip results in eventual hip dislocation in most of these children. It is in this group that surgical treatment of the hip is most controversial in terms of its influence on long-term ambulation preservation.

Patients with sacral level paraplegia have sufficient muscle control around the hip, the knee, and the ankle to provide the necessary stability. In theory, most sacral level patients could ambulate without orthotics. However, gait studies demonstrate that even patients with sacral level myelomeningocele ambulate most effectively with AFOs and crutches because of stresses at the knee and weakness in the foot and ankle [2, 4].

The force necessary to move forward is beyond the muscle contraction needed to control the joint. In normal individuals it is provided by the calf muscle, which pushes people forward into their next step, and the hip extensors, which pull forward after the foot hits the floor. Both of these muscles have sacral level innervation and are paralyzed in almost all children with myelomeningocele. In the thoracic and upper lumbar levels of paraplegia, the arms become the power producers to move forward. It takes increased energy to walk and the walking pace is much slower than normal. Eventually, most thoracic and upper lumbar level paraplegic patients discover that the wheelchair is a much more efficient means of transportation.

Finally, the orthopedic surgeon must assist in monitoring the neurologic status of the growing patient, since hydrocephalus, hydromyelia, or tethered cord syndrome secondary either to diastematomyelia or another anomaly, or to scarring at the original level of myelodysplasia, can occur. Any of these conditions can result in subtle deterioration in a patient's intellectual function and upper or lower extremity function.

General Principles of Orthopedic Management of Myelomeningocele

Latex Risk

Patients with spina bifida are at risk for the development of a serious allergy to latex [5-7]. Upwards of 40% of these children have serum antibodies to latex, and although fewer actually have a clinical allergy, fatal reactions have been reported. The allergy, an immunoglobulin E-mediated response, probably develops because of repeated early exposures to latex, especially in the first year of life [8, 9]. Risk factors for the presence of latex allergy include a history of prior allergic reactions and multiple previous surgeries [6].

Infection

Patients with myelomeningocele have a higher rate of complications, including postoperative infections, for almost all orthopedic surgical procedures, than patients undergoing similar procedures who do not have myelomeningocele [10]. The reason for the higher rate is multifactorial, with major factors being bladder paralysis and absence of protective pain perception. The former usually leads to the presence of bacteria in the urinary tract secondary to the bladder paralysis and its management. The diminished pain perception and skin insensitivity lead to more frequent wound breakdown and subsequent infection, either from unrecognized direct compromise of the wound under a cast, or from excessive swelling in patients who move, ambulate, or otherwise challenge the operated part in ways that a patient with normal sensation would not.

Pressure Sores

Pressure sores and frank ulcers are important issues in any population with sensory deficits, and children with myelomeningocele can have major skin problems. Pressure sores develop in as many as 60% of such children, typically on the feet and over the buttock, sacrum, the ischial tuberosities, and the greater trochanter [11]. These lesions can be very difficult to manage, especially if they are infected.

Pressure sores and ulcers are caused by unchecked pressure, usually over a bony prominence or prominent hardware. The pressure may be caused by normal sitting or positioning, or by an external brace, orthosis, or cast. Because of their deficient sensation and absence of motor power, children with myelomeningocele are unable to protect their skin. They do not feel ischemic pain, and they are unable to shift regularly the way neurologically intact people do without even thinking about it.

Aside from the obvious neurologic problems, children with myelomeningocele have other issues that contribute to the development and perpetuation of pressure sores and ulcers. The postural and positional problems that develop, including kyphosis, hip dysplasia and dislocation, and joint contractures, all lead to abnormally prominent bones. The bony prominences can tent the skin, placing it at high risk for breakdown. Also, many children have multiple scars from their many operations. The scars can be problematic with respect to initial healing and late breakdown. Finally, for children with fecal incontinence, urinary incontinence, or both, soiling of ulcers in the pelvic region can be a serious problem. When it occurs and infection cannot be controlled, temporary diverting ostomies of the bowel or genitourinary tract provide a means to keep the ulcers clean until they heal [10].

Upper Extremity Dysfunction

Problems in the upper extremities are ubiquitous in children with myelomeningocele, although they do not typically require orthopedic intervention. Arms, although not usually directly affected by the spinal lesion, can have problems related with strength and coordination. These difficulties are often secondary to brain damage resulting from hydrocephalus, and children with more shunt problems have been shown to have worse hand function [12]. If the upper extremity function appears to be deteriorating, a shunt blockage should be considered. An ascending syrinx is another possible cause of upper extremity dysfunction. The occupational therapist plays a central role in dealing with upper extremity problems in children with myelomeningocele.

Lower Extremity Deformity

Lower extremity problems are a major source of disability for children with myelomeningocele and frequently require orthopedic intervention. The following section outlines the basic deformities of the joints of the lower extremities in terms of etiology and treatment. The guiding principle for treatment of these deformities is to create a limb, via therapy or surgery, which can be placed in a functional position and held there with a brace (orthosis). The brace will supplement the dysfunctional muscles to maintain the proper position of the limb in order to facilitate mobility and the activities of daily living.

Foot and Ankle

Both congenital and developmental foot deformities are very commonly encountered in children with myelomeningocele [13-15]. Frawley and colleagues [14] reported foot deformity in 263 of 348 feet with lower lumbar or sacral level myelomeningocele, 64% of which required surgery. Similar to the hip, the development of foot and ankle deformities bears little relation to spontaneous motor activity. Broughton and colleagues [13] showed no correlation between neurologic level (excluding sacral level lesions) and the incidence or morphology of foot and ankle deformities. The authors found that nearly 90% of 124 children with thoracic and high lumbar lesions had foot deformities even though they had no voluntary motor activity in their feet. Equinus deformity was the most frequent, followed by calcaneus, valgus deformity, clubfoot, and vertical talus. Deformity present at birth, if symmetric, may be due to intrauterine positioning. In patients in whom deformity develops in childhood, reflex spasticity may play an etiologic role, although upward of 75% of deformities occur in the absence of spasticity [13].

The severe deformity of the leg and foot, limited ankle and subtalar motion, absent weak or spastic muscles, and the lack of sensation make it impossible for the foot to function normally by providing shock absorption, control of floor reaction forces, and the transfer of weight that is necessary for gait. Almost all of the myelomeningocele children require treatment of their feet. Even nonambulatory children require adequate positioning of the foot to accept shoe wear, placement on wheelchair foot rests, and prevent pressure sores. In Broughton's series, 78% of the nonambulatory children underwent corrective procedures for their feet [13]. Ambulatory children require an accurate correction of the foot deformity. They are unable to compensate for malpositioning of the foot because of weakness of the trunk, the hip, and the knee, which causes the weight-bearing line and the floor reaction force to fall outside the zone of stability of the hip, the knee, and the ankle. For example, a foot that has residual inward rotation produces a varus deformity at the knee and inward rotation of the leg during the stance phase of gait. Outward rotation of the foot causes a valgus deformity to the knee and an exaggerated outward rotation of the leg during stance. The foot must also be able to compensate for deformity of the knee. For example, a knee flexion contracture requires the ability of the ankle to dorsiflex so that the heel will contact the floor.

The correction of the foot deformity by itself is not sufficient. Muscle balance must also be achieved to prevent recurrence of the deformity. Muscle imbalance can be corrected either by removing the muscle force by excising the tendon or transferring the force to another location by tendon transfer. The preservation or removal of muscle activity must be considered carefully in relation to the function of the foot during walking. If the child needs an orthosis to walk then muscle control of the foot is of little importance, and the deforming forces should be eliminated; however, if the child has enough muscular control and sensation to walk without an orthosis, the muscle balance must be obtained by performing the appropriate tendon transfer.

The overall goals of treating foot and ankle problems in children with myelomeningocele are to create a braceable plantigrade foot to facilitate ambulation and positioning and to prevent skin problems.

The alignment of the foot should be corrected to allow transfer of the floor reaction force through the center of the ankle and to produce stability of the knee and hip during the stance phase of gait. The motion of the joints in the foot should be preserved to allow preservation of the shock-absorptive capacity of the foot and to lessen the possibility of joint degenerations. Subtalar arthrodesis or triple arthrodesis should be avoided because a rigid foot has a high incidence of ulceration even if the deformity has been corrected [1]. It is also important to avoid bony prominences in the weight-bearing area to lessen the likelihood of pressure sores.

In general, foot deformities in the infant should undergo a trial of gentle passive manipulation. This trial must be very judicious, as pressure sores or fractures may otherwise result. Even with early correction, recurrence is common, and surgery is ultimately needed on most feet. Deformities that may respond to passive manipulation alone include equinus contractures, mild or positional equinovarus and calcaneal positional deformity. Only the true clubfoot deformity that is not completely rigid should be casted between passive manipulations, and then only with great caution by an experienced physician, since pressure sores are likely otherwise. Surgical correction of severe deformities such as clubfoot or vertical talus, when required, should be delayed until the child is developmentally ready to be in the upright position. All major foot deformities in children with myelomeningocele have a high frequency of recurrence. To minimize early recurrence of the deformity, after the removal of postoperative casts, well-fitting orthoses should be applied immediately, and the child should be encouraged to stand or walk in them. Proceeding with surgery for foot deformity before the patient is ready to be fitted with orthoses for standing or walking will result in incurring a needless risk of recurrence before the child even begins to walk.

Equinus Deformity

Pure equinus contractures in patients with myelomeningocele are common [13, 14], but are not due to voluntary muscle imbalance, since the majority of patients have either flail feet or, in low lumbar level patients, tibialis anterior functioning. Positioning deformity, in utero or postnatally, and gastrosoleus spasticity account for some of the equinus contractures seen, and in some patients equinus will develop after tibialis anterior tendon transfer to the calcaneus.

Patients with positional neonatal equinus contractures associated with higher level paralysis can initially be treated with very gentle passive manipulation. If the equinus deformity persists when the child is ready for initial orthoses for standing and ambulation, percutaneous or open lengthening of the heel cord may be carried out. Resection of a segment, about 1 cm, of the Achilles tendon can also be considered to prevent the recurrent deformity. Careful postoperative casting for a few weeks should be followed by fitting of the orthoses required and standing or ambulation.

Clubfoot (Equinovarus) Deformity

The clubfoot, or equinovarus, is the most common deformity in children with myelomeningocele and occurs in well over 50% [1]. It is present in all levels of paraplegia, but the treatment differs at each level as a result of the muscle function that may be present. The typical clubfoot deformity in these children is truly teratologic, in that it is often present at birth and is quite rigid and recalcitrant to conservative treatment. In equinovarus deformity, the hindfoot is usually rigidly fixed in equinus and varus, often with midfoot cavus and forefoot adductus and supination (Fig. 27.1). Clubfeet can not only impair walking ability but can also create seating problems when the feet cannot sit properly on footrests. Left unchecked, this deformity can lead to the formation of pressure sores, especially on the dorsolateral aspect of the foot.

Patients with myelomeningocele and clubfoot deformity can be managed as other patients with idiopathic clubfoot deformity. Serial casting is still the first treatment to correct the deformity. A satisfactory position can be achieved at least in some of these children by manipulation and casting [16]. Currently, the Ponseti casting method is recommended for conservative management of the deformity, associated with percutaneous sectioning of the Achilles tendon in some cases, with good results (Fig. 27.2a) [17]. Occasionally, a limited posteromedial soft tissue release may be required, in addition to casting for complete correction of the deformity. However, most of these feet are rigid and the success rate with manipulation and casting has been poor. In addition, the absence of pain response or of protective sensation makes it very difficult to avoid pressure sores or fractures. Casting and manipulation must be stopped at least temporarily if swelling or skin necrosis develops. If satisfactory correction has been achieved by manipulation and casting then the child must be placed in splints to prevent recurrence of the deformity (Fig. 27.2b). The splints must be worn continuously until the age of standing.

Most often, conservative treatment will not prevent the patient from requiring surgical correction, and some surgeons defer all treatment until the time of surgical release [1]. Surgery should be delayed until the patient has developed to the point of being ready for brace fitting and ambulation or standing. The advantage of performing surgery at the time the child is ready to stand is that weight-bearing can be

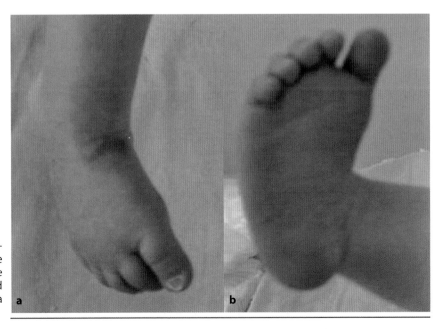

Fig. 27.1 a, b. Clubfoot (equinovarus) deformity. **a** Note the equinus and varus of the ankle (hindfoot) and **b** the adducted and supinated forefoot with a deep medial skin crease

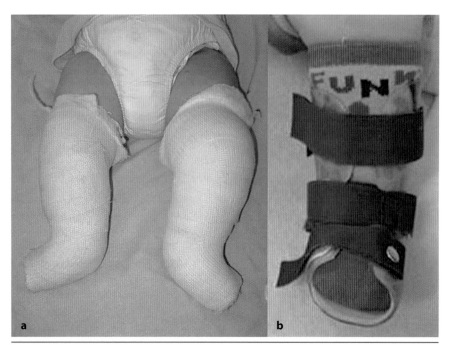

Fig. 27.2 a, b. a The initial treatment of clubfoot deformity includes manipulation and serial casting. **b** The child must be placed in splints to prevent recurrence of the deformity

used to maintain the correction along with the orthosis used for ambulation.

The surgical correction of the clubfoot is rarely accomplished by limited surgery. An extensive release, including tenotomies or excision of all contracted tendons to eliminate the deforming forces, is usually required. A radical complete circumferential subtalar release is necessary in order to allow the calcaneus to rotate sufficiently underneath the talus to align the axis of the foot to the axis of the ankle and knee [18]. Because of the deformity of the neck of talus, it is then necessary to displace the calcaneus medially beneath the talus so that the posterior facet and the anterior facets are reduced, in order to prevent the talar head from falling into a vertical position. It is important to repair the tibial calcaneal ligaments with nonabsorbable sutures to prevent lateral migration of the calcaneus into valgus. A plantar release and capsulotomy of the calcaneal cuboid joint is usually necessary as well.

Unless the child has a sacral level of paralysis, all of the contracted tendons should be resected rather than lengthened because they are spastic and nonfunctional. A simple cutting of the tendons often results in the tendon being caught in the scar, then acting as a tether as the foot grows. This causes recurrence of the deformity. Even though they are not contracted, the anterior tibialis and peroneal tendons should be released in the child with an L5 motor level to prevent a calcaneus deformity. It is better to have

a flaccid braceable foot than a deformed foot with muscle activity that is inappropriate for standing. This aggressive treatment gives a satisfactory result in the majority of patients [19]. Tendon transfer usually fails because the transferred tendon is out of phase, is weak owing to myelomeningocele, and loses a grade of strength in transfer.

Skin and incisional problems are common partly because of the severe nature of the deformity. Tension across the skin or closure must be avoided. If the skin is closed with excessive tension it will slough and heal by scar. This scar then contracts as the foot grows and causes recurrent deformity. None of the classical incisions used in clubfoot surgery, including Cincinnati, Turco or the two incisions described by Carroll, is free of complications in patients with myelomeningocele. Therefore, modified incisions such as carrying the medial arm of the incision over the dorsum of the foot, have been recommended to reduce tension on a medial skin bridge [1]. Tissue expanders and rotational pedicle flaps have also been described to address wound problems.

Postoperative splinting with orthotics is helpful in maintaining correction, but recurrences and reoperations are common. Recurrence of deformity may be treated by primarily bony procedures, including talectomy, talar enucleation, or triple arthrodesis [10]. Talectomy usually corrects hindfoot deformity but does not address forefoot deformity. On long-term follow-up, weight-bearing forces are not evenly distributed on the sole of the foot after talectomy, predisposing to the development of neurotropic ulcers [20]. Similarly, triple arthrodesis, even when the foot is clinically plantigrade, predisposes to the development of pressure sores on the foot in the myelomeningocele patient [21].

Calcaneus and Calcaneovalgus Deformities

Calcaneus deformity, an abnormal dorsiflexion of the foot (as opposed to equinus) commonly associated with ankle valgus, is another common abnormality in patients with myelomeningocele (Fig. 27.3a). About 30% of the children in this population have calcaneus deformity [22]. This deformity often results from a tibialis anterior muscle that is spastic or pulling against a weak or paralyzed gastrocnemius; thus this deformity is most frequently seen in children with L5- or S1-level paralysis. However, not all developmental calcaneal deformities can be explained solely on the basis of muscle imbalance or spasticity [13, 14].

Calcaneus deformity is usually progressive, and the calcaneus eventually becomes positioned vertically underneath the talus (Fig. 27.3b). This deformity prevents the forefoot from contacting the floor, interfering with balance, preventing the floor reaction force from stabilizing the knee, and causing the child to walk in a flexed-knee or crouched gait. Calcaneus deformity of the foot may make orthotic fit-

ting more difficult and less effective, and predisposes the patient to the development of a neurotrophic heel ulcer in the teenage years. The latter can be very difficult to eradicate and may progress to a recalcitrant calcaneal osteomyelitis.

Treatment varies with the rigidity of the deformity. Manipulations of the foot in the newborn period, and bracing as the child becomes older, may provide satisfactory position. However, in most cases the muscles continue to shorten, making brace and shoe wear difficult. Patients with persistent or progressive calcaneal deformities associated with unopposed tibialis anterior function will frequently require anterior release of the deformity, usually combined with posterior transfer of the tibialis anterior to the calcaneus to facilitate brace fitting and prevent the development of calcaneal plantar ulcers [15, 23-25]. At the time of surgery the deformity can be fully corrected; often the anterior tibial tendon is sectioned and then transferred. The remaining tight anterior structures including the peroneals, extensor hallucis longus, and extensor digitorum longus should also be released so that the foot can be brought into a satisfactory position for bracing [23, 25]. Although the posterior transfer of anterior tibial tendon is performed in the hope of providing enough ankle stability to make braces unnecessary, the transferred muscle is out of phase and has not been found to change bracing needs [26].

In children older than five years of age, soft tissue procedures rarely are sufficient. These patients also require osteotomy of the calcaneus with posterior displacement of the posterior fragment [1].

If the child has already developed ulceration underneath the calcaneus, the treatment must provide correction of the foot deformity, followed by removal of the prominent part of the calcaneus, excision of the ulcer, and primary closure by means of a local flap. To allow the ulcer to heal by secondary intention will not provide reconstruction of the normal weight-bearing fat pad. Repeat ulcerations may be seen. The weight-bearing skin and fat pad must be restored in order to prevent recurrence of the ulceration. Post-healing orthotic wear is essential.

In some cases, calcaneovalgus is caused by a vertical talus where the midfoot and forefoot are dorsiflexed on a rigid, plantar flexed talus (Fig. 27.4). Occasionally, this entity can be confused with a clubfoot if the forefoot is in equinus, but careful examination will reveal fixed calcaneus of the hindfoot [27]. Treatment of this condition consists of soft tissue releases combined with tendon transfers, fusion, or navicular excision.

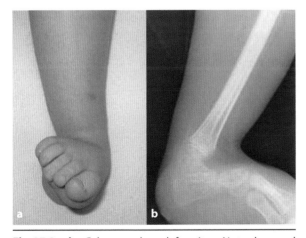

Fig. 27.3 a, b. Calcaneovalgus deformity. **a** Note abnormal dorsiflexion of the foot associated with ankle valgus. This deformity prevents forefoot from contacting the floor. **b** Lateral radiograph of the foot demonstrates vertically positioned calcaneus beneath the talus

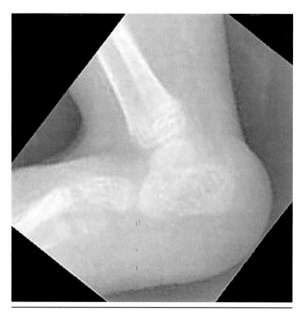

Fig. 27.4. Vertical talus may lead to calcaneovalgus deformity. Note the dorsiflexed midfoot on a plantar flexed talus

Valgus Deformity of the Foot and Ankle

Valgus without calcaneus is a common deformity in ambulatory patients with myelomeningocele, irrespective of the level of paralysis [10]. The deformity may arise from the distal tibia, the subtalar joint, or both. It is commonly associated with a flatfoot, the so-called planovalgus deformity (Fig. 27.5) [1]. The external appearance of the foot resembles that of a congenital vertical talus, but usually it is less rigid.

The cause of the deformity is undetermined, but is probably related to the floor reaction force during stance without the appropriate muscle control of the posterior tibial muscle. There usually is a lateral tilt to the ankle mortis with shortening of the fibula. The subtalar joint may be deformed as well. The location of the deformity can be determined by standing anteroposterior radiographs of the ankle mortis and foot. The outward rotation of the ankle axis in relation to the knee should be assessed. It may exceed 60 degrees. The most common sequela of valgus deformity is skin irritation or breakdown over the medial malleolus from excessive pressure against the orthosis.

Treatment depends on the rigidity and the specific location of the deformity. Flexible deformities can be treated with casting, manipulation, and bracing, although this rarely provides adequate long-term results. Most children will require surgical correction. A distal tibial valgus deformity that causes pressure sores in skeletally mature patients will require a distal tibial osteotomy and varus realignment [10]. Fixation can be done with crossed Steinmann pins, staples, an external fixator, or internal fixation with a dynamic compression plate. Delayed union, nonunion, or infection may be seen, particularly in adolescents. Recurrence of the deformity is also relatively common in the skeletally immature patient [1, 10]. Postoperatively, patients should be kept nonweight-bearing initially, since weight-bearing with diminished pain perception can lead to excessive swelling and motion.

Skeletally immature patients with minimal outward rotation of the ankle are candidates for either medial tibial hemiepiphysiodesis or Achilles tendon-fibular tenodesis [28]. The medial growth arrest can

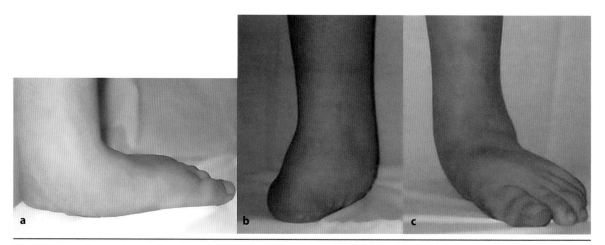

Fig. 27.5 a-c. Planovalgus deformity. **a** A flat arch and **b** a valgus heel characterize this deformity. **c** Also note external appearance of the foot. This deformity may lead to ulceration over the medial malleolus or head of the navicular from rubbing against the AFO component of the patient's orthosis

be performed by direct curettage, stapling of the medial side of the distal tibia, or insertion of a screw percutaneously from the medial malleolus proximally across the physis. The advantage of this technique is that usually immediate weight-bearing can be allowed and external immobilization is not necessary. Fibular-Achilles tenodesis is indicated in young patients with milder distal tibial valgus deformities who are considered too young for an epiphysiodesis of the distal tibia [10]. The rationale is that the valgus deformity is secondary to lateral compartment paralysis with subsequent underdevelopment of the fibula, and this lack of growth stimulation can be compensated for by tenodesis of a slip of the Achilles tendon to the fibula. With weight-bearing and ankle dorsiflexion, the tenodesis pulls downward on the fibula, leading to gradual correction of the deformity. However, stretching of the tenodesis is a major problem, and some authors recommend the addition of an anterior tibial tendon transfer to the calcaneus [1].

When radiographs reveal that most of the valgus deformity is in the subtalar region, an extensive subtalar release is required to allow reduction of the calcaneus beneath the talus [29]. This procedure includes resection of the Achilles tendon and the peroneal tendons, and division of the posterior ankle capsule along with the fibular calcaneal ligament. The anterior tibial tendon can also be resected. In most cases an extra-articular subtalar arthrodesis is needed [29, 30]. However, fusions in the foot, even when clinically plantigrade, predispose the patient to neurotrophic ulcers of the foot on long-term follow-up [21]. Thus, triple arthrodeses and subtalar fusions should be avoided whenever possible.

Cavus Deformity

Cavus deformity of the foot typically occurs in children with sacral level lesions [22]. This deformity is usually caused by unopposed pull of the tibialis anterior muscle and toe flexors, so clawing of the toes is a commonly associated deformity (Fig. 27.6a). The paralysis of the gastrocnemius-soleus muscles leaves the hindfoot in calcaneus position. These children have enough sensation and muscle control to walk without an orthosis, but frequently develop progressive deformity and ulcerations under their toes, their metatarsal heads, and their heels. Their gait is also abnormal, because of the lack of sufficient power in the gastrocnemius-soleus muscles. The cavus deformity is often progressive and may be associated with secondary varus deformity of the foot as the child attempts to use flexor hallucis and digitorum longus muscles to compensate for paralysis of the gastrocnemius-soleus muscles [1].

Flexible deformities can sometimes be contained in an ankle-foot orthosis. Brace compliance can be a problem because sacral level paraplegics are highly functional and will shed their braces, so most of these children will come to surgical correction.

Surgical treatment must include correction of the bone deformity and soft tissue contracture and restoration of the muscle imbalance [22]. In the young child with mild deformation, a plantar fascia release, followed by an ankle-foot orthosis, may provide satisfactory correction of the deformity. However, rigid deformities in older children may require a tarsal-metatarsal osteotomy associated with plantar release (Fig. 27.6b). If the deformity is due to the dorsiflex-

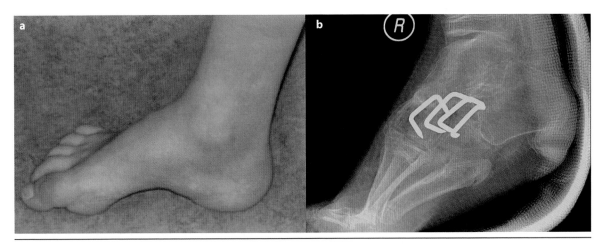

Fig. 27.6 a, b. This severe cavus deformity occurred in a young girl with a sacral level myelomeningocele. **a** Note the equinus deformity of the forefoot in relation to the hindfoot, resulting in an abnormally high arch along the medial border of the foot. **b** This deformity required tarsal-metatarsal osteotomy associated with plantar release

ion of the calcaneus, a calcaneal osteotomy is necessary to correct the cavus or cavovarus deformities [31].

Muscle-balancing procedures must consider the phase of the muscle during gait, the power of the muscle available, and the required muscle power necessary for walking [1]. The primary goal is to have a plantigrade braceable foot without recurrent deformity or pressure sores. An out-of-phase transfer of a muscle with a muscle power in the poor-to-fair range will not provide a functional foot, thus it is best to lengthen or resect the tendon of the deforming muscle and brace the foot. The tibialis anterior muscle is a swing-phase muscle, and cannot be made into a stance-phase muscle by being transferred to the calcaneus. In most circumstances it is better to lengthen the tibialis anterior and preserve its necessary function of foot clearance during swing. For a cavovarus deformity, a tibialis anterior transfer to the middle of the foot with or without a posteromedial release can be helpful. Muscle imbalance of the toes can be helped by transfer of the long extensor tendons to the metatarsal heads, with fusion of the interphalangeal joints. This transfer helps elevate the metatarsal heads and prevent recurrent cavus [10].

Rotational Deformities

Rotational deformities of the lower extremities are frequent in both ambulatory and nonambulatory patients with myelomeningocele [32-34]. Infants and young children tend to have internal tibial torsion. This deformity is usually either dynamic, secondary to medial hamstring dominance, or fixed, secondary to internal tibial torsion. In the ambulatory child, this torsion can lead to difficulty in walking and so needs surgical intervention. When dynamic internal rotational deformity is interfering with gait, Dias and colleagues [32] reported good results with transfer of the semitendinosus to the biceps and head of the fibula. Internal tibial torsion may also be treated by osteotomy of either the proximal or distal tibia and fibula. Distal tibial derotational osteotomy is a more commonly performed procedure and fixation can be done with staple, crossed Steinmann pins, or a dynamic compression plate.

External tibial torsion usually occurs after the age of six years and, in addition to being cosmetically displeasing to the family or patient, may also indirectly interfere with ambulation by making fitting or function of the AFO component of bracing more difficult. This deformity places the medial malleolus in the line of progression of the limb and may lead to constant skin breakdown due to rubbing against the AFO in this area. External tibial torsion is commonly asso-

ciated with a planovalgus foot which may aggravate the problem. As for the valgus ankle, treatment initially consists of orthotics management. When this modality fails, a derotational osteotomy (plus appropriate management of the ankle valgus) achieves the necessary correction. Distal tibial osteotomy can provide satisfactory results in the majority of the patients, however, significant complications such as delayed union or wound infections have been reported with this procedure in patients with myelomeningocele [33].

Knee

The function of the knee is important to a child with myelomeningocele. Function of the knee is dependent on both the absence of deformity and the presence of stability. It must be stable during stance to accept the weight of the child without buckling, and flex sufficiently during swing to clear the foot. However, it is possible to walk with a stiff knee, and stability is more important than motion [1]. Long-term studies in ambulatory patients with low lumbar or sacral level lesions suggest that knee instability, with or without pain, is present in about 25% [35].

The knee requires less surgery and clinical attention than the hip and foot in children with myelomeningocele, however, it can be a significant source of morbidity. Clinically significant knee arthropathy has been demonstrated in ambulatory young adults with myelomeningocele and is probably secondary to abnormal walking mechanics [35]. The three deformities that may seriously diminish the ambulatory ability are extension or hyperextension contractures, flexion contractures, and valgus rotational deformities.

Congenital Knee Deformities

Congenital Knee Flexion Contracture

Patients with myelomeningocele can be born with flexion contractures of the knee. Flexion contractures of less than 10 degrees will resolve by the time the patient is ready for ambulation, either spontaneously or with judicious passive stretching, even when the patient has no motor function across the knee. Knee flexion deformity may subsequently recur, particularly in patients with higher levels of paralysis [34].

Congenital Knee Hyperextension/Dislocation

Congenital knee hyperextension or dislocation may also occur in patients with myelomeningocele, most frequently in patients carried in the full breech position. Simple hyperextension deformity may respond to careful passive stretching and splinting. The treatment of congenital knee dislocation also begins with gentle stretching. The use initially of serial casts changed weekly, and subsequently, removable splints changed every two to three weeks, is often helpful, particularly in the milder forms. Once flexion beyond 90 degrees is obtained, it is unlikely that additional treatment will be needed. Those infants who do not respond to nonoperative treatment (failure to achieve knee flexion beyond more than 60 degrees) should be considered for surgical treatment consisting of a soft tissue lengthening of the extensor mechanism. This treatment should be performed well before the child reaches walking age, so that the postoperative knee-flexed position can be resolved before orthotics are required for ambulation [10]. In patients with myelomeningocele, treatment of congenital knee dislocation may result in some extension contracture, persistent hyperextension at the knee, and/or knee instability.

Developmental Knee Flexion Contracture

Knee flexion contractures are probably the most common knee deformity in patients with myelomeningocele. They develop in both ambulatory and nonambulatory children during growth, even in the face of normal quadriceps function. The development of such contractures does not appear to correlate with ambulatory status, level of paralysis, or the presence of spasticity [34, 36]. A small degree of contracture,

below 20 degrees, seems to be tolerated well, but contraction greater than 30 degrees decreases the likelihood that the child will continue to walk. Contractures over 20 degrees in the adult have a high incidence of patellofemoral pain [35].

The cause of knee flexion contracture is not always apparent. In some children, spasticity of the hamstrings or gastrocnemius can be implicated. In most middle or low lumbar paraplegic patients, the cause appears to be a co-contraction of the hamstring and the quadriceps during the entire stance phase of gait. This lack of coordinated activity appears to be related to brain stem abnormalities. The result is persistent knee flexion during stance and decreased knee flexion during swing [1].

In the neonatal period and in infancy, physical therapy may be helpful in decreasing the flexion contracture. Small contractures (less than 10 degrees) have also been treated successfully with well-padded serial casts. In those children who do not respond to conservative measures by 18 months to two years of age, surgical correction is indicated [22].

Normally, knee flexion deformities of 20 degrees or less are well tolerated in the ambulatory patient, either with or without bracing across the knee; nonambulatory patients will usually tolerate even more flexion contracture without interference to mobility status or transfers. If more deformity is present, careful thought must be given to the patient's ambulation level and the extent to which ambulation is being impeded by the flexion contracture. Severe contractures (greater than 30 degrees) that interfere with ambulation or transfers respond well to posterior soft tissue release, which hold up well over time (Fig. 27.7) [37, 38].

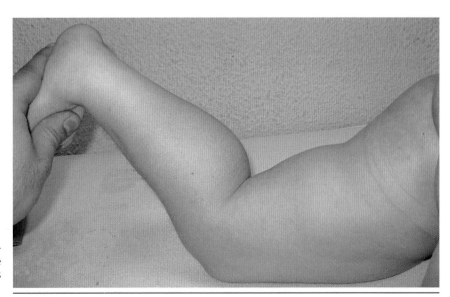

Fig. 27.7. Knee flexion contracture. Note severe knee flexion contracture in this child with total paralysis

If the child with flexion contractures has some voluntary function of the medial hamstrings, the hamstrings should be lengthened rather than sectioned. The biceps femoris and the posterior part of the iliotibial band can be sectioned. The gastrocnemius origin should be resected. A posterior capsulotomy should also be performed in almost all children with knee flexion deformity. Partial resection of the anterior cruciate ligament may also be required in some children, to allow the tibia to slide forward on the femur into extension [10].

Problems with wound closure and tightness of neurovascular structures may preclude a complete acute correction, and the soft tissue release may need to be followed by serial casting to obtain complete correction. Postoperatively, the patient must wear an above-the-knee orthosis for a prolonged period to prevent the development of knee instability.

In most children functioning at the low lumbar level, the hamstring muscles contract at the same time as the quadriceps muscle throughout the stance phase of walking. Biceps femoris and the semimembranosus muscles can be transferred to the cut end of the gastrocnemius muscle on the distal femur in these children [1]. This transfer will assist in extension without flexing the knee. The transfer can be performed at any age because the attachment to the distal femoral epiphysis will allow for future growth. By removing two of the hamstring muscles from the knee flexion, the quadri-

ceps usually will be able to maintain knee extension during stance.

In the child older than six or seven years, sufficient deformity may have developed in the femoral condyles to preclude satisfactory soft tissue correction of the contracture, and a distal femoral osteotomy is needed (Fig. 27.8) [22]. There is a tendency for recurrence of deformity with growth, and repeat surgery may be necessary.

Knee Extension Contracture

Another common knee problem in patients with myelomeningocele is extension contracture. Children with this deformity will have significant difficulty walking and sitting. Fortunately, the incidence of extension contractures is relatively low. The deformity is most commonly seen in children born with a breech presentation. Intrauterine compression forces may lead to hyperflexed hips, hyperextended knees and clubfoot in these children. In these infants with hyperextended knees, the hamstring tendons usually have displaced anterior to the knee axis, perpetuating the hyperextension deformity, although the child may be an L4- or L5-level paraplegic [1]. Knee extension contracture can be seen in the middle lumbar level paraplegic patient who has quadriceps function, but no perceptible knee flexors. Spastic quadriceps muscles in high level paraplegic patients may

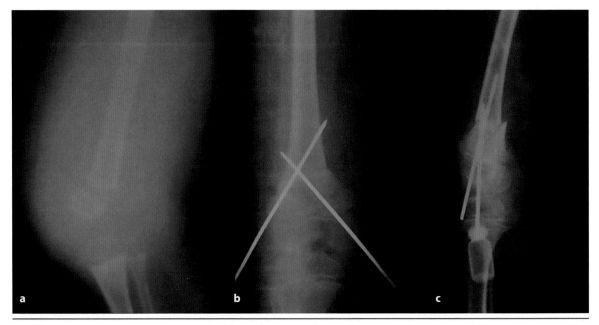

Fig. 27.8 a-c. Knee flexion contracture. In older children, satisfactory correction of severe knee flexion contracture frequently requires distal femoral extension osteotomy in addition to posterior soft tissue release

also result in knee extension contractures. Extension contractures may also occur as a consequence of extensive immobilization for repeated fractures of the femur and after treatment for flexion contracture or congenital knee dislocation.

Most of the patients with knee extension deformity can be treated by passive range of motion and splinting during the neonatal period of life. Although normal range of motion is rarely achieved, 60-70 degrees of flexion is common. In infancy, serial casting can be helpful to obtain 90 degrees of flexion [39]. For those paraplegic children who do not respond to physical therapy or casting, a soft tissue lengthening of the extensor mechanism is indicated. Several procedures have been described, including a Z-plasty of the extensor mechanism and a V-Y lengthening of the quadriceps [37]. If the child has voluntary function of the quadriceps, a modification of the V-Y plasty of the quadriceps tendons should be performed. This procedure is modified by detaching the vastus medialis and the vastus lateralis from the medial and lateral hamstrings, which slide posterior to the knee axis. This approach often restores the hamstring function, and the child develops both active flexion and extension of the knee. An anterior capsulotomy may also be required to obtain maximal correction. Patients without meaningful leg power may benefit from a simple patellar tendon release to facilitate seating [40]. With any surgical procedure, the patient should be immobilized in knee flexion only as long as necessary for the soft tissues to heal. This should be followed by a program of daily gentle passive and (if possible) active range of motion exercises of the knee.

Valgus and Rotational Deformities

Valgus and rotational deformities of the knee are unusual and primarily are caused by tightness of the iliotibial band and the forces of ambulation. During the Trendelenburg gait pattern, the shift of weight lateral to the hip joint, along with contraction of the adductors and fixed position of the foot to the floor, produce a valgus thrust to the knee. Knee valgus deformity rarely requires orthopedic intervention and can be treated by placing the child in a knee-ankle-foot orthosis to resist the valgus thrust to the knee [10]. Sectioning of the distal iliotibial band may be required if it is contracted. Rarely, contracture of the iliotibial band is associated with distal femoral valgus deformity, which may progress in spite of release. If this deformity becomes fixed, a distal femoral osteotomy is required to realign the knee.

Hip

Problems about the hip joint, ranging from joint contractures to subluxation to dislocation, are very common in myelomeningocele. The presence of hip deformity and dislocation is related to the neurologic level of the disorder, but not to muscle imbalance [41]. For example, despite the great muscle imbalance across a hip with an L4-level lesion (hip flexors function well but extensors and abductors are weak), there is a relatively low rate of dislocation. However, despite the complete paralysis across the hip seen in high lumbar or thoracic level lesions, there is a higher rate of hip subluxation and dislocation. For this reason, Menelaus [42] warns against prophylactic surgery to correct muscle imbalance, because it will not necessarily prevent hip dislocation. The approach to treatment of hip disorders in this population should be founded on maximizing a patient's function through consideration of current and predicted ambulatory status.

The most frequent hip problem in children with myelomeningocele is paralytic subluxation or dislocation. The presence of unopposed hip flexor and adductor muscle function in the growing child, as seen in patients with upper lumbar lesions and, to a lesser extent, in those with lower lumbar level lesions, leads almost inevitably to progressive hip subluxation and dislocation. The nature of the problem can be understood by evaluating the treatment of developmental dysplasia of the hip in patients with myelomeningocele compared to treatment in neuromuscularly intact patients. In the latter, Pavlik harness and closed reduction are the mainstays of treatment in patients before walking age. In patients with myelomeningocele, because of the associated muscle imbalance, such reduction inevitably is followed by recurrence of the dislocation, since there is no spontaneous improvement in the structural abnormalities of femoral and acetabular deformities which contribute to hip instability [10]. Specific treatment of a hip deformity depends on the neurological level, the specific deformity, and the individual child's function.

Thoracic and Upper Lumbar Paraplegia

The thoracic and upper lumbar level (L1-L2) paraplegic child does not have sensation or muscle control over the lower extremities. There is little, if any, meaningful strength across the hip in this group, and deformity is usually secondary to positioning and spasm. Although many of these children are able to walk early in life with extensive bracing and therapy, they can rarely do so after the age of ten. Nevertheless, some investigators believe that the psychological benefits of walking even temporarily can make the effort worthwhile [43].

Hip instability, even when unilateral, is not a source of disability in children with high level lesions and generally does not require treatment [44]. Without sensation and motor control, reduction of the hip is not necessary for sitting and walking using orthotic aids. However, these children need a functional range without contracture [45]. Surgical procedures should be used to provide range of motion so that the child can sit satisfactorily in a wheelchair, lie comfortably in bed, and use orthoses for standing and walking, if indicated.

Physical therapy and splinting play an important role in preventing and treating mild (greater than 20 degrees) hip flexion contractures. Soft tissue releases may be indicated for contractures greater than 20 degrees to maintain bracing and ambulation. An anterior hip release usually involves the iliopsoas, sartorius, rectus femoris, tensor fascia lata, and hip capsule. Treating hip contractures in paraplegics may be frustrating because many contractures return promptly, often to a worse degree than before surgical release [22]. It is important that prolonged bracing and physical therapy be used to maintain whatever motion has been obtained by surgery. Osteotomies, although rarely indicated, can be useful in treating severe flexion deformities (greater than 60 degrees) or treating pressure sores resulting from the hip deformity.

In addition to hip flexion contractures, abduction, adduction and external rotation contractures are also commonly seen in children with total paralysis across the hips and in the legs because of the posture they assume as infants (Fig. 27.9). Awareness of this problem and the use of prophylactic splinting and physical therapy can often prevent these deformities from becoming major problems. Soft tissue releases are useful for contractures that persist despite conservative measures, as described previously. Releasing the tensor fascia lata usually improves the abduction contracture. Subtrochanteric osteotomies may be required for persistent external rotation contractures. Adduction contractures can lead to pelvic obliquity and problems with ambulating, positioning, pressure sores, and perineal hygiene. When nonoperative measures fail, an open adductor release is indicated. The adductor longus and brevis and the gracilis are released through a transverse incision over the adductor longus.

Children with thoracic and high lumbar lesions have a relatively high rate of hip subluxation and dis-

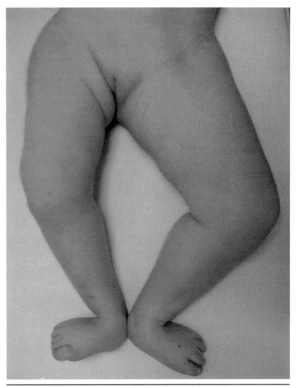

Fig. 27.9. External rotation contracture across the hip in thoracic or upper lumbar paraplegia. Note significant external rotation deformity across the left hip and the leg in this child with total paralysis

location (Fig. 27.10). If a hip is becoming dysplastic or is dislocating, the cause should be found and treated. Increased muscle tone or spasticity should be treated by muscle release, or perhaps by neurectomy. Pelvic obliquity caused by developing scoliosis should be treated. Attempts to reduce a dislocated hip are difficult and often unsuccessful. The principal risk of surgically reducing the hip is stiffness. Multiple surgical procedures should be avoided because the risk of stiffness increases with each surgical procedure [22]. It is better to have a supple dislocated hip than a stiff located hip.

The orthosis must provide pelvic, hip, knee, ankle, and foot stability. The standing frame, the parapodium, the swivel walker, and hip control orthosis all provide stability [46]. At approximately 18 to 24 months of age, if the child has developed head control and sitting balance, a standing orthosis is prescribed. Orthotic devices are needed to provide stability to the lower extremity. The child usually finds these devices to be confining because they are too slow, they require too much energy, and they are too difficult to apply. Consequently, most of these children give up walking by the time they are eight or nine years of age, and use a

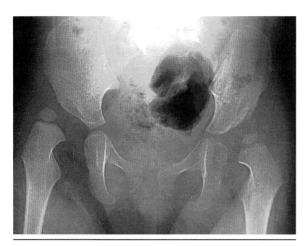

Fig. 27.10. Hip instability in thoracic or upper lumbar paraplegia. This pelvis radiograph demonstrates bilateral hip dislocation. Hip instability is not a source of disability in children with high level lesions and does not require treatment

wheelchair for their mobility. Two designs of orthotic devices, reciprocating orthosis and hip guidance orthosis, may change this prognosis for walking [47, 48]. These braces may be tried after the age of three years when the child is large enough to fit into the smallest size of the orthosis. However, these devices are quite expensive and need to be replaced frequently.

Middle and Lower Lumbar Paraplegia

The middle to lower lumbar paraplegic (L3-L5) patient has sensation to below the knee. Muscle function includes hip flexion and adduction, knee extension, and weak knee flexion. Foot dorsiflexion and eversion also may be present. These patients have the potential for control of the hip and knee, and therefore the potential for independent walking. Gait studies show almost normal sagittal plane motion, indicating that range of motion and control of the hip are probably the most important factors in walking for these children [1].

The hip in the middle to lower lumbar level paraplegic is a major source of deformity and disability. The natural history of the hip is to undergo progressive dysplasia and dislocation associated with hip flexion contracture, which becomes evident when the child begins to walk. Muscle imbalance is caused by strong hip flexors, adductors, and absent or weak hip abductors and extensors. This muscle imbalance is exaggerated by the forces of walking when the hip flexors and adductors are used to stabilize the hip during the stance phase of walking, instead of during

their typical function in the swing phase. Attempts to reduce the hip and correct the progressive deformity are unsuccessful unless there is correction of the forces around the hip [10].

Regardless of the cause, hip subluxation or dislocation complicates 50-70% of children with middle or lower lumbar paraplegia and is a source of controversy [22]. Studies have alternatively shown hip dysplasia to have a negative effect on ambulation [49] and to have no effect on ambulation [50]. Many recommend reserving surgical treatment for ambulatory children with a unilateral hip dislocation, strong quadriceps, and a stable neurological level [41, 51]. Unilateral dislocations are of greater concern because they interfere with ambulation by creating pelvic obliquity and leg length discrepancy (Fig. 27.11). Unilateral hip instability is also associated with scoliosis, but interestingly there is no correlation between the side of instability and the direction of the curve [52]. Bilateral dislocations have been shown not to have a negative effect on function, [53] so they do not typically warrant treatment unless they are associated with a significant fixed flexion contracture.

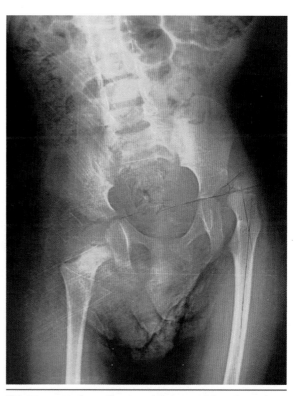

Fig. 27.11. Unilateral hip instability in middle or lower lumbar paraplegia. The pelvis radiograph demonstrates a left hip dislocation. Unilateral dislocations interfere with ambulation by creating pelvic obliquity and leg length discrepancy

Treating hip problems that develop in the first year of life is particularly challenging in children with myelomeningocele. Traditional bracing and surgical treatments are reported to have failure rates of 50% [54]. Many authors prefer to wait until the child is one year of age before carrying out hip reduction to avoid interfering with motor development [1]. If the child is between one and six years of age, an open reduction and capsular plication, associated with an anterior release, are carried out to produce a balanced, stable hip. If there is deformity of the femoral neck, a varus femoral shortening osteotomy is indicated. Pelvic osteotomy is indicated for severe acetabular dysplasia (Fig. 27.12) [55]. The type of pelvic osteotomy performed depends on the deformity and the surgeon's preference. The muscle transfers are then performed to help maintain reduction. The muscle transfers work better on a reduced hip than a dislocated one. Myotomies may improve balance, but they reduce stability.

The once popular transfer of the iliopsoas to the greater trochanter has fallen out of favor. The purpose of the tendon transfer was to produce an abduction force across the hip joint during the stance phase of gait, and thereby eliminate the deforming hip flexion force of the iliopsoas. Long-term studies have shown that this transfer is successful in maintaining hip reduction and decreasing the hip flexion contracture [56]. However, the iliopsoas is transferred out of phase to normal walking, and may decrease the necessary sagittal plane motion required for walking. In addition, it continues to contract during the flexion activity of the hip, and also may prevent the hip from flexing, leading to an extension contracture.

Transfer of the external oblique muscle from the abdomen to the greater trochanter, posterior transfer of the adductor longus, brevis, and gracilis to the ischium and transfer of the tensor fascia lata muscle posteriorly on the ilium and to the tendon of the gluteus maximus, have been used to control the hip [1]. Studies have shown the maintenance of hip reduction and improvement in the acetabular index and the centre-edge angle after those muscle transfers, similar to the results obtained with iliopsoas transfer. Transfer of the external oblique to the greater trochanter increases the extensor moment on the hip and has been shown to improve gait pattern and reduce or eliminate requirements for bracing. Combining this procedure with a transfer of the adductors and tensor fascia lata posteriorly may further improve results [57].

Although improvement in the hip indices can be produced by muscle transfers around the hip, they are not sufficiently forceful to correct major anatomic deformities. It is therefore necessary to reduce the hip and correct femoral and acetabular deformity at the time of, or prior to, the muscle transfer. Continued radiographic evaluation must be made following the reconstruction because recurrent dysplasia is possible.

Sacral Paraplegia

Sacral level paraplegics have intrinsic stability to their hip with sensation and motor control. These children are typically high functioning and have a low incidence of significant hip pathology. Hip dysplasia should be treated aggressively in this population, as it would be in an otherwise normal child, to best preserve their function (Fig. 27.13).

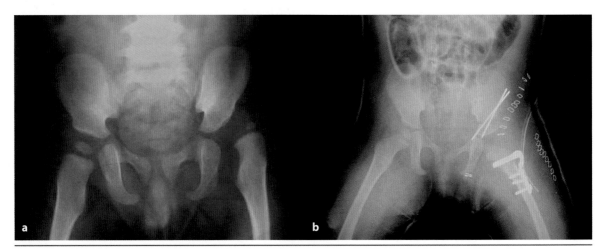

Fig. 27.12 a, b. Unilateral hip instability in middle or lower lumbar paraplegia. This 5-year-old boy with unilateral hip dislocation underwent open reduction, pelvic osteotomy, and proximal femoral varus osteotomy

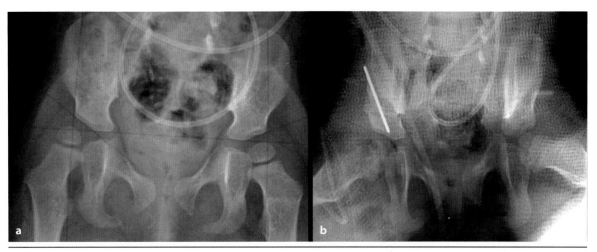

Fig. 27.13 a, b. Hip instability in sacral level paraplegia. This 2-year-old girl with unilateral hip dislocation was treated by open reduction and pelvic osteotomy. Hip instability should be treated aggressively in children with sacral level lesions

Pathologic Fractures

Wolff law states that bone forms in response to stress and, conversely, bone is resorbed when there is no stress. Therefore, the leg bones of paralyzed patients rapidly become thin and osteopenic when they are not loaded. The combination of sensory loss with osteopenic or outright osteoporotic bone is a setup for fracture in children with myelomeningocele. Barnett and Menelaus [58] report an overall incidence of about 20% for pathological fractures, with a much higher incidence in children with thoracic lesions (69%). These fractures do not occur in ambulatory patients with low level sacral lesions and can be delayed or prevented by encouraging other patients to bear weight. Quan and colleagues [59] assessed bone mineral density of the distal radius in an unselected group of patients with myelomeningocele. They found that all patients had a lower bone mineral density than the normal population, and patients with a history of fracture had densities lower than patients without a history of fracture.

The clinical symptoms of pathological fractures are similar to those of an infection, with a swollen, red limb, often associated with fever. Supracondylar femur fractures are the most common type and often manifest a warm, red, swollen knee (Fig. 27.14). The patient usually presents several days after the fracture, and there may be no history of trauma. Knowledge of these fractures is essential to prevent a delay in diagnosis with an unnecessary workup for infection. Any unexplained fever in association with a swollen warm leg that appears to be cellulitis should

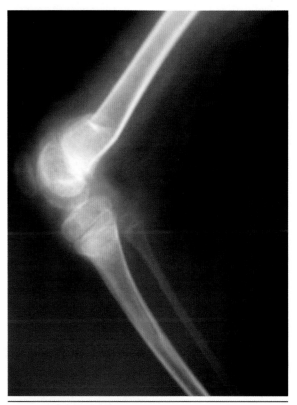

Fig. 27.14. Pathological supracondylar femur fracture in a child with myelomeningocele

be treated as a fracture in these children until radiographs prove otherwise.

Treatment consists of brief immobilization with a cast or fracture brace because these fractures usually heal quickly with exuberant callus (Fig. 27.15).

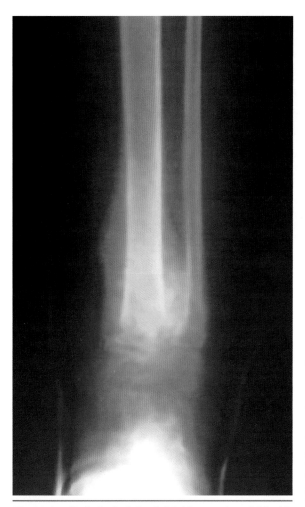

Fig. 27.15. Pathological distal tibial fracture in a child with myelomeningocele. The anteroposterior radiograph of the left distal leg demonstrates a several-week-old distal tibial fracture with exuberant callus formation

Fractures do not, however, invariably heal without incident, as malunion, delayed union, and physeal growth disturbance have all been reported [60, 61]. Therefore, adequate maintenance of alignment and immobilization is required. Physeal fractures may be slow to heal, and require reevaluation to detect subsequent growth disturbance [62].

Fracture following postoperative cast immobilization is common, and several studies have reported an incidence of 18-45% [1]. Prevention of fractures in the postoperative period includes starting the child on weight-bearing as soon as possible, and keeping the plaster immobilization time to a minimum. Once a fracture has occurred again it is best to carry out minimal immobilization and begin weight-bearing as soon as possible. Protective orthotics should be available when the cast is removed and cautious range of motion and weight-bearing exercises begun under supervision. Failure to follow these principles can lead to increased osteopenia and repeated fractures.

Charcot Arthropathy

Charcot, or neurotrophic, arthropathy is a progressive degeneration of a joint caused by a lack of protective sensation. It is a relatively uncommon complication in this population, with an incidence of about 1% [11]. Charcot arthropathy seems to occur in ambulatory children with a motor level at or below L4 and a sensory level slightly higher [63]. These patients often are able to stand and walk, but do not have protective sensation. The pathologic process begins following a minor initial traumatic episode. Following this initial traumatic episode, there usually is a considerable amount of swelling, redness and warmth around the joint (Fig. 27.16a). The appear-

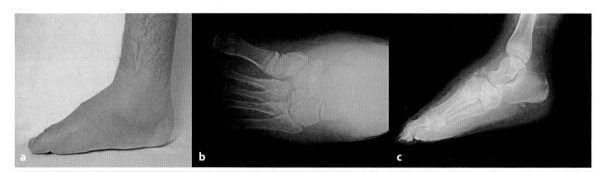

Fig. 27.16 a-c. Charcot arthropathy. **a** Note severe edema and erythema over the dorsal and medial aspects of the right foot. **b, c** The anteroposterior and lateral radiographs of the foot show degeneration in talonavicular and naviculocuneiform joints. Fragmentation can be seen in navicular

ance of the joint resembles an infection and cellulitis. Because of the lack of pain, the patient continues to walk on the joint, causing further microfractures to occur. Consequently, joint instability, leading to subluxation and occasionally dislocation develops. With this instability, the joint surfaces fragment, creating osteochondral bodies.

Initial radiographs often are unremarkable and the patient is often given antibiotics for the mistaken diagnosis of infection. Radiographic changes may become evident by several weeks or even months after the initial episode (Fig. 27.16b, c). Aggressive treatment of the suspected Charcot arthropathy after the initial traumatic episode with immobilization and non-weight bearing status offers the best chance for a successful outcome [1]. If the early treatment has been successful, radiographic changes may never be identified. The healing usually takes 6-8 weeks. However, if the diagnosis and treatment are delayed until the radiographs become positive for joint deformity or degeneration, prolonged immobilization and protection must be provided until the process has run its course. This may take 6-8 months or longer. The joint protection should be maintained until all skin changes resolve and there is radiographic evidence of healing. Once healed, continued protection with an orthosis is recommended to protect against further injury. Although the ankle is the most commonly affected joint, Charcot arthropathy has been described in the knee and hip in children with myelomeningocele [10].

Ambulation and Orthotic Devices

The goal of treatment of myelomeningocele foot is a braceable plantigrade foot. Only the sacral level paraplegic children have sufficient sensation and muscle control to gain stability of the foot and ankle without orthotic support. Most orthotics are applied to the lower extremities, and they are often used to facilitate gait. Therefore, one must have a working knowledge of normal gait to understand how different braces help children with myelomeningocele. A simplified summary of one gait cycle, commonly called a stride, follows.

The two main phases of the gait cycle are stance and swing, each of which can be broken up into several components. The stance phase describes any time a foot is on the ground and the swing phase, any time a foot is off the ground. By convention the gait cycle begins with stance phase, which is initiated by heel strike. In this phase, the ankle dorsiflexors (tibialis anterior muscle) are firing to hold the toes up to keep them from catching on the ground. After heel strike,

the limb begins to accept the weight of the body during loading response, as the ankle slowly plantar-flexes to meet the ground. Next is midstance, in which the center of gravity of the body is directly over the ankle and the foot is flat on the ground. Stance is completed by terminal stance as the ankle progressively dorsiflexes again to tension the plantar flexors in preparation for toe off, which requires plantar-flexion of the ankle to propel the body forward.

The swing phase consists of initial swing, midswing, and terminal swing. Initial swing requires hip flexion, knee flexion, and ankle dorsiflexion to keep the forefoot clear of the ground. In the midswing and terminal swing, the knee and hip begin to extend, moving the foot forward and down while the ankle dorsiflexors fire to keep the forefoot clear of the ground. When the heel strike occurs, swing phase ends and another cycle begins.

Obviously, this basic mode of locomotion, repeated thousands of times a day by most normal children from the age of one year, requires tremendous coordination of several major muscle groups, and problems in any one area will lead to a disturbance in gait that may manifest as a limp, a fall, or an inability to walk at all. Orthotics cannot correct a rigid deformity but rather are used to stabilize joints and replace muscles that are not functioning normally to improve, if not normalize, gait. Knowledge of the basic types of orthoses is important for all individuals involved in the care of children with myelomeningocele.

The AFO is one of the most commonly used braces in orthopaedics. There are many different types, but all AFOs essentially hold the foot in a neutral position (Fig. 27.17a). In accomplishing this goal, the AFO restricts motion at the ankle and subtalar joints. However, for the child with a weak tibialis anterior muscle (innervated by L4-L5), who cannot clear the floor during swing phase, this brace can greatly improve gait [64]. An AFO can also help children with weakness or absence of ankle plantar flexors by preventing the ankle from excessive dorsiflexion during the stance phase of gait, which could result in a crouch gait pattern.

Problems with the position of the subtalar joint, often resulting from an imbalance between the tibialis posterior, tibialis anterior, and peroneal muscles, can be aided with a foot orthosis. The University of California Biomechanics Laboratory (UCBL) shoe insert cups the heel and extends down to support the sole of the foot; this orthotic can help children with valgus ankles (Fig. 27.17b). Varus or valgus ankle can also be helped by placement of wedges in the shoe under half the ankle to make the foot roll into a more neutral position. For example,

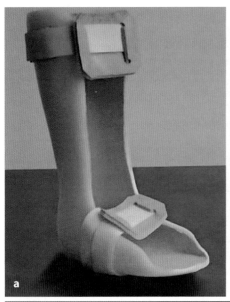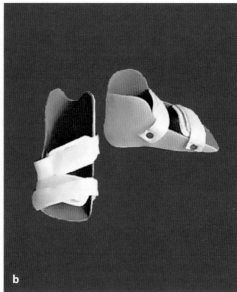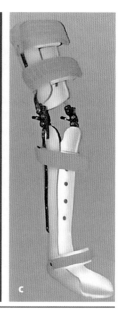

Fig. 27.17 a-c. Most orthoses are applied to the lower extremities to facilitate gait. **a** Ankle-foot orthosis (AFO) helps to control ankle equinus and, with the raised sides, can help to control ankle varus and valgus. **b** A valgus ankle can be helped by the University of California Biomechanics Laboratory (UCBL) shoe insert which cups the heel and extends down to support the sole of the foot. **c** A knee-ankle-foot orthosis (KAFO) can control both the knee and the ankle joints. The knee hinges can be locked or unlocked depending on the level of voluntary control of the knee

a heel in varus, if flexible, may be treated with a lateral heel wedge.

Children with weak quadriceps muscles (L3-L4) usually require help with knee stabilization and may benefit from a knee-ankle-foot orthosis (KAFO) (Fig. 27.17c). The quadriceps are important in gait both to extend the knee during the swing phase and to hold the knee straight during the stance phase. The KAFO can prevent unwanted knee flexion during stance with properly placed anterior pads and drop locks on the knee hinge [64].

The next stage of bracing is the hip-knee-ankle-foot orthosis (HKAFO). Such orthoses serve several functions. For the child with a low lumbar lesion and severe internal torsion of the legs, the HKAFO can help position the legs properly for ambulation, specifically heel strike and weight acceptance. For the same patient, the HKAFO can facilitate ambulation in the absence of torsional problems if the patient has difficulty with quadriceps weakness and proper placement of the leg with each stride. Weakness about the hip and a propensity toward hip flexion contractures in children with upper lumbar motor levels often make the HKAFO less functional. In these children, the reciprocating gait orthosis (RGO) is a better choice. The RGO has a mechanism that connects the motion of the two legs so that one hip passively extends as the other is actively flexed (hence the 'reciprocal').

Thoracic level paraplegics have no volitional control of any muscles of ambulation and require the cumbersome thoracic-hip-knee-ankle-foot orthosis if they are to walk. This brace supports the entire lower body and can be used as a stander or for walking if combined with Lofstrand crutches or a walker. Other options for these children are the RGO or, for children in whom arm use is impaired, the swivel walker. The swivel walker converts side-to-side movements of the thorax into forward motion by means of swiveling bases.

Conclusion

Myelomeningocele represents a fairly wide range of disease severity, from the highly functional, ambulatory child with a sacral level lesion, to the totally debilitated child with a thoracic level lesion. Treatment begins at, if not before, birth and requires constant vigilance from a multidisciplinary team that includes the orthopedic surgeon among its many members. Treatment of deformity in this population needs to be individualized to the patient. The patient's functional, intellectual, and emotional development must all be factored into the equation with the deformity when deciding on appropriate treatment. Surgery has a high complication rate in this population, but unfortunately nonoperative measures are not effective for many of their problems. Orthopedic surgery is often required to realign the limbs or spine into a functional position, one that can often be held with the assistance of an orthotic. Great care must be taken with the insensate skin of such children, for whom decubitus ulcers are a major preventable source of morbidity.

References

1. Lindseth RE (2001) Myelomeningocele. In: Morrissy RT, Weinstein SL (eds) Lovell and Winter's pediatric ortopaedics. Lippincott Williams & Wilkins, Philadelphia, pp 601-632
2. Lim R, Dias L, Vankoski S et al (1998) Valgus knee stress in lumbosacral myelomeningocele: a gait-analysis evaluation. J Pediatr Orthop 18:428-433
3. Thomson JD, Ounpuu S, Davis RB et al (1999) The effects of ankle-foot orthoses on the ankle and knee in persons with myelomeningocele: an evaluation using three-dimensional gait analysis. J Pediatr Orthop 19:27-33
4. Vankoski S, Moore C, Statler KD et al (1997) The influence of forearm crutches on pelvic and hip kinematics in children with myelomeningocele: don't throw away crutches. Dev Med Child Neurol 39:614-619
5. Banta JV, Bonanni C, Prebluda J (1993) Latex anaphylaxis during spinal surgery in children with myelomeningocele. Dev Med Child Neurol 35:543-548
6. Mazon A, Nieto A, Estornell F et al (1997) Factors that influence the presence of symptoms caused by latex allergy in children with spina bifida. J Allergy Clin Immunology 99:600-604
7. Tosi LL, Slater JE, Shaer C et al (1993) Latex allergy in spina bifida patients: prevalence and surgical implications. J Pediatr Orthop 13:709-712
8. Alenius H, Palosuo T, Kelly K et al (1993) Ig E reactivity to 14-kD and 27-kD natural rubber proteins in latex-allergic children with spina bifida and other congenital anomalies. Int Arch Allergy Immunol 102:61-66
9. Degenhardt P, Golla S, Wahn F et al (2001) Latex allergy in pediatric surgery is dependent on repeated operations in the first year of life. J Pediatr Surg 36:1535-1539
10. Herring JA (2002) Tachdjian's pediatric orthopaedics. WB Saunders Company, Philadelphia
11. Roye BD, Davidson RS (2004) Spina Bifida. In: Dormans JP (ed) Pediatric ortopaedics and sports medicine. The requisites in pediatrics. Mosby, Philadelphia, pp 417-436
12. Mazur JM, Menelaus MB, Hudson I et al (1986) Hand function in patients with spina bifida cystica. J Pediatr Orthop 6:442-447
13. Broughton NS, Graham G, Menelaus MB (1994) The high incidence of foot deformity in patients with high-level spina bifida. J Bone Joint Surg 76(B):548-550
14. Frawley PA, Broughton NS, Menelaus MB (1998) Incidence and type of hindfoot deformities in patients with low-level spina bifida. J Pediatr Orthop 18:312-313
15. Sharrard WJ, Grosfield I (1968) The management of deformity and paralysis of the foot in myelomeningocele. J Bone Joint Surg 50(B):456-465
16. Walker G (1971) The early management of varus feet in myelomeningocele. J Bone Joint Surg 53(B):462-467
17. Ponseti IV (1996) Congenital Clubfoot. Fundamentals of treatment. Oxford University Press, New York
18. Menelaus MB (1971) Talectomy for equinovarus deformity in arthrogryposis and spina bifida. J Bone Joint Surg 53(B): 468-473
19. de Carvalho Neto J, Dias LS, Gabrieli AP (1996) Congenital talipes equinovarus in spina bifida: treatment and results. J Pediatr Orthop 16:782-785
20. Sherk HH, Marchinski LJ, Clancy M et al (1989) Ground reaction forces on the plantar surface of the foot after talectomy in the myelomeningocele. J Pediatr Orthop 9:269-275
21. Maynard MJ, Weiner LS, Burke SW (1992) Neuropathic foot ulceration in patients with myelodysplasia. J Pediatr Orthop 12:786-788
22. Roye BD (2005) Neuromuscular Disorders. Myelomeningocele. In: Dormans JP (ed) Pediatric Ortopaedics. Core knowledge in orthopaedics. Elsevier Mosby, Philadelphia, pp 483-504
23. Bliss DG, Menelaus MB (1986) The results of transfer of the tibialis anterior to the heel in patients who have a myelomeningocele. J Bone Joint Surg 68(A):1258-1264
24. Fraser RK, Hoffman EB (1991) Calcaneus deformity in the ambulant patient with myelomeningocele. J Bone Joint Surg 73(B):994-997
25. Rogrigues RC, Dias LS (1992) Calcaneus deformity in spina bifida: results of anterolateral release. J Pediatr Orthop 12:461-464
26. Janda JP, Skinner SR, Barto PS (1984) Posterior transfer of tibialis anterior in low-level myelodysplasia. Dev Med Child Neurol 26: 100-103
27. Drennan JC, Sharrard WJ (1971) The pathological anatomy of convex pes valgus. J Bone Joint Surg 53(B):455-461
28. Burkus JK, Moore DW, Raycroft JF (1983) Valgus deformity of the ankle in myelodysplastic patients. Correction of stapling of the medial part of the distal tibial physis. J Bone Joint Surg 65(A):1157-1162
29. Aronson DD, Middleton DL (1991) Extra-articular subtalar arthrodesis with cancellous bone graft and internal fixation for children with myelomeningocele. Dev Med Child Neurol 33:232-240
30. Lee YF, Grogan TJ, Moseley CF (1990) Extra-articular subtalar arthrodesis in myelodysplasia. Orthop Trans 14: 590-594
31. Bradley GW, Coleman SS (1981) The treatment of the calcaneocavus foot deformity. J Bone Joint Surg 63: 1159-1166

32. Dias LS, Jasty MJ, Collins P (1984) Rotational deformities of the lower limb in myelomeningocele: evaluation and treatment. J Bone Joint Surg 66(B):215-223

33. Fraser RK, Menelaus MB (1993) The management of tibial torsion in patients with spina bifida. J Bone Joint Surg 75(B):495-497

34. Wright JG, Menelaus MB, Broughton NS et al (1992) Lower extremity alignment in children with spina bifida. J Pediatr Orthop 12:232-234

35. Williams JJ, Graham GP, Dunne KB et al (1993) Late knee problems in myelomeningocele. J Pediatr Orthop 13:701-703

36. Wright JG, Menelaus MB, Broughton NS et al (1991) Natural history of knee contractures in myelomeningocele. J Pediatr Orthop 11:725-730

37. Dias LS (1982) Surgical management of knee contractures in myelomeningocele. J Pediatr Orthop 2:127-131

38. Marshall PD, Broughton NS, Menelaus MB et al (1996) Surgical release of knee flexion contractures in myelomeningocele. J Bone Joint Surg 78(B):912-916

39. Menelaus M (1998). The knee. In: Broughton N, Menelaus M (eds) Menelaus' orthopaedic management of spina bifida cystica. WB Saunders, Philadelphia, pp 129-134

40. Sandhu PS, Broughton NS, Menelaus MB (1995) Tenotomy of the ligamentum patellae in spina bifida: management of limited flexion range at the knee. J Bone Joint Surg 77(B): 832-833

41. Broughton N (1998). The hip. In: Broughton N, Menelaus M (eds) Menelaus' orthopaedic management of spina bifida cystica. WB Saunders, Philadelphia, pp 135-144

42. Broughton NS, Menelaus MB, Cole WG et al (1993) The natural history of hip deformity in myelomeningocele. J Bone Joint Surg 75(B):760-763

43. Mazur JM, Shurtleff D, Menelaus M et al (1989) Orthopaedic management of high-level spina bifida: Early walking compared with early use of a wheelchair. J Bone Joint Surg 71(A):56-61

44. Fraser RK, Bourke HM, Broughton NS et al (1995) Unilateral dislocation of the hip in spina bifida: A long-term follow-up. J Bone Joint Surg 77(B):615-619

45. Menelaus MB (1980) Progress in the management of the paralytic hip in myelomeningocele. Orthop Clin North Am 11:17-30

46. Lough LK, Nielsen DH (1986) Ambulation of children with myelomeningocele-parapodium versus parapodium with Orlau swivel modification. Dev Med Child Neurol 28:489-497

47. McCall RE, Schmidt WT (1986) Clinical experience with the reciprocal gait orthosis in myelodysplasia. J Pediatr Orthop 6:157-161

48. Yngve DA, Douglas R, Roberts JM (1984) The reciprocating gait orthosis in myelomeningocele. J Pediatr Orthop 4:304-310

49. Lee EH, Carroll NC (1985) Hip stability and ambulatory status in myelomeningocele. J Pediatr Orthop 5:522-527

50. Bazih J, Gross RH (1981) Hip surgery in the lumbar level myelomeningocele patient. J Pediatr Orthop 1:405-411

51. Erol B, Bezer M, Kucukdurmaz F et al (2005) Surgical management of hip instabilities in children with spina bifida. Acta Orthop Traumatol Turc 39:16-22

52. Trivedi J, Thompson JD, Slakey JB et al (2002) Clinical and radiographic predictors of scoliosis in patients with myelomeningocele. J Bone Joint Surg 84(A):1389-1394

53. Heeg M, Broughton NS, Menelaus MB (1998) Bilateral dislocation of the hip in spina bifida: A long-term follow-up study. J Pediatr Orthop 18:434-436

54. Tosi LL, Buck BD, Nason SS et al (1996) Dislocation of hip in myelomeningocele. The McKay hip stabilization. J Bone Joint Surg 78(A):664-673

55. Canale ST, Hammond NL III, Cotler JM et al (1975) Pelvic displacement osteotomy for chronic hip dislocation in myelodysplasia. J Bone Joint Surg 57:177-183

56. Stillwell A, Menelaus MB (1984) Walking ability after transplantation of the iliopsoas-a long term follow up. J Bone Joint Surg 66:656-659

57. Phillips DP, Lindseth RE (1992) Ambulation after transfer of adductors, external oblique, and tensor fascia lata in myelomeningocele. J Pediatr Orthop 12:712-717

58. Barnett J, Menelaus M (1998) Pressure sores and pathological fractures. In: Broughton N, Menelaus M (eds) Menelaus' orthopaedic management of spina bifida cystica. WB Saunders, Philadelphia, pp 51-65

59. Quan A, Adams R, Ekmark E et al (1998). Bone mineral density in children with myelomeningocele. Pediatrics 102: E34

60. Drummond DS, Moreau M, Cruess RL (1981) Postoperative neuropathic fractures in patients with myelomeningocele. Dev Med Child Neurol 23:147-150

61. Kumar SJ, Cowell HR, Towsend P (1984) Physeal, metaphyseal, and diaphyseal injuries of the lower extremities in children with myelomeningocele. J Pediatr Orthop 4:25-27.

62. Parsch K (1991) Origin and treatment of fractures in spina bifida. Eur J Pediatr Surg 1:298-305

63. Nagarkatti DG, Banta JV, Thomson JD (2000) Charcot arthropathy in spina bifida. J Pediatr Orthop 20:82-87

64. Phillips D (1998) Orthotics. In: Broughton N, Menelaus M (eds) Menelaus' orthopaedic management of spina bifida cystica. WB Saunders, Philadelphia, pp 67-76

CHAPTER 28
Habilitation of Children and Young Adults with Spina Bifida

Giuliana C. Antolovich, Alison C. Wray

Spina bifida is a complex congenital condition that has far reaching complications and consequences for the affected child. There are implications for mobility and self-care, independence, sensory function continence, schooling and social functioning, and a range of medical complications that can also result in chronic illness [1-3].

Although the prevalence of this condition at birth has fallen [3, 4], there is still significant geographic and racial variation in prevalence and severity of the disease [3-5]. Additionally, improved medical care and hydrocephalus management has resulted in improved survival not only through childhood, but also into adulthood [6]. Survival in children with spina bifida, at the more severe end of the disease spectrum, has improved significantly, from about 10% survival in the 1950s to 90% survival by the 1980s [7].

The care of children and young adults with spina bifida extends beyond the management of their acute medical and surgical needs. Habilitation in children and young adults with physical or intellectual disabilities is the process of enhancing development, self-worth, and self-determination, in order to maximise independence, and physical and emotional well-being. Medical care includes both management of the neurological consequences of spina bifida and a holistic approach to address the substantial care needs of children and young adults with spina bifida. The complexity of the care of these children is increased, as up to one-third will have associated anomalies and 5% of cases occur in the setting of a genetic syndrome [8]. These patients are best managed by a coordinated team approach including a habilitation paediatrician and multidisciplinary therapy team to ensure both optimum health and quality of life, recognising that health is not just the absence of disease, but the presence of physical, mental and social well-being.

Introduction

The care and management of the child with spina bifida starts at the earliest point in their life, when the diagnosis is made (pre- or postnatally). The significant issues with respect to medical and psychosocial morbidity need to be addressed from the prenatal period, and continue throughout life.

The health impact of spina bifida is very significant: hydrocephalus, neurologic impairment especially relating to mobility and faecal and urinary incontinence, spasticity, contractures, deformity, scoliosis, epilepsy, visual impairment, constipation, renal impairment, hypertension, impairment of sexual function, cognitive impairment, school integration, socialisation, psychological issues, obesity, and chronic pain are all recognised. In addition, this group are exposed to multiple episodes of surgery (neurosurgical, orthopaedic, urological). These issues are life-long and have a substantial impact on quality of life [2, 9-11].

Frequently as practitioners caring for children with spina bifida we are asked at diagnosis (pre- or postnatally) to predict the health impact for a particular child. It is difficult to clearly determine the level of the spina bifida lesion, as it is often irregular. There is often discordance between the motor and sensory levels, and also variations from right to left. Nonetheless, in general terms, higher lesions (L2 and above), are more often associated with more significant disability and complications, with higher likelihood of associated hydrocephalus, and therefore with a higher risk of cognitive impairment (and low IQ scores) [2, 12]. This also has implications for functional independence. Higher level lesions and the presence of hydrocephalus are associated with poor functional outcomes, and higher dependence in all activities of daily living, including social functioning [11].

Quality of life studies also demonstrate that children with spina bifida who have higher levels of physical disability (including problems with continence) have poor reported quality of life [10, 13, 14]. Children with spina bifida also score lower on the Paediatric Evaluation of Disability Index (PEDI), which gives a good assessment of functional ability and engagement [15].

Chronic disability and chronic illness have a significant impact on all aspects of functioning and hence quality of life. Aside from the primary problems of sensory and motor disorders, there are additional burdens of psychological adjustments and poor self-esteem [16]. Social isolation is not uncommon as a consequence of poor mobility, poor self-esteem, and is compounded by continence issues [14]. Health-related quality of life scores are significantly lower in young adults with spina bifida compared to the general population [9]. Family functioning resources and supports are also critical in determining outcome and quality of life.

It is increasingly recognised that children and adolescents with spina bifida have complex long-term needs that are influenced by, and impact upon, their family dynamic. Family centred care, where the family works with the health care providers to make informed decisions about the intervention and support the child and family receive, is considered best practise for the care of these individuals. Family centred care encompasses three principles: that (1) the parents know the children best and want the best for their children; (2) families are unique and different; and (3) optimal child functioning occurs within a supportive family and community context [17].

This chapter will look at the range of potential impacts and discuss each in turn. The focus will be on infancy, childhood, adolescence, and encompass issues of early adulthood and transition.

Perinatal Care

Many cases of spina bifida are detected prenatally, raising the issue of the optimal route of delivery. For many years, delivery via elective caesarean section was recommended as it was thought to reduce the risk of further neurological injury, to reduce the risk of infection, and to ensure high quality neonatal care. There have been no randomised controlled trials of delivery routes (vaginal versus caesarean section); however, recent retrospective reviews [18, 19] have failed to detect any improvements in motor function or ambulation in children delivered via caesarean section, suggesting that a trial of labour in a tertiary centre should be allowed unless obstetric indications suggest otherwise. In many cases, however, this is academic as despite advances in prenatal detection some lesions remain undetected until after the delivery.

Protection of the exposed spinal cord and nerves, and reduction of the potential risk of infection are critical goals, and time to surgical repair has been associated with eventual motor function. Surgical repair is usually undertaken within the first 48 hours of life to provide protection to the cord, re-establish the integrity of the central nervous system (CNS) and to limit the loss of cerebrospinal fluid (CSF).

The next critical issue in the care of an infant with spina bifida is the early recognition of hydrocephalus and the early institution of hydrocephalus management. The impact on neurocognitive development of unrecognised hydrocephalus is considerable.

Postnatal Care

The postnatal management of children with spina bifida requires coordinated care from paediatricians, rehabilitation physicians, neurosurgeons, urologists, orthopaedic surgeons, physical occupational and speech therapists, orthotists and psychologists. Ideally these services are delivered via a multidisciplinary spina bifida clinic.

Neurosurgical Issues

Detailed neurosurgical care is beyond the scope of this discussion and is covered in other chapters in this book. The role of the neurosurgeon in the habilitative care of children and adults with spina bifida focuses on the early detection and management of hydrocephalus/shunt dysfunction and the associated conditions that may cause further sensorimotor dysfunction: Chiari malformation and tethered cord.

Shunt dysfunction is frequently insidious in presentation and should be considered with any regression or loss of previous function, particularly a decline in school performance. Cognitive outcome has been related to the presence of hydrocephalus but particularly to the number of shunt interventions, suggesting that control of hydrocephalus is necessary to realise neurocognitive potential.

Both clinical and radiological surveillance of these patients is recommended to detect early signs of cord or hindbrain dysfunction from either Chiari malformation or tethered cord.

Urinary Tract

Bladder function is usually altered in children with spina bifida, with problems of sphincter dysfunction, and bladder hyperreflexia (detrusor overactivity), or atonia – neuropathic bladder [20]. There are a number of secondary consequences including incontinence, urinary retention with the potential for hydronephrosis, urinary reflux, urinary tract infections, and ultimately renal impairment and associated morbidity.

The social consequences of bladder incontinence are important to young adults with spina bifida [21]. Better self-concept is associated with urinary continence, and poor self-esteem is associated with incontinence [22], with quality of life measures linked to urinary continence [10, 21]. However, it is of interest that another study did not demonstrate improvement in health-related quality of life following lower urinary tract reconstruction procedures [23].

Early identification of a urinary system under high pressure is critical to maintain normal renal function [24]. Ultrasound imaging of the renal tract, voiding cystourethrograms, and urodynamics testing are commonly employed to monitor and assess [24, 25].

Complete emptying of the bladder is important. In the past, techniques such as Crede's method (application of external pressure from the abdomen on the bladder to stimulate emptying) have been found to incompletely empty the bladder, and to increase the risk of refluxing urine into the upper part of the system, and also of maintaining the system at higher pressures.

Early institution of clean intermittent catheterisation (CIC) is a mainstay of management of the neuropathic bladder [26, 27]. CIC is now generally accepted as effective long-term management, maintaining some degree of continence, and resulting in protection of the urinary tract and reducing secondary morbidity due to infections and renal impairment [26, 27].

Initially the CIC is done by a parent, usually the mother. By about 6 years old most children years are able to self-catheterise. However, the ability to achieve this depends on sitting ability and stability, motor function and ability, cognitive ability, and is also affected by family function and support and the ability of the parent to transition responsibility for care to the child [26].

In a recent study [26], a number of practical and emotional challenges were identified in children learning to self-catheterise. However, if the children were well-prepared and supported, self-catheterisation was well-incorporated into the daily routine, pro-viding increased privacy and independence. One of the critical issues also identified in this study was that success was also linked to ensuring appropriate privacy and space to self-catheterise when the child was at school.

The majority of young people with spina bifida use CIC, although a recent survey suggested that incontinence is still common, and continence pads are frequently required [2, 28].

The use of bladder antispasmodics (both oral and intravesical, oxybutinin) is common and effective [27, 28], as the detrusor overactivity is neuropathic in origin [27].

A number of different surgical procedures have been employed in children and young adults with spina bifida with the aim of preserving and protecting renal function, and of achieving urinary continence. In many cases, surgical intervention is required because of failure of medical management to maintain a low pressure system [24].

Bladder reconstruction or augmentation (using bowel, or self-augmentation with detrusorotomy) has been used in patients with reduced functional bladder capacity, enabling patients to achieve continence with CIC [29]. Procedures that increase bladder outlet resistance have also been used (bladder neck closure, cinches, artificial sphincters, slings, or biomaterial injection [28, 29]. A number of both continent (e.g., Mitrofanoff) and incontinent (vesicostomy) urinary diversion procedures have been used in this group of children [28-30]. There is much controversy about the role of many of these procedures, and many reported complications have been described [28, 29, 31].

Newer techniques of reinnervation of the neurogenic bladder have been described in a limited series [32]. A review of Botulinum toxin A therapy for neurogenic bladder management has shown it to be useful in the management of detrusor overactivity in children with spina bifida [33].

However, it was noted by Lemelle et al. [9, 28] that frequency of incontinence alone may not be the most important criterion for surgical intervention of continence management in this group. This is supported by the MacNeily study, which suggests that there is no improvement in health-related quality of life following lower urinary tract reconstruction procedures [23].

The risk of urinary tract infection is significant, and common in this group of children and young adults [2] and urine analysis is an important part of the work-up of any febrile episode in children. The symptoms that in an older child will herald the onset of a urine infection, such as dysuria and frequency, will not be easy to identify in the incontinent child with impaired perineal sensation. However, fever, flank pain, and changes in urinary voiding patterns are considered reliable measures of a urinary tract infection [25]. Vomiting and fever may be cardinal features of an evolving urinary tract infection in a young child. Prompt and vigorous treatment of urinary infections is advocated; however, prophylactic use of antibiotics is not supported or indicated [2].

Methods for the surveillance of the urinary tract vary. The use of renal ultrasound is probably the most universal [25]. The role of DTPA and DMSA or MAG-3 scans should be considered on a case by case basis.

There is a risk of renal impairment and renal failure in children with spina bifida; however, active urological care, with appropriate use of CIC, anti-muscarinic agents and surgical intervention where required, it should be possible to preserve renal function and eliminate the risk of renal failure [27].

Bowel

The function of the bowel is invariably affected in the child with spina bifida. The recto-anal inhibitory reflex is often preserved; however, the urge for defecation is lost. The external anal sphincter is often paralysed, and when the internal sphincter relaxes, soiling is inevitable. Colonic transit time is prolonged, and there is inadequate peristaltic activity and poor muscle tone. Both the reflux contraction of the rectum upon distension with faeces, and the gastro-colic reflex are impaired. Compounding these issues, there is impaired sensation and reduced activity of the voluntary muscles required for defecation, which result in problems with constipation and faecal incontinence [34, 35].

Although the morbidity associated with faecal incontinence is not comparable to that associated with urinary incontinence, the impact of faecal incontinence is more psychologically devastating and damaging. Anger, depression and poor self-esteem have all been described [35].

The secondary complications of pain, poor appetite, and worsening of urinary function and control cannot be underestimated (personal observation). Recognition and active treatment of constipation in the young child is important. Early use of aperients and regular bowel clearance helps avoid longer-term problems (see below).

In older children, instruction on how to produce a bowel motion with contraction of abdominal musculature is important, but is more effective when there is some perineal sensation [35]. Biofeedback has also been used, but with mixed results [35, 36].

Medical management for faecal incontinence requires the development of a predictable bowel habit by creating a pattern of defecation to reduce accidental soiling. Prevention of constipation is also critical. Laxatives, softeners and bulking agents all have some benefits.

Regular use of aperients is the first line of management. In infants, prune juice can be helpful. Its mode of action is not clear [37], and it is rarely sufficient to maintain bowel function (personal observation). Paraffin oil is generally well-tolerated and has few side-effects [38], however, anal leakage is often seen at higher doses [39] and there is potential for fat-soluble vitamin malabsorption with long-term use. Lactulose, an osmotic laxative, can also alter the microflora of the bowel. It is effective, but sometimes causes abdominal cramps, and compliance can be a problem [38]. Bulking agents that add fibre can be helpful, but should be used with caution, as the increase in the volume of stool can lead to more problems with accidental soiling (personal observation).

The addition of stimulant laxatives may be required because of the poor peristalsis of the bowel – sennosides and bisacodyl are the most commonly used agents [39].

The newer polyethylene glycol agents (PEG 3350, macrogol 3350) are very promising for the management of constipation, as they are better tolerated than other osmotic aperients [36]. Polyethylene glycol has been shown to be more effective than other osmotic laxatives in children with spina bifida [40].

Oral laxatives are often used in combination with rectal enemas (bisacodyl), digital rectal stimulation, and digital evacuation [41].

Large volume rectal enemas aim to clear the bowel, and reduce the risk of accidental soiling. The enemas can be water, saline, saline/phosphate combinations, or saline polyethylene glycol combinations [41]. Care must be taken to avoid the use of hypotonic or hypertonic solutions, as there is very good absorption across the rectal mucosa and this can result in significant fluid shifts (personal observation).

There are limitations with the use of rectal enemas, as the child must have the physical and cognitive ability to self-administer. This is considerably more challenging than self-catheterisation, and invariably requires support from a carer [35]. Furthermore, the enema only clears the left side of the colon at best. In many cases, a continence pad is still required, although the use of anal plugs has also been successful in selected patients [42].

Surgical alternatives to manage both incontinence and intractable constipation are available. Currently, the most common procedure creates a stoma through which ante-grade colonic enemas can be given. This has the advantage of clearing the left and right side of the bowel, and offering independence to the child and young adult, as antegrade colonic enemas are more readily self-administered than rectal enemas. The two most common procedures are: (1) Malone antegrade colonic enema (MACE) and (2) Monti plasty to create a catheterisable neoconduit (umbilicus to transverse colon) [43]. Colostomy is rarely used or required [44].

Complications with antegrade colonic enema procedures are well-described [43, 45], with stoma stenosis the most common complication [45], and delayed emptying often described [41]. However, there are significant reported improvements in quality of life [43], and high levels of satisfaction [45] with antegrade colonic enemas.

Neurocognitive Function

Children with spina bifida have a range of recognised cognitive deficits [46, 47] that impact on their school and social functioning. This group of children have a unique neurocognitive profile, with higher verbal than performance IQ, better reading than mathematical function, and good grammatical language and vocabulary, with poor pragmatic language skills [47].

Difficulties with higher order language, inferential activities, and social discourse tasks have been described [48]. Additional problems include difficulties with visual spatial function, specific learning problems (mathematics), and significant attentional issues [49, 50]. In a recent study of a selected group of young adults with spina bifida (intact global function, normal verbal intelligence scores, no clinical depression), those with associated hydrocephalus had evidence of poor executive function [51]. It is noteworthy that this same group scored well on verbal intelligence and emotional intelligence tasks [51].

These problems have an impact on everyday function, and combined with the physical and medical morbidity experienced by young adults with spina bifida, have a negative impact on quality of life [49].

Significant morbidity associated with frequent hospitalisations, multiple medical and surgical procedures, and chronic pain (often under-recognised), are well-described in this group of children and young adults [2, 14, 52]. Additionally, challenges with mobility, independence, continence, sexual function, body image and cosmesis can also have a negative impact of the psychological function of children and young adults. Higher rates of depression and anxiety have been reported in this group than in age-matched peers [53].

Neuropsychological assessment is critical to support and understand the specific challenges of each child and young adult with spina bifida. An understanding of each individual's "higher order" cognitive abilities will help to identify strengths and weaknesses, support school success and ensure that appropriate vocational choices are available.

Strong support networks and connectivity are critical to support the young person as they move through adolescence [54].

Mobility

The ability to ambulate is determined by the neurological impairment of each child with spina bifida. The health benefits of ambulation, such as improved urinary drainage, bowel function and reduction in bone fractures and pressure sores, have been known since the 1970s [55, 56]. Additionally, ambulation allows improved socialisation and community participation, decreases unemployment and is an independent predictor of educational outcome in young adults with spina bifida [57].

Assistive technology can in many cases be used to facilitate ambulation in this population. For mobility, orthoses such as swivel walkers (± hoists) [58], the reciprocating-gait orthosis [59, 60], frames, crutches and braces may be employed. The success of this technology relies on careful ongoing assessment from the therapeutic team to assess the achievement of identified goals and to identify the appropriateness of ongoing therapy. As always the child needs to be assessed within the family and social context; not infrequently the positive benefits of assisted ambulation do not outweigh dissatisfaction with the appearance, cost and maintenance of the technology [61].

Musculoskeletal Complications, Skin Management and Bone Health

The neurological lesion of spina bifida has many implications for lower limb function and skin integrity.

Reduced sensation, paralysis and immobility are significant risk factors for injury to the skin and joints, and for the development of pressure areas.

Wound healing can be significantly impaired, and further complicated because of difficulties in changing position. Good seating, protective bedding, pressure control devices (cushions, shoes, orthoses), and frequent position changes are important to maintain skin integrity. Daily skin inspection is critical to ensure early management of skin lesions, prior to the development of deep wounds [2].

There is a risk of secondary infection, and spread to deeper tissues, including bone. Pressure care, frequent dressings, and debridement may also be required. Specialised procedures, including vacuum assisted closure of wounds [62] may be important in wound care management.

Management of continence stomas are also a critical part of wound and skin care management in this group of children and young adults, and high rates of complications are described [63].

The musculoskeletal problems experienced depend on the extent and level of the spinal lesion. There is a significant impact on mobility, with many individuals being largely wheelchair bound. Aids to support mobility and physical therapy are key management issues.

Both flaccid paralysis and spasticity can be observed. In some cases, spasticity management can be useful; this is predominantly to reduce pain and discomfort, however, and rarely does it prevent the development of deformity. Baclofen, a gamma-aminobutyric acid (GABA) agonist, has been shown to be efficacious in this group of children (personal observation).

Foot deformity is a very common problem. Rigidity of the foot leads to problems with pressure sores and ulceration, and difficulty in managing orthoses. Correction of the deformity to produce a flexible foot is the desired outcome [64]. Deformity and altered stresses at the knee joint are also an important cause of secondary arthritis and pain [64].

Hip dislocation affects 30-50% children and young adults with spina bifida, and congenital hip dislocation is not uncommon [2]. The secondary problems of pelvic obliquity, contractures, associated scoliosis, and pressure sores are significant. The aim of hip surveillance to avoid hip subluxation and dislocation is to maintain comfortable sitting posture, and avoid pain. There is some controversy as to treatment of hip dislocation in walkers [65]: a level pelvis and good range of motion at the hip are probably more important in maintaining good ambulation [66]. Importantly, in this population the low tone hip is at risk of subluxation and dislocation (personal communication Professor H.K. Graham, Orthopaedics, Royal Children's Hospital Melbourne). Ongoing sur-

veillance into adulthood is important as re-dislocation is not uncommon [65].

Scoliosis and kyphosis are also important management issues. Scoliosis affects 30-50% of children with spina bifida [67]. Corrective surgery has predominantly occurred in children and young adults who are non-ambulant. The aims of the surgery have been correction of deformity, and improvement of posture and therefore self-perception. The more significant issues relate to pain and sitting balance, which are found to be the case in those with higher level lesions [2]. A recent Canadian study suggested that young people with spina bifida did not have poor self-perception related to their posture, and that sitting balance was the most important aim for scoliosis correction [67]. This has implications as the risks associated with scoliosis surgery in this group are significant.

Bone health is also important to address, as this group of children have a number of significant risk factors for osteoporosis and secondary fractures. Ensuring good vitamin D status, and screening for osteoporosis with DEXA scan in this high risk group is suggested. The use of alendronate, an oral bisphosphonate, has been successful in children with spina bifida [68].

Transitional Care

Morbidity related to the underlying spina bifida lesion is high, as demonstrated by the above discussion. There is much evidence that these problems persist into the adult years [1], and the need for coordinated supportive services in adult care settings is critical for the long-term health management and quality of life.

From a patient and family perspective, one of the most difficult issues that occur at this time is the process of medical emancipation. Medical emancipation allows the individual to make his or her own decisions about medical treatment; because of the significant medical complications and chronic disability this process is often delayed [69]. Frequently this emancipation is thrust upon the adolescent by the rigid structures of the adult medical services. Transition involves facilitating and supporting the process of emancipation whilst still in paediatric services.

The identification of the key factors associated with the successful medical emancipation and transition of young adults with chronic health issues and developmental disabilities to adult services is a key future goal of care [70].

References

1. McDonnell GV, McCann JP (2000) Issues of medical management in adults with spina bifida. Childs Nerv Syst 16(4):222-227
2. Verhoef M et al (2004) Secondary impairments in young adults with Spina bifida. Dev Med Child Neurol 46:420-427
3. Kennedy DS et al (1998) Spina bifida. Med J Aust 169:182-183
4. Mitchell LE et al (2004) Spina bifida. Lancet 364:1885-1895
5. Williams LJ et al (2005) Decline in the prevalence of spina bifida and anencephaly by race/ethnicity 1995-2002. Pediatrics 116:580-586
6. Bowman RM et al (2001) Spina bifida outcome: a 25 year perspective. Pediatr Neurosurg 34:114-120
7. Dastgiri S et al (2003) Survival of children born with congenital anomalies. Arch Dis Child 88:390-394
8. The Consultative Council on Obstetric and Paediatric Mortality and Morbidity (2005) Annual report for the year 2004 incorporating the 43rd Survey of Perinatal deaths in Victoria. Melbourne
9. Lemelle JL et al (2006) Quality of life and continence in patients with spina bifida. Qual Life Res 15:1481-1492
10. Rendeli C et al (2005) Assessment of health status in children with spina bifida. Spinal Cord 43:230-235
11. Verhoef M et al (2006) Functional independence among young adults with spina bifida, in relation to hydrocephalus and level of lesion. Dev Med Child Neurol 48:114-119
12. Shurtleff DB, Lemire RJ (1995) Epidemiology, etiologic factors and prenatal diagnosis of open spinal dysraphism. Neurosurg Clin N Am 6:183-193
13. Padua L et al (2004) Relationship between the clinical-neurophysiologic pattern, disability, and quality of life in adolescents with spina bifida. J Child Neurol 19:952-957
14. Pit-ten Cate IM et al (2002) Disability and quality of life in spina bifida and hydrocephalus. Dev Med Child Neurol 44:317-322
15. Tsai PY et al (2002) Functional investigation in children with spina bifida – measured by the Pediatric Evaluation of Disability Inventory (PEDI). Childs Nerv Syst 18:48-53
16. Lavigne JV, Faier-Routman J (1993) Correlates of psychological adjustment to pediatric physical disorders: a meta-analytic review and comparison with existing models. J Dev Behav Pediatr 14:117-123
17. King S et al (2004) Family-centered service for children with cerebral palsy and their families: a review of the literature. Semin Pediatr Neurol 11:78-86
18. Lewis D et al (2004) Elective Cesarean delivery and long-term motor function or ambulation status in infants with meningomyelocele. Obstet Gynecol 103:469-473
19. Merrill DC et al (1998) The optimal route of delivery for fetal meningomyelocele. Am J Obstet Gynecol 179:234-240
20. Ab E et al (2004) Detruser over activity in spina bifida: how long does it need to be treated? Neurourol Urodyn 23:685-688
21. Verhoef M et al (2005) High prevalence of incontinence among young adults with spina bifida: description, prediction and problem perception. Spinal Cord 43(6):331-340
22. Moore C et al (2004) Impact of urinary incontinence of self-concept in children with spina bifida. J Urol 171:1659-1662
23. MacNeily AE et al (2005) Lower urinary tract reconstruction for spina bifida – does it improve health related quality of life? J Urol 174:1637-1643
24. Lee MW, Greenfield SP (2005) Intractable high-pressure bladder in female infants with spina bifida: clinical characteristics and use of vesicostomy. Urology 65:568-571
25. Elliott SP et al (2005) Bacteriuria management and urological evaluation of patients with spina bifida and neurogenic bladder: a multicenter survey. J Urol 173:217-220
26. Edwards M et al (2004) Neuropathic bladder and intermittent catheterization: social and psychological impact on children and adolescents. Dev Med Child Neurol 46:168-177
27. Dik P et al (2006) Early start to therapy preserves kidney function in spina bifida patients. Eur Urol 49:908-913
28. Lemelle JL et al (2006) A multicenter evaluation of urinary incontinence management and outcome in spina bifida. J Urol 175:208-212
29. Gonzalez R, Schimke CM (2002) Strategies in urological reconstruction in myelomeningocele. Curr Opin Urol 12:485-490
30. Shelby N et al (2005) Vesicostomy revisited: the best treatment for the hostile bladder in myelodysplastic children? B J Urol 97:397-400
31. Stein R et al (2005) Urinary diversion in children and adolescents with neurogenic bladder: the Mainz experience. Pediatr Nephrol 20:926-931
32. Xiao CG (2006) Reinnervation of neurogenic bladder: historic review and introduction of a somatic-autonomic reflex pathway procedure for patients with spinal cord injury or spina bifida. Eur Urol 49:22-28
33. Schurch B, Corcos J (2005) Botulinum toxin injections for pediatric incontinence. Curr Opin Urol 15:264-267
34. Rintala RJ (2002) Fecal incontinence in anorectal malformations, neuropathy, and miscellaneous conditions. Semin Ped Surg 119:75-82
35. Di Lorenzo C, Benninga MA (2004) Pathophysiology of pediatric fecal incontinence. Gastroenterology 126(1 Suppl 1):S33-40
36. Baker SS et al (2006) Evaluation and treatment of constipation in children: Summary of updated recommendations of the North American Society for Pediatric Gastroenterology, Hepatology and Nutrition. J Pediatr Gastroenterol Nutr 43:405-407

37. Stacewicz-Sapuntzakis M et al (2001) Chemical composition and potential health effects of prunes: a functional food? Crit Rev Food Sci Nutr 41:251-286
38. Urganci N (2005) A comparative study: The efficacy of liquid paraffin and lactulose in management of chronic constipation. Pediatrics Int 47:15-19
39. Biggs WS, Dery W (2006) Evaluation and treatment of constipation in infants and children. Am Family Phys 73:469-477
40. Rendeli C et al (2006) Polyethylene glycol 4000 vs lactulose for the treatment of neurogenic constipation in myelomeningocele children: a randomized-controlled clinical trial. Aliment Pharmacol Ther 23: 1259-1265
41. Lemelle JL et al (2006) A multicenter study of the management of disorders of defecation in patients with spina bifida. Neurogastroenterol Motil 18:123-128
42. Bond C et al (2007) Anal plugs for the management of fecal incontinence in children and adults – a randomized control trial. J Clin Gastroenterol 41:45-53
43. Perez et al (2001) Bowel management with ante grade colonic enema using a Malone or a Monti conduit – clinical results. Eur J Pediatr Surg 11:315-318
44. Krogh K et al (2001) Colorectal symptoms in patients with neurological diseases. Acta Neurol Scand 3:335-343
45. Curry JI et al (1999) The MACE procedure: experience in the United Kingdom. J Pediatr Surg 34:338-340
46. Barf HA et al (2003) Cognitive status of young adults with spina bifida. Dev Med Child Neurol 45:813-820
47. Dennis M et al (2006) A model of neuro cognitive function in spina bifida over the life span. J Int Neuropsychol Soc 12:285-296
48. Dise JE, Lohr ME (1998) Examination of deficits in conceptual reasoning abilities associated with spina bifida. Am J Phys Med Rehabil 77:247-251
49. Hetherington R et al (2006) Functional outcome in young adults with spina bifida and hydrocephalus. Childs Nerv Syst 22:117-124
50. Rose BM, Holmbeck GN (2007) Attention and executive functions in adolescents with spina bifida. J Pediatr Psychol 32:983-994
51. Iddon JL et al (2004) Neuropsychological profile of young adults with spina bifida with or without hydrocephalus. J Neurol Neurosurg Psych 75:1112-1118
52. Clancy CA et al (2005) Pain in children and adolescents with spina bifida. Dev Med Child Neurol 47:27-34
53. Appleton PL et al (1997) Depressive symptoms and self-concept in young people with spina bifida. J Pediatr Psychol 22:707-722
54. Barf HA et al (2007) Life satisfaction in young adults with spina bifida. Dev Med Child Neurol 49:458-63.
55. Carroll N (1974) The orthotic management of the spina bifida child. Clin Orthop 122:198-114.
56. Rose GK (1976) Surgical/orthotic management of spina bifida. In: Murdoch G (ed) The advance of orthotics. Edward Arnold, London, pp 403-414
57. Barf HA et al (2004) Educational career and predictors of type of education in young adults with spina bifida. Int J Rehabil Res 27:45-52
58. Stallard J et al (2003) New technical advances in swivel walkers. Prosthet Orthot Int 27:132-138
59. Gerritsma-Bleeker CL et al (1997) Ambulation with the reciprocating-gait orthosis. Experience in 15 children with myelomeningocoele or paraplegia. Acta Orthop Scan 68:470-473
60. Roussos N et al (2004) A long-term review of severely disabled spina bifida patients using a reciprocal walking system. Disabil Rehabil 23:239-244
61. Johnson KL et al (2007) Assistive technology use among adolescents and young adults with spina bifida. Am J Pub Health 97:330-336
62. Mendonca DA et al (2005) Vacuum-assisted closure to aid wound healing in foot and ankle surgery. Foot Ankle Int 26:761-766
63. Barqawi A et al (2004) Lessons learned from stomal complication in children with cutaneous catheterisable continent stomas. Br J Urol Int 94:1344-1347
64. Dias L (2004) Orthopedic care in spina bifida: past, present and future. Dev Med Child Neurol 46:5769
65. Smith PL et al (2005) Measuring physical function in children with spina bifida and dislocated hips. J Pediatr Orthop 25:273-279
66. Heeg M et al (1998) Bilateral dislocation of the hip in spina bifida; a long-term follow-up study. J Pediatr Orthop 18:434-436
67. Wai EK et al (2000) Assessing physical disability in children with spina bifida and scoliosis. J Pediatr Orthop 20:765-770
68. Sholas MG et al (2005) Oral Bisphosphonates to treat disuse osteopenia in children with disabilities. A case series. J Pediatr Orthop 25:326-331
69. Buran CF et al (2004) Adolescents with myelomeningocele: activities, beliefs, expectation, and perceptions. Dev Med Child Neurol 46:244-242
70. Binks JA et al (2007) What do we really know about the transition to adult-centered health care? A focus on cerebral palsy and spina bifida. Arch Phys Med Rehabil 88:1064-1073

CHAPTER 29
Independence in Mobility

Sharon Vladusic, David Phillips

Introduction

The recent integration of children and adults with disabilities into mainstream society has resulted in a renewed interest in their ability to be independent and to lead productive lifestyles. Advances in science and technology have enabled many with disabilities to achieve functional goals in activities of daily living, which include mobility.

Mobility has been defined as an individual's ability to move about effectively in his or her surroundings, without the assistance of other individuals, but where appropriate, in a wheelchair or with other assistive devices and aids [1]. Effective and efficient mobility allows a child to move from place to place to explore their environment, and stimulate their growth and development. Mobility and locomotion provide the means for learning, socialisation, and the development of cognition, independence and competence [2]. Locomotion is regarded as the major way in which a child's sense of initiative is achieved [3].

The need for efficient and effective mobility has become an increasingly important component in the medical management of children and adolescents with disabilities [2]. Mobility and ambulation signify independence and are important to the quality of life and lifestyle of the child with spina bifida and their family. Independence in mobility, which enables a child to fully participate in the activities of life, should be an important goal in the management of children with myelodysplasia.

The International Classification Model of Functioning, Disability and Health [4], also known as the ICF, has been developed by the World Health Organisation to provide a health status classification of disability and functioning due to the consequences of a health condition (Fig. 29.1, Table 29.1). The emphasis is on function, rather than on the health condition itself, and is structured around three components which are multifactorial, interactive and dynamic:

1. Body structures and function
2. Activities and participation
3. Environmental and personal factors

Myelomeningocele is considered 'the most complex treatable congenital anomaly of the central nervous system that is consistent with life' [5]. It is characterised by impaired mobility, which varies in severity from a mild motor deficit to complete lower limb paralysis.

Recent studies have emphasised that functional independence in mobility, self-care, and social cognition are important contributing factors to improving health-related quality of life (HRQOL) in adolescents with spina bifida [6, 7].

This chapter will discuss children and adolescents with myelodysplasia and the complex interaction between the components that influence a child's mobility and physical function, and their performance and involvement in life situations.

Activity and Participation

Our centre's philosophy is focused on assisting children with spina bifida to achieve their best possible functional outcome through independent mobility and good general strength and fitness. We encourage children in our centre to be physically active and fit, and involved in activities and exercise that can be incorporated into daily life (Fig. 29.2). Anecdotally, we find those children who participate in organised sport and regular activity are more confident, more social and appear to have fewer difficulties with self-esteem, particularly in their adolescent years. Recent evidence shows that activity and physical exercise stimulates brain processes, raises serotonin levels in the brain and

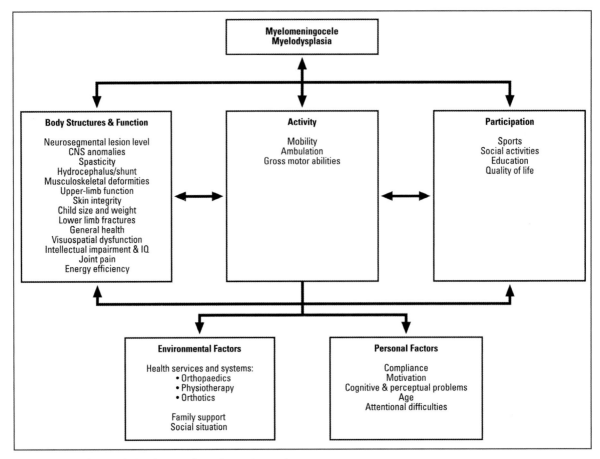

Fig. 29.1. ICF for myelodysplasia and myelomeningocele

Table 29.1. Definitions of the ICF Components (World Health Organisation, International Classification of Functioning, Disability and Health 2002 [4])

Body Functions are physiological functions of body systems (including psychological functions)

Body Structures are anatomical parts of the body such as organs, limbs and their components

Impairments are problems in body function or structure such as a significant deviation or loss

Activity is the execution of a task or action by an individual

Participation is involvement in a life situation

Participation Restrictions are problems an individual may experience in involvement in life situations

Environmental Factors make up the physical, social and attitudinal environment in which people live and conduct their lives

els of everyday physical activity, regardless of their ambulatory status [9-11]. This can result in a negative spiral of hypoactivity, causing a reduction in physical fitness and increased body fat, leading in turn to lower physical activity levels [11, 12]. Physical fitness has also been reported as subnormal in this population group [12-14]. Poor physical fitness combined with a sedentary lifestyle increases the risk of obesity and cardiovascular disease in the future [12, 15, 16].

There is evidence of the benefits of exercise for children and adolescents with disabilities [17-19]. Anecdotal evidence shows that involvement in sporting activities from a young age assists in personality development and level of independence, and the development of abilities to interact with peers [20]. Participation in sport also increases the trunk and upper limb strength, improves co-ordination and cardiovascular endurance, and boosts self-esteem and self-concept [17, 19, 21].

A balance between a child's educational and physical fitness needs is essential. The use of ambulation

can have a beneficial effect on a person's mood and behaviour [8].

Adolescents with myelomeningocele often have a more passive dependent lifestyle with lower lev-

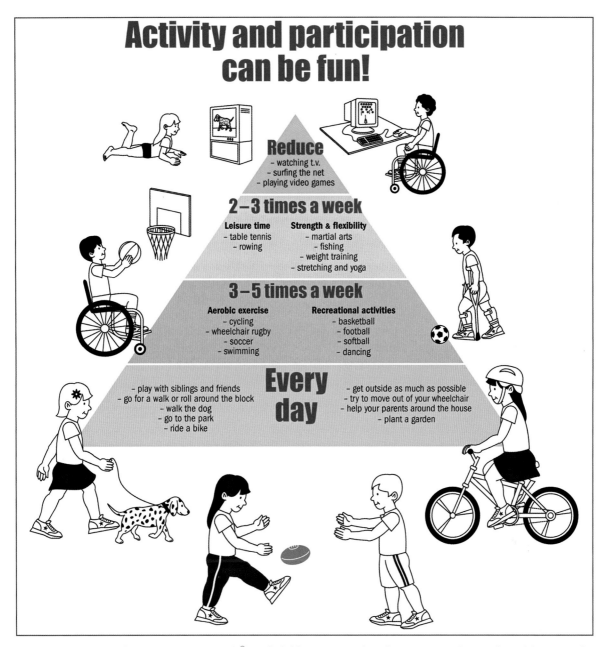

Fig. 29.2. Activity and Participation Pyramid. ©Royal Children's Hospital, Melbourne, Australia, as adapted from 'Aim for Activity' poster, with the permission of Dr. Gregory S. Liptak MD MPH, Golisano Children's Hospital at Strong University of Rochester Medical Centre

programs at school primarily for fitness may not be appropriate and alternative options may be required. A child with spina bifida should be encouraged to be involved in sporting and social activities with their peers, with modifications to activities as required. Children and adolescents with myelomeningocele benefit from creative and challenging physical fitness programs from an early age, and need to be taught to be responsible for their physical fitness, activity levels, nutrition and weight management.

Classification of Mobility

Different classification systems are used to describe both the neurological lesion level and motor function in children with myelomeningocele. The ICF classify mobility in children with spina bifida according to three dimensions:

- Body structures and function.
- Activity.
- Participation.

Body Structures and Function – Neurosegmental Lesion Level

The 'neurosegmental lesion level' is a term commonly referred to in the literature when discussing mobility and ambulation in children with spina bifida. The neurological level of lesion is classified according to the most caudal intact nerve root, determined by the motor function of the lower limbs. Lesion level is often defined as the lowest nerve root level with Grade 3 strength on manual muscle testing (MMT).

Detailed and accurate assessment of lower limb muscle power in children with spina bifida is performed through MMT, usually undertaken by physiotherapists. Serial examinations are undertaken on a six monthly or yearly basis, depending on a child's age and/or neurological status. MMT assesses the child's ability to actively contract a muscle or group of muscles against gravity or manual resistance [22].

The accuracy and predictive value of MMT has been questioned [23, 24], since the use of traditional muscle strength testing relies on a child's co-operation and ability to follow directions. Grading and methods of muscle testing in infants and young children require modification through the use of developmental and functional activities [21]. When testing neonates, the grading of muscle power into 'full/present', 'weak' or 'absent' categories, may be more accurate and easily understood [23].

Accurate assessment of lower limb muscle function is possible by three years of age, and this is verified by ongoing assessments throughout childhood [25]. MMT is most accurate and stable in children five years of age and older [24].

It is suggested that a classification system of the type of paralysis in the upper and lower limbs (i.e., flaccid paralysis versus spasticity) should be used in addition to grouping children according to their motor lesion level [26, 27].

In the literature, the most frequently used classifications of neurological lesion level are:
- Sharrard [28-31] (Fig. 29.3).
- Hoffer [32-35, 26].
- Lindseth [36-39].

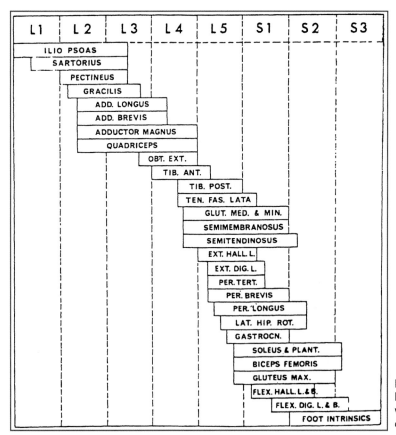

Fig. 29.3. The innervation of the lower limb muscles. Reproduced from [28], with permission from ©The Royal College of Surgeons of England

Two additional classification systems have been described in recent literature. Broughton et al. [40] uses a modification of Sharrard's neurosegmental levels. McDonald et al. [41] proposes grouping children with myelomeningocele according to specific muscle strength patterns. This is not to classify motor level, but rather to use lower limb muscle function to predict future ambulation capacities and establish 'ambulatory goals'.

The diagnosis of the neurological level of the lesion strongly influences a child's predicted ambulatory status, orthotics and therapy management and surgical intervention, with the level of motor function affecting the child's ability to perform functional activities.

Activity

Hoffer [32] categorised ambulation into four functional levels:

1. Community ambulators – walk indoors and outdoors for most of their activities, possibly with the use of orthotics and/or gait aides (e.g. crutches). They may use a wheelchair for long distances.
2. Household ambulators – walk indoors with orthotics and gait aides; sometimes use a wheelchair indoors. Use wheelchair for all outdoor and community activities.
3. Non-functional ambulators (therapeutic/exercise) – walk in therapy sessions only. Wheelchair for all other mobility.
4. Non-ambulators – use wheelchair indoors and outdoors.

There are often significant individual variations in clinical presentation and ambulatory abilities within a given neurological lesion level, particularly at lumbar levels of function. It has been suggested that the term 'functional motor level' be used when there are discrepancies between a child's motor level and motor function [42].

A variety of other ambulatory classifications are seen in the literature:

- Good, fair and poor walkers and sitters [43].
- 'Walkers' = community ambulators; and 'non-walkers' = household and non-ambulatory status [44, 45, 46].
- 'Useful walking' (can walk a 25 metre distance, walking within home/school/in community/to car) and 'non-useful walking' (walking with maximum support and of therapeutic use only) [47].
- Independently ambulant, ambulant with assistance, wheelchair-bound [48].

Parameters which evaluate and classify motor function, mobility and ambulatory status need to be easily understood by health professionals, parents and the general public. The term 'community ambulator' is frequently used in reference to a child's ambulation capacities, however this classification does not differentiate between those children who both ambulate and use a wheelchair, and those who only ambulate. Some classification systems tend to overestimate or underestimate the ability of children and adolescents with spina bifida categorised as community ambulators.

Children and parents may have a different perception of their ambulatory abilities, in comparison to health professionals. There are often discrepancies between reported and actual ambulation, with considerable variation in the distances and frequency of 'walking' by those children with spina bifida classified as community ambulators [49].

There is also little information about the effectiveness of methods used to classify mobility. Lerner-Frankiel [50] reported differences between actual mobility demands in community settings and the distance and speed criteria which were used to classify children with disabilities as 'functional community ambulators'.

Participation

It has been suggested that examining the distances a child can ambulate without stopping may better determine a child's true ambulatory status [49, 51]. The Functional Mobility Scale (FMS) is a simple assessment tool designed to measure a child's mobility within their various environments [52]. Functional mobility includes all the methods an individual uses to move and interact within the environment, ranging from independent walking to wheelchair use. The FMS rates a child's usual ambulation abilities over three distances, which represent home, school and community settings (Fig. 29.4). It includes the need for any assistive or mobility devices over these distances. The FMS has been shown to be both valid and reliable in children with cerebral palsy, but has also been used successfully in children with myelomeningocele in our centre.

The Timed Up and Go (TUG) test is a test of functional ambulatory mobility in adults that has recently been modified and examined for reliability and validity in normal children and children with disabilities [53]. Although the TUG test is not used for classification purposes, it provides a way of measuring a child's ability to integrate transitions of movement (e.g.

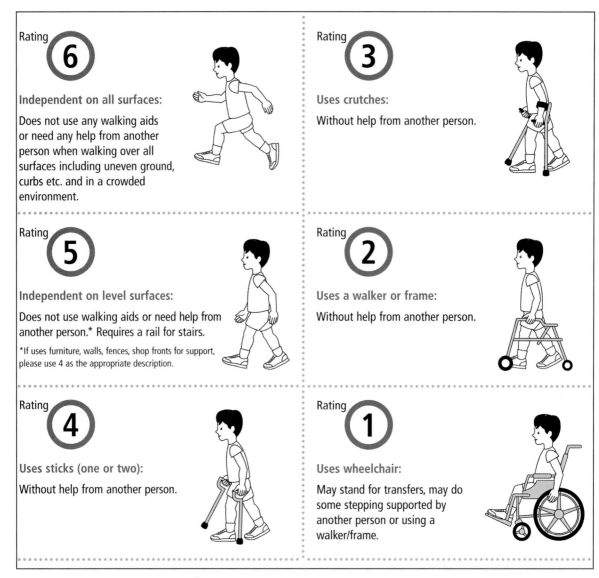

Fig. 29.4. Functional Mobility Scale. ©Royal Children's Hospital, Melbourne, Australia

sit to stand) and to move effectively [54]. While the number of children with disabilities tested in this study was small, the TUG test appears to be a reliable, valid, objective, quick and easy-to-use test of independence and functional mobility. Further studies of its use in the spina bifida population are recommended.

Assessment

Children and adolescents with spina bifida require thorough assessment, ongoing monitoring and lifelong surveillance by a multidisciplinary team of health professionals. In our centre, physiotherapists use an assessment tool known as the IMSG – International Myelodysplasia Study Group [55]. The IMSG project at the Royal Children's Hospital in Melbourne currently provides a core clinical and research physiotherapy service to children and adolescents with spina bifida across the state of Victoria in Australia.

The IMSG is a comprehensive, standardised assessment with objective measures for this complex and challenging condition. Qualitative and quantitative assessment is necessary to identify a child's strengths and difficulties, functional status, motor development, and to plan appropriate management. The assessment is repeated at regular intervals according to the child's age, needs and neurological status. Sequential examinations allow comparison to determine a child's progress, and the assessment includes the

ICF domains of body structures and function, activity and performance, as detailed below.

Body structures and function:
- Spine and posture.
- Joint range of movement and contracture management.
- Muscle strength testing of lower limbs on an expanded Oxford scale.
- Assessment of tone and sensation.
- Growth parameters (arm span, height, etc.).
- Upper limb function (gross measure of upper limb strength in using gait aides, grip strength, co-ordination).

Activity and Participation:
- Assessment of function using Hoffer's classification.
- Mobility – evaluate gait, wheelchair abilities, transfers, use of assistive devices, ambulation on different surfaces and environments, child's endurance.
- Gross motor skills – ability to move into/out of different positions, maintain positions, function within positions.
- Self-care – activities of daily living which include hygiene, feeding, dressing abilities and level of independence in such activities.

Standardised developmental tests, such as the Bayley Scales of Infant Development [56] and Motor Assessment of Infants (MAI) [57] can also provide quantitative objective information about motor abilities. When used for infants with spina bifida, they need to include modifications if the child uses adaptive equipment. When interpreting overall scores, the influence of motor level and associated orthopaedic and/or neurological problems should be considered.

The IMSG is a valuable clinical tool in allowing early detection of neurological deterioration, assisting in clinical decision-making and judging the effectiveness of interventions. The results of the initial and subsequent muscle strength testing of lower limbs are used to classify the neurosegmental level of lesion and possibly predict ambulation abilities and functional outcomes. Specific and realistic goals are formulated for each child from assessment results, aiming to maximise a child's function, independence and self-esteem, and minimise family stress.

Mobility versus Ambulation – Costs and Benefits

The term 'ambulation' refers to upright mobility, and includes the amount of assistance required to 'walk' in different environments (home, school, outdoors, stairs), both with and without assistive devices such as crutches or orthoses [58, 59]. The term 'ambulation', rather than 'walking', is used when referring to spina bifida gait, as it describes a variety of gait patterns used in this population, rather than just reciprocal stepping.

In today's world with the competitive nature of the health dollar and the need for evidence-based practice, the question is raised-should extensive resources be put into encouraging upright ambulation in the young child with a high level myelomeningocele when it is deemed unlikely that they will be a 'community walker' in the future? Are there benefits and advantages of upright ambulation that outweigh the costs and possible disadvantages, even if the child ambulates for a limited time?

In the ICF multidimensional approach to function and disability, mobility is considered in the context of how it assists a disabled child's participation in society during childhood, adolescence and adulthood. Upright ambulation is a component of mobility that may be a stepping-stone to a child's involvement in life situations such as education, sport and future vocation. The questions posed above perhaps should include:
- Does ambulation in childhood contribute to the quality of life of a child with spina bifida and their family in the immediate and long-term future?
- Are there benefits of ambulation in childhood that contribute to a child's increased participation in society and involvement in life situations in adulthood (regardless whether they are a long-term community ambulator or wheelchair user as adults)?

Treatment philosophies regarding mobility and ambulation differ from centre to centre. Some have a vigorous approach with large investments in therapy, orthotics, assistive devices and orthopaedic surgery to try and achieve and maintain the highest levels of ambulation. In contrast, an eclectic approach offers a variety of mobility options to encourage independence, but does not aggressively strive for upright ambulation. Children have limited gait training, limited physiotherapy, and orthopaedic care is aimed at good seating posture for wheelchair and activities of daily living.

The well-intentioned advocates of each approach cite many physiological benefits to support their management. Children with high level lesions who ambulate in early childhood have been reported as having significantly few lower limb fractures and pressure sores and increased independence in adolescence at home and school, compared to children who have always used a wheelchair for mobility [60].

In contrast, advocates for wheelchair mobility suggest that ambulation should be discouraged in children with high level myelomeningocele lesions, who should learn to use a wheelchair early in life [61]. They maintain that these children learn skills in activities of daily living earlier, and that they move faster, compete better in physical activities and are more likely to be independent and continent in bladder and bowel function [62].

In our centre, most children are given the opportunity to achieve a goal of functional ambulation, using therapy, orthotics and surgery. We firmly believe that children with spina bifida benefit from opportunities to move from different positions and it is important to look at a variety of approaches to meet the different mobility needs of each individual child with myelodysplasia [2]. Normal children are encouraged to be active and experience a variety of postures and activities, and we believe the approach to children with spina bifida should be similar. Different activities and positions also allow the sharing of general 'wear and tear' on joints. Anecdotally, we believe that children who ambulate in childhood are better wheelchair users, have greater upper limb strength, and less lower limb joint contractures, and this contributes to their independence in mobility and self-care skills in their later years.

The benefits and costs of ambulation are difficult to measure objectively, and there are variable and often conflicting opinions in the literature on the mobility management of children with myelomeningocele. Most researchers agree that children with low lumbar and sacral lesions should be encouraged to ambulate. The question of whether children with high lumbar and thoracic lesions should be given similar opportunities and encouragement is still controversial.

The issues of early ambulation versus early wheelchair use are discussed under the following headings relating to the domains of the ICF:

Body Structures and Function
- Joint pain and deformity – lower limb, upper limb
- Fractures and bone mineral density
- Energy efficiency
- Joint contractures
- Obesity and growth
- Skin
- Bowel and bladder

Participation
- Quality of life (QOL)

Personal factors
- Psychological
- Cognitive

Body Structures and Function

Joint Pain and Deformity

Recent concerns have been raised over early joint degeneration and joint pain in the spina bifida population. Since a primary goal of care of children with myelodysplasia is the preservation of ambulatory status and the maintenance of mobility into adulthood, joint pain is an important consideration associated with ambulation. Arthritic pain of knees, elbows and shoulders is emerging as significant problems for adults who were encouraged to ambulate supposedly 'beyond their neuromuscular capacities' [63]. It is suggested that repetitive movements of wheelchair propulsion can lead to early onset repetitive strain injuries of the upper limbs [63]. This could also result from high stress placed on upper limb joints through use of crutches [64]. Chronic low back pain and instability is a reported concern for young adults with spina bifida [65, 66].

There is limited literature regarding pain experienced by children and adolescents with spina bifida, with most reports of joint pain and degenerative joint changes occurring in adults. A recent study investigating the nature and prevalence of pain in children and adolescents with spina bifida found that lesion level and ambulatory status were not associated with any of the pain variables [67]. Lower back pain has also been demonstrated in 53% of adults with myelomeningocele, regardless of changes in ambulatory status [51]. Back and lower limb pain can also be caused by tethered cord syndrome [68, 69] and should always be a consideration.

Lower Limb Joint Pain

There are limited reports describing Charcot arthropathy in the spina bifida population. The widely accepted cause is the 'neurotraumatic' theory, which proposes that minor traumatic injuries to unprotected joints with abnormal sensory innervation results in rapid joint destruction [70].

Computerised gait analysis has improved our understanding of the complex gait patterns in patients with spina bifida [71, 72]. Specific gait patterns have been identified in symptomatic patients with low lumbar and sacral lesions. Those with low lumbar lesions exhibit a common gait pattern due to hip abductor and calf weakness, characterised by an abductor lurch with knee valgus and external tibial torsion. This, in combination with excess pelvic obliquity and trunk motion, places abnormal and increased stress on the knee ligaments and articular cartilage and may result in anteromedial instability and associated degenerative arthritis of the knee [73-76].

The incidence of neuropathic arthropathy in young adults with spina bifida has been reported at 1 in 100, with community ambulators (L4 and L5 lesion levels) at highest risk, and the knee and ankle joints most commonly affected [77]. Other studies have reported up to a 30% incidence of knee pain in young adults with myelomeningocele classified as either community ambulators or with sacral level lesions [78, 79]. This is possibly due to a 'crouch' or 'flexed knee gait', and increased instability in the knee resulting from decreased muscle strength.

The early detection of neuropathic arthropathy with regular clinical and radiographic examination is essential and avoiding any arthrodesis of lower limb joints is recommended [77]. Other centres also recommend the use of specific orthoses, or modification of current lower limb orthoses to control increased valgus knee stress and protect and support the involved joint/s [77, 80]. Several authors have proposed prophylactic management, including early surgical correction of rotational deformities of the lower limb for those children who have the potential to be community ambulators [81, 82].

There is also recent evidence suggesting the early use of crutches is beneficial for those deemed at risk of developing knee problems [83]. Crutches allow a more even weight bearing distribution between upper and lower limbs and produce a more normal gait pattern. The early introduction of crutches to children with lumbosacral lesion levels (between 3-4 years old) is recommended in order to encourage their use during adolescent and adult years. Forearm crutches should be used when ambulating long distances and outdoors, in order to reduce abnormal knee stresses and maintain joint integrity. Although our centre has adopted this practice, it is very hard to convince active children (and their parents) to use crutches during gait, in order to prevent pain that may occur later in life.

Upper Limb Joint Pain

The problem of shoulder pain related to weight bearing and overuse is well documented in patients with spinal cord injuries (SCI) [84]. The age of onset of wheelchair use appears to be a variable associated with shoulder pain in patients with SCI, but it is currently unknown whether this theory can be applied to the spina bifida population with respect to early ambulation versus wheelchair use. There are no reported studies as to whether different methods of ambulating with crutches cause more stress on shoulder, elbow and wrist joints.

The prevalence of shoulder pain in adults who had been wheelchair users since early childhood has been compared to those who began using their wheelchairs as adults (after 16 years of age) [84]. The majority of the childhood onset group had spina bifida, while the entire adult-onset group had traumatic SCI. The adult onset wheelchair group experienced greater shoulder pain than the childhood onset wheelchair users, despite having similar lifestyles and activity levels. It was proposed that the immature paediatric skeleton had a greater capacity to remodel and adapt to manage forces imposed from wheelchair propulsion.

Bone Mineral Density and Fractures

Children with spina bifida are at increased risk of osteoporosis and pathological fractures due to motor and sensory deficits, disuse of the lower limbs and lower levels of everyday activity compared to their able-bodied peers [85-90]. It has been demonstrated that children with myelomeningocele have a bone mineral density (BMD) one to two standard deviations below the mean of the normal population [91]. Bone mineral density correlates with the incidence of fractures and bone strength [92].

Studies have shown conflicting results in the incidence of fractures in children who ambulate compared to those who use wheelchairs [38, 60, 62, 91, 93]. There have also been conflicting results in studies looking at the association of ambulatory status, neurological level of lesion and bone mineral density [38, 94-96].

Children with spina bifida who have had multiple fractures have been noted to have a significantly lower bone density compared to those children who have no history of fractures [91]. The urinary calcium excretion is higher in non-ambulators than in children who ambulate, and it is thought that this may contribute to decreased bone density.

There is a widely-held theory that children with neuromuscular impairments should be encouraged to weight bear and ambulate, in order to prevent osteoporosis [95, 97]. The use of orthoses or adaptive equipment to provide weight bearing in standing or assisted ambulation has been an accepted method of practice in children with myelomeningocele. The efficacy of standing and ambulation programs on bone development and bone mineral density, however, has not been thoroughly examined. There are few studies that provide guidelines for standing and ambulation programs, and hence clinicians base their frequency, duration and orthotic devices used on their clinical experience or intuition.

Physical inactivity may have a systemic effect on bone mineralisation, since reductions in bone density mineralisation have been seen in both upper and lower limbs of children with myelomeningocele, regardless of whether they were ambulators or non-ambulators [38, 96]. Direct and indirect factors, as well as localised and systemic factors, appear to affect total bone mineralisation in children with myelomeningocele. Further research is required in order to determine the appropriate amount of ambulation necessary to maintain or increase bone mineral density in this population, without undue stress to the musculoskeletal system.

Energy Efficiency

Previous studies have demonstrated the increased relative effort required for walking in adults with physical impairments [98]. Normal and disabled people naturally attempt to walk at speeds that are most energy efficient and as a result, those with disabilities move more slowly. The more abnormal the gait patterns, the greater energy expenditure and slower speed used [99, 100]. Walking with aids (e.g., crutches, orthotics, etc.) increases energy cost and decreases speed, regardless of the individual's age or type of disability [98].

The issue of energy costs is often raised in regards to mobility in children and adolescents with spina bifida, particularly those children with thoracic and high lumbar lesion levels. Studies show the energy requirements for ambulation in children with spina bifida are significantly higher than the energy costs expected for the normal population [13, 100-104].

The increased energy costs of ambulation with crutches in children with thoracic and high lesions compared to wheelchair propulsion have been verified in many studies [13, 49, 102]. Using a wheelchair is as fast and energy efficient as normal walking and helps prevent fatigue. In children with low lumbar myelomeningocele (L3-4 level), a swing-through gait with crutches, rather than reciprocal gait, has been shown to be a more energy efficient ambulation pattern [105].

Even when walking at their slowest speed, the required energy demands for children with thoracic and high lumbar lesions is equal to their maximum aerobic capacity [13]. Children with L3-4 lesions require 85% of their maximal aerobic capacity to ambulate, in comparison to 30% maximum aerobic capacity during normal walking. Using ambulation for ther-

apeutic purposes appears equivalent to a heavy exercise session, and naturally, the child with a high level lesion myelomeningocele will fatigue.

It has been proposed that the high-energy cost of ambulation-assisted devices may have a potentially negative effect on certain aspects of a child's academic performance [106]. Although evidence is inconclusive, studies suggest that fine motor performance, cognitive tasks and visual attention may be affected by submaximal exercise [102, 107-109]. Educators, parents and health professionals need to be aware that fatigue from excessive ambulation may have a significant impact on classroom performance.

Mobility goals need to be made in the appropriate social and educational perspective, with a comprehensive outlook at the child's total function and participation in their different environments. This is particularly relevant in the high school environment where the physical demands change and the adolescent is expected to move between classrooms quickly on a more frequent basis. There are increasing demands on the child to 'keep up' with their able bodied peers. This differs from the primary school setting, where the child often stays in one classroom for most of the day.

The cost-benefit ratio of ambulation needs to be advantageous to the child with myelomeningocele, with mobility options available for these children, e.g., periods of assistive device ambulation, alternated with wheelchair propulsion. Performing short walking distances in everyday life with frequent breaks may keep the heart rate and energy expenditure at a comfortable level [110].

Bleck's [111] opinion is one to be carefully considered with regards to a child with spina bifida and ambulation: '... how impractical it is to encourage (or force) disabled children to walk long distances with assistive devices. They need to avoid undue fatigue in order to accomplish other tasks of daily living as well as school work, learning, social life and community integration'.

Joint Contractures

Children with spina bifida who ambulate full-time have been found to have minimal hip and knee contractures, when compared to those who have never ambulated and had severe lower limb joint contractures [13]. Full-time ambulation, rather than motor function level, is reported as an important factor in maintaining normal joint range of movement in the lower limbs. Non-ambulatory or minimal ambulatory subjects are more susceptible to the formation of lower limb joint contractures, since 'form follows function' and habitual sitting results in formation of fixed flexion deformities [32, 93, 112].

Obesity and Growth

Many children and adolescents with spina bifida considered to be obese are often non-functional ambulators. Obesity in this population is thought to be related to the neurological level of lesion, activity levels, increasing age, decreasing ambulation abilities and the increasing use of a wheelchair in adolescence [9, 13, 33, 37, 113-115].

By subjective assessment, however, many children with myelomeningocele appear obese [116]. Body mass index (BMI) can overestimate obesity, especially in children and adolescents with high level lesions, due to short stature and underestimated height from musculoskeletal deformities, such as kyphoscoliosis and lower limb joint contractures [114, 116-120].

Studies suggest that children with spina bifida are at increased risk of obesity due to a decreased basal metabolic rate and basal energy expenditure, resulting from atrophy of paralysed muscles and lower levels of physical activity [121-123]. Obesity has been reported as more prevalent in females with spina bifida, children and adolescents with high level neurological lesion levels and this is further complicated for those who are wheelchair users for mobility [9, 116, 124, 125].

Children and adolescents with myelomeningocele also differ from the standard population in terms of body composition and growth, especially those with high level lesions [114, 121]. In early childhood, body composition is similar to normal values, however increased adipose tissue is acquired with increasing age and decreasing ambulatory activity [118]. The use of the limbs in functional activities, including methods of ambulation, influences limb growth and development and body composition [114, 118].

Ambulation, however, should not be considered as a protection against obesity [126]. While weight has direct impact on function, mobility, orthotics, wheelchair fit, self-care skills and independence in transfers, good food choices and regular exercise from an early age are important. An emphasis on weight control and prevention of obesity through family counselling, diet, and exercise is recommended in an approach to weight reduction [127]. Further studies into the effect of ambulatory activity on obesity and growth in children with myelomeningocele are required [118].

Skin

Children with spina bifida who ambulate have been reported as having fewer pressure sores than wheelchair users [60]. However, other studies have found no difference in the incidence in pressure sores in children with spina bifida who used only a wheelchair for mobility [62]. The pattern of skin breakdown correlated with the mobility device used [62, 126]. Wheelchair users had more pressure sores on ischeal, sacral and perineal areas, while those who ambulated had pressure sores on lower limbs.

Bowel and Bladder Function

Upright ambulation is said to promote urinary tract drainage and thereby reduce complications such as urinary tract infections and hydronephrosis [33, 38, 93]. It is also believed to decrease constipation through the effect of increased gravity [128].

There are other studies that report no difference in renal health or continence between ambulators and wheelchair users [62], and no correlation between renal function and ambulatory status [37]. Stress incontinence can be a problem for those children who ambulate, and braces can interfere with self-toileting [61].

Participation

Quality of Life (QOL)

Neurophysical examination is often used to predict physical and cognitive function in children with spina bifida and their future health-related quality of life (HRQOL). 'Quality of life' is an all-inclusive concept, involving many factors affecting an individual's life. There are limited studies on QOL in adolescents with spina bifida and their families, and little is known about the associated or predictive factors of QOL in this population group.

Factors associated with perceived QOL include limitations imposed on the adolescent and family due to physical disabilities. The degree of physical impairment appears to have minimal association with the extent of behavioural and/or social problems in adolescents with myelomeningocele. Parental support, family resources and socioeconomic variables, rather than mobility and physical impairments, appear to be important factors associated with positive outcomes for this population group [9, 129-131].

Studies have found that positive parental attitudes and parental hope are closely associated with QOL in children and adolescents with spina bifida, more so than a child's current mobility, physical function and deficits [9, 129]. Interventions that influence this parental hope have an impact on adolescent outcomes [131]. One cannot deny the great joy and pride parents have when their child with myelomeningocele takes their first 'steps' and is able to 'walk'. Could early ambulation have an influence on parental hope, and thus affect their child's QOL?

Maximising functional independence in self-care, mobility and social cognition are important contributing factors to HRQOL in patients with myelomeningocele [6, 7]. Only one study has demonstrated an association between HRQOL and functional ambulation in children and adolescents with myelomeningocele [7].

Although research in this area is limited, health professionals should consider the findings and be careful when attempting to predict an individual child's HRQOL based purely on physical signs and symptoms. Families and patients are often the best judges of their own QOL, especially since attempts to predict future HRQOL are always from an outsider's perspective [7, 129].

Personal

Psychological

Each approach believes it best meets the developmental needs of the child with spina bifida. Those promoting ambulation report upright posture stimulates intellectual development, permits better social interaction, improves self-esteem and the child with myelomeningocele is perceived more favourably by their peers [38, 60]. In contrast, advocates of wheelchairs argue that the children move faster and are more independent in their skills of daily living, also resulting in an improved self-image and better social interactions [2, 132].

Gaff et al. [47] reported that while most children with high lumbar and thoracic lesion levels were 'non-useful walkers' by their adolescent years, both parents and children felt the efforts put into assisting their ambulation had been of benefit. They reported the satisfaction and increased self-morale gained by being able to stand upright and take limited steps.

The impact of disability on a young person's feelings of self-esteem and self-worth are difficult to assess. It is expected that ambulation status and difficulties with mobility would have a negative impact on self-esteem and self-concept [133, 134], however no studies have demonstrated an association [135].

Cognitive

Myelomeningocele is associated with cognitive disorders, language disorders and intellectual impairment, particularly in those children with hydrocephalus and higher lesion levels [136-144]. Rendeli et al. [145] tested the theory that locomotion improved the cognitive profile of children with myelomeningocele, using IQ and neuropsychological assessment and neuroimaging. They found a significant performance-related difference between ambulatory children and those children who were wheelchair-dependant.

Mobility Across the Lifespan

'Will my child walk?' is a question commonly asked by new parents of a baby with myelomeningocele. Most parents associate their child's walking with independence, health and success, and future walking potential is often a major focus in their child's early years of life.

Studies over the past 35 years consistently show that the most significant factor determining ambulation status in children with myelomeningocele is the neurological level of lesion [32-35, 37, 39, 43, 45, 146-149]. There is a general consensus that children with myelomeningocele achieve their maximal ambulatory abilities by nine years old [32, 43, 44, 49, 150] and changes in ambulatory status are expected between the ages of ten to twenty [32, 33, 49].

Mobility and ambulatory function and outcomes are dependent on many variables and these are often complex and interactive. Seldom is one factor responsible for ambulatory status or changes in ambulatory function. The factors influencing ambulation in children with myelomeningocele can be summarised under the ICF domains of body structures and function, environmental, personal factors and activity (see Table 29.2). Many investigators have attempted to determine which factors correlate with ambulatory ability and the predictive factors of future ambulatory status in children with myelomeningocele, however studies remain somewhat inconclusive and sometimes contradictory.

Children with high level lesions will often use a wheelchair for childhood mobility and are unlikely to ambulate long-term compared to those with low-

Table 29.2. Factors influencing ambulation and mobility

Domain of ICF	Factor	References
Body Structures and Function	Neurological level of lesion	Hoffer et al. 1973 [32]; De Souza and Carroll 1976 [33]; Feiwell et al. 1978 [34]; Stillwell and Menelaus 1983 [35]; Asher and Olsen 1983 [37]; Samuelsson and Skoog 1988 [39]; Huff and Ramsey 1978 [43], Swank and Dias 1994 [45]; Banta et al. 1983 [146]; Taylor and McNamara 1990 [147]; Fraser et al. 1992 [148]
	Child's size and weight	Agre et al. 1987 [13]; De Souza and Carroll 1976 [33]; Asher and Olsen 1983 [37]; Gaff et al. 1984 [47]
	Central nervous system anomalies	Mazur et al. 1986 [26], Mazur and Menelaus 1991 [30]; Samuelson and Skoog 1988 [39]; Vinck et al. 2006 [136]
	Hydrocephalus and associated upper limb neurological abnormalities	Hoffer et al. 1973 [32], Asher and Olsen 1983 [37], Iddon et al. 2003 [137]; Wallace 1973 [184]; Minns et al. 1977 [185]
	Upper limb function and hand strength	Asher and Olsen 1983 [37]; Norrlin et al. 2003 [161]; Wallace 1973 [184]; Minns et al. 1977 [185]; Muen 1997 [186], Turner 1986 [187], Aronin and Kerrick 1995 [188]; Mazur et al. 1986 [189]
	Spasticity in upper limb and lower limb	Mazur et al. 1986 [26], Hoffer et al. 1973 [32], Bartonek et al. 1999 [51]; Bartonek and Saraste 2001 [190]
	Neurological deterioration (recurrent shunt problems, tethered cord syndrome, syringomyelia)	Samuelson and Skoog 1988 [39]; Swank and Dias 1992 [44]; Vinck et al. 2006 [136]; Brinker et al. 1994 [191]
	Musculoskeletal deformities (notably scoliosis, hip flexion contractures, unilateral hip dislocation)	Hoffer et al. 1973 [32]; De Souza and Carroll 1976 [33]; Stillwell and Menelaus 1983 [35]; Asher and Olsen 1983 [37]; Samuelsson and Skoog 1988 [39]; Huff and Ramsey 1978 [43]; Carstens et al. 1995 [192]; Schiltenwolf et al. 1991 [193]
	Lower limb muscle strength (particularly hip flexors, quadriceps and hip abductor muscle groups)	Schopler and Menelaus 1987 [25]; Mazur and Menelaus 1991 [30]; Hoffer et al. 1973 [32]; De Souza and Carroll 1976 [33]; Stillwell and Menelaus 1983 [35]; McDonald et al. 1991 [41]; Huff and Ramsey 1978 [43]; Gaffe et al. 1984 [47]; Mazur et al. 1989 [60]; Lee and Carroll 1985 [194]
	Low postural tone (associated with brainstem dysfunction)	Norrlin et al. 2003 [161]
	Functional motor level	Swank and Dias 1992 [44]
	Balance in sitting and standing	Asher and Olsen 1983 [37]; Swank and Dias 1994 [45]; Bartonek and Saraste 2001 [190]
	Lower limb fractures	Hoffer et al. 1973 [32]
	Age of achieving early gross motor milestones	Findley et al. 1987 [49]
	Amputations, osteomyelitis	Brinker et al. 1994 [191]
	Poor skin integrity, pressure sores	Asher and Olsen 1983 [37]; Gaffe 1984 [47]; Taylor and McNamara 1990 [147]; Brinker et al. 1994 [191]; Schiltenwolf et al. 1991 [193]
	Energy expenditure	Butler et al. [2]; Vankoski et al. 1997 [83]; Duffy et al. 1996 [104]; Bartonek et al. 2001 [190]
Environment	Availability of physiotherapy services and intervention	Charney et al. 1991 [149]
	Social situation, parental compliance, family support	Hoffer et al. 1973 [32]; Charney et al. 1991 [149]
	Type of orthotics	Knutson and Clark 1991 [42]; Taylor and McNamara 1990 [147], Rose et al. 1983 [195], Thomas et al. 1989 [196]; Flandry et al. 1986 [197]
	Problems with orthotics	Asher and Olsen 1983 [37]; Gaffe et al. 1984 [47], Taylor and McNamara 1990 [147], Schiltenwolf et al. 1991 [193]

continued →

→ continue

Domain of ICF	Factor	References
	Major surgical interventions/medical events	Swank and Dias 1992 [44]; Bartonek et al. 1999 [51]
	Periods of immobilisation and deconditioning secondary to fractures/orthopaedic surgery	Findlay et al. 1987 [49]
Personal	Cognitive and perceptual problems	Blum and Pfaffinger 1994 [9]; Friedrich et al. 1991 [138], Wills 1993 [139]; Casari and Fantino 1998 [140]; Lindquist et al. 2004 [141]; Norrlin et al. 2003 [161]
	Motivation of child and family	De Souza and Carroll 1976 [33]; Asher and Olsen 1983 [37]; Bartonek et al. 1999 [51]; Schiltenwolf et al. 1991 [193]
	Visuospatial dysfunction	Friedrich et al. 1991 [138]; Wills 1993 [139]; Ito et al. 1997 [198]
	Attentional difficulties, impaired executive function	Wills 1993 [139], Fletcher et al. 1996 [142], Burmeister et al. 2005 [143]; Ito et al. 1997 [198]
	Intellectual impairment and IQ	Blum and Pfaffinger 1994 [9]; Hoffer et al. 1973 [32]; Findlay et al. 1987 [49]; Mapstone et al. 1984 [144]; Charney et al. 1991 [149]
	Age of child	Hoffer et al. 1973 [32]
	Motivation of child and family	De Souza and Carroll 1976 [33]; Asher and Olsen 1983 [37]; Swank and Dias 1994 [45]; Taylor and McNamara 1990 [147]; Schiltenwolf et al. 1991 [193]
Activity	Gross motor delays	Swank and Dias 1992 [44]; Findley et al. 1987 [49]; Williams et al. 1999 [150]; Wolf 1992 [158]

er neurological lesions [59, 147, 150]. There is less uniformity in the level of ambulation achieved in those children with lumbar level lesions [32]. Children with L3 lesion levels present a variable picture and are a very transitional group in terms of being able to predict future ambulatory status [45]. Children and adolescents with low lumbar lesion levels (L4-5) tend to maintain their ambulatory abilities, with 50-95% maintaining community ambulatory status as adults [9, 35, 39, 51, 151]. It is a general expectation that most children (89-100%) with sacral level lesions will function at or near normal levels, have few complications and will be long-term community ambulators [9, 32, 34, 35, 37, 39, 45, 49, 60, 147, 152]. It has been proposed that patients with sacral myelomeningocele be classified into high and low sacral groups in order to provide a clearer clinical picture and assist in management [152].

Ambulation is not always strictly determined by physical abilities. There are often discrepancies between the assigned neurological level of lesion, lower limb muscle strength and the ambulation levels and abilities achieved by children with myelomeningocele. A child with spina bifida may have the capacity to ambulate with assistive devices, but their actual functional performance may be influenced by other factors. This potential discrepancy needs to be considered when making appropriate management goals for mobility and ambulation. For example, the motivation of a child and their family is a factor that is difficult to assess, and is unable to be directly controlled or measured. Often, despite their neurological patterns and/or orthopaedic surgery, a child with spina bifida with motivation can achieve higher than expected or predicted levels of ambulation. Some children with spina bifida simply have a 'joy of walking'.

Decisions regarding clinical management and mobility are made on an individual basis, and may require modification as a child grows. Ambulation may not be a realistic goal for some children with spina bifida. The focus on achieving ambulation should not be at the expense of teaching a child other skills of a functional significance that are necessary for them to attain independence in activities of daily living, mobility, transfers and schooling.

The functional nature of ambulation ultimately determines the long-term mode of ambulation of the child with spina bifida. The ability to ambulate in childhood does not guarantee the same ability in adulthood. Ambulation in adolescence and adulthood is again strongly related to neurologic level, with the high level lesions (thoracic) predominantly using wheelchairs and being non-ambulatory, and those with low lesions (sacral) being community ambulators [32, 33, 35, 153]. The link between neurological lesion and adolescents who are household or therapeutic ambulators is less clear. Children with spina bifida who achieve only household ambulation tend not continue to ambulate into adulthood [35].

As children with thoracic and high lumbar lesions grow older, they are more likely to use a wheelchair for mobility. This change in ambulation status may come as an anticipated development or big disappointment for the parents and child with spina bifida, depending on the approach taken with the family regarding prognosis during early childhood. Some families regard the use of a wheelchair as a symbol of being 'crippled', or 'regressive' and discourage its use for their child [63]. The decision of whether to continue ambulation or opt for full-time wheelchair use is best made by the family and adolescent, based on lifestyle and abilities.

A wheelchair is an aid to mobility, not a 'failure in management', and can serve to increase self-confidence, independence in mobility and allow the child to participate in activities with their peers. Using a wheelchair for mobility is often for reasons of convenience and not necessarily evidence of neurological deterioration or 'laziness' [48]. Adolescents and adults with spina bifida report a wheelchair is faster and easier than ambulating with orthoses. It is also more acceptable socially, both in the cosmetic sense and in terms of the clothing that can be worn [147].

'Downward transitions' of ambulatory function can also be associated with neurological deterioration. [51]. Neurological patterns and presentations can change due to associated central nervous system anomalies, including hydrocephalus and repeated shunt revisions, syringomyelia, tethered cord syndrome, and Arnold-Chiari malformations [153, 154]. It is important to assess and monitor children and adolescents with myelomeningocele on a regular basis, since detailed serial neurological examinations are essential in identifying early changes in neurological function [155, 156]. The clinical manifestations which suggest alteration of neurological function are variable and children with spina bifida usually present with one or more symptoms, which may include:

- Motor deficit or dysfunction.
- Sensory deficit.
- Lower limb and/or back pain.
- Spasticity in upper or lower limbs.
- Deterioration in gait.
- Progressive foot deformities.
- Increased hip/knee fixed flexion deformities.
- Progressive scoliosis, kyphosis or lordosis, bladder and bowel dysfunction.

Health Services and Systems (Environmental Factors)

Adolescents with spina bifida and their families require a multidisciplinary and holistic approach to the management of their health in order to achieve optimal outcomes. The concept of development of the 'total child' with myelomeningocele includes cognitive, personality and emotional development [20]. Myelodysplasia is a complex condition and the individual variation seen in clinical presentation means management and treatment will often differ significantly between children. It is essential to have a multidisciplinary, co-ordinated approach to the mobility management of children and adolescents with spina bifida, involving the family, an orthopaedic surgeon, physiotherapist and orthotist.

Orthopaedics

The principle aim of orthopaedic management is to establish and maintain stable posture through minimal surgery and bracing, and to establish a pattern of motor development which is as close to normal as the neurosegmental level of lower limb paralysis allows [30, 157]. The orthopaedic management of children with spina bifida is discussed in Chapters 24 and 25.

Physiotherapy

Children with myelomeningocele have delays in the development of their gross motor skills due to hypotonia and abnormalities of postural control, delayed development of automatic reactions and delays in integrating primitive reflexes [158]. Brainstem and central nervous system anomalies and medical problems such as shunt difficulties, also contribute to problems with postural control, limited mobility and gross motor skills delays [61, 159, 160].

Gross motor delay is more prevalent in children with high level lesions, but is also significant in children with minimal lower limb paralysis [150]. The higher the motor lesion, the greater loss of lower limb motor function, and the greater delays are expected in mobility and the first onset of ambulation [44]. There are also differences in the quality of early movement and motor skills in many infants with myelomeningocele, regardless of lesion level, when compared to normal infants [158].

Cognitive, attentional and visuospatial dysfunction also interfere with mobility with regards to the child's ability to judge spatial distances, difficulties in gaining a comprehensive picture of their surroundings, and difficulties in planning complex movement [161].

It is important to facilitate the development of gross motor milestones from an early age in infants with spina bifida. They need to be challenged and learn to move without assistance, in order to encourage the achievement of independent mobility and their maximum participation in life activities.

It is essential to focus on the positive aspects of what the child can and will be able to do, rather than focus on their limitations and disabilities. Parents of a child with spina bifida need to have realistic expectations for their child, but to also to encourage and value independence for their child. The needs of the individual child, their family and the level of function must always be considered when discussing and setting goals of treatment and management.

An infant with spina bifida should experience a variety of positions (prone, supine, side lying) in order to stimulate the development of head and trunk control, and strengthen innervated muscle groups. Parents should be encouraged to assist their child in early exploration, by providing them with a stimulating home environment – this gives a child motivation to move and helps them interact with their environment in a purposeful way.

Supported sitting in an upright position at an age appropriate time assists in improving the infant's head control and developing posture and balance reactions. The use of a beanbag, cushions or the corner of the couch can provide initial support for sitting to encourage two-handed play. A corner chair (Fig. 29.5) or Tumbleform chair may be more appropriate for the infant with significant delays in head and trunk control. Once static sitting balance is achieved, activities that encourage weight shift, reaching and propping assist in developing dynamic sitting balance.

Children with spina bifida will move on the floor in a variety of ways depending on their level of paralysis and the degree of deformity or contractures. They will use the method of mobility that is easiest for them, ranging from rolling to commando crawling or bottom shuffling. A scooter board, prone trolley or chariot (Fig. 29.6) may also be used to facilitate independent mobility from an early age.

It is essential to teach rigorous skin care practice to parents and children with spina bifida from an early age, as poor skin integrity will have an impact on the child's ambulation abilities. Ensure good skin care practice is integrated into everyday care, with practical applications, such as:

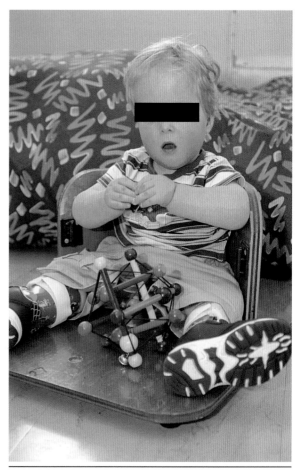

Fig. 29.5. Child with high lumbar myelomeningocele using a corner chair for supported sitting

- The child always wears socks and pants when crawling on carpet and wears shoes when walking outside.
- The child wears protective footwear in the pool and at the beach to avoid skin abrasions from rough pool surfaces and sand.
- The child does not carry hot foods on their lap at any time.
- Shoes and splints are removed and cleaned out after playing in a sandpit.

Assisted standing is commenced after the first year of age when the child with spina bifida is demonstrating some floor mobility and is showing an interest in pulling up to a standing position (Fig. 29.7). The level of support and orthotics or equipment required will depend on the neurological level of lesion. This may be provided through a standing frame, long leg calico splints, supportive ankle boots and/or ankle–foot orthoses (AFO). A child requires maximum security and support in this initial

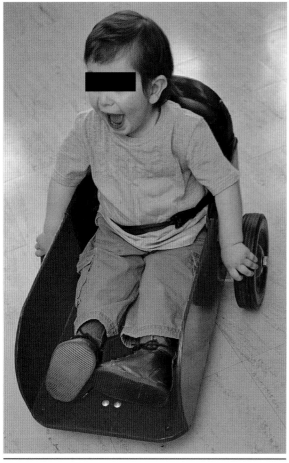

Fig. 29.6. Child with high lumbar myelomeningocele using a chariot for mobility

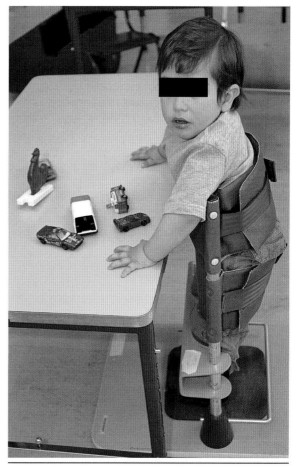

Fig. 29.7. A standing frame is used for supported standing for a child with a high lumbar myelomeningocele

stage to promote their confidence, and temporary over-bracing with subsequent reductions is acceptable. Once static standing is achieved, the child increases their standing endurance and learns skills in side-to-side and diagonal weight shift in preparation for ambulation.

There are a wide variety of techniques, aids and assistive devices available to supplement and enhance the mobility and upright ambulation of children and adolescents with myelodysplasia. These include orthotics, crutches, K-walkers, modified trikes, bikes and wheelchairs.

Independent mobility by ambulation is a goal in early childhood, however many children with spina bifida require a wheelchair to access their environment. Controversy exists regarding the timing of introducing a wheelchair to children deemed unlikely to be community ambulators in the future. A wheelchair can enhance mobility and independence and allow a child to participate in activities and keep up with their peers. Others argue that the early introduction of a wheelchair limits ambulation potential. Mazur et al. [60] found the timing of introducing a wheelchair made no difference in the ultimate level of ambulation or activities of daily living and wheelchair skills achieved by children with spina bifida.

A wheelchair for a child with spina bifida needs to be correctly prescribed to fit the child (not 'child to fit the chair'), with postural modifications and support customised to their needs [162]. A lightweight wheelchair allows maximum efficiency and propulsion method at an appropriate mechanical advantage, and anti-tip bars and a seatbelt are strongly recommended. A seat cushion is essential to reduce pressure and sheer forces, with its early introduction allowing preventative measures of skin care. The paediatric wheelchair requires regular review and ongoing monitoring to ensure it continues to fit correctly with growth of the child.

Orthotic Management

The role of orthoses in myelomeningocele is primarily to augment the absent function of the major locomotive musculature. In those with high sacral lesions, this may mean the plantarflexors only, while in thoracic lesions the plantarflexors, knee and hip extensors need support. Orthoses have several other roles, which often overlap with one another:

- To provide support to prevent the body falling against gravity.
- To protect joints from damaging pathomechanics.
- To increase efficiency of gait.
- To prevent or reduce the development of joint contractures.
- To maintain bony or joint alignment following surgery.
- To provide an alternative form of mobility to a wheelchair.

When prescribing orthoses, many factors need to be taken into account by the clinical team. Biomechanical assessment provides us with most of the information in regard to prescription, but other factors will often determine one design of orthoses over another. These other structural, environmental and personal factors, such as level of cognition, surgical events and clinical goals, are mentioned in Table 29.2.

Patients with myelomeningocele present the orthotist with challenging problems. Not only must the orthotist contend with the individual's biomechanical deficits but also with insensate skin that is prone to skin breakdown with undue pressure or shear stress. Poorly designed or ill-fitting orthoses are able to cause damage to skin and subcutaneous tissues that can severely restrict mobility while the injury heals. Education in regards to regular self-examination for skin problems will prevent occurrences of skin breakdown, as orthoses can be adjusted before any medical treatment is required.

Precluding factors for ambulation include lack of motivation, lack of upper limb strength, obesity, significant spinal deformity, significant hip or knee flexion contractures and decreased cognition [163, 164]. If resources allow, trialling patients with used orthoses will help to give the clinical team a good insight into the child's potential for ambulation [165].

Technological Considerations

Materials used in the prosthetic and orthotic industry are constantly evolving and improving, giving the orthotist more design options to transfer loads to limb segments. The adoption of thermoplastic materials in the 1970s was a great step forward in improving outcomes for patients, both functionally and aesthetically. The next step may involve the use of composite materials and silicones, which are currently expensive and difficult to work with but show great potential in their engineering properties when correctly applied [166].

Polypropylene, high-density polyethylene and copolymer are the thermoplastic materials of choice for most orthoses, as they are inexpensive, durable and are able to be modified for growth. Common interface materials include polyethylene foams, low-density ethyl-vinyl acetate (EVA) foams and urethane foams. Silicone gel liners, such as those used for prosthetic socket liners, make excellent interfaces for bony or high-load areas due to their shear-absorbing properties, although the materials are difficult to work with.

Metal components in orthoses are made from high tensile aluminium, stainless steel or titanium. A variety of different metal ankle, knee and hip joints are available for a range of functions. Metal components to bracing can be fixed externally to plastic sections or can be incorporated underneath the plastic for a more cosmetic appearance. External mounting is preferred, as it requires less time in alteration for the orthotist as the child grows.

Plastic sections of orthoses for spina bifida patients are mostly manufactured from plaster-of-paris or fibreglass casts of the body segment. The mould can be taken using various techniques according to the orthotist's preference.

Loading of the tissues to simulate biomechanical effects on the limb from the orthosis should be included in the cast if possible. Great care needs to be taken to position the joints in their optimum alignment, as modifications made to the negative cast will affect the final fit of the orthosis. Knee and ankle angle adjustments to a negative cast are more anatomically accurate than sub-talar or mid-tarsal adjustments, thus it is better to position the foot accurately than trying to correct ankle and knee position at the same time. Long leg casts can be done in sections, first to position the foot and ankle and then a further wrap to position the knee in optimal alignment. For a knee-ankle-foot orthoses (KAFO), hip knee-ankle-foot orthoses (HKAFO), or reciprocating gait orthosis (RGO), careful measurements and tracings are also taken to facilitate a good anatomical/mechanical alignment.

The manufacturing process for a thermoplastic orthosis occurs as follows: a dental plaster slurry is poured into the sealed, modified (if necessary) negative cast and a steel tube positioned into the plaster to allow the cast to be later held in a vice. Once the plaster is set, the negative mould is stripped away and the positive model is modified to set the tolerances of the orthosis. Bony or pressure sensitive areas are unloaded in favour of pressure tolerant areas that are able to bear load. When pressure sensitive areas coincide with biomechanical load areas, the appropriate skin interface must be incorporated into the design, otherwise pressure or shear damage to the skin may occur.

Heated plastic is vacuum-formed or laminated to the modified cast. The plastic shell is later removed from the cast and trimmed to the appropriate shape for the design of the brace. Straps, metal componentry, and any extra pads are fabricated and attached and the orthosis is ready for fitting. Complex orthoses such as RGOs can take two or three fittings to achieve a satisfactory result.

It is essential for the best fit of an orthosis that the orthotist, rather than an orthotic technician, should always make the modifications to the positive plaster model. The orthotist who takes the negative cast will have a better "feel" of how much tolerance should be given to different tissues. Supervision of negative cast correction before cast filling is also vitally important.

Indications for Orthotic Use (Table 29.3)

Foot Orthoses

Foot orthoses of various designs are prescribed prophylactically to distribute plantar pressures. The weakness of intrinsic muscles of the foot can cause toe deformities or cavus, leading to increased plantar pressures and occasionally ulceration of the metatarsal heads or heel. Paraesthesia of the plantar surface of the foot gives no warning of any accumulating damage until visual signs of skin breakdown appear. The most common and versatile designs are semi-rigid orthoses utilising varying densities of EVA foam. Multi-density orthoses can be accurately fabricated to unload areas of high pressure identified by palpation, hyper-keratinosis and examination of footwear. It is unlikely that orthoses will prevent the ultimate formation of toe deformities, as the long flexor/extensor muscles have a much greater influence, unchecked by the lack of intrinsics.

When there are foot deformities present, such as cavo-varus/valgus, abducto-valgus and planus, an improvement in the posture of the feet may be maintained through the use of University of California Biomechanics Laboratory (UCBL) shoe inserts [167]. The UCBL utilises a combination of calcaneal grip, medial and lateral longitudinal arch support and extended medial and/or lateral walls to the metatarsal heads. Correction of deformity can only be attempted with flexible feet, as an attempt to force stiff joints into a better posture will result in skin breakdown.

Ankle-Foot Orthoses (AFOs)

Weak or absent plantarflexors commonly seen in children with lower lesion levels cause an unrestrained second ankle rocker and markedly reduced power generation in late stance, effectively ablating the third rocker. Dorsiflexion in stance also causes the ground reaction force to move posteriorly to the knee, increasing the external knee flexion moment (GRF),

Table 29.3. Details according to lesion level, resulting muscle weakness and appropriate orthoses

Lesion Level	Low Sacral	High Sacral	Low Lumbar	High Lumbar	Thoracic
Muscle weakness:	Foot Intrinsics---				
		Plantarflexors--			
		Hip extensors---			
			Dorsiflexors/Inverters/Evertors---		
			Hip Abductors--		
Orthoses:	Foot orthoses		Knee Flexors--		
	UCBLs			Knee extensors--------------------------	
		Solid-Ankle AFOs		Hip Adductors--------------------------	
		Twister HKAFOs			Hip Flexors------------
			KAFOs/HKAFOs		Abdominals
			HKAFOs/RGOs		
					THKAFOS

producing a characteristic crouch gait (Fig. 29.8). The solid AFO has been the standard orthosis of choice for many years now in this situation, as it can increase energy efficiency [168], improve kinematics and kinetics [168-172] and reduce heel pressure sores by normalising the centre of pressure [171].

Solid AFO design varies slightly from centre to centre but the design principles are the same. The AFO is designed so as to support medio-lateral instabilities/deformities of the foot and ankle, with total contact rigid plastic with trimlines anterior to the malleoli, and either a wide pre-tibial strap or shell (floor-reaction AFO) (Fig. 29.9). The footplate is usually extended to the end of the toes, both for toe protection and to increase the lever arm for dorsiflexion resistance.

There have been several studies confirming the beneficial use of solid AFOs [168, 169, 171] for patients with low lumbar and high sacral spina bifida. The solid AFO performs several important biomechanical functions:
- Prevents excessive tibial advancement in stance. The design of the solid AFO provides a braking force to the tibia as it advances over the planted foot. The angle the AFO is set as well as the strength and shape of the material around the ankle determines the amount of resistance applied.
- Decreases the energy cost of walking [168, 173, 174].
- Moves the centre of pressure from the heel to the forefoot in late stance. In unbraced gait, the centre of pressure remains at the heel for the entire

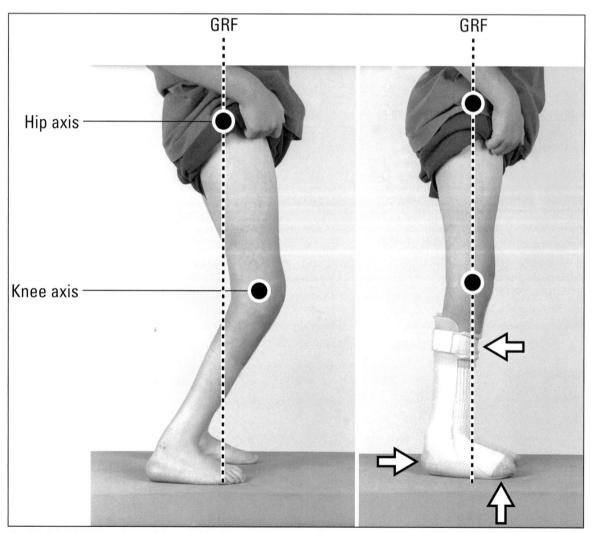

Fig. 29.8. Reduction of crouch in a child with sacral myelomeningocele using solid AFOs (Reprinted from [113], with permission from Elsevier

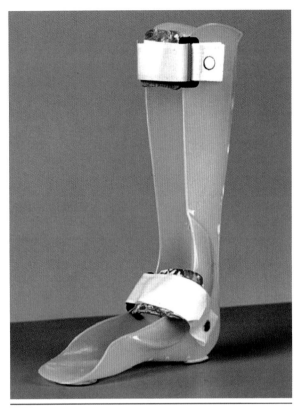

Fig. 29.9. Solid ankle foot orthosis (AFO)

cycle [171]. AFOs also help in distributing pressure around the plantar surface of the foot, lessening the chance for pressure sores on the heel.

- Decreases the external knee flexion moment. As the second ankle rocker is blocked by the AFO, the GRF moves anteriorly towards the knee centre. This decreases the amount the knee extensors must work to maintain weight bearing. Interestingly, little difference is reported in the energy cost with improved GRF about the knee [168]. Although energy cost of a flexed knee gait may not be raised as high as was once thought, there is little doubt that a flexed knee gait, combined with valgus knee stress and external rotation stress will ultimately result in knee pain in a large proportion of patients [73-76].
- Walking speed is increased with AFOs [173].
- Improves power generation in late stance. There is some evidence that AFOs provide some increase to power generation due to storage of energy in the AFO [168]. As the AFO comes under dorsiflexion strain, it will flex to some degree, releasing that energy as the limb advances in late stance. This power generation would appear to be the consequence of the material choice and design of the

AFO. Thomson et al. [169] found a reduction in power generation with AFOs, but an improvement in ankle and knee kinematics in contrast to that found by Duffy et al. [168]. The more rigid AFOs used in the study by Thomson et al. [169], however, seemed to cause an increase in rotational knee motion when compared to barefoot, which was unchanged in the study by Duffy et al. [168]. It would seem that there is a need for an AFO design that allows torsional stresses to dissipate through the material while being rigid enough to provide an increased plantarflexion-knee-extension couple and providing some energy return.

Disadvantages to the gait of plantarflexor deficient patients when using AFOs may include:

- First and third rockers are blocked. At initial contact, there is a strong knee flexion moment observed in patients using a solid AFO. The normal plantarflexion occurring at initial contact is prevented and as a result the knee is thrust forward. This effect can be reduced somewhat by using shoes with a soft heel such as a running shoe, or by modifying the shoe by adding a rocker sole, allowing a more fluid transition of weight onto the foot and then allowing tibial progression in late stance. At late stance, third rocker is prevented by the rigid AFO, decreasing any propulsive force.
- Increased external rotation moment at the knee for patients with high sacral lesions [169]. Second rocker can be restricted too far into the gait cycle, making it difficult to 'roll over' the grounded foot. This may cause the patient to find it difficult to walk with any speed unless they externally rotate the limb to reduce the lever arm of the AFO footplate. Patients with spina bifida also often have external tibial torsion which frustrates the attempt for an increased plantarflexion-knee extension couple [172].
- Progressive weakening of remaining plantarflexor power.

Ground Reaction Ankle-Foot Orthoses (GRAFO)

GRAFOs (Fig. 29.10) are often mentioned in discussions involving support for crouch gait. The GRAFO differs to a solid AFO only in that it has a pre-tibial shell placed more proximally than a standard solid AFO tibial strap. The pre-tibial shell is continuous with the rest of the AFO and is donned by placing the foot through the proximal circumferential opening. The solid AFO is in reality a ground-reaction AFO as it increases the knee extension moment at midstance by restraining the

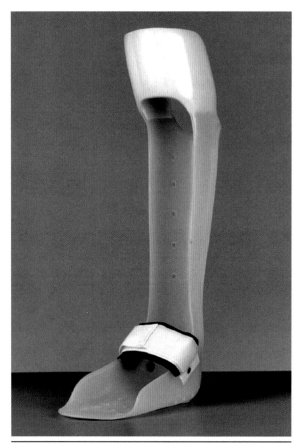

Fig. 29.10. Ground reaction ankle foot orthoses (GRAFO)

second ankle rocker. The term GRAFO has come to describe a solid-ankle AFO that provides more of a knee extension moment than a regular AFO by the use of longer lever arms and perhaps a stiffer material.

Above-Knee Bracing

Above-knee bracing includes Knee-Ankle-Foot Orthoses (KAFOs), Hip-Knee-Ankle-Foot Orthoses (HKAFOs) and Thoracic-Hip-Knee-Ankle-Foot Orthoses (THKAFOs).

Foot placement can be a problem in children with lower lesion spina bifida. The lack of hip abductor control, tibial torsion deformities and valgus/rotated knees can cause poor foot placement. Internal rotation past ninety degrees to the line of progression is quite possible. For foot positioning, the use of twister cables linking AFOs to a pelvic band has some merit. The cable can be pre-tensioned to provide an internal or external torque onto the AFO. KAFOs with single uprights and dynamic knee strapping or a HKAFO with single up-

rights and free knee joints can also be used to provide better foot placement.

The knee can be protected from valgus stresses incurred from weak abductors and increased pelvic motion by simple three-point pressure application through a KAFO [75]. Rotational forces about the knee can be reduced at the expense of some mobility: increased coronal plane motion of the body is the main propulsive force for patients without plantarflexors and hip abductors and extensors [173]. Orthotic control of rotational stresses is difficult to achieve without crossing the hip joint due to soft tissue deformation around the femur. Thus mobility may be sacrificed for joint control.

In children with higher lesion levels, the absence of plantarflexors, hip extensors and weakness or absence of knee extensors preclude an unbraced gait. Children with L3 lesions with quadriceps strength are able to ambulate with AFOs or GRAFOs but rely very heavily on assistive devices. Lumbar lordosis is increased as these children struggle to keep the centre of mass over the feet. Without quadriceps function, ambulation is only possible with high level bracing and the use of crutches or a walker. KAFOs can be prescribed to prevent knee flexion, but the problem of lack of hip extension remains.

Orthoses that cross the hip include HKAFOs, THKAFOs, the RGO [175] and its derivatives, and the Hip Guidance Orthosis or Parawalker [176]. The RGO derivatives include the isocentric or rocker-bar RGO, the horizontal cable RGO and the Advanced RGO or ARGO.

HKAFOs and THKAFOs link a pelvic and/or thoracic support to a pair of KAFOs. This will provide upper body support to prevent the child flexing at the hip. Most children with thoracic lesion levels will need the longer lever arm of the THKAFO to stand with stability as it takes a lot of trunk control to maintain balance in an HKAFO.

The RGO types are similar in function to one another as flexion of one hip causes contralateral hip extension. The decision to use one or the other RGO finally comes down to the orthotist's preference.

To be able to stand without the major anti-gravity muscles, patients require four points of opposing forces to prevent collapse: a posteriorly directed force at the chest, an anteriorly directed force at the hip, a posteriorly directed force at the knees and an anteriorly directed force at the heels (Fig. 29.11). Standing frames and parapodiums allow upright weight bearing with the upper limbs free; but for any active mobility, forearm crutches or a walker are essential. The only exception to this is the swivel walker [177] which allows limited hands free mobility. The swiv-

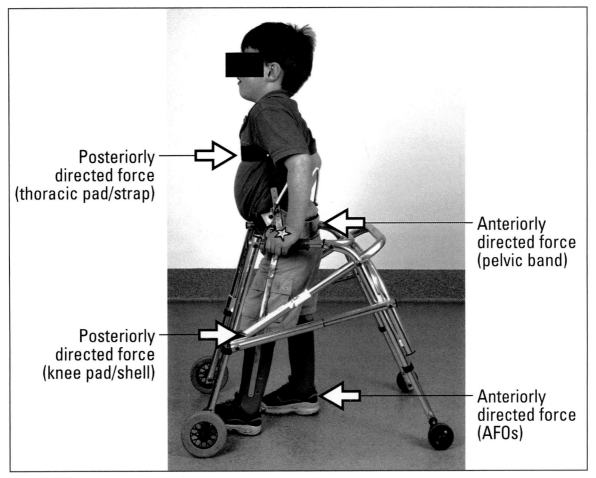

Fig. 29.11. Reciprocating gait orthoses (RGO) demonstrating four points of opposing forces

el walker may be the only choice of upright mobility when upper limb strength is inadequate for other reciprocating orthoses and is used mostly for pre-reciprocal training [178].

Patients who require higher bracing will ambulate with either a swing-through or reciprocal gait. HKAFOs or THKAFOs with locked hip and knee joints will not allow a reciprocal gait pattern, and are used for swing-through gait.

The preference for either gait depends on the desired velocity of ambulation and perhaps economic factors. A swing through gait will provide a faster velocity than a reciprocal gait [179] and the orthoses for swing through gaits are cheaper and easier to manufacture. If speed is more important to the patient, as in school age children who want to keep up with their peers, a swing through gait will be more appropriate.

There is some confusion as to the energy costs between swing-through or reciprocal patterns. Several studies done on energy costs and velocity of children using HKAFOs and RGOs show conflicting results [163, 174, 175, 180, 181]. It would appear, however, that the greater velocity of swing-through gait requires increased energy expenditure than does the reciprocal gait. Moderately small sample sizes in the studies and the number of physiological and biomechanical factors that affect the proficiency of ambulation would seem to confuse the data.

Reciprocal gait is possible in patients with inactive hip flexors. Trunk extension with a diagonal weight-shift from a gait aid to free the swing–limb from the ground allows forward motion.

In addition to muscle paralysis, children with higher lesions have other disadvantages in order to achieve gait as the preferred method of locomotion. Knee and hip flexion contractures are common. Hip dislocation will cause a significant limb inequality but will not preclude walking. Hip dislocation itself is not a factor that disqualifies walking ability [182]. Hip and knee flexion contractures can be accommodated into a brace by shaping the metal components to follow the alignment of the patient. The associated leg length inequality from a hip dislocation is managed by shoe modifications. When manufacturing high level orthoses for patients with contractures, deformities and dislocations, the orthotist must try to set up a brace so that the centre of gravity remains over the feet when standing.

Compromises between desired biomechanical goals and functional reality must often be made.

Children with high level myelomeningocele present the clinical team with great difficulties to overcome in order to achieve the goal of standing and walking. The social, therapeutic and even financial benefits of ambulation [178] must be weighed against the time and effort required to achieve ambulation. It must be recognised that most children with thoracic lesions will cease walking before adulthood. There is encouraging data from Roussos [178] showing that the average age of ceasing ambulation was 17.8 years, but other studies show earlier discontinuation [165, 183]. The primary mode of mobility for children with high level lesions will always remain the wheelchair, for reasons of energy efficiency, speed and convenience.

Conclusion

Advances and improvement in the management of children with spina bifida have resulted in their increased life expectancy. There has been an added interest in ways to improve the mobility and functional outcomes of children with spina bifida, and the levels of activity and participation they can achieve in today's society.

A goal-oriented approach to the mobility management of children and adolescents with spina bifida allows the optimum fulfilment of a child's potential for adult living. Children and adolescents with spina bifida need to achieve developmental independence and self-management skills in order to be successful in adulthood. Maintaining and improving their mobility status and functional abilities is an important component of this.

Adulthood is the longer lifespan beyond childhood and '...a disabled child is a growing person who will become a disabled adult suffering the same condition, albeit modified by therapy and surgical and orthotics interventions.... Daily we see evidence that efficient self-produced mobility is critical to independence and self-esteem, to making and keeping friends, to achieving the least restrictive educational environment, and to grow into a productive adult' [182].

References

1. World Health Organisation (1980) International classification of impairments, disabilities and handicaps. Geneva, pp 181-194
2. Butler C (1991) Augmentative mobility: why do we do it? Physical Med and Rehab Clinics of N America 2(4):801-815
3. McDermott JF, Akina E (1972) Understanding and improving the personality development of children with physical handicaps. Clin Pediatr 11:134
4. World Health Organisation (2002) International classification of functioning, disability and health. Geneva, pp 1-22
5. Bunch WH (1976) Myelomeningocele. Instr Course Lect 25:61-65
6. Bier JB, Prince A, Tremont M, Msall M (2005) Medical, functional and social determinants of health-related quality of life in individuals with myelomeningocele. Dev Med Child Neurol 47:609-612
7. Schoenmakers MA, Uiterwaal CS, Gulmans VA et al (2005) Determinants of functional independence and quality of life in children with spina bifida. Clin Rehabil 19:677-685
8. Meeusen R (2005) Exercise and the brain: insight in new therapeutic modalities. Ann Transplant 10(4):49-51
9. Blum RW, Pfaffinger K (1994) Myelodysplasia in childhood and adolescence. Pediatr Rev 15(12):480-484
10. Bandini LG, Schoeller DA, Fukagawa NK et al (1991) Body composition and energy expenditure in adolescents with cerebral palsy or myelodysplasia. Pediatr Res 29:70-77
11. Van den Berg-Emons HJ, Bussmann JB, Brobbel AS et al (2001) Everyday physical activity in adolescents and young adults with meningomyelocele as measured with a novel activity monitor. J Pediatr 139(6):880-886
12. Van den Berg-Emons HJ, Bussmann JB, Meyerink HJ et al (2003) Body fat, fitness and level of everyday physical activity in adolescents and young adults with myelomeningocele. J Rehabil Med 35(6):271-275
13. Agre JC, Findley MD, McNally MC et al (1987) Physical activity capacity in children with myelomeningocele. Arch Phys Med Rehabil 68(6):372-377
14. Sherman MS, Kaplan JM, Effgen S et al (1997) Pulmonary dysfunction and reduced exercise capacity in patients with myelomeningocele. J Pediatr 131(3):413-418
15. Francis K (1996) Physical activity in the prevention of cardiovascular disease. Phys Ther 76:456-468

16. Baranowski T, Bouchard C, Bar-Or O et al (1992) Assessment, prevalence and cardiovascular benefits of physical activity and fitness in youth. Med Sci Sports Exerc 24(6 suppl):S237-S247

17. O'Connell D, Barnhart R (1995) Improvement in wheelchair propulsion in paediatric wheelchair users through resistance training: a pilot study. Arch Phys Med Rehabil 76:368-372

18. Fragala-Pinkham MA, Haley SM, Rabin J, Kharasch VS (2005) A fitness program for children with disabilities. Phys Ther 85(11)1182-1200

19. Andrade CK, Kramer J, Garber M, Longmuir P (1991) Changes in self-concept, cardiovascular endurance and muscular strength in children with spina bifida aged 8 to 13 years in response to a 10-week physical activity program: a pilot study. Child Care Health Dev 17:183-196

20. Drennan JC, Banta JV, Bunch WH, Linseth RE (1987) Symposium: Current concepts in the management of myelomeningocele. Contemp Orthop 19(1):63-88

21. Ryan KD, Ploski C, Emans JB (1991) Myelodysplasia – the musculoskeletal problem: habilation from infancy to adulthood. Phys Ther 71(12):935-946

22. Daniels L, Worthington C (1980) Muscle testing: Techniques of manual evaluation. 5th edn, WB Saunders, Philadelphia

23. Murdoch A (1980) How valuable is muscle charting? Physiotherapy 66(7):221-223

24. McDonald CM, Jaffe KM, Shurtleff DB (1986) Assessment of muscle strength in children with myelomeningocele: accuracy and stability of measurements over time. Arch Phys Med Rehabil 67:885-861

25. Schopler SA, Menelaus MB (1987) Significance of the strength of the quadriceps muscles in children with myelomeningocele. J Pediatr Orthop 7(5):507-512

26. Mazur JM, Stillwell A, Menelaus MB (1986) The significance of spasticity in lower and upper limbs in myelomeningocele. J Bone Joint Surg 68-B(2):213-218

27. Bartonek A, Saraste H, Knutson LM (1999) Comparison of different systems to classify the neurological level of lesion in patients with myelomeningocele. Dev Med Child Neurol 41:796-805

28. Sharrard WJW (1964) The segmental innervation of the lower limb muscles in man. Ann R Coll Surg Engl 35:106-122

29. Stark GD, Baker GC (1967) The neurological involvement of the lower limbs in myelomeningocele. Dev Med Child Neurol 9:732-744

30. Mazur JM, Menelaus MB (1991) Neurologic status of spina bifida patients and the orthopaedic surgeon. Clin Orthop Relat Res 264:54-63

31. Duffy CM, Hill AE, Cosgrove AP et al (1996) The influence of abductor weakness on gait in spina bifida. Gait Posture 4:34-38

32. Hoffer MM, Feiwell E, Perry R, Bonnett G (1973) Functional ambulation in patients with myelomeningocele. J Bone Joint Surg 55:137-148

33. De Souza LJ, Carroll N (1976) Ambulation of the braced myelomeningocele patient. J Bone Joint Surg 58:112-118

34. Feiwell E, Sakai D, Blatt T (1978) The effect of hip reduction in patients with myelomeningocele. J Bone Joint Surg 60-A:169-173

35. Stillwell A, Menelaus MB (1983) Walking ability in mature patients with spina bifida cystica. J Pediatr Orthop 3:184-190

36. Lindseth RE (1976) Treatment of the lower extremity in children paralysed by myelomeningocele (birth to 18 months). Instr Course Lect 25:76-82

37. Asher M, Olsen J (1983) Factors affecting the ambulatory status of patients with spina bifida cystica. J Bone Joint Surg 65:350-356

38. Rosenstein BD, Greene WB, Herrington RT, Blum AS (1987) Bone density in myelomeningocele: the effects of ambulatory status and other factors. Dev Med Child Neurol 29:486-494

39. Samuelsson L, Skoog M (1988) Ambulation in patients with myelomeningocele: a multivariate statistical analysis. J Pediatr Orthop 8:569-75

40. Broughton NS, Malcolm BM, Cole WG, Shurtleff DB (1993) The natural history of hip deformity in myelomeningocele. J Bone Joint Surg 75-B:760-763

41. McDonald C, Jaffe K, Mosca V, Shurtleff DB (1991) Ambulatory outcome of children with myelomeningocele: effect of lower-extremity muscle strength. Dev Med Child Neurol 33(6):482-490

42. Knutson LM, Clark DE (1991) Orthotic devices for ambulation in children with cerebral palsy and myelomeningocele. Phys Ther 71:947-960

43. Huff CW, Ramsey PL (1978) Myelodysplasia: the influence of the quadriceps and hip abductor muscles on ambulatory function and stability of the hip. J Bone Joint Surg 60-A:432-443

44. Swank M, Dias L (1992) Myelomeningocele: a review of the orthopaedic aspects of 206 patients treated from birth with no selection criteria. Dev Med Child Neurol 234:1047-1052

45. Swank M, Dias LS (1994) Walking ability in spina bifida patients: a model for predicting future ambulatory status based on sitting balance and motor level. J Pediatr Orthop 14:715-718

46. Smith PL, Owen JL, Fehlings D, Wright JG (2005) Measuring physical function in children with spina bifida and dislocated hips: the spina bifida hips questionnaire. J Pediatr Orthop 25(3):273-279

47. Gaffe JE, Robinson JM, Parker PM (1984) The walking ability of 14 to 17-year-old teenagers with spina bifida – a physiotherapy study. Physiotherapy 70:473-474

48. Dawnette L, Tolosa JE, Kaufmann M et al (2004) Elective cesarean delivery and long-term motor function or ambulation status in infants with myelomeningocele. ACOG Educ Bull 103(3):469-473

49. Findley TW, Agre JC, Habeck RV et al (1987) Ambulation in the adolescent with myelomeningocele I: Early childhood predictors. Arch Phys Med Rehabil 68:518-522

50. Lerner-Frankiel MB, Vargus S, Brown M et al (1986) Functional community ambulation: what are your criteria? Clin Manage Phys Ther 6:12

51. Bartonek A, Saraste H, Samuelsson L, Skoog M (1999) Ambulation in patients with myelomeningocele: a 12 year follow-up. J Pediatr Orthop 19(2):202-206

52. Graham HK, Harvey A, Rodda J et al (2004) The Functional Mobility Scale (FMS). J Pediatr Orthop 24(5):514-520

53. Williams EN, Carroll SG, Reddihough DS et al (2005) Investigation of the timed 'Up and Go' test in children. Dev Med Child Neurol 47:518-524

54. Williams EN (2004) An investigation of the Timed 'Up and Go' test in children. Thesis. Master of Physiotherapy, The University of Melbourne.

55. Shurtleff DB (1991) Computer databases for paediatric disability: Clinical and research applications. Physical Med and Rehab Clinics of N America 2:665-687

56. Bayley N (1993) The Bayley scales of infant development manual. Second Edition. Psychological Corporation, San Antonio, Texas

57. Chandler LS, Andrews MD, Swanson MW (1980) Movement assessment of infants: a manual. Published by the authors, Rolling Bay, Washington

58. Burns Y, Gilmour J, Kentish M, Mac Donald J (1996) Physiotherapy management of children with neurological, neuromuscular and neurodevelopmental problems. In: Burns Y and Mac Donald J (eds) Physiotherapy and the growing child. WB Saunders, London, pp 374-413

59. Bax M (1991) Walking: Editorial. Dev Med Child Neurol 33:471-472

60. Mazur JM, Shurtleff D, Menelaus MB, Colliver J (1989) Orthopaedic management of high level spina bifida: early walking compared with early use of a wheelchair. J Bone Joint Surg 71:56-61

61. Shurtleff DB (1986) Mobility. In: Shurtleff DB (ed) Myelodysplasia and exstrophies: Significance, prevention and treatment. Grune & Stratton, New York, pp 313-356

62. Liptack GS, Shurtleff DB, Bloss J et al (1992) Mobility aids for children with high level myelomeningocele: parapodium versus wheelchair. Dev Med Child Neurol 34:787-796

63. Hayden PW (1985) Adolescents with myelomeningocele. Pediatr Rev 6 (8):245-252

64. Ito JA (2001) Issues for young adults with spina bifida. In: Sarwark JF, Lubicky JP (eds) Caring for the child with spina bifida. American Academy of Orthopaedic Surgeons, Illinois, pp 609-625

65. Duffy CM, Hill AE, Cosgrove AP et al (1996) Three-dimensional gait analysis in spina bifida. J Pediatr Orthop 16(6):786-791

66. Broughton N, Menelaus MB (1998) General considerations. In: Broughton N, Menelaus MB (eds) Menelaus' orthopaedic management of spina bifida cystica. 3rd edn, WB Saunders, London, pp 1-18

67. Clancy CA, McGrath PJ, Oddson BE (2005) Pain in children and adolescents with spina bifida. Dev Med Child Neurol 47:27-34

68. Hendrick EB, Hoffman HJ, Humphreys RP (1982) The tethered spinal cord. Clin Neurosurg 30:457-463

69. Johnson DL, Levy LM (1995) Predicting outcome in tethered cord syndrome: a study of cord motion. Pediatr Neurosurg 22:115-119

70. Alpert SW, Koval KJ, Zuckerman JD (1996) Neuropathic arthopathy: review of current knowledge. J Am Acad Orthop Surg 4:100-108

71. Duffy CM, Hill AE, Cosgrove AP et al (1996) Three-dimensional gait analysis in spina bifida. J Pediatr Orthop 16(6):786-791

72. Gutierrez EM, Bartonek A, Haglund-Akerlind Y, Saraste H (2003) Characteristic gait kinematics in persons with lumbosacral myelomeningocele. Gait Posture 18: 170-177

73. Vankoski S, Sarwark JF, Moore C, Dias L (1995) Characteristic pelvic, hip and knee kinematic patterns in children with lumbosacral myelomeningocele. Gait Posture 3:51-57

74. Gupta RT, Vankoski S, Novak RA, Dias S (2005) Trunk kinematics and the influence of valgus stress in persons with high sacral level myelomeningocele. J Pediatr Orthop 25(1):89-94

75. Ounpuu S, Thomson J, Davis R, DeLuca P (2000) An examination of the knee function during gait in children with myelomeningocele. J Pediatr Orthop 20:629-635

76. Moore C, Dias L, Vankoski S et al (1995) Valgus stress at the knee joint in lumbo-sacral myelomeningocele: a gait analysis evaluation. Dev Med Child Neurol 28(suppl):2-3

77. Nagarkatti DG, Banta JV, Thomson JD (2000) Charcot arthropathy in spina bifida. J Pediatr Orthop 20:82-87

78. Williams JJ, Graham GP, Dunne KB, Menelaus MB (1993) Late knee problems in myelomeningocele. J Pediatr Orthop 13:701-703

79. Selber P, Dias L (1998) Sacral-level myelomeningocele long-term outcome in adults. J Pediatr Orthop 18:423-427

80. Gutierrez EM, Bartonek A, Haglund-Akerlind Y, Saraste H (2005) Kinetics of compensatory gait in persons with myelomeningocele. Gait Posture 21:12-23

81. Dunteman R, Vankoski SJ, Dias LS (2000) Internal derotation osteotomy of the tibia: pre- and postoperative gait analysis in persons with high sacral myelomeningocele. J Pediatr Orthop 20:623-628

82. Lim R, Dias L, Vankoski S et al (1998) Valgus knee stress in lumbosacral myelomeningocele: a gait-analysis evaluation. J Pediatr Orthop 18(4):428-433

83. Vankoski S, Moore C, Statler KD et al (1997) The influence of forearm crutches on pelvic and hip kinematics in children with low lumbar level myelomeningocele: don't throw away the crutches. Dev Med Child Neurol 39:614-619

84. Sawatzky BJ, Slobogean GP, Reilly CW et al (2005) Prevalence of shoulder pain in adult-versus childhood-onset wheelchair users: a pilot study. J Rehabil Res Dev 42(3):1-8

85. James CC (1970) Fractures of the lower limbs in spina bifida cystica: a survey of 44 fractures in 122 children. Dev Med Child Neurol 22(suppl):88-93

86. Anschuetz RH, Freehafer AA, Shaffer JW, Dixon MS (1984) Severe fracture complications in myelodysplasia. J Pediatr Orthop 4:22-24

87. Barnett JS, Menelaus MB (1998) Pressure sores and pathological fractures. In: Broughton NS, Menelaus MB (eds) Menelaus' orthopaedic management of spina bifida cystica. 3rd edn, WB Saunders, London, pp 51-65

88. Quilis AN (1974) Fractures in children with myelomeningocele. Acta Orthop Scand 45:883-897

89. Cuxart A, Iborra J, Melendez M, Pages E (1992) Physeal injuries in myelomeningocele patients. Paraplegia 30:791-794

90. Lock TR, Aronson DD (1989) Fractures in patients who have myelomeningocele. J Bone Joint Surg 71:1153-1157

91. Quan A, Adams R, Ekmark E, Baum M (1998) Bone mineral density in children with myelomeningocele. Pediatrics 102:E34

92. Chan GM, Hess M, Hollis J, Book LS (1984) Bone mineral status in childhood accidental fractures. Am J Disease Child 138:842-845

93. Rosen N, Spira E (1974) Paraplegic use of walking brace: a survey. Arch Phys Med Rehabil 55:310-314

94. Greene WB, Carter MD, DeMasi RA, Herrington RT (1991) Bone mineral density in myelomeningocele:effect of growth and other factors. Dev Med Child Neurol (suppl) 64:18

95. Thompson CR, Figoni SF, Devocelle HA et al (2000) Effect of dynamic weight bearing on lower extremity bone mineral density in children with neuromuscular impairment. Clin Kinesiol 54(1):13-18

96. Valtonen KM, Goksor L, Jonsson O et al (2006) Osteoporosis in adults with meningomyelocele: an unrecognized problem at rehabilitation clinics. Arch Phys Med Rehabil 87:376-382

97. Stuberg WA (1992) Considerations related to weight-bearing programs in children with developmental disabilities. Phys Ther 72(1):35-40

98. Waters RL, Mulroy, S (1999) The energy expenditure of normal and pathologic gait. Gait Posture 9:207-231

99. Fisher SV, Gullickson G Jr (1978) Energy cost of ambulation in health and disability: literature review. Arch Phys Med Rehabil 59:124-133

100. Bare A, Vankoski SJ, Danduran M, Boas S (2001) Independent ambulators with high sacral myelomeningocele: the relation between walking kinematics and energy consumption. Dev Med Child Neurol 43:16-21

101. Galli M, Crivellini M, Fazzi E, Motta F (2000) Energy consumption and gait analysis in children with myelomeningocele. Funct Neurol 15(3):171-175

102. Williams LO, Anderson AD, Campbell J (1983) Energy costs of walking and of wheelchair propulsion by children with myelodysplasia: comparison with normal children. Dev Med Child Neurol 25:617-624

103. Evans EP, Tew B (1981) Energy expenditure of spina bifida children during walking and wheelchair ambulation. Z Kinderchir 34:425-427

104. Duffy CM, Hill AE, Cosgrove AP et al (1996) Energy consumption in children with spina bifida and cerebral palsy: a comparative study. Dev Med Child Neurol 38:238-243

105. Moore CA, Bahareh N, Novak RA, Dias LS (2001) Energy cost in low lumbar myelomeningocele. J Pediatr Orthop 21(3):388-391

106. Franks CA, Palisano RJ, Darbee JC (1991) The effect of walking with an assistive device and using a wheelchair on school performance in students with myelomeningocele. Phys Ther 71(8):570-579

107. Salmela JH, Ndoye OD (1986) Cognitive distortions during progressive exercise. Percept Mot Skills 63:1067-1072

108. Spano JF, Burke EJ (1976) Effects of three levels of work intensity on performance of a fine motor skill. Percept Mot Skills 42:63-66

109. Gupta VP, Sharma TR, Jaspal SS (1974) Physical activity and efficiency of mental work. Percept Mot Skills 38:205

110. Bartonek A, Eriksson MC, Saraste H (2002) Heart rate and walking velocity during independent walking in children with low and midlumbar myelomeningocele. Pediatr Phys Ther 14(4):185-190

111. Bleck EE (1987) Goals, treatment and management. In: Bleck EE (ed) Orthopaedic management in cerebral palsy: Clinics in developmental medicine No 99-100. JB Lippincott, Philadelphia, p 174

112. Kottke FJ, Pauley DL, Ptak RA (1966) The rationale for prolonged stretching for correction of shortening of muscle tissue. Arch Phys Med Rehabil 47:345-352

113. Broughton N, Menelaus MB (1998) General considerations. In: Broughton N, Menelaus MB (eds) Menelaus' orthopaedic management of spina bifida cystica. 3rd edn, WB Saunders, London

114. Roberts D, Shepherd RW, Shepherd K (1991) Anthropometry and obesity in myelomeningocele. Paediatr. J Paediatr Child Health 27:83-90

115. Mita K, Akataki K, Itoh K et al (1993) Assessment of obesity in children with spina bifida. Dev Med Child Neurol 35(4):305

116. Shurtleff DB, Lamers J, Goiney T, Gordon L (1982) Are myelodysplastic children fat? Anthropometric measures: a preliminary report. Spina Bifida Ther 4(1):1-21

117. Shurtleff DB, Duguay S, Cardenas DD, Walker WO (2005) Obesity and myelomeningocele: Anthropometric measure of patients with myelomeningocele. Society for Research into Hydrocephalus and Spina Bifida, Barcelona, Hospital Universitari Vall d'Hebron, Spain

118. Shepherd K, Roberts D, Golding S et al (1991) Body composition in myelomeningocele. Am J Clin Nutr 53:1-6

119. Hayes-Allen MC (1972) Obesity and short stature in children with myelomeningocele. Dev Med Child Neurol 14 (suppl 22):59-64

120. Charney EB, Rosenblum M, Finegold D (1981) Linear growth in a population of children with myelomeningocele. Z Kinderchir 34:415-419

121. Littlewood, RA, Trocki O, Shepherd RW et al (2003) Resting energy expenditure and body composition in children with myelomeningocele. Pediatr Rehabil 6(1):31-37

122. Bandini LG, Schoeller DA, Fukagawa NK et al (1990) Body composition and energy expenditure in adolescents with cerebral palsy or myelodysplasia. Pediatr Res 29(1):70-77

123. Shurtleff DB (1986) Dietary Considerations. In: Shurtleff DB (ed) Myelodysplasia and exstrophies: Significance, prevention and treatment. Grune & Stratton, New York, pp 285-311

124. Hayes-Allen MC, Tring FL (1972) Obesity: Another hazard for spina bifida children. Br J Prev Soc Med 27:192-196

125. Shurtleff DB, Dunne K (1986) Adults and adolescents with myelomeningocele. In: Shurtleff DB (ed) Myelodysplasia and exstrophies: Significance, prevention and treatment. Grune & Stratton, New York, pp 433-448

126. Brown JP (2001): Orthopaedic care of children with spina bifida: you've come a long way baby! Orthop Nurs 20(4):51-58

127. Dietz WH (1983) Childhood obesity: susceptibility, cause and management. J Pediatr 103:676-686

128. Carroll N (1974) The orthotics management of the spina bifida child. Clin Orthop 102:108-114

129. Kirpalani HM, Parkin PC, Willan AR et al (2000) Quality of life in spina bifida: importance of parental hope. Arch Dis Child 83:293-297

130. Pit-ten Cate IM, Kennedy C, Stevenson J (2002) Disability and quality of life in spina bifida and hydrocephalus. Dev Med Child Neurol 44:317-322

131. Sawin KJ, Brei TJ, Buran CF, Fastenau PS (2002) Factors associated with quality of life in adolescents with spina bifida. J Holist Nurs 20(3):279-304

132. Liptak GS, Bloss JW, Briskin H et al (1988) The management of children with spinal dysraphism. J Child Neurol 3(1):3-20

133. Appleton PL, Minchom PE, Ellis NC et al (1994) The self-concept of young people with spina bifida: a population-based study. Dev Med Child Neurol 36:198-215

134. Thomas AP, Bax MC, Smyth DP (1989) The health and social needs of young adults with physical disabilities. Blackwell Scientific Publications, Oxford

135. Minchom PE, Ellis NC, Appleton PL et al (1995) Impact of functional severity on self concept in young people with spina bifida. Arch Dis Child 73(1):48-52

136. Vinck A, Maassen B, Mullaart R, Rotteveel J (2006) Arnold-Chiari malformation and cognitive functioning in spina bifida. J Neurol Neurosurg Psychiatry 77:1083-1086

137. Iddon JL, Morgan DJR, Ahmed R et al (2003) Memory and learning in young adults with hydrocephalus and spina bifida: specific cognitive profiles. Eur J Pediatr Surg 13:S28-S46

138. Friedrich WN, Lovejoy MC, Shaffer J et al (1991) Cognitive abilities and achievement status of children with myelomeningocele: a contemary sample. J Pediatr Psychol 4:423-428

139. Wills KE (1993) Neuropsychological functioning in children with spina bifida and/or hydrocephalus. J Clin Child Psychol 2:247-265

140. Casari EF, Fantino AG (1998) A longitudinal study of cognitive abilities and achievement status of children with myelomeningocele and their relationship with clinical types. Eur J Pediatr Surg 8:52-54

141. Lindquist B, Carlsson G, Persson E, Uvebrant P (2005) Learning disabilities in a population- based group of children with hydrocephalus. Acta Paediatrica 94:878-883

142. Fletcher JM, Brookshire BL, Landry SH et al (1996) Attentional skills and executive functions in children with early hydrocephalus. Developmental Neuropsychology 12:53-76

143. Burmeister R, Hannay HJ, Copeland K et al (2005) Attention problems and executive functions in children with spina bifida and hydrocephalus. Child Neuropsychology 11:265-283

144. Mapstone TB, Rekate HL, Nulsen FE et al (1984) Relationship of CSF shunting and IQ in children with myelomeningocele. Child's Brain 11(2):112-118

145. Rendeli C, Salvaggio E, Cannizzaro GS et al (2002) Does locomotion improves the cognitive profile of children with myelomeningocele? Child's Nervous System 18:231-234

146. Banta JV, Casey JM, Bedell L, Morgan J (1983) Long-term ambulation in spina bifida. Dev Med Child Neurol 110 (abstract)

147. Taylor A, McNamara A (1990) Ambulation status of adults with myelomeningocele. Z Kinderchir 45(1):32-33

148. Fraser RK, Hoffman EB, Sparks LT, SS Buccimazza (1992) The unstable hip and mid-lumbar myelomeningocele. J Bone Joint Surg 74-B(1):143-146

149. Charney EB, Melchionni RN, Smith DR (1991) Community ambulation by children with myelomeningocele and high level paralysis. J Pediatr Orthop 11:579-582

150. Williams EN, Broughton NS, Menelaus MB (1999) Age-related walking in children with spina bifida. Dev Med Child Neurol 41:446-449

151. Selber P, Pauleto AC, Dias L (1997) The adult low lumbar and sacral level myelomeningocele. Proceedings from the American Orthopaedic Association Annual Meeting. Colorado Springs, CO, USA

152. Selber P, Dias L (1998) Sacral-level myelomeningocele: long-term outcome in adults. J Pediatr Orthop 18:423-427

153. Park TS, Cail WS, Maggio WM, Mitchell DC (1985) Progressive spasticity and scoliosis in children with myelomeningocele. J Neurosurg 62:367-375

154. Peterson MC (1992) Tethered cord syndrome in myelodyplasia: correlation between level of lesion and height at time of presentation. Dev Med Child Neurol 34:604-610

155. Just M, Schwarz, Ermert JA et al (1988) Magnetic resonance imaging of dysraphic myelodysplasia: findings in 56 children and adolescents with postrepair meningomyelocele. Childs Nerv Syst 4:149-153

156. Banta JV (1991) The tethered cord in myelomeningocele: should it be untethered? Dev Med Child Neurol 33:173-176

157. Menelaus MB (1976) Orthopaedic management of children with myelomeningocele: a plea for realistic goals. Dev Med Child Neurol 37(18 suppl):3-11

158. Wolf LS, McLaughlin JF (1992) Early motor development in infants with myelomeningocele. Pediatr Phys Ther 4:12-17

159. Sousa JC, Telzrow RW, Holm RA et al (1983) Developmental guidelines for children with myelodysplasia. Phys Ther 63:21-29

160. Dahl M, Ahlsten G, Carlson H et al (1995) Neurological dysfunction above cele level in children with spina bifida cystica: a prospective study to three years. Dev Med Child Neurol 37:30-40

161. Norrlin S, Strinnholm M, Carlsson M, Dahl M (2003) Factors of significance for mobility in children with myelomeningocele. Acta Paediatr 92:204-210

162. Gilmour J, Kentish M (1996) Aids and orthotics. In: Burns Y and Mac Donald J (eds) Physiotherapy and the growing child. WB Saunders, London

163. Guidera KJ, Smith S, Raney E et al (1993) Use of the reciprocating gait orthosis in myelodysplasia. J Paed Orth 13:341-348

164. Diaz L, Lopis I, Bea Munoz M et al (1993) Ambulation in patients with myelomeningocele and high-level paralysis. J Paed Orth 11:579-582

165. Katz-Leurer M, Weber C, Smerling-Kerem J et al (2003) Prescribing the reciprocal gait orthosis for myelomeningocele children: A different approach and clinical outcome. Paed Rehab 7(2)105-109

166. Polliack AA, Elliot S, Caves C et al (2001) Lower extremity orthoses for children with myelomeningocele: User and orthotist perspectives. J Prosthet Orthot 13(4):123-129

167. Henderson WH, Campbell JW (1969) UC-BL shoe insert: Casting and fabrication. Bull Prosthet Res 10:215-235

168. Duffy CM, Graham HK, Cosgrove AP (2000) The influence of ankle-foot orthoses on gait and energy expenditure in spina bifida. J Paed Orth 20(3):356-361

169. Thomson JD, Ounpuu S, Davis RB, DeLuca PA (1999) The effects of ankle-foot orthoses on the ankle and knee in persons with myelomeningocele: An evaluation using three-dimensional gait analysis. J Paed Orth 19(1):27-33

170. Freeman D, Orendurff M, Moor M (1999) Case study: Improving knee extension with floor-reaction ankle-foot orthoses in a patient with myelomeningocele and 20 degree knee flexion contractures. J Prosthet and Orthot 11(3):63-68

171. Hullin MG, Robb JE, Loudon IR (1992) Ankle-foot orthosis function in low-level myelomeningocele. J Paed Orth 12(4):518-21

172. Vankoski SJ, Michaud S, Dias L (2000) External tibial torsion and the effectivness of the solid ankle-foot Orthoses. J Paed Orth 20(3):349-355

173. Duffy C, Barwood S, Graham HK (1998) Energy studies in spina bifida. Course notes. Clinical gait analysis: a focus on interpretation. Melbourne, Australia

174. Thomas SS, Buckon CE, Melchionni J et al (2001) Longitudinal assessment of oxygen cost and velocity in children with myelomeningocele: a comparison of the hip-knee-ankle-foot orthosis and the reciprocating Gait Orthosis. J Paed Orth 21:798-803

175. Yngve DA, Douglas R, Roberts JM (1984) The reciprocating gait orthosis in myelomeningocele. J Paed Orth 4:304-310

176. Rose GK (1979) The principles and practice of hip guidance articulations. Prosthet Orthot Int 3:37-43

177. Motloch WM, Elliott J (1966) Fitting and training children with swivel walkers. Artif Limbs 10:27-38

178. Roussos N, Patrick JH, Hodnett C, Stallard J (2001) A long-term review of severely disabled spina bifida patients using a reciprocal walking system. Disabil Rehabil 23(6):239-244

179. Cuddeford TJ, Freeling RP, Thomas SS et al (1997) Energy consumption in children with myelomeningocele: a comparison between reciprocating gait orthosis and hip-knee-ankle-foot orthosis ambulators. Dev Med Child Neur 39:239-242

180. Katz DE, Haideri N, Song K, Wyrick P (1997) Comparative study of conventional hip-knee-ankle-foot orthosis versus reciprocating gait orthosis for children with high-level paraparesis. J Paed Orth 17:377-386

181. McCall RE, Schmidt WT (1986) Clinical experience with the reciprocal gait orthosis in myelodysplasia. J Paed Orth 6:157-161

182. Broughton N, Menelaus MB (1998) The hip. In: Broughton N, Menelaus MB (eds) Menelaus' orthopaedic management of spina bifida cystica, 3rd edn. WB Saunders, London, pp 135-144

183. Phillips DL, Field RE, Broughton NS, Menelaus MB (1995) Reciprocating orthoses for children with myelomeningocele: a comparison of two types. JBJS (Br) 77-B:110-113

184. Wallace SJ (1973) The effect of upper limb function on mobility of the children with myelomeningocele. Dev Med Child Neurol 29:84-91

185. Minns RA, Sobkowiak CA, Skardoutsou A et al (1977) Upper limb function in spina bifida. Z Kinderchir 22(4):493-506

186. Muen WJ, Bannister CM (1997) Hand function in subjects with spina bifida. Eur J Paediatr Surg (7 suppl I):18-22

187. Turner A (1986) Upper limb function of children with myelomeningocele. Dev Med Child Neurol 28:790-798

188. Aronin PA, Kerrick R (1995) Value of dynamometry in assessing upper extremity function in children with myelomeningocele. Pediatr Neurosurg 2:7-13

189. Mazur JM, Menelaus MB, Hudson I, Stillwell A (1986) Hand function in spina bifida cystica. J Pediatr Orthop 6:442-447

190. Bartonek A, Saraste H (2001) Factors influencing ambulation in myelomeningocele: a cross-sectional study. Dev Med Child Neurol 43:253-260

191. Brinker M, Rosenfeld S, Feiwell E et al (1994) Myelomeningocele at the sacral level: long-term outcomes in adults. J Bone Joint Surg 76-A:1293-1300

192. Carstens C, Rohwedder J, Berghof R (1995) Orthotic treatment and walking ability in patients with myelomeningocele. Z Orthop 133:214-221

193. Schiltenwolf M, Carstens C, Rohwedder J, Grundel E (1991) Results of orthotics treatment in children with myelomeningocele. Eur J Pediatr Surg (1 suppl):50-52

194. Lee E, Carroll NC (1985) Hip stability and ambulatory status in myelomeningocele. J Pediatr Orthop 5:522-527

195. Rose GK, Sankarankutty J, Stallard J (1983) A clinical review of the orthotics treatment of myelomeningocele patients. J Bone Joint Surg Br 65(3):242-246

196. Thomas SE, Mazur JM, Child ME, Supan TJ (1989) Quantitative evaluation of AFO use with myelomeningocele children. Z Kinderchir 44(1):38-40

197. Flandry F, Burke S, Roberts JM et al (1986) Functional ambulation in myelodysplasia: the effect of orthotics selection on physical and physiologic performance. J Pediatr Orthop 6:661-665

198. Ito J, Saijo H, Araki A et al (1997) Neuroradiological assessment of visuoperceptual disturbance in children with spina bifida and hydrocephalus. Dev Med Child Neurol 3:385-392

Section VI
UROLOGY

Chapter 30
Neuro-Urological Management of the Neuropathic Bladder in Children with Myelodysplasia

Tufan Tarcan, Stuart Bauer

General Principles and Goals of Neuro-Urological Management in Children With Myelodysplasia

Myelodysplasia, a Urological Disease?

Myelodysplasia, which refers to developmental anomalies of the spinal cord caused by closure defects of the neural tube, is the leading cause of neurogenic bladder dysfunction (NBD) in children. Myelomeningocele (MMC), the most common form of open spinal dysraphism, constitutes at least 90% of neural tube defects compatible with life leading to NBD. Classification and terminology of neural tube defects is beyond the scope of this chapter and is discussed elsewhere in this book.

As a result of improvements in the neurosurgical management of children born with MMC, this disorder is a neuro-urological disease today. Until the early part of the twentieth century, the mortality of children born with MMC reached almost 100%, with 80-90% of deaths occurring within the first year of life [1]. The development of surgical repair techniques of the primary defect at the end of the nineteenth century created a chance for survival in those children with good general health status and no co-morbidities or associated anomalies [2]. Throughout the nineteenth century, hydrocephalus was a contraindication to primary surgical repair, as was paralysis of the lower extremities [3]. According to these criteria, only one third of children were found to be suitable for surgical intervention [4]. Primary closure of the spinal defect was not performed until the lesion was epithelialized and the hydrocephalus resolved [3]. Even under these circumstances, at the end of the nineteenth century the surgical mortality was 50%. Whether or not an individual was operated on, hydrocephalus and infection were the most common reasons for mortality until the 1950s. Since then, the

mortality rate has dropped to 10%, due to improvements in shunting techniques for hydrocephalus and the discovery of broad spectrum antibiotics [5, 6]. Today, early closure of the primary spinal defect with improved neurosurgical techniques and ventricular peritoneal shunting significantly increases the survival rate of children with an open lesion and shifts the chief causes of morbidity and mortality from central nervous system infection and hydrocephalus to long term urological complications such as pyelonephritis, hypertension and chronic renal failure (CRF) [7].

Early Neurosurgical Intervention after Birth Improves the Neuro-Urological Prognosis

Early closure of the primary defect is crucial not only for survival, but also for a favorable neuro-urological outcome of children with MMC. A recent study of 129 children with MMC has shown that urological follow-up data at three years of age revealed a significantly increased incidence of febrile urinary tract infection (UTI), vesicoureteral reflux (VUR), hydronephrosis and secondary tethering of the spinal cord in children who were operated on more than 72 hours after birth, as compared to those children who were operated on before that time [8]. In addition, early intervention was associated with a significantly higher cystometric bladder capacity and a lower detrusor leak point pressure (DLPP) [8]. A subgroup analysis comparing children who underwent repair before 24 hours and between 24-72 hours following delivery failed to demonstrate any significant difference in terms of febrile UTI, VUR, hydronephrosis and secondary tethering, whereas mean bladder capacity was significantly higher and mean DLPP was lower in children undergoing repair within 24 hours of delivery [8]. This study has offered the best evidence so far that the timing of primary neurosurgical repair has a significant impact on the prognosis of bladder function in children with MMC, whereas closure of the spinal lesion on the first day of life appears to provide the best chance for favorable lower urinary tract function.

Dynamic Character of the Disease and Basic Goals of Neuro-Urological Management

Neurologic denervation of the detrusor smooth muscle and urethral sphincter due to abnormal development of the spinal canal leads to a wide variety of voiding abnormalities. Debilitating issues such as urinary incontinence (UI), UTI, VUR and CRF can be complications of NBD. CRF is the most serious complication of this spectrum, especially affecting children with an upper motor neuron lesion associated with detrusor-sphincter dyssynergia (DSD), seen in about one third of all affected children [9]. A smaller percentage of children with a synergic sphincter and normal detrusor activity, who usually do not have a significant lower extremity motor deficit, constitute the opposite end of the spectrum and have a much more favorable outcome. However, even this latter group of children with initially normal neurourological findings is at risk due to secondary tethering of the spinal cord. One study has shown that secondary tethering can occur in 32% of this group, especially during the first six years of life [10].

Independent of the type of the neurogenic deficit present, neuro-urological management of children with myelodysplasia has two basic goals: 1) to protect the urinary tract, especially the kidneys, but also the urinary bladder, urethra and ureters from irreversible functional and morphological damage; and 2) to increase the quality of life of children by treating or minimizing their lower urinary tract symptoms and/or by bringing the child into a socially adaptable situation in terms of their lower urinary tract symptoms (LUTS).

Dynamic Character of the NBD in Myelodysplasia Warrants Close Urological Surveillance

Achieving these goals is not always an easy task. A proactive approach is often needed, stemming from the unpredictable and dynamic nature of the disease process and its associated anomalies. First of all, in contrast to spinal cord trauma, the type and prognosis of the NBD in MMC is not determined by the level of the spinal defect; rather it is due to the specific neural elements that are incorporated within the sac, as well as the dynamic process of the elongating vertebral bodies and the spinal cord itself, that defines the ultimate extent of the neurogenic impairment [7, 11]. An Arnold-Chiari malformation, which may be present in 85% of cases, includes herniation of cerebellar tonsils through the foramen magnum, obstructing the fourth ventricle and inhibiting the passage of cerebrospinal fluid into the subarachnoid space [12]. Hydrocephalus caused by this deformity may have additional effects on the central nervous system (CNS) centers of micturition in the pons, brainstem and cerebral cortex that further impinge on the NBD. In 20% of children with lumbosacral MMC, a secondary vertebral or intraspinal abnormality at a more cephalad level may accompany the primary defect. In addition to these factors, the differential longitudinal growth of bony vertebra and the spinal cord adds a dynamic character to the disease process. In more than one third of cases, neuro-urological findings change within the first several years of life [13]. In half the children this change is associated with worsening of the NBD, whereas the other half has re-innervation of their bladder and external sphincter [12]. This change cannot be predicted by any radiological, laboratory or urodynamic examination performed at birth or at the first evaluation of the child. In this sense, one of the aims of proactive treatment is to monitor the neuro-urological picture closely in order to denote any change in the function of the lower urinary tract in this early period and take appropriate action once signs of potential deterioration are evident.

As mentioned above, secondary tethering of the spinal cord, which may be seen in about one third of children with MMC, is the major reason for the dynamic character of this disease [10]. If not treated judiciously, secondary tethering may significantly worsen the prognosis of NBD. The patho-physiology of this process is believed to be due to mechanical damage and ischemic injury caused by spinal cord tethering [14]. The differential growth rates between the vertebral bodies and the elongating spinal cord leads to mechanical stretching of the spinal cord when the conus medullaris is fixed to the lower end of the spinal canal. The fixation of the conus medullaris is encountered most commonly as a consequence of adhesions after primary closure or infections of the spinal cord. Fetal surgery does not seem to protect the individual from this consequence [15]. The mechanical stretching of the spinal cord results in a compromise of its blood supply and subsequent ischemia of neural tissue, causing progressive neurological deficits [14]. These deficits normally include weakness and sensory loss of the lower limbs producing a muscle imbalance that leads to deformities of the feet. However, NBD may represent the only initial symptom of secondary tethering in a substantial number of cases [10, 16].

Unfortunately, the diagnostic criteria for secondary tethering of the spinal cord in children with myelodysplasia are not well defined. Urological, neurological or orthopedic deterioration during follow-up remains the only indicator for the diagnosis of this condition. Urological deterioration may be defined as new onset upper urinary tract dilation or VUR on radiological imaging, urodynamic deterioration, such as a decrease in bladder compliance and/or increase in DLPP, recurrent febrile UTI and new onset or worsening of UI during appropriate management with clean intermittent catheterization (CIC), despite the use of anticholinergic medication and/or antibiotic prophylaxis (Table 30.1) [16].

The outcome from detethering surgery is not always predictable either. The success of any secondary detethering surgery strongly depends on its timing. The outcome is most favorable when it is performed before ischemia-related irreversible changes in the innervation of the lower urinary tract have occurred. Therefore, close urological surveillance remains the most valuable tool for early diagnosis and a more favorable outcome. A recent study of 401 children with MMC supporting this hypothesis revealed secondary

tethering in 56 (14%) based on urological and neuro-orthopedic deterioration in 58% and 42% of the tethered spinal cords, respectively [16]. When compared to preoperative urological findings, postoperative assessment at six months revealed urodynamic and clinical improvement in all children, which was more significant when the diagnosis was made and treatment instituted before the age of seven years.

Basic Information About the Lower Urinary Tract Function

Urologic morbidity of myelodysplasia develops secondary to pathological innervation of the lower urinary tract and it is therefore essential to understand the basic physiology of the urinary bladder and the urethral sphincter mechanisms that constitute the functional lower urinary tract.

The Urinary Bladder

The urinary bladder is composed of mucosa, the detrusor smooth muscle and adventitia. Smooth muscle fibers are organized irregularly and are surrounded by connective tissue rich in collagen. Compliance of the bladder is determined by the tone of the detrusor. Smooth muscle fibers are capable of increasing their length four-fold going from an empty to a full bladder.

The urinary bladder can be divided into two parts – the base and the dome – that have different embryological and functional properties. The detrusor muscle of the dome is richly innervated by the parasympathetic pelvic nerve originating from the S2-S4 nuclei of the spinal cord. A full and coordinated contraction of the detrusor muscle is needed to empty the bladder. The detrusor muscle contracts when stimulated by the pelvic nerve via release of the neurotransmitter, acetylcholine, acting on muscarinic type 2 and 3 receptors in the detrusor muscle. The detrusor muscle is also innervated by the sympathetic iliohypogastric nerve that relaxes the detrusor muscle via the action of the neurotransmitter, noradrenaline, on beta-3 adrenergic receptors. The density of muscarinic receptors is much more intense in the fundus of the bladder compared to adrenergic receptors and thus, the effect of a cholinergic stimulus on the detrusor muscle is much more pronounced compared to an adrenergic stimulus. The non-adrenergic and non-cholinergic (NANC) systems affecting detrusor contractility may include neuro-

Table 30.1. Neuro-urological clues of re-tethered cord syndrome

New onset upper urinary tract dilation on radiologic studies

New onset or worsening grade of VUR

New febrile and/or recurrent UTI episodes

New onset of urinary leakage between clean intermittent catheterizations

Deterioration of urodynamic findings:
- New onset detrusor over-activity
- Worsening bladder compliance
- New onset bladder hyposensitivity with detrusor weakness and high post-voiding residual urine
- New onset detrusor sphincter dyssynergia

New onset of lower urinary tract symptoms in children who void and who are over five years of age:
- Increased frequency
- Urgency
- Urinary incontinence
- Interrupted voiding
- Incomplete emptying with increased postvoid residual urine

transmitters or pathways such as the ATP-purinergic system, vasoactive intestinal polypeptide (VIP), cyclo-oxygenase and lipo-oxygenase products, nitric oxide and serotonin, etc. Although the NANC innervation seems to play a minor role in the regulation of normal bladder contractility, it may play a more pivotal role in pathological states, but this is still not completely understood.

The base of the bladder consists of the trigone and bladder neck, which are innervated by the iliohypogastric nerve originating from sympathetic nuclei at the T10-12 levels of the spinal cord. Its neurotransmitter, noradrenaline, stimulates alpha adrenergic receptors and contracts the smooth muscle fibers in the trigone. Here, there is a greater concentration of alpha-1A adrenergic receptors than muscarinic receptors. Thus, the effect of adrenergic stimulation may be quite intense. The smooth muscle fibers of the trigone further constitute the internal urethral sphincter mechanism around the bladder neck.

The Urethral Sphincters

In humans, there are two urethral sphincter mechanisms – the internal and external urethral sphincters – located around the bladder neck and at the membranous urethra, respectively. The internal urethral sphincter is an involuntary and functional sphincter composed of smooth muscle fibers. The tone of the internal urethral sphincter is under the control of the autonomic nervous system. It is innervated via the adrenergic iliohypogastric nerve and contracts due to noradrenalin acting on alpha-1A adrenergic receptors. The role of the internal urethral sphincter mechanism in the maintenance of continence in both genders has not been fully established. However, in men the internal urethral sphincter plays an important role during the ejaculatory phase of orgasm. Damage to the internal urethral sphincter mechanism, the iliohypogastric nerve, or the thoracolumbar sympathetic chain can lead to retrograde ejaculation.

The external urethral sphincter is a true voluntary sphincter muscle composed of striated smooth muscle fibers. It is innervated by the pudendal nerve originating from the S2-4 somatic nuclei in the spinal cord. The pudendal nerve also innervates the external anal sphincter and therefore any damage to the pudendal nerve will decrease the tone of both the external urethral and anal sphincters. For this reason, assessment of anal sphincter activity during physical examination or anal sphincter electromyography (EMG) provides information about the innervation of the external urethral sphincter. The external ure-

thral sphincter is the only organ of our voiding machine that is under volitional control; urinary continence directly depends on a healthy external urethral sphincter mechanism.

Sacral and Central Controls of Micturition

The spinal micturition center is located at the S2-4 levels of the spinal cord and it supplies motor innervation to the bladder. Motor innervation of the pelvic floor and the external urethral sphincter is received from Onuf's nucleus, located at the S2-3 levels of the spinal cord. Bladder sensations of pain, heat and mucosal stretching are transferred via afferent pelvic and hypogastric sensory nerves to the spinothalamic tract and then to the thalamus. Proprioceptive impulses originating from the detrusor and the external urethral sphincter reach the nucleus tegmentolateralis dorsalis in the pontine mesencephalic center through the posterior spinal columns. The sacral spinal micturition center is under the control of pontine and suprapontine centers.

The Center of Barrington, located in the anterior pons, is the center of impulses facilitating a detrusor contraction. It can be suppressed by other brain centers such as the cerebellum, basal ganglia, thalamus and hypothalamus. Any suprapontine damage or dysfunction of these suppressor centers will lead to neurogenic detrusor overactivity. The upper medial segments of the frontal lobes and the genu of the corpus callosum are involved in micturition and have an inhibitory effect on a contracting detrusor. Neurotransmitters responsible for this effect are thought to be gamma-aminobutyric acid (GABA) and glycine.

The Storage and Emptying Phases of Bladder-Sphincter Function

The function of the lower urinary tract can be characterized as having two phases: the storage phase and the emptying phase.

Storage Phase

This phase corresponds to the period between two micturitions. The urinary bladder has the ability to store urine at a low and constant intravesical pressure (less than 10 cmH$_2$O), despite gradually increasing volumes of intravesical urine during the storage phase. This phenomenon is known as the compliance of the bladder. It is calculated as the ratio of a change in intravesical volume to a change in detrusor pressure ($\Delta V/\Delta P$) during the storage or filling phase during a urodynamic study (UDS). The compliance of the bladder is related to the viscoelastic properties of the bladder wall and the arrangement of detrusor muscle bundles that allow for an increase in intravesical urine volume. The viscoelastic properties include elastin and collagen fibers, lamina propria and mucosa of the bladder wall, which allow for accommodation as the bladder fills. The tone of the detrusor muscle decreases in parallel to the increasing volume of intravesical urine. This phenomenon is supplemented by increased sympathetic impulses activating beta-3 adrenergic receptors while inhibiting cholinergic receptors. Compliance of the bladder may diminish due to neurogenic detrusor overactivity or fibrosis of the bladder wall from chronic infection or in response to increased bladder outlet obstruction. This then leads to high intravesical pressures during the storage phase. The non-compliant bladder is a major risk factor for upper urinary tract damage.

During the storage phase, a closed bladder outlet is needed to prevent urinary leakage. To maintain closure of the bladder outlet, the tone of the two urethral sphincters increases in parallel to the increase in intravesical pressure. This is called the guarding reflex. However, the major component of bladder outlet resistance is the resistance generated by the external urethral sphincter. Denervation of the internal and external urethral sphincter mechanisms is the most common reason for urinary incontinence in children with myelodysplasia. In addition to sphincter tone, urethral mucosal coaptation passively adds to the outlet resistance. Urethral denervation as commonly seen in children with myelodysplasia may lead to urethral atrophy and loss of mucosal coaptation.

During the storage phase the detrusor muscle should not generate unstable or premature contractions, i.e., detrusor overactivity, that can be of neurogenic or non-neurogenic etiology. The premature detrusor contractions in children with myelodysplasia indicate neurogenic detrusor overactivity which can lead to LUTS such as increased frequency and incontinence and decreased compliance of the bladder.

Emptying Phase

A normal emptying phase depends on three factors: first, a coordinated and sustained contraction of the detrusor muscle; second, complete relaxation of both sphincters; and third, a urethra free of intraluminal obstruction.

Any damage to the pelvic nerves or sacral micturition center will decrease the cholinergic stimulus to the bladder and decrease detrusor contractility. When complete denervation is present the detrusor muscle cannot contract and the bladder cannot empty. Structural degeneration of the bladder wall (e.g., secondary to long term bladder outlet obstruction due to DSD or fibrosis of the external sphincter) may be another factor impairing normal detrusor contractility in children with myelodysplasia. During micturition, the urethral sphincters must relax in concert with a decrease in bladder outlet resistance. Coordination between the detrusor muscle and the sphincter mechanisms is under control of the pontine mesencephalic micturition center, and involves spinal neural pathways and the sacral spinal micturition arc. DSD refers to non-relaxation of either or both of the urethral sphincters during micturition. It is typically caused by an upper motor neuron lesion breaking the connection between the detrusor and the sphincter muscles and the central nervous system. About one third of children with MMC have an upper motor neuron lesion leading to DSD-related infravesical obstruction. These children carry the highest risk for upper and lower urinary tract damage. For a healthy emptying phase, the urethra must also be free of other causes of infravesical obstruction such as posterior urethral valves and urethral and meatal strictures.

Urodynamic Evaluation and Initial Neuro-Urological Management of Children with MMC

Initial urological management of children with MMC (Fig. 30.1) should start in the newborn period, as soon as possible after the primary closure of the spinal defect has been performed. Apart from the physical examination, the first evaluation should include a urine analysis and culture, renal function measurements, ultrasound visualization of the urinary tract and video-urodynamic studies. Circumcision in boys is advocated to prevent UTI and to facilitate CIC. Undescended testis is seen more commonly in children with MMC, when compared with the normal population, and thus a careful scrotal examination in newborn boys is warranted [17].

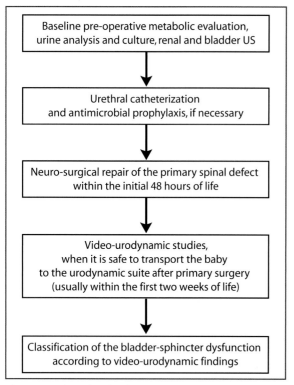

Fig. 30.1. Algorithm for the neuro-urological management of newborns with MMC

UDS is the gold standard evaluation method to understand lower urinary tract function and dysfunction. This study investigates the pressure-volume relationship during storage and emptying phases of the bladder, together with the assessment of pelvic floor (anal or urethral sphincter) EMG. Video-UDS, which combines a standard voiding cystogram with conventional UDS, is considered the gold standard for urodynamic evaluation. The purpose of the initial urodynamic evaluation is to classify the NBD and to differentiate the group of children who carry the highest risk for urinary tract deterioration.

There are several arguments regarding the timing of UDS. Some authors advocate UDS prior to primary closure of the back in order to avoid the effects of spinal surgery that may produce spinal shock (3-5%) and a change in innervation. However, implementing this can be very difficult in a clinical setting because surgical intervention is usually undertaken immediately after birth and UDS may increase the risk of infection of the open lesion in MMC. Furthermore, one study which compared pre- and post-closure urodynamic studies has shown a significant difference in findings in only 5%, with spinal shock seen as the only major consequence of the closure [18]. Therefore, UDS can be safely performed after

the primary surgical repair when the back wound has healed and the child is able to be transferred to the urodynamic suite [13].

Although the majority of reports in the literature support the use of UDS shortly after birth to predict which newborns are at risk for upper tract deterioration in the future, some authors advocate that routine UDS in the newborn period is not necessary, suggesting instead that it should be reserved only for those babies with evidence of urinary retention on physical examination, new onset hydronephrosis or febrile urinary tract infection, or for an evaluation to achieve continence. For example, Hopps and Kropp [19] followed 84 infants with MMC, where only 18 infants with hydronephrosis or evidence of retention were placed into a high risk group and underwent UDS. The remaining 66 were classified as the low risk group and were followed up in two to four month intervals without performing UDS. After a mean follow-up of 10.4 years, 29 children (42%) from the low risk group converted to the high risk group and underwent urodynamic evaluation and further appropriate treatment. In total, renal deterioration was found in only 1.2% of the renal units. In another study, Teichman et al. [20] presented an even more conservative approach where they screened patients shortly after birth with ultrasound, urine culture and serum creatinine, and then followed them at three to six month intervals with similar studies, reserving urodynamics evaluation following any adverse change in clinical status or ultrasound features [20]. These authors reported a rate of renal deterioration of 5% that was associated with a statistically significant incidence of UTI and VUR, but not with abnormal urodynamic findings. Despite these favorable results in terms of renal deterioration, the authors of this approach advocate early urodynamic evaluation and follow-up of children with periodic UDS, depending on their initial risk for deterioration. UDS is the best method to understand the lower urinary tract dysfunction in children with myelodysplasia and also to monitor the patho-physiological changes in the lower urinary tract that are due to secondary tethering of the spinal cord. Early UDS provides an opportunity to start CIC and/or anticholinergic medication in the high risk group before morphologic and radiologic changes can be detected. It should be kept in mind that these changes may not always be reversible and that the definition of renal deterioration may differ from study to study. Furthermore, other endpoints such as urinary incontinence or bladder compliance/capacity should also be assessed. Large scale randomized studies are needed to compare proactive therapy with this conservative approach to determine the safest, most efficient and least invasive way to manage children with MMC.

Basic UDS that are performed to define the NBD in newborns with MMC generally include a cystometrogram (CMG) with anal or urethral sphincter EMG. Pressure-flow studies and free uroflowmetric studies can be employed in children who volitionally void and can empty their bladder. CMG evaluates the storage function of the urinary bladder by measuring pressure-volume relationships. For this purpose, a double lumen cystometry catheter is used to fill the bladder with sterile saline at a controlled rate through one port while measuring the real-time intravesical pressure through the other port. The CMG provides important information about bladder capacity, bladder compliance, detrusor activity and DLPP that are essential in describing, classifying and treating the NBD. Decreased bladder compliance, detrusor overactivity and high DLPP are strongly associated with upper urinary tract deterioration, which may lead to CRF. DSD may be best demonstrated by combining video-CMG with sphincter EMG.

EMG of the external urethral sphincter can be assessed with needle electrodes during the CMG and pressure flow studies. Although external urethral sphincter EMG is more sensitive, it is invasive and more difficult to interpret compared to anal sphincter EMG, which is simple and non-invasive. For this reason, anal sphincter EMG is used more routinely in clinical practice. In older children who can void volitionally, free uroflowmetry combined with anal sphincter EMG is a non-invasive but very informative study. Besides these complicated and mostly invasive UDS, two simple tests, namely post-voiding residual urine (PVR) measurement and bladder diaries, may provide important information about lower urinary tract function. A high PVR is usually associated with decreased detrusor contractility. It can be measured during UDS or ultrasound examination of the bladder. Bladder or voiding diaries, which are simple and almost cost-free, may be utilized in children who void or who are on CIC. Bladder diaries can accurately predict the cystometric capacity and may assess lower urinary tract function.

Initial UDS reveal neurological impairment of the lower urinary tract in more than 90% of newborns with a MMC [21]. Fortunately, renal function is normal in greater than 90% of these infants. Radiologic assessment demonstrates an abnormal finding in about 10-15% [22]. Among these abnormal findings, hydroureteronephrosis due to spinal shock is seen in 3-5%, whereas other radiologic abnormalities are the result of infravesical obstruction due to NBD during fetal life [23]. For instance, vesicoureteral reflux is diagnosed in 4% of all newborns but is invariably seen in those with DSD detected on UDS in the newborn period. If left untreated, the incidence of a radiological abnormality such as hydronephrosis, VUR and/or bladder distension rises to 50% when these children reach five years of age [7]. This finding clearly indicates urologic deterioration of the NBD with time in about half of the children with MMC. The etiology of radiological deterioration is apparently related to the effect of high hydrostatic pressure within the urinary tract. Possible causes include undiagnosed and/or untreated DSD, reinnervation of the sphincter muscle with the development of DSD, fibrosis of the denervated external urethral sphincter leading to increased bladder outlet obstruction, and to secondary tethering of the spinal cord that produces an overactive detrusor.

Different classification systems have been proposed to describe the NBD in children with myelodysplasia. For example, it has been shown that 43% of children with MMC have an areflexic bladder, whereas the rest (57%) have detrusor activity [24]. The areflexic bladder is sub-classified according to its compliance as either normal (25%) or decreased (18%). According to another classification system, 47% of children with MMC had an intact sacral reflex arc, with 24% and 29% having partial and complete denervation (lower motor neuron lesion), respectively [25]. Bauer et al. [24] have proposed a classification system combining bladder contractility with external sphincter activity resulting in three main groups of NBD in children with myelodysplasia [24]:

1. Synergic group: This group of children with myelodysplasia and an intact sacral spinal arc has the most favorable outcome and corresponds to 10-15% of the whole cohort. It is characterized by a synergic sphincter and a contractile detrusor. Although the upper urinary tract is less at risk compared with the other two groups, 17% of children with a synergic sphincter develop upper urinary tract damage in the long term due to the dynamic character of the process, as described above (Fig. 30.2).

2. Dyssynergic group: This is defined by non-relaxation of the external urethral sphincter at cystometric capacity, or during micturition or leakage (DSD) secondary to an upper motor neuron lesion. In urodynamic studies, these children typically have increased detrusor pressure during emptying but not necessarily during filling. Bladder compliance, however, is usually diminished.

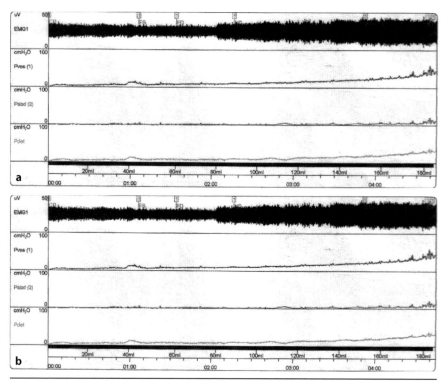

Fig. 30.2 a, b. Synergic group. A cystometrogram and uroflowmetry analysis with anal sphincter EMG in a 4-year old walking child with a sacral level MMC in the synergic group. **a** CMG reflects normal detrusor activity and normal compliance with normal bladder capacity. It is important to note that the anal sphincter activity increases in conjunction with increasing intravesical volume, which is described as the 'guarding reflex'. **b** Uroflowmetry shows decreasing EMG activity during a normal void. These children with synergic sphincters and normal detrusor activity have the most favorable outcome and a very low risk of urinary tract deterioration. However, even in this group there is a risk of secondary tethering that can lead to urological complications

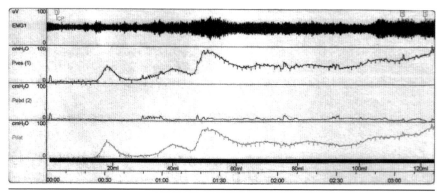

Fig. 30.3. Dyssynergic group. CMG of 5-year old girl with an upper motor neuron lesion due to MMC reflecting a poorly compliant (2.1 ml/cmH$_2$O), reduced capacity (113 ml) bladder and significant neurogenic detrusor overactivity. Urinary leakage was noted at 113 ml infused volume with a detrusor leak point pressure of 67 cmH$_2$O. The high DLPP is due to a dyssynergic sphincter. This group of children has the greatest risk of urinary tract deterioration. Treatment includes CIC and anticholinergic drugs

If left untreated, the risk of upper urinary tract damage in this group can reach 100% in five years (Figs. 30.3, 30.4).

3. Areflexic bladder: This group is defined by a complete lower motor neuron lesion, which is seen in about one third of children. It is characterized by complete external urethral sphincter and detrusor muscle denervation. Although the risk of urinary tract deterioration is lower compared to the dyssynergic group, one study has found hydroureteronephrosis to develop in 23% of these children in the long term [12]. The reason for upper urinary tract damage over time is partially due to infravesical obstruction secondary to fibrosis of the denervated external urethral sphincter (Fig. 30.5).

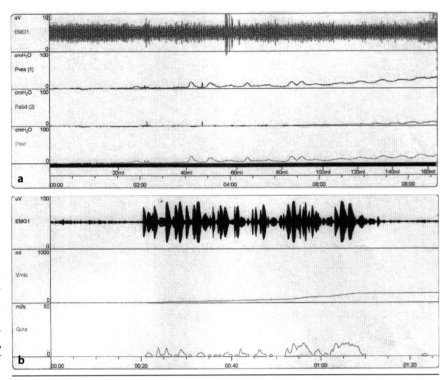

Fig. 30.4 a, b. Another 5-year old girl in the dyssynergic group with a partial upper motor neuron lesion. **a** CMG reflects detrusor overactivity in a highly compliant (9.6 ml/cmH$_2$O) bladder with reduced capacity (164 ml). No leakage was observed during the CMG. Treatment includes primarily CIC with anticholinergic drugs added if incontinence between CIC is problematic. **b** The child can initiate voiding. Uroflowmetry with anal sphincter EMG shows an interrupted voiding pattern with a low flow rate and increased EMG activity, suggesting bladder sphincter dyssynergy

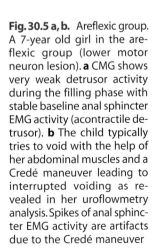
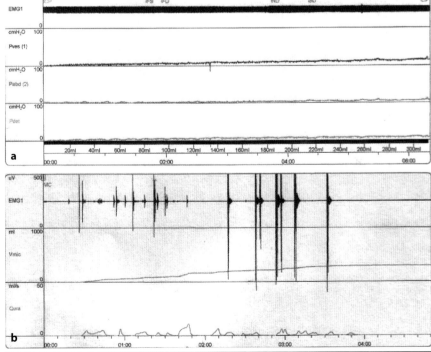

Fig. 30.5 a, b. Areflexic group. A 7-year old girl in the areflexic group (lower motor neuron lesion). **a** CMG shows very weak detrusor activity during the filling phase with stable baseline anal sphincter EMG activity (acontractile detrusor). **b** The child typically tries to void with the help of her abdominal muscles and a Credé maneuver leading to interrupted voiding as revealed in her uroflowmetry analysis. Spikes of anal sphincter EMG activity are artifacts due to the Credé maneuver

Management of NBD and its Complications in Children with Myelodysplasia

As mentioned above, the first goal of neuro-urological management is to protect the upper urinary tract from any damage resulting from high hydrostatic pressure. It has been shown that DLPP higher than 40 cmH$_2$O is a major risk factor associated with urinary tract damage and children who are found to have higher DLPP during UDS need further management [26]. Experience with long term follow-up of ten to 20 years has revealed that supravesical diversion does not always protect the upper urinary tract [27]. In 1971, Lapides introduced the concept of CIC, which created a revolution in the management of children with myelodysplasia by preventing major urinary tract complications such as hydronephrosis, VUR and chronic renal failure [28]. As many as 30-60% of children with urinary incontinence benefit from CIC [7]. Today, CIC with or without anticholinergic medication is the first choice in treating children with DSD or an acontractile detrusor with incomplete emptying. CIC should be started in infants even before the initial UDS, if the infant cannot spontaneously void or has a PVR greater than 5 ml after attempting to empty the bladder with a Credé maneuver. Bladder emptying with Credé can be utilized until UDS is performed if the bladder does not empty spontaneously. However, Credé should never be applied or continued in children who have VUR or DSD [29]. If the initial UDS reveals a DLPP greater than 30 cmH$_2$O, CIC should be started. If a repeat UDS performed four weeks later shows a non-compliant bladder with a high DLPP, CIC should be combined with anticholinergic medication. This primary management of newborns with MMC can successfully control the hydrostatic pressure within the entire urinary tract and prevent complications in a majority of children so that additional surgical intervention such as urethral dilatation and vesicostomy is rarely required (8-10% of the time). Following this regimen, bladder augmentation in early childhood is almost never needed.

It is important to stress that even children in the synergic group need close attention due to the dynamic nature of the disease process. The intensity of the follow-up protocol depends on the risk of potential complications from the disease (Table 30.2).

Urinary Incontinence

Until five years of age, neuro-urological surveillance should focus on having (low) normal pressures during filling and emptying of the urinary bladder, and families should be informed that UI is not the primary target of treatment in early childhood. For families, however, UI is usually the main concern. It is obvious that management of NBD in these children is challenging for families and physicians. It has been shown that families who do not adhere to this program due to psychological, financial and/or social reasons or as a result of problems stemming from the health care system, may adversely impact the quality of neuro-urological follow-up and treatment these children get, especially when CIC is needed but not satisfactorily performed [30]. In order to increase compliance in families, the importance and the aims of neuro-urological follow-up should be clearly and periodically explained to parents who may frequently find this treatment modality overwhelming.

Treatment of UI becomes another major target of neuro-urological surveillance in children with myelodysplasia after four years of age. UI may result from neurogenic detrusor overactivity or sphincteric insufficiency, or both. Therefore, its management should target the underlying etiology. Neurogenic detrusor overactivity can be managed by anticholinergic medication, intravesical therapies such as Botulinum neurotoxin injection, neuromodulation techniques and finally by bladder augmentation surgery. Sphincteric insufficiency may be man-

Table 30.2. Follow-up surveillance in children with MMC should be dictated by the type of NBD and risk of urinary tract deterioration until the child is five years old. *Voiding cystourethrogram (VCUG) should be performed separately only if video-urodynamic studies are not available

	Dyssynergic sphincter	Areflexic bladder	Synergic sphincter
Urine analysis and cultures	Every 3 months	Every 3 months	Every 6 months
VCUG*	Every 6 months	Every year	Every year
Renal ultrasound	Every 6 months	Every 6 months	Every 6 months
(Video)-urodynamic studies	Every 6 months	Every year	Every year
PVR measurement	Every 3 months	Every 3 months	Every 6 months

aged by alpha-sympathomimetic agents, periurethral injections of bulking agents, artificial sphincter implantation, bladder neck reconstruction and finally, continent urinary diversion with closure of the bladder outlet. CIC also helps to achieve continence in children with high PVR who experience overflow incontinence.

Vesicouretral Reflux Secondary to NBD

VUR is seen in 3-5% of newborns with MMC (Fig. 30.6), but this rate increases to 40-50% at five years of age if not properly managed [31]. VUR in myelodysplasia is related to detrusor overactivity or DSD [24]. Children with low or moderate grades of VUR who have a synergic sphincter and normal bladder filling and emptying pressures can be followed with only antimicrobial prophylaxis. However, children with higher grades of VUR and/or high intravesical pressure are at risk for renal damage; thus, additional measures should be undertak-

en [31, 32]. Treatment strategies of VUR associated with high intravesical pressure during filling or emptying should focus on increasing compliance of the bladder and decreasing its emptying pressure. It should be stressed again that a Credé maneuver is contraindicated in children with VUR and/or DSD [29]. CIC with anticholinergic medication is the first step in the management of VUR. With this treatment, VUR resolves in about half of the cases by five years of age. If conservative measures fail or CIC cannot be performed easily, vesicostomy should be considered [33]. Bladder augmentation combined with or without antireflux surgery is the treatment of choice when the aforementioned strategies fail (Fig. 30.7) [34]. Antireflux surgery alone should never be performed when intravesical pressure is high and efficient bladder emptying has not been achieved. The indications for antireflux surgery alone to treat VUR in children with myelodysplasia are as follows: 1) recurrent febrile UTI in a normally compliant bladder despite appropriate antimicrobial prophylaxis and CIC; 2) per-

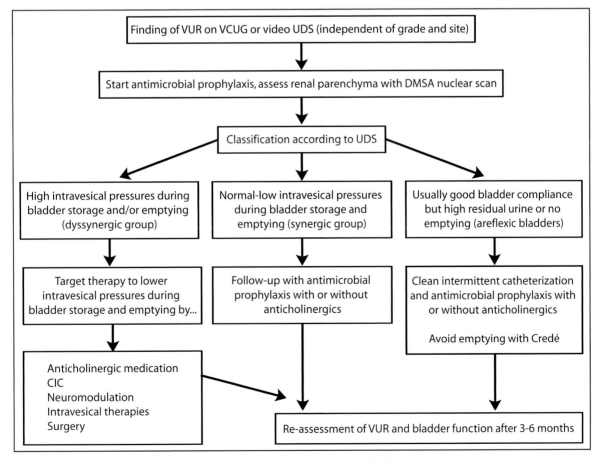

Fig. 30.6. Algorithm for the initial management of VUR in children with MMC

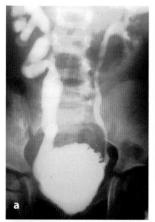

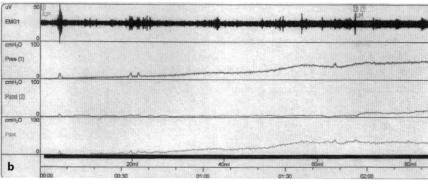

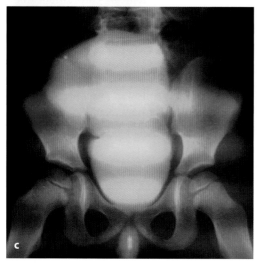

Fig. 30.7 a-c. a Voiding cystourethrogram in a 5-year old boy with MMC who is on anticholinergic medication and clean intermittent catheterization shows significant trabeculation and diverticula formation as well as a poorly compliant bladder ('christmas tree' appearance) and bilateral high grade vesicoureteral reflux. The morphological deterioration and VUR occurs secondary to elevated hydrostatic pressure within the bladder, which may be secondary to neurogenic detrusor overactivity and/or a dyssynergic sphincter. **b** CMG in the same boy reflects a bladder with very low compliance (1.7 ml/cmH$_2$O) and reduced capacity (67 ml). Urinary leakage was noted at 64 ml infused volume with a detrusor leak point pressure of 51 cmH$_2$O, despite anticholinergic treatment. **c** His VCUG one year after bladder augmentation surgery (ileocystoplasty) and bilateral ureteroneocystostomy reveals that the VUR has resolved and the bladder capacity is significantly increased

sisting VUR or hydronephrosis despite efficient bladder emptying and normal intravesical pressure; 3) VUR associated with an anatomic abnormality at the ureterovesical junction; and 4) VUR persisting into puberty.

With the recent popularity of bulking agents and the ease of treating reflux effectively with a simple outpatient procedure, these indications may change with experience and endoscopically acceptable results.

Conclusion

Myelodysplasia is associated with pathologic innervation of the urinary bladder and urethral sphincters, which may lead to significant urological complications such as inability to empty, UTI, VUR, UI and CRF. In an open spinal dysraphism such as MMC, early primary closure of the spinal defect should be followed by proactive neuro-urological surveillance in order to minimize the risk of urological complications. The management strategies of children with myelodysplasia differ according to the specific nature of the existing NBD and the risk of urinary tract deterioration, which is primarily revealed by UDS. Proactive conservative management with CIC and anticholinergic treatment has been shown to significantly reduce the incidence of upper urinary tract deterioration and need for surgical intervention such as bladder augmentation surgery [35]. Efforts at fetal closure of MMC so far have not revealed a better urological outcome, but are associated with a higher incidence of complete denervation of the external urethral sphincter and detrusor overactivity as compared to postnatal closure [15]. Therefore, even this group of children should undergo urodynamic studies in the immediate newborn period and should be under close postnatal surveillance to document possible tethering of the spinal cord, urinary incontinence and increased detrusor pressures. In summary, independent of the type of primary lesion and surgical technique employed to correct it, all children with myelodysplasia, even those with very low sacral lesions who can walk without difficulty and who have apparent normal urinary tract function, should be followed regularly because of the dynamic nature of the disease and the not insignificant risk of secondary tethering of the spinal cord.

References

1. Sharpe N (1915) Spina bifida. An experimental and clinical study. Ann Surg 61:151-165
2. Mayo-Robson AW (1885) A series of cases of spina bifida treated by plastic operation. Trans Clin Soc Lond 18:210-220
3. Beckman EH, Adson AW (1917) Spina bifida: Its operative treatment. St Paul Med J 19:357-363
4. Siris IE (1936) Spina bifida: Treatment and analysis of 84 cases. Ann Surg 103:97-123
5. Ingraham FD, Swan H (1943) Spina bifida and cranium bifidum. I: A survey of five hundred forty-six cases. N Eng J Med 228:559-563
6. Lorber J (1973) Early results of selective treatment of spina bifida cystica. Br Med J 4:201-204
7. McGuire EJ, Bloom DA, Ritchey ML (1993) Myelodysplasia. Problems in urology. Vol 7(1) part 2:1-14
8. Tarcan T, Önol FF, İlker Y et al (2006) Early primary repair improves the neurourological prognosis significantly in infants with myelomeningocele. J Urol 176:1161-1165
9. Kaefer M, Pabby A, Kelly M et al (1999) Improved bladder function after prophylactic treatment of the high risk neurogenic bladder in newborns with myelomeningocele. J Urol 162:1068-1071
10. Tarcan T, Bauer SB, Olmedo E et al (2001) Long-term follow up of newborns with myelodysplasia and normal urodynamic findings: Is follow up necessary? J Urol 165:564-567
11. Bauer SB, Labib KB, Dieppa RA et al (1977) Urodynamic evaluation in a boy with myelodysplasia and incontinence. Urology 10:354-362
12. Bauer SB (1992) Neurogenic vesical dysfunction in children. In: Walsh PC, Retik AB, Stamey TA, Vaughan ED (eds) Campbell's urology. WB Saunders, Philadelphia, pp 1634-1668
13. Bauer SB (1988) Early evaluation and management of children with spina bifida. In: King LR (ed) Urologic surgery in neonates and young infants. WB Saunders, Philadelphia, pp 252-264
14. Yamada S, Iacono RP, Andrade T et al (1995) Pathophysiology of tethered cord syndrome. Neurosurg Clin N Am 6:311-323
15. Koh C, DeFilippo R, Bauer SB et al (2006) Lower urinary tract function after fetal closure of myelomeningocele. J Urol 176:2232-2236
16. Tarcan T, Önol FF, İlker Y et al (2006) Does surgical release of the secondary spinal cord tethering improve the prognosis of neurogenic bladder in children with myelomeningocele? J Urol 176:1601-1606
17. Yücel S, Ertuğrul A, İlker Y et al (2000) The incidence of undescended testis in children with myelodysplasia and its relation with spinal level of the lesion. Turk J Urol 26:328-331
18. Kroovand RL, Bell W, Hart LJ et al (1990) The effect of back closure on detrusor function in neonates with myelodysplasia. J Urol 144:423-425
19. Hopps CV, Kropp KA (2003) Preservation of renal function in children with myelomeningocele managed with basic newborn evaluation and close followup. J Urol 169:305-308
20. Teichman JM, Scherz HC, Kim KD et al (1994) An alternative approach to myelodysplasia management: aggressive observation and prompt intervention. J Urol 152(2 Pt 2):807-811
21. Stark G (1968) The pathophysiology of the bladder in myelomeningocele and its correlation with the neurological picture. Dev Med Child Neurol (Suppl) 16:76-86
22. Bauer SB (1985) The management of spina bifida from birth onwards. In: Whitaker RH, Woodard JR (eds) Pediatric urology. Butterworth & Co, London, pp 87-112
23. Chiaramonte RM, Horowitz EM, Kaplan GA et al (1986) Implications of hydronephrosis in newborns with myelodysplasia. J Urol 136:427-429
24. Bauer SB (1984) Myelodysplasia: Newborn evaluation and management. In: McLaurin RL (ed) Spina bifida: A multidisciplinary approach. Praeger, New York, pp 262-267
25. Spindel MR, Bauer SB, Dyro FM et al (1987) The changing neuro-urologic lesion in myelodysplasia. JAMA 258:1630-1633
26. McGuire EJ, Woodside JR, Borden TA et al (1981) Prognostic value of urodynamic testing in myelodysplastic patients. J Urol 126:205-209
27. Shapiro SR, Lebowitz R, Colodny AH (1975) Fate of 90 children with ileal conduit urinary diversion a decade later: analysis of complications, pyelography, renal function and bacteriology. J Urol 114:289-295
28. Lapides J, Diokno AC, Silber SJ et al (1972) Clean intermittent self-catheterization in the treatment of urinary tract disease. J Urol 107:458-461
29. Barbalias GA, Klauber GT, Blaivas JG (1983) Critical evaluation of the Credé maneuver: A urodynamic study of 207 patients. J Urol 130:720-723
30. Tarcan T, Önol FF, Tanıdır Y et al (2007) Are myelodysplastic children receiving sufficient health care in Turkey? An analysis of the problems in primary management and their impact on neurourological outcome. J Ped Urol 3:19-23

31. Bauer SB (1984) Vesico-ureteral reflux in children with neurogenic bladder dysfunction. In: Johnston JH (ed) International perspectives in urology, Vol 10, Williams & Wilkins, Baltimore pp 159-177

32. Joseph DB, Bauer SB, Colodny AH et al (1989) Clean intermittent catheterization in infants with neurogenic bladder. Pediatrics 84:78-82

33. Mandell J, Bauer SB, Colodny AH, Retik AB (1981) Cuteneous vesicostomy in infancy. J Urol, 126:92-93

34. Kaplan WE, Firlit CF (1983) Management of reflux in myelodisplastic children. J Urol 129:1195-1197

35. Edelstein RA, Bauer SB, Kelly MD et al (1995) The long-term urological response of neonates with myelodysplasia treated proactively with intermittent catheterization and anticholinergic therapy. J Urol 154:1500-1504

Section VII
PSYCHOSOCIAL ASPECTS

CHAPTER 31
Sexuality, Sex, Pregnancy, and Spina Bifida

Ann de Vylder

During the last 40 years, more and more myelo-meningocele (MMC) patients have survived to adulthood, and since the 1980s there is growing interest in the sexual functioning of these patients. However, most of what is known about the impact of MMC on sexual functioning pertains to males. There are several reasons for this bias. First, much of the research in which the issues associated with sexuality of MMC patients have been examined consists of self-report questionnaire studies. Because males have protruding external genitalia and visible sexual responses, they are more likely to be aware of physical sexual responsiveness and thus can seemingly respond more accurately to questionnaires. Secondly, there appears to have been a societal bias that has limited research in females with MMC to studies that focus primarily on reproductive issues, thus more or less avoiding areas as sexual activity and its difficulties.

We have reviewed the literature pertaining to female and male sexuality and MMC with regard to sexual activity, dysfunction, sexual knowledge and education, pregnancy and delivery, and future trends, especially with regard to new diagnostic techniques and possible treatments [1].

Neuroanatomy of Female Sexual Functioning

Neurological control of lubrication and erection of the clitoris and vestibular bulbs is both central and peripheral. The primary central nervous system components believed to be involved with female sexual arousal are the medial preoptic- and the anterior hypothalamic area and the related limbic-hippocampal structures. In animals, activation of these centers rapidly transmits impulses through the autonomic parasympathetic pathway (pelvic nerves), causing relaxation of clitoral and vaginal smooth muscle and an increase in vaginal length and luminal diameter, especially in the distal two thirds of the vagina [2].

Vascular engorgement of the vagina enables plasma transudation, which results in vaginal lubrication. Finally, an increase in clitoral cavernosal arterial inflow and intracavernosal pressure results in tumescence and elevation of the clitoral glans.

The somatic sensory pathway arises from the dorsal nerve, a branch of the pudendal nerve. Following research in rats, an additional functional sensory pathway involving the vagus nerve has been proposed, which may account for sexual responses (menstrual cramping, orgasm) in females with complete spinal cord injury [3]. Practice shows that MMC females may also have erogenous zones in the periumbilical areas and the nipples by which they could acquire sexual pleasure and even orgasm, so the absence of genital sensation does not preclude physical enjoyment of sex.

In females with MMC, the abnormal conditions of the vertebral column variably affect spinal cord function, especially with regard to sensory dysfunction in a sexual perspective. The sensation of touch, light pressure, and vibration are conducted by the dorsal column of the spinal cord and the large myelinated fibers in the peripheral nerves. The small fiber system and its central connections in the spinothalamic tracts mediate modalities of temperature and pain, but these are probably less relevant for sexual functioning.

Female Sexual Activity and Dysfunctions

In 1977 Dorner reported on sexual functioning in 63 adolescent MMC patients aged 13 to 19 years old [4]. Almost all of his subjects denied sexual activity: only one 19-year-old female acknowledged intercourse in the total group of 63. However, sexual history was obtained in the presence of parents or, in some cases, solely from a parent.

Gender-specified data about the sexual life of adult patients with MMC were published in the 1970s

Table 31.1. Studies of sexual activity and sexual difficulties of adult female MMC patients. Reprinted from [1], with permission from Elsevier

	Shurtleff et al.	Wabrek et al.	Perez et al.	Cass et al.	Hirayama et al.	Vroege et al.	Sawyer et al.	Total
Pts (n)	23	10	17	35	24	1	27	137
Age	16-72	–	18	16-19 4 20-29 22 30-39 9	(25.2) (18-42)	–	18	
Masturbation	–	2 (20%)	1 (6%)	7 (20%)	–	100%	–	
Intercourse	12 (57%)	1 (10%)	4 (24%)	17(49%)	8 (33%)	0 (0%)	10	52 (38%)
Problems with:								
Genital sensitivity	–	1 (10%)	–	6 (17%)	19 (81%)	–	–	
Genital pain	1 (4%)	–	–	–	–	–	–	
Present orgasm	–	–	–	13 (31%)	–	–	10(37%)	23 (16%)

by Shurtleff et al. [5] and Wabrek et al. [6], in the 1980s by Perez-Marrero et al. [7] and Cass et al. [8], and in the 1990s by Hirayama et al. [9], Vroege et al. [10] and Sawyer et al. [27].

Together these authors investigated about 137 female patients. Considering the response rates, the patients in these studies probably do not form a representative sample. Moreover, the authors studied different aspects of their patients' sexual lives and reported these in varying degrees of detail. Table 31.1 therefore does not give more than a rough indication of the results of these studies.

Sexual activity related to functional motor level from the series of Cass et al. is summarized in Table 31.2.

The Japanese study showed that 83% of the MMC females had 'interest' in the opposite sex and 75% had sexual desire. Just as in Cass' series, one third had had intercourse. Only 19% of them felt pelvic or perineal ecstasy upon this activity. In this Japanese series, sexual functioning was neither correlated with age nor with the degree of lower extremity paralysis or bladder/sphincter activity [9].

However, sexual dysfunctions that young females with MMC encounter are in theory related to the level of their spinal defect. According to Shurtleff, MMC patients can be divided into three groups, defined by functional motor level, as follows: lesions at or above the L2 level, with function of intercostal, abdominal, hip flexor and adductor muscles (essentially all wheelchair-bound patients); lesions between the L3 and L5 levels, with additional muscle strength in quadriceps and hamstrings given stronger hip flexion, and adduction with knee flexion (weak) and extension (most of these patients walk effectively with aid, surgical procedures and bracing); and lesions at or below the S1 level, with additional muscle strength around the

ankle, and variable degrees of hip abduction and extension [5].

MMC patients with lesions at or below S1 level typically have minimal neurological defects and may have normal sexual function. Those who have lesions between L3 and L5 may have variable sexual function, but according to Woodhouse sexual function is often more common than would be expected in theory or from investigations of MMC adolescents alone [11].

Those with lesions at or above L2 are essentially all wheelchair-bound and have gross neurological and anatomical abnormalities due to MMC. Although they are assumed to be asexual, the neurological and social consequences of MMC obviously do not prevent these patients from having interest in sex [9].

With regard to females, only vulval sensation and orgasm were described (Table 31.2), while vaginal lubrication and erection of the clitoris and vestibular bulbs were not investigated.

Dryness of the vagina at intercourse is incidentally discussed, but in fact there is a lack of data re-

Table 31.2. Sexual activity related to functional motor level female patients. Modified from [1], with permission from Elsevier

Cass et al.	L2 and above	L3-L5	S1 and below	Totals
No. pts	8	15	12	35
Vulval sensation	4	14	11	29
Orgasm*	1 (+5)	6 (+4)	6 (+2)	13 (+11)
Intercourse	0	5	7	12

*Numbers in parentheses indicate number not known (no sexual activity)

lated to this issue and Shurtleff's predictions still have to be confirmed in MMC females [12].

According to Joyner et al. [13], orgasm may cause particular problems in MMC patients with hyperreflexia. In this population, orgasms that occur when the bladder is empty may provoke excruciatingly painful contractions. An orgasm with a full bladder may cause urinary incontinence. Unfortunately, there are no scientific data on this issue, so these findings still have to be elucidated.

Many MMC patients, who in the past were encumbered with external devices to collect urine, are now dry and infection-free with a combination of medication and intermittent self-catheterization, with or without augmentation enterocystoplasty and bladder neck reconstruction. These procedures have been available since the mid 1980s. They have revolutionized the ileal conduit and its attendant drainage bag. Although never investigated, these treatments have undoubtedly enhanced the sexual appeal and improved sexual functioning in female MMC patients. For psychosexual development as well as hygiene reasons, most pediatric urologists advocate continence surgery to be completed prior to the menarche.

Regarding future trends, the diagnostic techniques used in the evaluation of female sexual dysfunction are evolving and will continue to be refined and improved. Vaginal photoplethysmography is one of the older techniques [13, 14]. It provides quantitative data on the extent of vasocongestion in the vaginal capillaries. In fact, this test measures vaginal mucosal engorgement and vaginal blood volume, good indicators of sexual function in the arousal phase of the sexual response, including the motor pathways.

In general, female sexual dysfunction due to neurological causes is currently unexplored. MMC as well as multiple sclerosis, peripheral neuropathy and lumbar neuropathy can cause abnormal innervation of the female genital organs. Today, thermal and vibratory thresholds of both the vaginal and clitoral region seem to be clinically feasible, valid and repeatable, so in the near future these tests will be applied as a diagnostic tool to assess neurogenic sexual dysfunction more adequately [15].

A variety of oral agents are now available to treat male sexual dysfunction. However, only one study addresses male MMC patients with promising results [16]. With regard to female sexual dysfunction, oral agents, including sildenafil, are still undergoing trials in the general population to assess their efficacy and safety.

Neuroanatomy of Male Sexual Functioning

The neurological control of the erection is central and peripheral. The CNS centers controlling the erection are the septal portion of the hippocampus, the anterior cingulated gyrus, the anterior thalamic nuclei, the mammillothalamic tract and the mammillary bodies [13, 17].

These centers are intact in MMC patients, where the problem is peripheral, more specifically the thoracolumbar and sacral erection centers. Axons from these two centers extend ventrally to join the inferior hypogastric and pelvic plexuses. Nerve bundles from these plexuses innervate the bladder, the prostate, the rectum and the penis [13, 18]. The autonomic nervous system controls the vascular events of erection and detumescence [13, 17].

Erections can be divided into reflex and psychogenic erections. Reflex erections occur as a result of direct stimulation and mostly within a local spinal cord reflex arc. Some patients with sacral defects may even be able to ejaculate. The sensory input from the penis may pass to the sacral or thoracolumbal erection center, inducing a reflexogenic erection. Alternatively, sensory input can travel through the ascending spinal tracts to the thalamus and the brain for sensory perception. This sensory input is the afferent arm of the bulbocavernous reflex [13, 17].

Psychogenic erections arise from a central mechanism through visual or auditory input, and are transmitted through the corticospinal tract from the anterior horn cells of S2-S4. From here they go to the pudendal nerves, which give spontaneous erections without direct stimulation of the genitalia [13].

Male Sexual Activity and Dysfunction

Sexual function is related to the level of the neurological defect (Table 31.3). The classical Shurtleff study divided the male MMC patients into three groups. Lesions at or below L1 have normal sexual function. Lesions between L3 and L5 have variable sexual function. Lesions at or above L2 result in asexuality. This is the MMC group which is wheelchair-bound and with gross anatomical and neurological malformations [5]. This division is repeated in later publications. Shurtleff's predictions were confirmed in Cass' study (Table 31.4), which showed that the majority of the male MMC patients with lesions lower than L3 had more penile sensation, erections and ejaculations than those with lesions above L2 [8].

Table 31.3. Studies of sexual activity and sexual difficulties in adult male MMC patients

	Shurtleff et al.	Wabrek et al.	Perez et al.	Cass et al.	Hirayama et al.	Vroege et al.	Sawyer et al.	Total
Pts (n)	28	9	13	12	22	8	24	116
Age	16-72	18-31	18 (med.)	16-39	24 (18-50)	19-44	14-23	
Sexual fantasies, %	–	–	–	–	–	75	79	
Masturbation,%	–	67	31	–	–	50	–	
Intercourse, %	18	–	31	50	18	62	13	
Problems with:								
Genital sensitivity, %	–	–	–	33	–	–	12	
Erection, %	14	11	31	8	14	–	12	
Ejaculation, %	–	11	15	8	33	–	33	

Table 31.4. Sexual activity related to functional motor level

Male pts Cass et al.	L2 and above	L3-L5	S1 and below	Totals
Pts (n)	3	5	4	12
Penile sensation	1	4	3	8
Orgasm*	2 (+1)	3 (+1)	4	9 (+2)
Ejaculation*	2(+1)	3(+1)	4	9(+2)
Erection (n partial)	3 (1)	4	4	11(1)

* Numbers in parentheses indicate number not known (no sexual activity)

In the study of Cass, 10/15 subjects has subjective glans sensitivity, which, when measured objectively is reduced to 2/15. Glans sensitivity is related to the possibility of erections [8].

In the Sandler study, 10/15 men had some glans sensation on physical examination. The number of nocturnal erections was related to sensory level [19].

Males with a spinal defect at T11-L2 usually have neither psychogenic, nor reflex erections and may be candidates for therapy.

Erections are related to the neurological defect, but there is also a bias relating to purely reflex erections. These can occur in all patients with a positive anocutaneous reflex, in 64% of those with a negative reflex and a sensory level at or below the sympathetic outflow (D10 to L2). Only 14% of males with higher lesions and absent reflex had erections [11, 12]. Sandler et al. evaluated erectile function in an objective manner using a standardized physical examination and the use of the Rigiscan. Eleven of fifteen young men reported erections with stimulation. Rigiscan data showed that two men with sacral

level lesions experienced normal number and duration of erection, while seven others had abnormally brief and infrequent nocturnal erections and six had none [20].

Erectile function can be an unwanted side-effect of neurosurgical untethering [21].

Orgasm and ejaculation occurred in seven of nine men with a sensory level at L3 or below. Only three men with higher levels were studied and although two of them had ejaculations, only one had sexual sensation [8].

Infertility can be due to failure to penetrate, failure to ejaculate, ductal obstruction and failure of spermatogenesis. Erectile dysfunction was discussed earlier. 20% of MMC patients with normal bladder function have normal ejaculation. However, there is also failure of spermatogenesis. It has been shown in one study that ten men with spina bifida requiring electroejaculation therapy were azoospermic and showed primary testicular failure on biopsy.

Concerning erectile dysfunction, pharmacotherapy (sildenafil) was administered in a small population of MMC patients (17 patients) with erectile dysfunction, and was successful in 80% of the patients. Only lower doses were administered (25 and 50 mg), because men with neurological erectile dysfunction have the tendency to require lower doses for therapeutic success and a greater risk of priapism [17, 22].

Self-injection therapy with papaverine, prostaglandine E1 or combinations of papaverine and phentolamine has also been used. Eighty to 90% of neurogenic impotence patients respond to this therapy [13]. Possible problems are priapism, infection and fibrosis of the corporal tissue.

Vacuum constriction devices give good results in a large series patients (effective intercourse in 92% of patients) [13].

Penile prostheses can also offer a solution; there is the choice between semi-rigid and inflatable prostheses, each of which has advantages and disadvantages [13]. Ejaculation disorders can be treated by electroejaculation and vibrator stimulation can be helpful.

The artificial urinary sphincter given for urinary incontinence has the advantage of facilitating antegrade seminal emission by sphincter occlusion of the bladder neck [23]. Concerning penile sensitivity, a small study was published in which males with a lesion at L3, L4 and L5 had a bypass from the ilio-inguinal nerve to the ipsilateral dorsal nerve of the penis, resulting in excellent sensibility in the glans penis. This could be promising for future therapeutic options [24].

Knowledge of Sexuality and Education

There is little information regarding knowledge of sexuality of MMC patients. Hayden et al. [25] reported that adolescents with MMC had 'less knowledge of sex' than a matched control group, but no quantitative measurement was performed.

In the early 1990s, 91 adult MMC patients, aged 16-25 years, were interviewed about their sexual knowledge and experience by Blackburn et al. [26]. Answers were compared to those received from 71 able-bodied adults of similar age and socio-economic status.

In 1998, a group of 51 Australian MMC patients (27 females and 24 males) were interviewed about the subject of general and MMC-specific sex education. There was a discrepancy between the high percentage of received general sex education versus the spina bifida-specific sex education, which was perceived as poor or extremely poor. Of these patients, 39% had never discussed sexual issues such as fertility, heredity, pregnancy and the oral contraceptive pill with a doctor. Ninety-three percent of those patients who did not discuss these items felt that they would have discussed it if only these topics had been addressed by the physician [27].

Cromer et al. [28] explored the level of knowledge, attitude and activity related to sexuality in a group of adolescents and young adults with MMC, a group of matched controls and a group of adolescents with cystic fibrosis. Slightly more than half of the study sample were female, the mean age was 17.2 years. Twenty-eight percent of the MMC group reported previous sexual activity, compared with 60% of the control group and 43% of the group with cystic fibrosis. Most of the disabled adolescents expressed a desire to marry and have children, but fewer than 20% had sought information from their physician. Among those sexually active, 60% of the controls and 67% of those with cystic fibrosis had used contraception, compared with 16% of the MMC group. The authors concluded that sex education and screening for contraceptive need is indicated for adolescents with chronic disabilities such as MMC.

Females with MMC usually have normal internal and external genitalia, but they tend to be short for their age, wheelchair-bound and restricted by their kyphoscoliosis. This means that inserting and removing vaginal mechanical devices might be difficult for them. Considering the other options, it should be remembered that many MMC patients have severe, often life-threatening latex allergy and should use only non-latex condoms.

Precocious puberty is common and more pronounced in the MMC females than in the MMC males. The high incidence of hypothalamic and pituitary dysfunction is probably secondary to hydrocephalus, which leads to an early release of gonadotrophins. The beginning of puberty typically occurs around age six to nine, one and a half to two years earlier than normal. On the other hand, girls with MMC may have delayed psychosexual development and not be prepared to handle the challenges of puberty adequately. Many of them lack the independence of their more adroit and mobile counterparts. As a result, they remain too dependent upon their parents to serve as their care-takers, teachers and even their friends. According to Blum et al. [29], there is a noticeable absence of adolescent-parent conflict, a conflict which is necessary to shift the mid-adolescent away from the parent-centered and toward the peer-centered relationship.

Counseling of the patients as well as their parents should help in these cases. However, we found no data about the results and outcome of such an approach.

Pregnancy and Delivery

Females with MMC are thought to have normal fertility. Combined series have shown an increased risk of MMC as high as 4% in the offspring of MMC patients. The risk is the same whether the affected parent is male or female, but daughters have a 1 in 13 incidence while the risk for sons is only 1 in 50 [30]. The risk can be reduced by treating the potential mother with folic acid supplement for three months before pregnancy and continuing to week 12.

For females in general and for girls with MMC in particular, one of the great success stories of the last 20 years has been the discovery of this prophylactic role of folic acid, even though the incidence of all neural tube defects in babies in the Western world had already diminished before this discovery. In a recent study from the United Kingdom it was shown that the incidence of MMC started to decrease about 18 years before the use of folic acid became popular [31].

The Department of Health in the United Kingdom now recommends that women who are at high risk of conceiving a baby with a neural tube defect should take 5 mg folic acid daily [32]. This therapy would include all females who are affected and normal females married to an affected male. In The Netherlands it is recommended that every pregnant female take 0.5mg folic acid daily, even when affected, except where one offspring already has MMC, when 5mg of folic acid is advised.

Despite this prophylaxis there remains a small risk of neural tube defects due to inborn error of folic acid metabolism. In addition, females relying on increased folic acid in their diet may get suboptimal prophylaxis. There appears to be a better absorption of synthetic folic acid (pills or fortified food) than natural folic acid in food [33].

Pregnant MMC patients can be monitored for neural tube defect by fetal ultrasound and by measuring maternal alpha-fetoprotein. A program of selective termination can largely eliminate MMC, but in many countries this still is not allowed [34]. Recently, a large majority of the Dutch professors of pediatric neurology advocated terminating the pregnancy in the case of spina bifida aperta, up until the 24th week of pregnancy.

Only small studies of pregnancies in females with MMC have been published [8, 35, 36].

Although good outcomes have been reported, especially with liberal use of cesarean section, several specific problems have been identified. Kidney function can be compromised by recurrent pyelonephritis, whether or not it is based on obstruction by uteral enlargement. In order to prevent this, periodic controls of kidney function and of urine are mandatory. All infections should be treated at an early stage in order to prevent premature labor and the sequelae of pyelonephritis. Serum creatinine should be checked monthly and, if increased, hydronephrosis should be ruled out by renal ultrasound.

In the case of enterocystoplasty, false positive proteinuria is possible due to mucus secretion of the used intestinal segments. To detect pre-eclampsia, serum uric acid analysis should be carried out. Urinary tract infections are almost invariable, bladder function often deteriorates, and a small deformed pelvis makes accommodation of the fetus difficult, leading to premature labor and increased need for caesarean section.

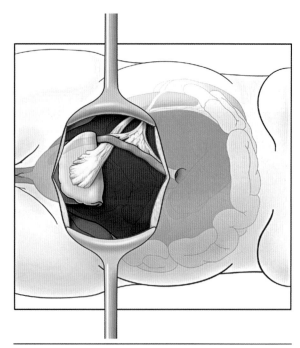

Fig. 31.1. The altered anatomy after ileocystoplasty as encountered at the sectio caesarea. Reprinted from [40], with permission

As the possibilities for reconstruction in cases of neurogenic bladder dysfunction increase (e.g., enterocystoplasty with or without continent stoma or bladder neck reconstruction), the number of females with a desire to become pregnant also increases. It is also possible that incontinence will result due to either pregnancy or delivery.

To avoid the potential for disrupting the continence mechanism during vaginal delivery, some authors have suggested that all patients who have had augmentation enterocystoplasty with or without bladder neck reconstruction should deliver by caesarean section [37, 38]. Others advocate vaginal delivery or an individual assessment for caesarean section, based on obstetrical indication [39]. Every attempt should be made to do so selectively, so that care can be taken to avoid injury to the cystoplasty and its blood supply. Before opening the uterus the augmented bladder may have to be taken down and the mesentery (with the vessels to the neobladder) be pushed aside (Fig. 31.1). This should be taken care of by an urologist who is familiar with the altered anatomy.

Myelomeningocele is nowadays not a contra-indication for pregnancy. Patients should be counseled prior to conception in order to assess renal function and radiological dimensions of the pelvis without risks for the fetus.

References

1. de Vylder A, van Driel MF, Staal AL et al (2004) Myelomeningocele and female sexuality: An Issue? Eur Urol 46:421-427

2. Munarizz RM, Berman JR, Goldstein I (2000) Female sexual dysfunction: new frontiers in diagnosis and therapy. Cont Urol 6:55

3. Komisaruk BR, Whipple B (1995) The suppression of pain by genital stimulation in females. Annual Review of Sex Research 6:151

4. Dorner S (1977) Sexual interest and activity in adolescents with spina bifida. J Child Psychol Psychiatry 18:229

5. Shurtleff DB, Hayden PW, Chapman WH et al (1975) Myelodysplasia. Problems of long-term survival and social function. West J Med 122:199

6. Wabrek AJ, Wabrek CJ, Burchell RC (1978) The human tragedy of spina bifida: spinal meningomyelocele. Sex Disabil 1:210

7. Perez-Marrero R, Young M, Stitzel D (1984) A sexuality survey of young adults with spina bifida. J Urol 131:104A

8. Cass AS, Bloom BA, Luxenberg M (1986) Sexual function in adults with meningomyelocele. J Urol 136:425

9. Hirayama A, Yamada K, Tanka Y, Hirata N, Yamamoto Suemori T, Momose H, Shiomi T, Hirao Y (1995) Evaluation of sexual function in adults with meningomyelocele. Hinyokika Kiyo 41:985

10. Vroege JA, Zeijlemaker BY, Scheers MM (1998) Sexual functioning of adult patients born with meningomyelocele. Eur Urol 34:25

11. Woodhouse CR (1994) The sexual and reproductive consequences of congenital genitourinary anomalies. J Urol 152:645

12. Diamond DA, Rickwood AM, Thomas DG (1986) Penile erections in myelomeningocele patients. Br J Urol 58:434-435

13. Joyner BD, McLorie GA, Jhoury AE (1998) Sexuality and reproductive issues in children with meningomyelocele. Eur J Pediatr Surg 8:29

14. Novelly RA, Perona PJ, Ax AF (1973) Photoplethysmography: system calibration and light history effects. Psychophysiology 10:67

15. Geer JH, Morokoff P, Greenwood P (1974) Sexual arousal in women: the development of a measurement device for vaginal blood volume. Arch Sex Behav 3:559

16. Vardi Y, Gruenwald I, Sprecher E et al (2000) Normative values for female sensation. Urology 56:1035

17. Palmer JS, Kaplan WE, Firlit CF (2000) Erectile dysfunction in patients with spina bifida is a treatable condition. J Urol 164 (3 Pt 2):958-961

18. Donatucci CF, Lue TF (1993) Pathophysiology of sexual dysfunction in males with physical disabilities. Clin Exp Hypertens 291-310

19. Lue TF, Zeineh SJ, Schmid RA, Tanagho EA (1984) Neuroanatomy of penile erection: its relevance to iatrogenic impotence. J Urol 131:273-280

20. Sandler AD, Worley G, Leroy EC et al (1996) Sexual function and erection capability among young men with spina bifida. Dev Med and Child Neur 38:823-829

21. Boemers TM, Van Gool JD, de Jong TP (1995) Tethered spinal cord: the effect of neurosurgery on the lower urinary tract and male sexual function. B J Urol 76:747-751

22. Lue TF, Broderick G (1998) Evaluation and non-surgical management of erectile dysfunction and priapism. In: PC Walsh, AB Retik, ED Vaughan jr et al (eds) Campbell's urology, vol 2, 7th edn. WB Saunders Co, Philadelphia, pp 1181-1214

23. Jumper BM, McLorie GA, Churchill BM et al (1990) Effects of the artificial urinary sphincter on prostatic development and sexual function in pubertal boys with meningocele. J Urol 144:438-442

24. Overgoor ML, Kon M, Cohen-Kettenis PT et al (2006) Neurological bypass for sensory innervation of the penis in patients with spina bifida. J Urol 173(3):1086-1090

25. Hayden RW, Davenport SLH, Campbell MM (1979) Adolescents with myelodysplasia: impact of physical disability on emotinal maturation. Ped 64:53

26. Blackburn M, Bax MCO, Strehlow CDS (1991) Sexuality and disability. Eur J Pediatr Surg 1(Suppl 1):37

27. Sawyer SM, Roberts KV (1999) Sexual and reproductive health in young people with spina bifida. Dev Med Child Neurol 41:671-675

28. Cromer BA, Enrile B, McCoy K et al (1990) Knowledge, attitudes and behavior related to sexuality in adolescents with chronic disability. Dev Med Child Neurol 32:602

29. Blum RW, Resnick ME, Nelson R, St Germaine A (1991) Family and peer issues among adolescents with spina bifida and cerebral palsy. Ped 88:280

30. Laurence KM, Beresford A (1975) Continence, friends, marriage and children in 51 adults with spina bifida. Dev Med Child Neurol 17:123

31. Kadir RA, Sabin C, Whitlow B et al (1999) Neural tube defects and periconceptional folic acid in England and Wales: retrospective study. B Med J 319:92

32. Loyd J (1992) Folic acid and the prevention of neural tube defects. Department of Health, London

33. Neuhouser ML, Beresford SA, Hickok DE et al (1998) Absorption of dietary and supplemental folate in women with prior pregnancies with neural tube defects and controls. J Am Coll Nutr 17:625

34. Chan A, Robertson EF, Haan EA et al (1993) Prevalence of neural tube defects in South Australia 1996-91: effectiveness and impact of prenatal diagnosis. B Med J 307:703

35. Richmond D, Zahariefski I, Bond A (1993) Management of pregnancy in mothers with spina bifida. Eur J Obst Repro Biol 25:341

36. Rietberg CC, Lindhout D (1993) Adult patients with spina bifida cystica: genetic counselling, pregnancy and delivery. Eur J Obstet Reprod Biol 52:63

37. Hill DE, Kramer SA (1990) Management of pregnancy after augmentation cystoplasty. J Urol 144:457

38. Kennedy AW, Hensle TW (1993) Pregnancy after orthotopic continent urinary diversion. Surg Gynaecol Obstet 177:405

39. Quenneville V, Beurton D, Thomas L, Fontaine E (2003) Pregnancy and vaginal delivery after augmentation cystoplasty. B J Urol 91:893

40. Breeuwsma AJ, de Vylder AAM, van Driel MF et al (2004) Pregnancy and delivery after augmentation cystoplasty. Ned Tijdschr voor Obstetrie en Gynaecologie 117(10):292-293

CHAPTER 32
Intellectual Outcome in Spina Bifida

Pietro Spennato, Luciano Savarese, Giuseppe Cinalli

In most of the series in the literature [1-4], the mean intelligence quotient (IQ) of patients with open spina bifida has been reported to be within the normal range, but usually lower than that of the general population. In a recent case-control study, Nejat et al. [1] found a statistically significant correlation between having a myelomeningocele and having a lower IQ. However, this data may be inaccurate, as typically only one aspect of cognitive functioning, namely nonverbal visuospatial reasoning, was assessed. Other skills that may better reflect the difficulties encountered by these patients, such as verbal responses or skilled manipulative ability were often not tested.

Several factors are implicated in intellectual outcome; these include hydrocephalus, Chiari malformation, incidence of shunt revisions/infection, level of the lesion, poor mobility, epilepsy and associated brain malformations. These have all been investigated for their role in intellectual outcome, with often conflicting results. Genetic predisposition, family care and support, nutrition, home environment and the presence of other morbidities, such as gait disturbance or paraplegia, genitourinary dysfunction and ophthalmological complications, may similarly affect the affected child's physical, social, emotional, and cognitive development.

In this chapter we review the cognitive profile of the typical spina bifida patient and the factors implicated in intellectual outcome.

Typical Profile of a Spina Bifida Patient

In congenital disorders such as spina bifida, cognitive and motor processes develop in a brain in which multiple components have been damaged and the normal connectivity among brain regions has been permanently changed. Neuronal reorganization therefore potentially plays a significant role in the processes that support learning and development. This reorganization may differ from that in the adult brain, with the brain of a child with spina bifida supporting fractionation of preserved and deficient skills based on the relative preservation or dissolution of particular brain regions [5]. Outcomes thus may be better for some skills than for others and are variable, dependent upon the degree to which reorganization occurs in different children [5]. Like the patterns of brain anomalies, the cognitive profiles of spina bifida patients are uneven. Brain malformations and hydrocephalus lead to disruption of higher cortical functions, particularly involving motor, spatial, and nonverbal skills. As a group, these children appear to be stronger in language and weaker in visual-spatial and motor skills [6, 7]. The discrepancy between Verbal IQ (VIQ) score, typically in the average range, and Performance IQ (PIQ), which is usually reduced, is reported by several authors [8-10]. These children have difficulty with higher order language, inferencing, and social discourse tasks [11].

Degenerative changes involving the posterior subcortical brain regions, commonly observed in hydrocephalus, may result in a functional disconnection with the frontal regions of the brain, leading to additional executive deficits [12, 13]. This may have a critical impact on the acquisition and consolidation of new skills and knowledge as the young child moves toward adulthood [13]. A wide spectrum of deficits have been reported in the spina bifida patient, including attention problems [14]; material specific memory deficits [9, 15]; impaired spontaneous retrieval and delayed recall [15, 16]; deficiencies in aspects of executive skills [12, 14], poorer performance on tasks tapping spelling and arithmetic skills [3, 4, 17].

In a recent paper, Fletcher et al. [5] focused on the language development of such children. They concluded that in the language domain many children with spina bifida demonstrate good development of grammar and lexicon, showing that the form and content of their language is normal. Other children demonstrate more pervasive impairments of language. For nearly all children, regardless of cognitive level, there are significant difficulties in the construction of meaning and in pragmatic communication, both of which require flexible language processing in real time [5]. Their observations did not confirm earlier studies of speech that noted a fluent language, even if accompanied by poor content of speech with chunks of stereotyped phrases [18]. In their cases spina bifida was associated with dysfluency; ataxic dysarthria (articulatory inaccuracy, prosodic excess and phonatory-prosodic insufficiency) and slowed speech rate.

In the study of Vachha and Adams [19] children with spina bifida and shunted hydrocephalus (excluding those with a prior diagnosis of mental retardation and a history of shunt complications) demonstrated a significantly impaired memory span. Children remembered fewer words overall irrespective of the value (higher or lower) of the words. This deficit of working memory entails a selective learning disability, due to the lack of the "the ability to temporarily maintain and manipulate information that one needs to keep in mind" [20].

These learning problems, associated with preserved reading ability, may produce a specific math disability [21]. This may also be related to the impairment in visuospatial skills, which are important for the spatial organization and manipulation of numerical information.

In conclusion, a typical spina bifida patient, despite a normal IQ, usually presents neuropsychological deficits in visual perception and specific academic difficulties in mathematics.

This cognitive profile appears to persist into adulthood [10, 22], even if early research suggests stable or improving abilities over time [4].

Concerning the academic careers of such patients, in 2001 the group of McLone [23] reported 20- to 25-year outcome for a group of patients aggressively treated between 1975 and 1979. At the time of the review, 85% of the 71 available patients (of the initial cohort, 28 had died and 19 were lost to follow up) had been attending or had graduated from high school: 63% attended regular classes, whereas 37% required at least some special educational classes. Forty-five percent were actively employed and five young adults provided their services as volunteers.

Cognitive Difficulties in Children with Spina Bifida: Global or Selective?

In 2001 Jacobs et al. [13] published a longitudinal prospective study on long-term cognitive outcomes in 19 children with myelomeningocele who were shunted for hydrocephalus within the first year of life. In comparison to a healthy control group matched for age and gender, patients in the clinical sample were found to have globally compromised cognitive skills. Myelomeningocele patients demonstrated impairments in most of the cognitive and memory domains investigated, including IQ, educational achievement, memory and learning, organization and higher level language and speed of processing. Few intact skills were identified. Moreover, there was a significant decrease in abilities across childhood, from infancy to later childhood, suggesting a failure to acquire cognitive skills within the expected time frame and an increasing discrepancy between these children and their age peers. Of interest, the commonly reported difference between verbal and nonverbal abilities (i.e., VIQ-PIQ discrepancy) [9, 24, 25] was not present in this study. In contrast, children demonstrated globally depressed intellectual abilities.

This pattern of deficits is consistent with Dennis' developmental model of outcome [25] following early brain insult. Her model would argue that the earlier the cerebral insult, the fewer established cognitive skills, and the greater the resultant impairment. A congenital condition, such as myelomeningocele, would be predicted to have a global impact on skill acquisition, with no areas of cognitive development escaping the effects of brain dysfunction.

These difficulties may not always be initially apparent, but emerge some time later as children are required to function more independently.

Hydrocephalus and Shunt Complications

Hydrocephalus is commonly associated with myelomeningocele and develops in 80-90% of patients with this anomaly. In the pre-shunt era, hydrocephalus was by far the most important factor affecting outcome. Often these patients were considered at birth as having such a poor prognosis that treatment was not offered at all [26-28]. The invention of the cerebrospinal fluid (CSF) shunt in the 1950s saved the lives of many hundreds of babies with spina bifida. However, when the results were reviewed by Laurence in 1974 he noted that the surviving children had a lower intelligence and greater disability than those few cases who had survived without a shunt [27], suggesting that shunt-dependent children had a worse outcome than shunt independent-children.

Several authors confirmed these data, noting that when patients with or without hydrocephalus were similarly matched, those with hydrocephalus scored lower on intelligence tests [4, 29, 30]. Some authors suggested that shunt placement and its related complications (infection, obstruction, and the need for shunt revision surgery) may play a greater role in the decreased mean IQ than the hydrocephalus itself [31]. Thereafter, the relationship between specific treatment parameters (e.g., number of shunt revisions), developmental factors (e.g., age at which the child develops hydrocephalus), and cognitive skills have been investigated, in an attempt to determine specific risk factors for poor outcome. Early researchers tended to examine single predictors. For example, studies by Badell-Ribera et al. [32] and Raimondi and Soare [33] document a linear relationship between the number of shunt revisions and intellectual outcome. Hunt et al. [34] observed the best outcome in those patients who had not required a shunt, followed by those whose shunts were never revised. The worst outcome was seen in patients who had needed revisions of their shunts after the age of 2 years and in any who had had symptoms of raised intracranial pressure.

However, recently researchers have taken a more multidimensional approach, investigating interactions among risk factors. Using this method, Donders et al. [24] identified a link between complications that occurred in the first 12 months of life and poorer intellectual outcome [13]. In more recent literature [1, 2, 35] no correlation was found between the IQs of patients with myelomeningocele who had undergone shunt placement and those who had not. However, almost all these patients, even if they did not have shunt infections, revisions or any other complications, scored lower on IQ tests than those of developmentally normal children. This would suggest that IQ is affected predominantly by the presence of the disease process itself and not by its associated complications [1, 2, 35].

Comparing different causes of hydrocephalus, it has been reported that myelomeningocele patients have at least as good an intellectual outcome as patients with aqueductal stenosis [11, 28].

Chiari II Malformation and Supratentorial Abnormalities

In the last decade it has been noted that cognitive impairments in spina bifida could not be explained by hydrocephalus and its complications alone, raising the importance of the role of the Chiari II malformation in motor and cognitive impairment [36]. In particular, cognitive functions subserved by cerebellar structures such as automation, verbal fluency

and visual processing may be impaired as a consequence of the cerebellar dysmorphology associated with spina bifida [37, 38].

Chiari II malformation is present in virtually all patients with open spina bifida. This malformation involves the entire brain and the surrounding structures (meninges and bones), but especially the posterior fossa. The most characteristic finding is hindbrain herniation, i.e., the caudal displacement of the cerebellar tonsils and vermis, together with the caudal brainstem (medulla and occasionally the pons) through an enlarged foramen magnum into the cervical spinal canal [39].

Vinck et al. [39] administered a complete battery of neuropsychological tests, including tests for cerebellar cognitive functions, to two groups of children with spina bifida: those with Chiari malformation and those without. Results showed that the group of patients affected by Chiari II malformation had a significantly lower PIQ than the other group, even after excluding the confounding effect of global cognitive impairment. In the nonretarded group (total IQ > 70) the patients with and without Chiari matched well on VIQ, which is not supposed to be associated with cerebellar dysfunction. In terms of cognitive profile, the Chiari malformation group performed particularly poorly on tests requiring visual analysis and synthesis, verbal memory, and verbal fluency.

This study confirmed the recent observations by Rapoport et al. [40] on the role of the cerebellum in cognition and behaviour. The cerebellum should be part of a cerebrocerebellar network contributing to motor processes and also to cognitive functions. The pattern of cognitive impairment of patients affected by Chiari II malformation is consistent with that reported in patients with tumoral or ischemic cerebellar damage [39-41].

Due to the coexistence of hydrocephalus and Chiari malformation in spina bifida patients, it is difficult to attribute a pattern of cognitive impairment to either factor alone. The study of Vinck and coworkers [39], however, suggests that impaired visual analysis and synthesis seems to be related to both the hydrocephalus and the Chiari malformation, whereas deficiencies in verbal memory and fluency may be attributed to cerebellar dysfunction only.

Chiari II malformation is associated with a high incidence of several supratentorial abnormalities such as polymicrogyria, cortical heterotopia and corpus callosal dysgenesis [42, 43].

The real contribution of these additional malformations is not known due to the lack of studies correlating anatomical neuroimaging data with cognitive measures [39].

Subependymal heterotopias, the most frequent form of heterotopias in spina bifida, are generally thought to have the fewest clinical manifestations [44]: regardless of primary etiology, the intellectual and motor development of affected children are normal or only mildly impaired. On the other hand, focal subcortical heterotopias are associated with developmental delay in more than 50% of cases.

The clinical presentation of patients with polymicrogyria is variable and depends on the severity of involvement and its location. The outcome is worse in those children with a smaller head size and more extensive polymicrogyria. In patients with spina bifida/Chiari II malformation, polymicrogyria is generally limited to the parieto-occipital regions; moreover, the cortex is often histologically normal, with the six layered lamination preserved. Thereafter the exact role of such a malformation in the pathogenesis of mental retardation is under debate.

The co-existence of corpus callosal dysgenesis with neural tube closure defects is well recognized since Gross' description [45], it is also known that even if congenital isolated anomalies of the corpus callosum may be completely silent, callosal dysgenesis is often associated with deficits in idiomatics, figurative and syntactic-pragmatic language. Recently, Huber-Okrainec et al. [46] addressed the presence of neuropsychologic problems, involving language, strictly related to the grade of dysgenesis of the corpus callosum in patients with spina bifida. Corpus callosum agenesis, causing interhemispheric transfer deficits, should impair figurative language comprehension.

Communication between hemispheres, which in most individuals takes place along the corpus callosum, is a very important step in the achievement of sophisticated tasks. In the absence of the corpus callosum, alternative hierarchically vicarious commissural patterns develop during fetal life. However, primary neural tube defects associated with corpus callosum in myelomeningocele hinders the development of the alternative commissural pathways of interhemispheric data transfer. During embryonic and fetal life the same pathological process may alter cortical development leading to loss of function from some cerebral areas, which cannot be offset through normal communication between the hemispheres. Therefore, corpus callosum dysgenesis, habitually silent, may cause a true disconnection syndrome in children with myelomeningocele [47].

Level of the Spinal Lesion

The correlation between the spinal level of the myelomeningocele and outcome has been the object of several studies, often with controversial conclusions. Poorer medical and cognitive outcomes have been reported in upper-level spinal lesions [2, 48, 49]. Some authors found no correlation between IQ and spinal lesions [50]; others found the correlation between lower IQ and thoracic spine lesions [30, 49]; others between IQ and lesions above L2 [51, 52]. Nejat et al. [2] noted that among patients harboring lesions at high locations in the spine, the proportion of children with normal intelligence is lower than those harboring lesions at lower spinal locations. In no case was a comprehensive explanation of such observations given. Lorber [49] suggests that differences in IQ that vary according to lesion level are due to the association of perinatal complications with higher lesion levels. Lonton [48] found that children with thoracic lesions had thinner cortical mantles than those with lumbar and sacral lesions, and Badell-Ribera et al. [32] found more brain defects in children with thoracic lesions. Akar [53] reported a higher incidence of hydrocephalus for lesions located higher in the spine.

In a recent paper, Fletcher et al. [54] analyzed magnetic resonance imaging of the head and assessed handedness, intelligence, academic skills and adaptive behaviour in a large series of patients affected by myelomeningocele (268 children), subdivided into two groups according to the level of the spine lesion (above T12, below L1). Their findings indicate that children with upper- and lower level spinal lesions differ in terms of both anomalous brain development and behavioral outcomes; upper-level lesions were associated with significantly more compromise. Children with upper-level lesions had more anomalous brain development in the midbrain, tectum, and corpus callosum than those with lower-level lesions. Moreover, quantitative analysis of the cerebrum and cerebellum revealed that both were smaller in children with upper-level lesions. For the cerebrum, the differences reflected less gray and white matter in those with upper-level defects with no regional specificity other than a tendency to be more reduced in the right than left hemispheres. The authors concluded that "the higher the lesion, the more malformed the brain, and the more malformed the brain, the poorer the neurobehavioral outcome" [54].

Social Factors and Co-morbidities

The presence of neurological deficits such as paraplegia and incontinence may interfere with the development of cognitive skills, because physical disabilities may restrict the capacity to interact efficiently with the environment. Further, visual and auditory deficits may impact on the ability to process information efficiently for learning and acquiring new skills. However, in the only study where IQ was correlated with ambulatory/continence status [2], no significant differences were found between the mean IQ of ambulatory and nonambulatory children, or continent and incontinent children.

Generic illness factors such as school absence and living with chronic illness are also insufficient to explain the severity of cognitive problems in spina bifida patients [13].

In their study on spinal level lesion and cognitive outcome, Fletcher et al. [54] found a relationship between the environmental factors related to socio-economic status and ethnicity, which make it more likely that economically disadvantaged cohorts experienced more frequent upper-level defects and poorer intellectual outcome. Dietary factors may be especially critical as a factor related to the heritability of spina bifida and lesion level [55]. Nevertheless, poverty and socio-economic factors did not account for the overall pattern of effects of lesion level in Fletcher's study [54].

Even if the effects of poverty on language and cognitive development are well known, in the study of Nejat et al. [2] no statistically significant correlation was found between the mean IQ and the education levels of the parents or the socioeconomic level of the families.

Additional Factors

Often parents of children born with myelomeningocele ask whether their children will have normal mental cognitive development or will need to attend a school for special needs. Many variables at birth, including ventricular size, head size, duration of gestation, prenatal problems, aspect and site of the back wound, date of primary shunting and presence of cranial defects (such as lückenschädel or craniolacuna) have been correlated with cognitive outcome. Most studies reveal that ventricular size, open arch above vertebra lumbar 3, a very small or a very large head may be accompanied by a lower IQ [1, 48, 56].

In a recent paper, Beeker et al. [1], computing the linear relationship between the outcome IQ and the data at birth in a large cohort of patients, found a significant linear relationship between outcome IQ and three variables, two neuroanatomical (size of ventricle and level of arch defect) and one anthropomorphic (quotient of length [L] by circumference occiput-frontal [COF]). It was observed that a very high concentration of patients (> 80%) with an IQ > 85 were present in the area with a supine length (L) between 49 and 51 cm, and a COF between 335 and 365 mm at birth. This result produced the new variable L/COF. The authors formed an equation with the multiple linear regression using these three variables, calculating a predicted IQ. The predicted IQ at birth was the same or nearly the same as the measured IQ in 92% of cases. This study indicates that the loss of IQ may be already present at birth and that the source of the intellectual handicap in myelomenigocele children should be considered a congenital defect in most cases.

Nevertheless, in developed countries there is a consensus that children with myelomeningocele should be treated aggressively and that such treatment will benefit most, if not all, affected children [2]. In older patients with shunts there is a widespread belief that normal intelligence can be assured if the shunt functions satisfactorily, and in some centers blocked shunts have been revised for this purpose even in asymptomatic patients [56]. Matarò and coworkers [57] reported their experience in 23 young adult patients with spina bifida meningomyelocele, Chiari malformation and increased but stable ventriculomegaly. None of the patients had overt clinical signs or symptoms of increased intracranial pressure (ICP). These patients underwent ICP monitoring. In no cases a diagnosis of arrested hydrocephalus was confirmed, but all patients showed mean ICP above 12 mmHg or the presence of abnormal ICP waves. Neuropsychological assessment demonstrated poor performance on visual memory, visuoconstructive and frontal functions, and fine motor speed. Shunt surgery in this group of patients improved neuropsychological functioning. Significant improvements were obtained in verbal and visual memory, motor coordination, and attention and cognitive flexibility.

Under the assumption that shunt history and related complications could affect the intellectual development of these children, every effort to minimize the burden of shunt-linked complications must be made through a policy aiming to rigorously rule out every episode of shunt-failure and where appropriate to consider the current alternative to shunting, i.e., endoscopic third ventriculostomy (ETV). This technique appears to be effective in controlling hydrocephalus in case of aqueductal stenosis, especially in patients presenting with shunt malfunction [58]. Further studies are required to assess the effect of ETV on cognitive outcome in spina bifida patients.

References

1. Beeker TW, Scheers MM, Faber JA, Tulleken CA (2006) Prediction of independence and intelligence at birth in meningomyelocele. Childs Nerv Syst 22:33-37

2. Nejat F, Kazmi SS, Habibi Z et al (2007) Intelligence quotient in children with meningomyeloceles: a case-control study. J Neurosurg (2 Suppl Pediatrics) 106:106-110

3. Wills KE, Holmbeck GN, Dillon K, McLone DG (1990). Intelligence and achievement in children with myelomeningocele. J Pediatr Psychol 15:161-176

4. Tew B, Laurence KM (1975) The effects of hydrocephalus on intelligence, visual perception and school attainment. Dev Med Child Neurol 35:129-134

5. Fletcher JM, Barnes M, Dennis M (2002) Language development in children with spina bifida. Semin Pediatr Neurol 9(3):201-208

6. Barnes MA, Dennis M (1998). Discourse after early-onset hydrocephalus: Core deficits in children of average intelligence. Brain Lang 61:309-334

7. Fletcher JM, Dennis M, Northrup H et al (2004) Spina bifida: Genes, brain, and development. In: Glidden LM (ed) Handbook of research on mental retardation, Vol 28. Academic Press, San Diego, pp 63-117

8. Evans DR, Cope MA (1989) Manual for the quality of life questionnaire. Multi-Health Systems Inc., Toronto

9. Fletcher JM, Bohan TP, Brandt ME et al (1992) Verbal and nonverbal skill discrepancies in hydrocephalic children. J Clin Exp Neuropsychol 14:593-609

10. Hetherington R, Dennis M, Barnes M et al (2006) Functional outcome in young adults with spina bifida and hydrocephalus. Childs Nerv Syst 22:117-124

11. Dennis M, Futz M, Netley C et al (1981) The intelligence of hydrocephalic children. Arch Neurol 38:607-615

12. Fletcher JM, Brookshire BL, Landry SH et al (1996) Attentional skills and executive functions in children with early hydrocephalus. Dev Neuropsychol 12(1):53-76

13. Jacobs R, Northam E, Anderson V (2001) Cognitive outcome in children with myelomeningocele and perinatal hydrocephalus: a longitudinal perspective. J Dev Phys Disabil 13:389-405

14. Loss N, Yeates KO, Enrile BG (1998) Attention in children with myelomeningocele. Child Neuropsychol 4:7-20

15. Cull C, Wyke M (1984) Memory function of children with spina bifida and shunted hydrocephalus. Dev Med Child Neurol 26:177-183

16. Yeates KO, Enrile BG, Loss N et al (1995) Verbal learning and memory in children with myelomeningocele. J Pediatr Psychol 20(6):801-815

17. Shaffer J, Friedrich WN, Shurtleff DB, Wolf L (1995) Cognitive and achievement status of children with myelomeningocele. J Pediatr Psychol 10(3):325-336

18. Taylor EM (1961) Psychological appraisal of children with cerebral defects. Harvard Press, Cambridge

19. Vachha B, Adams RC (2005) Memory and selective learning in children with spina bifida-myelomeningocele and shunted hydrocephalus: a preliminary study. Cerebrospin Fluid Res 2:10

20. Budson AE, Price BH (2005) Current concepts: memory dysfunction. N Eng J Med 352:692-699

21. Barnes MA, Wilkinson M, Khemani E et al (2006) Arithmetic processing in children with spina bifida: calculation accuracy, strategy use, and fact retrieval fluency. J Learn Disabil 39:174-187

22. Taylor HG, Alden J (1997) Age-related differences in outcomes following childhood brain insults: An introduction and overview. J Int Neuropsychol Soc 3:355-567

23. Bowman RM, McLone DG, Grant JA, Tomita T (2001) Spina Bifida outcome: a 25-year prospective. Pediatr Neurosurg, 34:114-120

24. Donders J, Canady AI, Rourke BP (1990) Psychometric intelligence after infantile hydrocephalus. Child Nerv Syst 6:148-154

25. Dennis M (1989) Language and the young damaged brain. In: Boll T, Bryant B (eds) Clinical neuropsychology and brain function: Research, measurement and practice. American Psychological Association, Washington, pp 85-123

26. Jansen J (1985) A retrospective analysis 21 to 35 years after birth of hydrocephalic patients born from 1945 to 1955. An overall description of the material and the criteria used. Acta Neurol Scand 71:436-447

27. Laurence KM, Coates S (1962) The natural history of hydrocephalus. Detailed analysis of 182 unoperated cases. Arch Dis Child 37:345-362

28. Sgouros S (2004) Hydrocephalus with myelomeningocele. In: Cinalli G, Maixner WJ, Sainte-Rose C (eds) Pediatric hydrocephalus. Springer-Verlag, Italy, pp 133-144

29. Casari EF, Fantino AG (1998) A longitudinal study of cognitive abilities and achievement status of children with myelomeningocele and their relationship with clinical types. Eur J Pediatr Surg 8:52-54

30. Soare PL, Raimondi AJ (1977) Intellectual and perceptual-motor characteristics of treated myelomeningocele children. Am J Dis Child 131:199-204

31. Cohen AR, Robinson S (2001) Early management of myelomeningocele. In: McLone DG (ed) Pediatric neurosurgery: Surgery of the developing nervous system, 4th edn. WB Saunders, Philadelphia, pp 241-260

32. Badell-Ribera A, Shulman K, Paddock N (1966) The relationship of non-progressive hydrocephalus to intellectual functioning in children with spina bifida cystica. Pediatrics 37(5):787-793

33. Raimondi AJ, Soare P (1974) Intellectual development in shunted hydrocephalic children. Am J Dis Child 127(5):664-671

34. Hunt GM, Oakeshott P, Kerry S (1999) Link between the CSF shunt and achievement in adults with spina bifida. J Neurol Neurosurg Psychiatry 67:591-595

35. Mirzai H, Ersahin Y, Mutluer S, Kayahan A (1998) Outcome of patients with meningomyelocele, the Ege University experience. Childs Nerv Syst 14:120-123

36. Dennis M, Hetherington R, Spiegler BJ et al (1999) Functional consequences of congenital cerebellar dysmorphologies and acquired cerebellar lesions of childhood. In: Broman SH, Fletcher JM (eds) The changing nervous system—neurobehavioural consequences of early brain disorder. Oxford, New York

37. Dennis M, Edelstein K, Hetherington R et al (2004) Neurobiology of perceptual and motor timing in children with spina bifida in relation to cerebellar volume. Brain 127:1292-1301

38. Huber-Okrainec J, Dennis M, Brettschneider J et al (2002) Neuromotor speech deficits in children and adults with spina bifida and hydrocephalus. Brain Lang 80:592-602

39. Vinck A, Maassen B, Mullaart R, Rotteveel J (2006) Arnold-Chiari-II malformation and cognitive functioning in spina bifida. J Neurol Neurosurg Psychiatry 77:1083-1086

40. Rapoport M, van Reekum R, Mayberg H (2000) The role of the cerebellum in cognition and behavior: a selective review. J Neuropsychiatry Clin Neurosci 12:193-198

41. Leggio MG, Silveri MC, Petrosini L et al (2000) Phonological grouping is specifically affected in cerebellar patients: a verbal fluency study. J Neurol Neurosurg Psychiatry 69:102-106

42. Gilbert JN, Jones KL, Rorke LB et al (1986) Central nervous system anomalies associated with meningomyelocele, hydrocephalus, and the Arnold-Chiari malformation: Reappraisal of theories regarding the pathogenesis of posterior neural tube closure defects. Neurosurgery 18(5):559-564

43. Kawamura T, Morioka T, Nishio S et al (2001) Cerebral abnormalities in lumbosacral neural tube closure defect: MR imaging evaluation. Childs Nerv Syst 17:405-410

44. Cho WH, Seidenwurm D, Barkovich AJ (1999) Adult-onset neurologic dysfunction associated with cortical malformations. AJNR Am J Neuroradiol 20:1037-1043

45. Gross H, Jellinger K, Kaltenbac E (1974) Progressive hydrocephalus associated with spina bifida caused by a peculiar cerebellum-brain stem syndrome. Presented at the VIIth International Congress of Neuropathology, Budapest, Hungary

46. Huber-Okrainec J, Blaser SE, Dennis M (2005) Idiom comprehension deficits in relation to corpus callosum agenesis and hypoplasia in children with spina bifida meningomyelocele. Brain Lang 93:349-368

47. Kawamura T, Nishio S, Morioka T, Fukui K (2002) Callosal anomalies in patients with spinal dysraphism: correlation of clinical and neuroimaging features with hemispheric abnormalities. Neurol Res 24:463-467

48. Lonton AP (1977) Location of the myelomeningocele and its relationship to subsequent physical and intellectual abilities in children with myelomeningocele associated with hydrocephalus. Z Kinder 22:510-519

49. Lorber J (1971) Results of treatment of myelomeningocele. An analysis of 524 unselected cases, with special reference to possible selection for treatment. Dev Med Child Neurol 13:279-303

50. Mapstone TB, Rekate HL, Nulsen FE et al (1984) Relationship of CSF shunting and IQ in children with myelomeningocele: a retrospective analysis. Childs Brain 11:112-118

51. Friedrich WN, Lovejoy MC, Shafer J et al (1991) Cognitive abilities and achievement status of children with myelomeningocele: a contemporary sample. J Pediatr Psychol 16:423-428

52. Hunt GM (1990) Open spina bifida: outcome for a complete cohort treated unselectively and followed into adulthood. Dev Med Child Neurol 32:108-118

53. Akar Z (1995) Myelomenincele. Surg Neurol 43:113-118

54. Fletcher JM, Copeland K, Frederick JA et al (2005) Spinal lesion level in spina bifida: a source of neural and cognitive heterogeneity. J Neurosurg (Pediatrics 3) 102:268-279

55. Volcik KA, Blanton SH, Tyerman GH et al (2000) Methylenetetrahydrofolate reductase and spina bifida: evaluation of level of defect and maternal genotypic risk in Hispanics. Am J Med Genet 95:21-27

56. Hunt GM (1999) Non-selective intervention in newborn babies with open spina bifida: the outcome 30 years on for the complete cohort. Eur J Pediatr Surg 9 (Suppl 1):5-8

57. Mataró M, Poca MA, Sahuquillo J et al (2000) Cognitive changes after cerebrospinal fluid shunting in young adults with spina bifida and assumed arrested hydrocephalus. J Neurol Neurosurg Psychiatry 68:615-621

58. O'Brien DF, Javadpour M, Collins DR et al (2005) Endoscopic third ventriculostomy: an outcome analysis of primary cases and procedure performed after ventriculoperitoneal shunt malfunction. J Neurosurg (5 Suppl Pediatrics) 103:393-400

CHAPTER 33

A Family-Centered Evaluation of Psychosocial Agendas in Spina Bifida

Mehmet Kemal Kuşcu, Banu Cankaya

Introduction

Care patterns and parenting quality have an important effect on the infant-caregiver relationship, as well as on the developmental outcomes of children [1]. High quality care is linked to higher cognitive ability and higher social competence in children [2]. Especially in the case of disability, families and other close networks gain a pivotal role as the main caregivers for the child [3]. Currently, the role and needs of families attract considerable attention due to the growing amount of evidence regarding their participation in the illness process and the attached psychosocial outcomes.

Spina bifida (SB) is a congenital birth defect that has debilitating and chronic health consequences for individuals across different levels of functioning, including biological, neurological, psychological, and cognitive development. Individuals with SB need intensive treatment and care that requires the involvement of their families. Thus, as with many other chronic health problems, SB has serious implications for many aspects of families' lives, not only in terms of the increased demands for intensive care, but also in terms of the families' psychological status across different levels, including the family as a whole, marital, parental, and sibling subsystems, and at the level of individual functioning.

Children with SB have varied problems with their physical, neuropsychological, and psychological functioning. The severity of SB depends on the level of the spinal lesion and the associated neurological deficits. Families need to constantly adjust their care arrangements according to these deficits, as well as to those that arise due to complications. At the biological level, aside from health problems including either weakened or paralyzed lower extremities, sphincter disturbance, and hydrocephalus, children with SB are likely to experience precocious puberty [4]. In most cases, early puberty does not coincide with the age of social development of these children, leading to increased stress on these children and their families [5]. In addition to biological functioning, children with SB also exhibit neurological and cognitive problems. These problems include various levels of difficulties with attention capacity [6] and executive functions, such as deficits in logical thinking, planning ability, and organizational skills [7].

Studies have also shown that children with SB have various psychological adjustment problems, including higher risk of social isolation [6, 8], internalization of symptoms and low self-esteem, compared to their peers without chronic health problems [9, 10, 11]. Furthermore, Holmbeck et al. [6] found that pre-adolescent children with SB were more likely to rely on the guidance of adults, and were less likely to be assertive about their viewpoints or make their own decisions.

As discussed above, children with SB experience deficits in their physical capabilities, neuropsychological functioning, and psychological adaptation. Due to the chronic nature and severity of these deficits, children with SB are likely to have their families as the main sources of support for their physical rehabilitation and psychological well-being. Families coping with SB are faced with challenges that are very different to those that are faced by families who are raising able-bodied and normally-developing children. One of the stressors that families of children with SB experience is the need for continuous interaction with medical care agencies. Families of these children need to make constant changes to their lives as a result of frequent hospitalizations and medical visits, compliance with strict treatment regimens, and decision making related to medication, physiotherapy, and more intrusive types of interventions. They are also under increased levels of financial stress due to frequent involvement with the health care system and the purchase of equipment necessary for the maintenance of function. Furthermore, the attention and resources allocated to the needs of children with SB can lead to difficulties in marital and sibling relationships. For instance, Quittner and Opipari [12] pointed out how families of children with chronic illness engage in "differential attention" to siblings in the family, and how this affects the sibling's psychological functioning. Overall, families of children with SB are under a lot of strain, and several studies have supported the conclusion that families of children with SB experience more stress than families of able-bodied children [13, 14].

Understanding the family functioning of children with SB is very important for multiple reasons, one of which is to find ways to help families better adjust to a chronic illness and consequent changes in their lives. Another purpose is to help the psychological as well as the physical adjustment of children with SB via intervening in family functioning. It has been shown that adaptive coping skills and healthy psychological adjustment in children are related to healthy parenting behavior and the family environment [15, 16]. For instance, children were shown to be more likely to use adaptive coping strategies such as problem-focused coping skills [17], if their family was cohesive [18], responsive to the needs of their children, and demanding in terms of asking for mature behavior [16].

Psychological Functioning of Families with SB-Affected Children

Families of children with SB have been examined with regards to their psychological status across different levels of functioning. The level of analyses includes family systems or global functioning variables (e.g., family cohesion, conflict, life events), parental and marital functioning (e.g., parental stress, parenting style, parenting satisfaction, marital satisfaction), sibling relationships, and individual functioning (e.g., perceived stress, psychological symptoms). A limitation of this research is that none of the studies on family functioning has included factors that are disease/SB-specific, such as health care management, decision-making processes, or medication adherence [19]. However, despite this limitation, findings have provided valuable information that helps our understanding of and interventions for families of children with SB.

Developmental Framework

A developmental perspective has been suggested as an important framework for better understanding the impact of SB on family functioning. The developmental perspective takes into account how having a child with SB affects family functioning differently depending on the transitional development periods in both the family's and child's life [19]. Unfortunately, little research has been carried out using a longitudinal design or measures of developmental processes for children with SB or other types of chronic illnesses [5].

Adolescence has been suggested as a critical stage of development that needs to be taken into consideration when studying factors related to both chronically ill and healthy children's psychological adjustment. During this stage of development, children go through a lot of changes in the biological, psychological, cognitive, and social spheres of life, and these changes call for new adjustments in their treatment and care, thus potentially leading to increased levels of stress in family functioning and relationships. Furthermore, Holmbeck [5] referred to adolescence as critical for the development of adaptive behaviors in different areas of a child's life, including attitude toward health care.

During adolescence, in comparison with children without physical disabilities or chronic illness, families need to remain involved in the lives of children with SB. Furthermore, children with SB are likely to have a limited social/interpersonal network that mainly includes the family and the health care system. Thus, for children with SB, family functioning is of particular importance during adolescence because family relationships are most likely to be the targets and means with which they will meet their new needs and demands in their development. Just like children without SB, children with SB make the transition to adolescence and have an increased desire for involvement with peers, autonomy, control, and privacy, although within the limitations of their physical and neurological disability [20]. Also, a child with a normal progression to adolescence has increased capacities for problem-solving and planning for the future with an understanding of consequences of actions. Children with SB, depending on the level of their executive functioning, may also require more autonomy from their families and may want to monitor their lives and illness, for instance by sharing more responsibility in their treatment and intervention.

During adolescence and, for children with SB who mature early, even during preadolescence, parents may struggle between their need for protection and care, and the child's developing need for autonomy [21]. Anderson and Coyne [20] called it "miscarried helping" when parents cannot adjust their level of protection and involvement in their child's life as a result of the development of their cognitive sophistication and need for autonomy. Other researchers referred to and studied this phenomenon using the term "overprotection" [21]. Findings indicated that higher levels of parental control during this transitional developmental period were associated with lower levels of autonomy and higher levels of externalizing behaviors.

Given the lack of a developmental approach to examining psychological status of families of children with SB, the following review was organized in terms of the impact of SB on psychological status of families across different levels of functioning, without much reference to the developmental phases of these children. How families and children with SB struggle during different stages of their lives and how this affects their psychological status will be fruitful avenues for future research.

Global Family Functioning

In terms of family functioning at the global level, several studies [9, 22] looked at the general functioning using the Family Assessment Device [23] and found that approximately 12-13% of families of children with SB experience clinically significant levels of general family "dysfunction." These results were lower than the results found for families with children who have cerebral palsy [22]. In another study, parents of children with SB did not report any significant effects of SB on their general family functioning [24, 25]. Families of children with SB showed problems other than a general dysfunction within the family system, such as difficulties with maintaining boundaries in roles and responsibilities [9, 22].

When more specific SB-related factors were examined, the impact of factors related to the health status and severity of SB on family adjustment were equally represented. Several studies have shown that higher severity and more problems related to SB-specific conditions lead to problems in family functioning [26–28]. According to one study, good family functioning was best predicted by decreased levels of parental perception of the child's daily living and self-care limitations, and fewer problems related to the child's health condition [26]. Other important disease-related factors were resources of care, such as number of adults

at home, insurance, frequency of doctor visits, and employment status of fathers [26]. In a study of 19 children with SB [27], it was shown that mothers who rated their children's condition as more severe also reported higher family functioning difficulties in daily life. Furthermore, in several studies, higher lesion level was related to more adverse effects of SB on family functioning [28]. On the other hand, in a study of 65 children and adolescents with SB [29], higher lesion level was found to be related to lower levels of family conflict as reported by the mothers of children with SB. Likewise, for families of children with SB, early puberty was either not related or positively related to family cohesion and conflict over time in families of children with SB, while early puberty was found to be related to lower cohesion and higher conflict for the families of able-bodied children [30]. These discrepancies in findings suggest that there is a need to explore and examine moderating and mediating variables that lead some families to be more vulnerable and some to be more resilient to problems in their functioning.

In addition to the general functioning of the family, in a study carried out by Holmbeck et al. [5], family conflict, cohesion, and stressful life events in families of children with SB were examined, and three aspects of the relationships between these family system factors and function were tested. One was the resilience-disruption hypothesis, originally described for families with children who have mental retardation [31]. It was hypothesized that families of children with chronic illness inevitably experience disruptions within the family system as a function of having a child with numerous physical and neuropsychological problems. On the other hand, these families show resiliency to high levels of stress and thus do not necessarily experience increased levels of dysfunction at the family and individual level.

A second aspect of the psychological status of families of children with SB is that family functioning and relationships may be challenged by a potential clash between the parents' tendency to overly control their children with SB and the child's need for autonomy. On one hand, the parents' tendency to control the lives of their children may serve as an adaptive function for children with chronic illness or disability, more so than for the child without a chronic condition [20, 32]. On the other hand, children with SB may transition into adolescence earlier than healthy children, and thus have needs for autonomy and differentiation from their families. Children with SB may want to, for instance, independently make decisions about their treatment and manage their medications as they grow older [14]. From this point of view, families of children with SB, compared to families of able-bodied children, may have more difficulties in relinquishing control due to concerns about their children's health. These difficulties may lead to increased levels of tension in the parent-child relationship, more conflicts, and less cohesion within the family.

Another aspect proposed by Holmbeck et al. was that a significant proportion of children with chronic illness tend to depend on their parents for their health care due to limitations imposed by their cognitive, behavioral, and physical development. Due to sharing the same goal of meeting the needs of their children, families of children with SB may feel closer to each other, be more cohesive, and have less conflict.

Overall, the results of Holmbeck et al. study [14] showed that families of children with SB, in comparison with families of able-bodied children, have less family cohesion and less agreement between the mother and the child with SB with respect to activity preferences. However, there were no differences between these families in terms of the level of family conflict and stressful life events. Apart from health status, socioeconomic status (SES) was found to have a significant impact on the functioning of families of children with and without SB. Lower SES was found to be related to lower family cohesion, higher conflict, and higher stress levels. Findings suggested that if families of children with SB have low levels of SES, they have more difficulties with family cohesion. Furthermore, children's verbal IQ was found to account for almost half of the differences observed between the families of children with SB and without SB. Holmbeck et al. [14] suggested that these results supported a resilience-disruption hypothesis, showing that families of children with SB have disruptions (i.e., less cohesion) as well as resilience (no elevations in conflict or stressful life events). The factors of low SES and limitations in cognitive functioning were found to be potential moderators and mediators, respectively, to be examined and considered in future research and family interventions.

Marital and Parental Functioning

Family functioning at the level of marital and parental relationships has been examined in terms of satisfaction, distress, and conflict. Holmbeck et al. [13], in their study of 55 families of preadolescent children with SB and a matched control group, found that the most salient factor that differentiated families of preadolescents with SB from those with able-bodied children was parenting role satisfaction, with the former group being less satisfied. Furthermore, in contrast to fathers, mothers of children with SB perceived themselves as less competent and more socially isolated in their parenting role. An alternative study [33] comparing reports of 59 mothers of children with SB, 19 fathers with SB, and a normative group, showed no differences between the parents of children with SB and the normative group in terms of competency and satisfaction with parenting. These conflicting results may indicate that specific factors related to parents' lives other than the health status of children may make a difference to parents' satisfaction in their parenting role. In a study of 50 mothers of children with SB [34], having an adult companion and higher social support was related to higher ratings of maternal satisfaction. In addition, better general family functioning was found to be a predictor of higher maternal competence and psychological well-being. In this study, African-American and Latino mothers showed more difficulties in their parenting role, indicated by lower satisfaction compared to Caucasian mothers. In another study [35], maternal parenting stress was found to be related to maternal age, but not to demographic variables such as SES and maternal education level, medical severity, and family support.

In terms of marital functioning, there has been consistent evidence for the lack of differences in marital satisfaction of parents of children with SB and with able-bodied children [13, 25, 36]. In a study of 46 families [36], marital quality was reported to be higher for mothers of female children with SB who are younger than five years old, in comparison with mothers of male children with SB who are older than five years old. Furthermore, increases in parenting stress, maternal symptoms of anxiety, depression, global distress, and ambulatory problems were found to be related to maternal reports of lower levels of marital quality [36, 37]. In another study of 56 families of children with SB and a matched sample of families of children without SB [38], maternal and paternal reports of lower marital satisfaction were found to be associated with higher illness severity.

Parenting style is another factor examined in families of children with SB. A study with 55 families of children with SB and a matched sample of families with able-bodied children [39] showed that parents of children with SB were highly demanding and directive, but not particularly responsive toward their children (i.e., higher authoritarian control), in comparison with parents of able-bodied children. The non-democratic style of parenting was more apparent in families of children with SB who were also of low SES.

Different sets of parenting styles (i.e., behavioral and psychological control) were examined in mothers of preadolescents with SB and able-bodied children [40]. It was shown that mothers of children with SB showed higher levels of psychological control over their children than mothers of children without SB. In other words, mothers of children with SB were more likely to exert control over their children which would affect their psychological development, including thinking style, emotional expression, and attachment. For both the children with SB and able-bodied children, parental psychological control was related to various negative psychosocial outcomes for children.

Differences between parents of children with SB in terms of their attempts to control their child's behavior were examined as a function of disease-related features, such as lesion level. Within a sample composed of only mothers of children with SB [29], mothers of children with SB who have higher level lesions are likely to grant more behavioral autonomy to their children, in comparison with the mothers of children with lower level lesions. In another study of 19 children with SB [27], mothers who gave higher severity ratings to their child's condition reported greater perceived restrictions on their child's behavior.

In a study with 68 families of children with SB and a matched sample of 68 families of able-bodied children [21], mothers and fathers of children with SB showed higher levels of overprotection, in comparison with parents of able-bodied children. The cognitive functioning of the children partially explained the difference in the tendency to overly protect their children. For the families of children with SB, lower perceived levels of behavioral autonomy of these children accounted for the relationship between the child's increased levels of externalizing behavior problems and the parents' higher level of overprotection.

Overall, investigation of different parenting styles of parents with SB-affected children suggest that these parents exert more psychological control over their children and are more overly protective of their child's behavior, relative to parents with able-bodied children. In terms of behavioral control, mothers of children with SB may not be different from the mothers of able-bodied children in the extent to which they control their child's behaviors. Findings

suggest that within the families with SB-affected children, SB-specific factors such as cognitive functioning, lesion level and general severity of illness are likely to make a difference in the parenting styles with respect to behavioral control and the behavioral autonomy granted to their children.

Individual Functioning

Paternal and Maternal Functioning

Paternal and maternal functioning has been studied mainly in terms of perceived stress, psychological symptoms, and coping skills. In terms of the level of perceived global distress by parents, findings have been equivocal. Across several studies, no differences were found between the level of perceived distress of parents of children with SB and able-bodied children [25, 33]. On the other hand, a study comparing 60 parents of children with SB, cerebral palsy, and children with limb deficiencies [22], showed that 41% of parents of children with SB have experienced stress at a clinical level, compared to 48% of parents whose children were diagnosed with cerebral palsy and 37% of parents of children with limb deficiencies.

In a study of 66 mothers of children with SB [41], factors related to medical conditions caused the most stress for mothers. Likewise, Kazak and Clark [38] showed a relationship between the severity of SB and maternal reports of perceived stress. However, regardless of severity ratings, both mothers' and fathers' stress levels fell within the normal range. In a study of 111 mothers of children with cerebral palsy, SB, or diabetes, maternal hope was found to be a moderator of the relationship between levels of stress and maternal psychological adjustment. Accordingly, with high levels of stress, mothers who had higher levels of hope experienced less adjustment problems [42].

In addition to the level of stress experienced by parents, parents' psychological symptoms were examined as a function of having a child with SB. In a study of 55 families of preadolescent children with SB and a matched control group [13], none of the parents in the general sample were within the dysfunctional range in terms of their functioning. Nevertheless, fathers of children with SB had more psychological symptoms than fathers of able-bodied children, while mothers of children with SB and without SB did not differ in terms of the level of psychological symptoms. In a study of mothers of children with SB [37], maternal psychological status was related to factors such as increased levels of family support, better marital functioning, lower levels of emotion regulation through the use of friends, and lower levels of control and conflict within the family.

In terms of parental coping styles, Holmbeck et al. [13] found differences between parents of children with SB and able-bodied children. Accordingly, mothers of children with SB reported using less active coping strategies and more denial when they experienced stressful events. Also, mothers of children with SB were less likely to be adaptable to change in different areas of their lives such as their own development, occupation, finances, and the development of their children. Fathers of children with SB, on the other hand, indicated using the coping strategy of venting more frequently than fathers of able-bodied children.

Holmbeck et al. [13] suggested that the differences between parents of SB and able-bodied children in terms of their coping and adaptability to change may result from coping strategies that are more situation-specific, thus only adaptive for SB-specific conditions. For instance, it may be adaptive for mothers of children with SB to use denial and be less active when managing uncontrollable stressors and challenges related to having a child who is chronically and severely ill. Furthermore, lower levels of adaptability to change may be adaptive for parents of children with SB who need strict schedules for treatments and interventions [43].

Particular coping strategies were found to be maladaptive for both parents of children with SB and without SB [13]. Disengagement and emotion-focused coping were related to negative psychological outcomes for both groups. Similarly, another study [44] confirmed that all forms of maladaptive coping strategies, with avoidant coping in particular, were related to negative outcomes in maternal psychological outcomes (e.g., lower levels of adjustment, higher threats to self-esteem).

Contrary to the findings of Holmbeck et al. [13], Bower and Hayes [45] did not find any difference among the coping styles of mothers of children with SB and Down's syndrome, and able-bodied children. As with many other areas of research, more studies on SB and family functioning are warranted for a better understanding of the different types of coping skills that families of children with SB need to acquire for healthier functioning.

In terms of the cognitive factors related to parental psychological status, mothers of children with SB were found to be less optimistic than mothers of children with able-bodied children [44]. Maternal future expectations were also examined [46]. Findings showed that the expectation of mothers of children with SB was that their children would learn more adaptive skills within the next five years. However, the relationship between higher expectations of these mothers and psychosocial outcomes was not examined.

Social support has been found to be strongly related to maternal psychological adaptation [27, 42], unrelated to the presence of SB [44]. Furthermore, for both mothers and fathers, psychological well-being was related to higher levels of family-centered caregiving, which involved higher levels of support, involvement, and information exchange from professionals [47].

Siblings

In a study of 56 families of children with SB and a matched control group without SB [38], no significant differences were found between the self-image of siblings in the two groups of families. When differences among siblings in families of children with chronic illnesses such as SB were examined, better maternal mood and general family functioning were found to be significantly related to higher perceived support by siblings, and higher scores in self-esteem and mood of siblings [48]. In another study with 252 parents and healthy siblings of children with chronic illness or disability including SB [49], SES was found to be the strongest factor that impacted sibling adaptive behavior. Siblings' attitude toward the chronic illness or disability was associated with general family functioning indicated by family cohesion, siblings' self-esteem, and siblings' knowledge about the illness. Siblings who have a better attitude toward illness had better mood states. Furthermore, siblings' self-esteem was also associated with multiple factors that involved siblings' mood, perceived social support, and family cohesion.

Suggestions for Intervention

As it was indicated in the review of Holmbeck et al. [19], there are no empirically studied treatments specific for families of children with SB. Nevertheless, recommendations for intervention can be made by drawing from the research findings on the psychological status of families of children with SB and treatment research with families of children with other chronic illnesses.

Given the findings of increased levels of stress in families of children with SB, skills to modulate emotions and cope with stressors could be targeted in interventions for these families. Furthermore, issues related to medical adherence may also be another important target of treatment [19]. Failures in medical compliance lead to increased problems in the health of the children with SB, which in turn challenges families who have already been struggling to maintain a status quo in order to function at an optimal level. Non-compliance could be addressed in specific interventions aimed at families' attitude toward the illness and involve psycho-education of the parents in terms of the consequences of medical non-compliance.

Another treatment target for families of children with SB could be the asynchrony between the child's needs for autonomy and the parents' protectiveness. Interventions targeting parenting skills could help these families to acknowledge and deal with this conflict of interest. Issues related to autonomy may also be conceptualized from the point of view of family systems. In a parenting skills training or family systems intervention, one of the areas of focus of therapy may be how children and parents could collaborate to manage medications and make decisions about interventions. Problems related to desires for autonomy of children with SB has been discussed with respect to medical compliance and choice of treatment [19]. In several studies of children with chronic illnesses, it has been shown that when children transition into adolescence, medical compliance decreases [50]. The goal would be to support the independence of the child with SB while keeping parents involved in their treatment without being intrusive or overly protective of them. A family environment that is supportive of the child's need for autonomy is likely to decrease their risk for psychosocial problems such as externalizing disorders [21].

Given the evidence for decreased levels of cohesion in the families of children with SB, family cohesion may be another target of intervention that could be addressed using family systems or structural therapy. Family cohesion could be targeted by clarifying the boundaries between different subsystems in the family such as parental and marital, and helping family members to be more flexible in terms of their role in the caregiving process. Rather than one family member assuming the caregiver role, family cohesion and increased resilience may be achieved by having more flexibility around the roles of caregiving, particularly when new health-related demands and difficulties arise for children with SB. The ben-

efits of increased involvement of other parties in the care of children have received support from a cross-sectional study with couples who have children with chronic illness [51]. In this study, higher involvement of fathers in the management of illness was found to be associated with lower levels of maternal psychopathology, less impact on family functioning in general, and higher marital satisfaction. Though this finding awaits support via longitudinal studies, families in which mothers are the sole caregivers may benefit from interventions that target increased paternal involvement in the care of their children.

Parallel to the idea of extending the network of caregivers, as with increased paternal involvement in disease management [51], family-centered caregiving was studied as a potential protective factor for the well-being of parents of children with disabilities [47]. Family-centered caregiving was defined by the increased involvement of health professionals in the care of the child. This was achieved by supporting partnership in child care, being available as sources of information about the child, and providing coordinated and comprehensive care for the child, while respecting and supporting the autonomy of the family in decision making about disease management [52]. Results of this study showed that more family-centered caregiving was related to decreased levels of perceived stress and better parental emotional well-being, particularly less depression. Furthermore, as family functioning was better and the social support was increased, parents' well-being also improved.

In another study of 56 caretakers of children with SB [35], caregivers, mainly mothers, who had a dysfunctional parent-child interactions, were less likely to use resources or support systems, in comparison with mothers with lower levels of dysfunctional parent-child interaction. A clinical implication of these studies is that increasing the network of care is an important treatment consideration for increasing the well-being of parents of children with chronic illnesses or disabilities [47]. This can be achieved by educating health care providers to approach the treatment of chronic illness in children from a family-centered point of view that involves maintaining respect for the parents, increasing support, exchange of information, and creating "partnerships" with parents [53]. Better outcomes for the families of these children are likely to be achieved by increasing availability of and access to resource and support centers for parents, and coordinating the efforts of these centers with the service provided by a team of health care professionals. There is little information regarding extended family systems and wider family networks in the literature. Further studies on this is-sue within its cultural context, especially in countries with limited formal resources, are also needed.

Several characteristics such as low SES, low so-cial support network, and belonging to a minority cul-ture also need to be considered when planning in-terventions for families of children with SB. Never-theless, studies examining these factors are scarce. More studies are thus warranted to explore the risks and the protective factors related to resilience and dis-ruptions in these families. Depending on these fac-tors, the risk of psychological adaptation problems may be increased for some families, and interven-tions may need to be adjusted accordingly.

Despite the growing literature on SB and family functioning, data on family intervention is still lack-ing. The pivotal role of the family in SB provides an opportunity to design supportive care programs focusing on the families' resilience and coping strate-gies. Especially in a long lasting process such as SB management, structured family-centered approach-es, starting early from the postpartum period, will support both clinical and rehabilitation efforts and the coping capacities of the families.

References

1. Hungerford A, Cox MJ (2006) Family factors in child care research. Eval Rev 30:631-655
2. NICHD (2003) Does quality of child care affect child outcomes at age 41/2? Dev Psychol 39:451-469
3. Jansen LM, Ketelaar M, Vermeer A (2003) Parental experience of participation in physical therapy for chil-dren with physical disabilities. Dev Med Child Neu-rol 45(1):58-70
4. Greene SA, Frank M, Zachman M, Prader A (1985) Growth and sexual development in children with meningomyleocoele. Eur J Pediatr 144:146-148
5. Holmbeck GN (2002) A developmental perspective on adolescent health and illness: An introduction to the special issues. J Pediatr Psychol 27:409-416
6. Holmbeck GN, Westhoven VC, Philips WS et al (2003) A multi-method, multi-informant, and multi-dimen-sional perspective on psychosocial adjustment in pre-adolescents with spina bifida. J Consult Clin Psychol 71:782-796
7. Fletcher JM, Dennis M, Northrup H (2000) Hydro-cephalus. In: Yeates KO, Ris MD, Taylor HG (eds) Pe-diatric neuropsychology: Research, theory, and prac-tice. Guilford Press, New York, pp 25-46
8. Blum RW, Resnick MD, Nelson R, St Germaine A (1991) Family and peer issues among adolescents with spina bifida and cerebral palsy. Pediatrics 88:280-285
9. Ammerman RT, Kane VR, Slomka GT et al (1998) Psychiatric symptomatology and family functioning in children and adolescents with spina bifida. J Clin Psy-chol Med Sett 5:449-465
10. Appleton PL, Minchom PE, Ellis NC et al (1994) The self-concept of young people with spina bifida: A pop-ulation-based study. Dev Med Clin Neurol 36:198-215
11. Appleton PL, Ellis NC, Minchom PE et al (1997) De-pressive symptoms and self-concept in young people with spina bifida. J Pediatr Psychol 22:707-722
12. Quittner AL, Opipari LC (1994) Differential treatment of siblings: Interview and diary analyses comparing two family contexts. Child Dev 65:800-814
13. Holmbeck GN, Gorey-Ferguson L, Hudson T et al (1997) Maternal, paternal, and marital functioning in families of preadolescents with spina bifida. J Pediatr Psychol 22:167-181
14. Holmbeck GN, Coakley RM, Hommeyer J et al (2002) Observed and perceived dyadic and systemic func-tioning in families of preadolescents with a physical disability. J Pediatr Psychol 27:177-189
15. Hardy DF, Power TG, Jaedicke S (1993) Examining the relation of parenting to children's coping with everyday stress. Child Dev 64:1829-1841
16. McKernon WL, Holmbeck GN, Colder CR et al (2001) Longitudinal study of observed and perceived family influences on problem-focused coping behaviors of preadolescents with spina bifida. J Pediatr Psychol 26(1):41-54
17. Hollahan CJ, Valentiler DP, Moos RH (1995) Parental support, coping strategies, and psychological adjust-ment: An integrative model with late adolescents. J Youth Adolesc 24:633-648
18. Kliewer W, Lewis H (1995) Family influences on cop-ing processes in children and adolescents with sickle cell disease. J Pediatr Psychol 20:511-525
19. Holmbeck GN, Greenley EN, Coakley RM et al (2006) Family functioning in children and adolescents with spina bifida: An evidence-based review of research and evidence. J Dev Behav Pediatr 27(3):249-277
20. Anderson BJ, Coyne JC (1993) Family context and compliance behavior in chronically ill children. In: Krasnegor NA, Epstein L, Johnson SB, Yaffe SJ (eds) Developmental aspects of health compliance behavior. Lawrence Erlbaum Associates, Hillside, pp 77-89
21. Holmbeck GN, Johnson SZ, Wills K et al (2002) Observed and perceived parental overprotection in relation to psychosocial adjustment in pre-adoles-cents with a physical disability: The mediational role of behavioral autonomy. J Consult Clin Psychol 70:96-110
22. Wiegner S, Donders J (2000) Predictors of parental dis-tress after congenital disabilities. J Dev Behav Pedi-atr 21:271-277
23. Epstein NB, Baldwin LM, Bishop DS (2000) Family Assessment Device (FAD). In: Handbook of psychi-

atric measures. American Psychiatric Association, Washington, DC

24. Loebig M (1990) Mothers' assessments of the impact of children with spina bifida on the family. MCN Am J Mat Child Nurs 19:251-265

25. Spaulding BR, Morgan SB (1986) Spina bifida children and their parents: A population prone to family dysfunction? J Pediatr Psychol 11:359-374

26. McCormick MC, Charney EB, Stemmler MM (1986) Assessing the impact of a child with spina bifida on the family. Dev Med Child Neurol 28:53-61

27. Havermans T, Eiser C (1991) Mothers' perceptions of parenting a child with spina bifida. Child Care Health Dev 17:259-273

28. Bier JB, Liebling JA (1996) Parents' and pediatricians' views of individuals with meningomyelocele. Clin Pediatr 35:113-118

29. Holmbeck GN, Faier-Routman J (1995) Spinal lesion level, shunt status, family relationships, and psychosocial adjustment in children and adolescents with spina bifida myelomeningocele. J Pediatr Psychol 20:515-529

30. Coakley RM, Holmbeck GN, Friedman D et al (2002) A longitudinal study of pubertal timing, parent-child conflict, and cohesion in families of young adolescents with spina bifida. J Pediatr Psychol 27:461-473

31. Costigan CL, Floyd FJ, Harter KSM, McClintock JC (1997) Family process and adaptation to children with mental retardation: Disruption and resilience in problem-solving interactions. J Fam Psychol 11:515-529

32. Seiffge-Krenke I (1998) The highly structured climate in families of adolescents with Diabetes: Functional or dysfunctional for metabolic control? J Pediatr Psychol 23:313-322

33. Lemanek KL, Jones ML, Lieberman B (2000) Mothers of children with spina bifida: Adaptational and stress processing. Child Health Care 29:19-35

34. Fagan J, Schor D (1993) Mothers of children with spina bifida: Factors related to maternal psychosocial functioning. Am J Orthopsychiatry 63:146-152

35. Macias MM, Clifford SC, Saylor CF, Kreh SM (2001) Predictors of parenting stress in families of children with spina bifida. Child Health Care 30(1):57-65

36. Cappelli M, McGrath PJ, Daniels T et al (1994) Marital quality of parents of children with spina bifida: A case-comparison study. J Dev Behav Pediatr 15:320-326

37. Kronenberger WG, Thompson RJ (1992) Dimensions of family functioning in families with chronically-ill children: A higher order factor analysis of the Family Environment Scale. J Clin Child Psychol 19:380-388

38. Kazak AE, Clark MW (1986) Stress in families of children with myelomeningocele. Dev Med Child Neurol 28:220-228

39. Seefeldt T, Holmbeck GN, Belvedere MC et al (1997) Socioeconomic status and democratic parenting in families of preadolescents with spina bifida. Psi Chi J Undergrad Res 2:5-12

40. Holmbeck GN, Shapera WE, Hommeyer JS (2002) Observed and perceived parenting behaviors and psychosocial adjustment in preadolescents with Spina Bifida. In: Barber BK (ed) Intrusive parenting: How psychological control affects children and adolescents. APA, Washington, pp 191-234

41. Kronenberger WG, Thompson RJ (1992) Medical stress, appraised stress, and the psychological adjustment of mothers of children with myelomeningocele. J Dev Behav Pediatr 13:405-411

42. Horton TV, Wallander JL (2001) Hope and social support as resilience factors against psychological distress of mothers who care for children with chronic physical conditions. Rehabil Psychol 46:382-399

43. Kazak AE (1989) Families of chronically ill children: A systems and social ecological model of adaptation and challenge. J Consult Clin Psychol 57:25-30

44. Barakat LP, Linney JA (1995) Optimism, appraisals, and coping in the adjustment of mothers and their children with spina bifida. J Child Fam Stud 4:303-320

45. Bowers AM, Hayes A (1998) Mothering in families with and without a child with disability. Int J Disabil Dev Educ 45:313-322

46. Edwards-Beckett J (1995) Parental expectations and child's self-concept in spina bifida. Child Health Care 24:257-267

47. King G, King S, Rosenbaum P, Goffin R (1999) Family centered caregiving and well-being of parents of children with disabilities: Linking process with outcome. J Pediatr Psychol 24:41-53

48. Williams PD, Williams AR, Graff JC et al (2002) Interrelationships among variables affecting well siblings and mothers in families of children with a chronic illness or disability. J Behav Med 25:411-424

49. Williams PD, Williams AR, Hanson S et al (1999) Maternal mood, family functioning, and perceptions of social support, self-esteem, and mood among siblings of chronically ill children. Child Health Care 28:297-310

50. Anderson B, Ho J, Brackett J et al (1997) Parent involvement in diabetes management tasks: Relationships to blood glucose monitoring adherence and metabolic control in young adolescents with insulin dependent diabetes mellitus. J Pediatr 130:257-265

51. Gavin L, Wysocki T (2005) Associations of paternal involvement in disease management with maternal and family outcomes in families with children with chronic illness. J Pediatr Psychol 31(5):481-489

52. King S, Rosenbaum P, King G (1996) The Measure of Processes of Care (MPOC): A means to assess family-centered behaviors of health care providers. Hamilton, Ontario, Canada: McMaster University and Chedoke-McMaster Hospitals, Neurodevelopmental Clinical Research Unit

53. Rosenbaum P, King S, Law M et al (1998) Family-centered service: A conceptual framework and research review. Phys Occup Ther Pediatr 18:1-20

Chapter 34
Endocrine Aspects of Neural Tube Defects

Abdullah Bereket

Children with open neural tube defects (NTDs) are prone to several endocrine problems. Short stature and precocious puberty are the most common endocrine sequelae of NTDs; however, abnormalities in thyroid hormone and prolactin (PRL) have also been reported. Thus, multidisciplinary evaluation and management of NTDs should also include a thorough endocrine evaluation.

Short Stature in Neural Tube Defects

Short stature (SS) is by far the most common endocrine sequela of NTDs. The etiology of SS in patients with NTDs is multifactorial. Underdevelopment of the lower limbs and spinal deformities due to neurological deficits are a major factor in the small size of these patients. Disordered shape and growth of vertebrae in children with myelomeningocele (MMC) results in a shortened sitting height [1]. Presence of a tethered spinal cord contributes to scoliosis and may explain some of the apparent SS. In addition, endocrine dysfunction is frequently encountered in children with NTDs and further compromises growth of the child. In a study investigating height and growth velocities of non-referred children with shunted hydrocephalus, 31% were below the fifth percentile, 34% were short for target height, and 25% were short for siblings [2]. Slow growth velocity was present in 41% of children. SS was present in 40% of patients who had concurrent medical problems, and in 24% with no such problems. Medical problems with increased risk of SS included spina bifida or MMC, Dandy Walker syndrome, brain tumor, cerebral palsy, epilepsy, impaired vision, mental retardation, and pulmonary disorders. Finally, history of premature birth, seen in 31%, led to a higher incidence of SS for target height (54%) than did term birth (28%). Children with NTDs, and especially those with hydrocephalus, are at increased risk for SS, slow growth velocity, or accelerated growth. The presence of pre-cocious puberty, or accelerated or slow growth velocity should prompt an endocrine evaluation.

Adult Stature in Patients with Neural Tube Defects

Although little data exists on adult stature and anthropometric measurements in patients with NTDs, adults with spina bifida are exceedingly small. In one study, the recumbent length for females was 141.9 cm, with an expected length of 167 cm in normal females [3]. Males were 152 cm, with a mean expected length of 182 cm. Recumbent length correlated with weight, level of lesion, arm span and arm length, but most strongly with sitting height (r: 0.87). Arm length of adults with NTDs was also significantly less than the 50th percentile for normal males and females, indicating that etiology of shortness is not solely a function of orthopedic and neurological abnormalities, but also due to endocrine reasons.

Reasons for altered endocrine function in open NTDs are several. Anterior midline defects such as septo-optic dysplasia, cleft palate and transsphenoidal encephalocele have been associated with pituitary hormone deficiencies, the most common being growth hormone (GH) deficiency [4-6]. Increased intracranial pressure of any etiology is known to cause GH neurosecretory dysfunction. Arnold-Chiari deformity, which is associated with abnormalities of the midbrain and ventricles, is frequently observed in these patients. Shunt catheters necessary to control hydrocephalus may impinge on the third ventricle with possible injury to several hypothalamic nuclei.

Growth Hormone Deficiency in Children with Neural Tube Defects

Alterations in the frequency and amplitude of GH secretion in children with open NTDs were first reported in 1989 [7]. In a 12 hour nocturnal sampling study, Rotenstein et al. [7] demonstrated that in seven children with NTDs and an average height 28 cm less than expected for age and sex, the mean nocturnal GH value was diminished (1.88 ng/ml). Only one GH peak above 7 ng/ml was observed in NTD children, whereas four to five peaks are expected in this time frame, indicating subnormal GH secretion in NTD children. Response to GH treatment was good in these patients, as growth rate increased from 1.7 cm/year to 7.9 cm/year after GH treatment for six months. Delayed bone age (1.3-3.0 years) observed in these children further supports the hypothesis that GH deficiency contributes to short stature [7].

Bone age alterations in children with NTDs are dependent upon age and sex. In a study including 98 patients with NTDs, males younger than 9.9 years of age had significant short stature and bone age delay [8]. Males older than 9.9 years had normal bone maturation. Females younger than 9.2 years also had significant short stature and bone age delay, whereas females older than 9.2 years had significantly advanced bone age and short stature most likely related to rapid progression of puberty in females with NTDs.

Insulin-like growth factor 1 (IGF-1) and IGF binding protein-3 (IGFBP-3) are GH dependent peptides and are used as clinical markers of GH secretory status. The prepubertal children with hydrocephalus (including children with spina bifida) had been shown to have lower IGF-1 and IGFBP-3 concentrations than controls, and pubertal children had four times lower basal GH concentrations. There was a correlation between height standard deviation score (SDS) and IGF-1 levels in the total patient population, clearly indicating that reduced GH secretion may contribute to the pattern of slow linear growth and reduced final height observed in these patients [9]. Furthermore, IGF-1 levels significantly increased during growth hormone treatment in children with NTDs [7].

It is extremely difficult to obtain accurate standing height measurements in children with NTDs due to lower extremity paralysis, and the frequent necessity of braces and appliances. Furthermore, orthopedic problems (vertebral deformities, scoliosis and underdevelopment of lower extremities) make recumbent length also less useful in evaluating hormonal problems in linear growth. Arm span is a valuable anthropometric measurement to assess linear growth in children with NTDs. A normal arm span indicates adequate growth of long bones and makes a GH problem less likely. Trollmann et al. [10] in-

vestigated auxo-logical and laboratory parameters to differentiate short stature due to neurological deficits from short stature caused by growth hormone deficiency (GHD) in a group of 38 prepubertal patients with MMC and hydrocephalus aged 3.8-11.0 years. Patients with normal supine length (n=15) had normal arm span. Serum IGF-1 and IGFBP-3 levels were normal (≥ 10th percentile) in 14 of 15 patients. Twenty-three MMC patients had short stature (height SDS <–2), 11 of 23 patients had reduced arm span (SDS <–2), and 12 of 23 had normal arm span. Serum IGF-1 and IGFBP-3 levels were normal in 10 of 12 of short statured patients with normal arm span, but low (<10th percentile) in those patients with reduced arm span. GH secretion was investigated in 7 of 11 short statured MMC patients with reduced arm span and low serum IGF-1 and IGFBP-3 levels. All had a disturbed GH secretion (GHD: n=4; neurosecretory dysfunction: n=3). The researchers concluded that arm span, serum IGF-1 and IGFBP-3 levels are appropriate screening parameters for GHD in patients with MMC. Initiating GH therapy in children with NTDs should be considered not only according to endocrine findings, but also with respect to neurological and orthopedic anomalies.

Arm span measurements in GHD MMC patients are found to be almost identical to height measurements in idiopathic GHD patients both before and during human GH therapy. The physical condition of children with MMC makes reproducible longitudinal height measurements difficult. Routine determinations of arm span measurements for children with MMC will assist in recognizing growth failure as well as monitoring treatment results in a more reliable and reproducible way [11].

In a similar study, Hochhaus et al. [12] evaluated 108 patients with hydrocephalus and/or MMC aged between 3 and 17.8 years. Growth was documented on the basis of arm span measurements. Short arm span was found in 44% of children with hydrocephalus and/or MMC. Mean arm span was –2.0 SDS (–6.4 to +0.8) in 43 girls and –1.4 SDS (–5.6 to +1.3) in 65 boys. Detailed endocrine evaluation was performed in those children with growth deficiency or early sexual maturation. Levels of serum IGF-1 and IGFBP-3 were low in 34% of the patients. GHD and GH neurosecretory dysfunction was detected in 11 and 5% of the patients, respectively. Precocious puberty or early onset of puberty associated with elevated luteinizing hormone (LH) and follicle stimulating hormone (FSH) concentrations after stimulation with luteinizing hormone-releasing hormone was found in 13 of 108 (12.0%) patients (7-9 years of age). Free thyroxine was abnormally low in two of 62 (3.2%) patients. Cortisol was within the normal range in all 62 (100%) tested patients.

Loppanen et al. [13] compared anthropometric measures and the degree of physical maturation in children with shunted hydrocephalus (including children with spina bifida) to those in healthy children. One hundred fourteen patients (62 male) and 73 healthy subjects (38 male) from 5 to 20 years of age were analyzed for growth data and current auxology, stage of puberty, and bone age. They found that boys with hydrocephalus were shorter than control boys during their first eight years of life, and no catch-up growth was observed until puberty. Girls with hydrocephalus were of the same size at birth as the control girls, but their linear growth was retarded during the first years of life, leading to reduced relative height between the ages of five to eight years. The pubertal growth spurt occurred earlier in boys with hydrocephalus (age at midgrowth spurt: 12.1 vs. 13.3 years), and a similar trend was seen in girls (10.0 vs. 10.7 years). The final height was again reduced, especially in boys. Patients with hydrocephalus were more obese than control subjects, girls more often than boys. Relative bone age was retarded in prepubertal and accelerated in pubertal patients.

Systematic endocrine evaluation of 46 prepubertal and 10 pubertal subjects with MMC showed that more subtle abnormalities in pituitary hormone secretion exist in these patients. Three patients presented with precocious puberty. Six subjects had modest elevations of serum thyroid-stimulating hormone (TSH) together with normal free thyroid hormone levels. In three cases, TSH responses to thyrotropin-releasing hormone (TRH) were significantly exaggerated and prolonged, while in two patients TSH responses were delayed. The mean basal plasma FSH level in females with a ventriculo-peritoneal shunt was significantly higher than in controls. In six cases, FSH responses to gonadotropin-releasing hormone (GnRH) were significantly higher than in controls. Both basal and stimulated PRL levels were elevated in patients with shunts; in patients without shunts, basal PRL was normal, but peak PRL levels following TRH stimulation were elevated. These findings reinforce the importance of physical examination, hormonal evaluation and follow-up of pubertal development in patients with MMC [14].

Endocrine abnormalities in children with NTDs are not limited to those children with spina bifida. A retrospective review of 84 patients with frontoethmoidal encephalomeningocele demonstrated 64% of patients had heights below the mean height of normal children. The incidence of hypothy-roidism (1:28), central diabetes insipidus (DI) (1:42) and GHD (1:42) were higher than that in the general population [6].

In summary, short arm span in children with hydrocephalus and/or MMC is frequently accompanied by GHD or neurosecretory GH dysfunction. Early onset of puberty is another frequent finding. Both hormonal disorders may be the consequence of damage to the hypothalamus or the pituitary gland caused by raised intracranial pressure. Short-arm span and slow growth are the key points in diagnosing GHD, however, these can be normal in children with GHD and precocious puberty. The presence of inappropriate advancement of bone will alert the clinician in these rare cases.

Response to Growth Hormone Treatment

Children with MMC and SS respond to treatment with recombinant human growth hormone (rhGH) with an acceleration in growth. However, controlled long-term studies investigating the effect of GH treatment on adult height of children with NTDs and SS are scarce. Early, short-term studies have demonstrated increased growth rate from 3.3-8.4 cm/year in height and from 4.8-8.6 cm in arm span in children with MMC and GHD/neurosecretory dysfunction [15]. Height SDS increased by 1.2 SDS at the end of one year of treatment with GH.

Trollmann et al. [16] reported their experience in 52 patients with NTDs treated with GH in the KIGS database. The three year longitudinal growth was analyzed in 21 patients, all of whom were pre-pubertal at the commencement of and during GH therapy. Height SDS improved from –2.97 (start of GH) to –2.01. Body mass index (BMI) SDS was in the normal range and remained unchanged during GH therapy. No major side effects of GH were recorded.

Rotenstein et al. [17] followed GHD children with MMC to near-adult height. Retrospective evaluation of 20 patients who were consistently measured using recumbent length and who had achieved more than 90% of their adult stature on GH treatment were analyzed. Pretreatment scoliosis was present in 13 patients (<30 degrees); 16 patients had a lesion at the lumbar level, while four were sacral; 19 of 20 had a ventriculoperitoneal shunt. During GH treatment, two girls were successfully treated with leuprolide acetate for precocious puberty, two patients were concurrently treated for hypothyroidism and were euthyroid. SDS for recumbent length at near adult stature increased in comparison to the general adult population and untreated adults with MMC (–2.6 to

−1.4 and +0.6, respectively). Fifteen of 20 patients at near adult stature were above the third percentile of current United States growth charts. These patients were less overweight as their BMI was less than untreated shorter adults with MMC. Scoliosis did not progress. The authors concluded that near adult stature for GH-treated children with MMC is significantly greater than untreated adults with MMC. Relative obesity is decreased with significant improvement of BMI.

These studies demonstrate that GH is helpful in ameliorating short stature in NTDs. Furthermore, GH increased both height and arm span similarly, suggesting that body proportions are not negatively affected by GH treatment. Growth velocity increased in supine length from 3.3 cm/year (−2.1 SDS) to 8.4 cm/year (+2.4 SDS) and in arm span from 4.8 cm/year (−1.3 SDS) to 8.6 cm/year (+3.1 SDS) during GH treatment. Linear correlation between SDS growth velocity supine length and SDS growth velocity arm span during one year of treatment was excellent (r=0.65, p<0.0025) in MMC patients [15].

Growth evaluation in GH-treated and non-treated children before and after tethered spinal cord release (TCR) showed that TCR significantly increased the growth rate compared with matched controls; however, TCR and rhGH in combination provided an increased gain in growth rate and L-SDS over TCR alone [18].

Precocious Puberty in Children with Myelomeningocele

In patients with MMC, central precocious puberty (CPP) is also increased compared to normal children. Furthermore, average age of menarche is early in patients with myelomeningocele (10.3 years), compared to their mothers (11.9 years) and sisters (12.3 years) [19]. Of a group of 79 patients (45 males, 34 females) with MMC (52 with hydrocephalus), three of the hydrocephalic patients were found to have precocious sexual development. Hydrocephalus is known to be associated with precocious puberty (incidence ranging between 6-11%) [12, 20-21].

Sexual precocity in patients with MMC is usually seen in those patients with associated hydrocephalus [21]. Early/precocious puberty (E/PP) in girls with MMC is strongly associated with raised intracranial pressure, particularly during the perinatal period. Proos et al. [22] demonstrated that 20 of 32 girls with MMC had early or precocious puberty. In the girls who had reached the age of 9.2 years,

the incidence of E/PP was at least 52%. Girls with E/PP had a higher incidence of hydrocephalus, were treated with intraventricular shunts more often, and had a significantly higher frequency of raised intracranial pressure during the perinatal period. The girls who developed E/PP were also more severely disabled with respect to motor and urological function and had more shunt revisions. Therefore, particular attention should be paid to children with NTDs associated with hydrocephalus, as even patients with arrested hydrocephalus have been shown to develop precocious puberty.

The pathogenesis of precocious puberty in patients with hydrocephalus is not well understood. It is seen in cases of both congenital and acquired hydrocephalus and is felt to be due to the adverse effect of raised intracranial pressure on the hypothalamus-pituitary region. However, precocious puberty has also been reported in patients with arrested hydrocephalus. It is thought that even small increases in intraventricular pressure may cause dysfunction of neurons that tonically inhibit the onset of puberty.

Treatment of precocious puberty is indicated for the following reasons:

- Accelerated bone maturation in children with precocious puberty causes early closure of epiphyses with consequent short stature. Treatment of precocious puberty slows down skeletal maturation thus preventing loss in adult height.
- Early development of breasts, pubic hair and menstruation in children with precocious puberty causes psychological distress, and menstruation in children with mental retardation may cause problems with hygiene.

Central precocious puberty is effectively treated with GnRH analogues. These agents desensitize pituitary gonadotropin receptors by constant stimulation. GnRH analog treatment leads to complete suppression of the gonadotroph axis, inhibiting the gonadotropin response to GnRH and lowering FSH, LH and sex steroid levels after an initial brief stimulation. As a result, arrest or regression of pubertal findings is observed. Accelerated growth rate and bone maturation return to the normal prepubertal rate, resulting in an improved adult height [23].

Literature is scarce in regard to the final height of patients with NTDs and precocious puberty and the effect of GnRH treatment in these patients. Due to growth disturbances and difficulties in obtaining standardized measurements, MMC patients have been excluded from GnRH analog studies in the past. Reports of small numbers of MMC, hydrocephalus, and CPP patients who were treated with GnRH analogues – triptorelin intramuscularly (n=5) or leuprorelin subcutaneously (n=3) – demonstrated that elevated gonadotropin levels and sex steroid levels decreased during treatment, although complete suppression to prepubertal levels was not attained [24]. Progression of pubertal development and menses stopped in all patients. The tempo of bone age (BA) acceleration (deltaBA:deltaCA) decreased, but no significant improvement in height SDS BA and predicted adult height resulted. No side effects during treatment were observed. CPP in MMC patients needs to be recognized as early as possible in order to enable early diagnosis and treatment. Further prospective studies on the effects of GnRH analogs in MMC patients are necessary.

Reproductive Issues

Few studies have adequately examined the unique issues of women with spina bifida as they enter their reproductive years. Most studies are anecdotal, retrospective case studies that contribute little to our understanding of the physiological effects of the disability on the reproductive system and, conversely, the effects of the reproductive endocrine changes on the woman's disability. A recent review of more than 150 articles on the reproductive issues facing female adolescents and women concluded that the level of evidence is poor and future controlled prospective research studies are needed to examine issues related to pubertal, sexual and gynecologic issues in these patients [25].

In addition, a high incidence (15%) of cryptorchidism was found in males with MMC [21].

Obesity in Neural Tube Defects

Assessment of weight and BMI in children with NTDs demonstrated that weight was no different than expected for age and sex. However, BMI was signifi-

cantly greater than expected. The increased BMI correlated significantly with bone age and Tanner stage, suggesting the advent of puberty may be a factor in the increased BMI [3, 8, 26]. In adults, anthropometric data on 110 MMC subjects demonstrated that in 52 subjects, indices of obesity were validated against body composition analysis of total body fat using body potassium and body water techniques. Most subjects were short and light compared to reference data and became relatively shorter and heavier with age. Overall trunk growth was not affected by the level of lesion, but sitting height was affected by kyphoscoliosis. Arm spans were similar to reference data, but were significantly greater in wheelchair users. Leg length was greatest in those who walked. Body composition data showed excess adiposity in many MMC subjects, with this tendency increasing with age.

Conclusion

Children with NTDs may have several endocrine problems. Short stature, in addition to orthopedic problems, are frequently caused by GHD. Precocious puberty is another common disorder in children with NTDs and hydrocephalus. Together, these factors result in a reduced final height. An increase in relative weight emerges in the preadolescent period, and this phenomenon is accentuated after puberty, leading to an increased prevalence of obesity. GH treatment and GnRH analog treatment seem to ameliorate SS caused by GHD and precocious puberty respectively in children with NTDs. However, further controlled studies will be necessary to determine if therapeutic intervention with respect to growth and pubertal progression will increase final stature with minimal complications. Through various endocrine interventions, puberty that is closer to normal duration, decrease in adiposity and taller adult stature may aid this group on an emotional and functional level as they strive toward self-sufficiency.

References

1. Charney EB, Rosenblum M, Finegold D (1981) Linear growth in a population of children with myelomeningocele. Z Kinderchir 34:415-491
2. Klauschie J, Rose SR (1996) Incidence of short stature in children with hydrocephalus. J Pediatr Endocrinol Metab 9:181-187
3. Rotenstein D, Adams M, Reigel DH (1995) Adult stature and anthropomorphic measurements of patients with myelomeningocele. Eur J Pediatr 154:398-402
4. Hoyt WF, Kaplan SL, Grumbach MM (1970) Septo-optic dysplasia and pituitary dwarfism. Lancet 1:893-894
5. Rudman D, Duns T, Priest JH et al (1978) Prevalence of growth hormone deficiency in children with cleft lip or palate. J Pediatr 93:378-382
6. Wacharasindhu S, Asawutmangkul U, Srivuthana S (2005) Endocrine abnormalities in patients with frontoethmoidal encephalomeningocele. A preliminary study. Horm Res 64:64-67

7. Rotenstein D, Flom LL, Reigel DH (1989) Growth hormone treatment accelerates growth of short children with neural tube defects. J Pediatr 115:417-420

8. Rotenstein D (1990) Endocrine aspects of open neural tube defects. Neuroscience Journal 12:21-23

9. Lopponen T, Saukkonen AL, Serlo W et al (1997) Reduced levels of growth hormone, insulin-like growth factor-I and binding protein-3 in patients with shunted hydrocephalus. Arch Dis Child 77:32-37

10. Trollmann R, Strehl E, Wenzel D, Dorr HG (1998) Arm span, serum IGF-1 and IGFBP-3 levels as screening parameters for the diagnosis of growth hormone deficiency in patients with myelomeningocele-preliminary data. Eur J Pediatr 157:451-455

11. Satin-Smith MS, Katz LL, Thornton P et al (1996) Arm span as measurement of response to growth hormone (GH) treatment in a group of children with meningomyelocele and GH deficiency. J Clin Endocrinol Metab 81:1654-1656

12. Hochhaus F, Butenandt O, Schwarz HP, Ring-Mrozik E (1997) Auxological and endocrinological evaluation of children with hydrocephalus and/or meningomyelocele. Eur J Pediatr 156:597-601

13. Lopponen T, Saukkonen AL, Serlo W et al (1995) Slow prepubertal linear growth but early pubertal growth spurt in patients with shunted hydrocephalus. Pediatrics 95:917-923

14. Perrone L, Del Gaizo D, D'Angelo E et al (1994) Endocrine studies in children with myelomeningocele. J Pediatr Endocrinol 7:219-23

15. Hochhaus F, Butenandt O, Ring-Mrozik E (1999) One-year treatment with recombinant human growth hormone of children with meningomyelocele and growth hormone deficiency: a comparison of supine length and arm span. J Pediatr Endocrinol Metab 12:153-159

16. Trollmann R, Bakker B, Lundberg M, Doerr HG (2006) Growth in pre-pubertal children with myelomeningocele (MMC) on growth hormone (GH): the KIGS experience. Pediatr Rehabil 9:144-148

17. Rotenstein D, Bass AN (2004) Treatment to near adult stature of patients with myelomeningocele with recombinant human growth hormone. J Pediatr Endocrinol Metab. 17:1195-1200

18. Rotenstein D, Reigel DH, Lucke JF (1996) Growth of growth hormone-treated and nontreated children before and after tethered spinal cord release. Pediatr Neurosurg 24:237-241

19. Furman L, Mortimer JC (1994) Menarche and menstrual function in patients with myelomeningocele. Dev Medicine and Child Neurol 36:910-917

20. De Luca F, Muritano M, Rizzo G et al (1985) True precocious puberty: a long term complication in children with shunted non-tumoral hydrocephalus. Helvetica Paediatrica Acta 40:467-472

21. Meyer S, Landau H (1984) Precocious puberty in myelomeningocele patients. J Pediatr Orthop 4:28-31

22. Proos LA, Dahl M, Ahlsten G et al (1996) Increased perinatal intracranial pressure and prediction of early puberty in girls with myelomeningocele. Arch Dis Child 75:42-45

23. Kaplan S, Grumbach M (1990) Pathophysiology and treatment of sexual precocity. J Clin Endocrinol Metab 71:785-789

24. Trollmann R, Strehl E, Darr HG (1998) Precocious puberty in children with myelomeningocele: treatment with gonadotropin-releasing hormone analogues. Dev Med Child Neurol 40:38-43

25. Jackson AB, Sipski ML (2005) Reproductive issues for women with spina bifida. J Spinal Cord Med 28:81-91

26. Roberts D, Shepherd RW, Shepherd K (1991) Anthropometry and obesity in myelomeningocele. J Paediatr Child Health 27:83-90

Section VIII
OCCULT SPINAL DYSRAPHYSM

CHAPTER 35
Anterior and Lateral Meningoceles

James L. Frazier, George I. Jallo

Introduction

Spinal meningoceles are protrusions or expansions of one or more layers of the thecal sac through a canal or foramen of the spinal column in which there is a defect. They are frequently found in a posterior location with the dysraphic vertebrae over the thoracolumbar region. Spinal meningoceles are most commonly observed at birth and constitute approximately 10% of all patients with spina bifida [1, 2]. Although non-dysraphic anterior, lateral, and anterolateral meningoceles in the cervical, thoracic, and lumbar spine are very rare and frequently characterized by the absence of a congenital defect of the vertebrae, they are usually associated with neurofibromatosis 1 (NF-1) or Marfan's syndrome [1-8]. However, anterior lumbosacral meningoceles are a rare form of spinal dysraphism because of a bony defect. Their embryologic origin remains unclear, although there are several hypotheses [2]. Thoracic and/or lumbosacral spinal levels are the most common, with cervical localization being very rare [5-7, 9-11].

Clinical Presentation

Anterior and lateral spinal meningoceles occur as a manifestation of generalized mesenchymal dysplasia such as NF-1 or Marfan syndrome and rarely as an isolated defect [1, 8, 12, 13]. In addition, these lesions have been linked to syndromes such as Currarino's triad and lateral meningocele syndrome. Unlike posterior spinal meningoceles that are associated with dysraphic vertebrae and frequent skin manifestations allowing for prenatal diagnosis or earlier detection after birth, anterior and lateral meningoceles are non-dysraphic and usually demonstrate no dermatologic manifestations unless associated with NF-1 [1, 14]. Therefore, these meningoceles tend to have an initial presentation along a spectrum ranging from infancy to adulthood. The symptomatology is usually caused by mass effect on the surrounding anatomical structures in the vicinity, prompting radiologic studies that lead to diagnosis.

Anterior and lateral meningoceles in the cervical region are rare, and clinical presentation is dictated by the nerve roots involved [1, 5, 7, 9, 10]. Symptoms can include neck pain, radicular pain, hypoesthesia, and/or weakness. Thoracic meningoceles are often asymptomatic or produce radicular intercostal pain, but can have clinical manifestations that are usually associated with their size and surrounding anatomical distortion [2, 15]. These may include back pain, paraparesis from spinal cord compression, or shortness of breath, coughing, and palpitation by compression of the lung and mediastinal structures [2]. Progressive hydrothorax caused by rupture of thoracic meningoceles has been documented in the literature [2, 16]. Otherwise, asymptomatic patients in the setting of small meningoceles may have an incidental diagnosis on a routine chest radiograph. Most thoracic meningoceles have been reported to be either lateral or anterolateral, but a true anterior thoracic meningocele has been reported, in which the lesion herniated into the thoracic cavity through a vertebral bone defect [2].

Similarly, anterior and lateral meningoceles in the lumbosacral spine also have clinical presentations associated with their size and mass effect upon surrounding structures but may be found incidentally. Anterior sacral meningoceles may be detected as early as infancy because of intractable constipation that eventually leads to radiographic studies [17]. If detected in the neonatal period, this lesion is usually associated with the caudal regression syndrome, known as Currarino syndrome, and is associated with an imperforate anus [14, 18-20]. Infants with chronic constipation may need a rectal biopsy to exclude Hirschsprung's disease. Otherwise, anterior sacral meningoceles more commonly present in adolescents and adults [14, 18, 21, 22]. They are often found incidentally on radiographic studies or as a smooth mass on rectal or pelvic examination [14, 23]. Chronic constipation is a common manifestation and some patients may present with back pain [24]. Women may experience difficulty with intercourse secondary to mass effect upon anatomical structures in the pelvic region [18, 21]. Also, headaches may develop secondary to intracranial hypotension that results from accumulation of cerebrospinal fluid within the meningocele.

Currarino's Triad

Currarino's triad is a rare hereditary condition comprised of an anorectal malformation (anal stenosis or agenesis), sacral bony defect, and a presacral mass, such as an anterior meningocele, teratoma, dermoid cyst, lipoma, hamartoma, or enteric cyst [19, 25-29]. An anterior meningocele is found in approximately 60% of patients with this syndrome. The triad was first described by Kennedy in the case of a neonate in 1926 [30]. In 1981, Currarino et al. [31] recognized these disorders as a syndrome of developmentally related defects predicated upon a common mechanism occurring during embryogenesis. The three anomalies characterizing the syndrome have been proposed to be caused by a common developmental defect of the notochord in the early phases of embryogenesis [29]. A more recent postulation considers the anomalies to arise through a failure of dorsoventral separation of the caudal eminence from the hindgut endoderm during late gastrulation [26].

This syndrome is an autosomal dominant disorder with incomplete penetrance and variable expressivity. A familial pattern of transmission in 50% of cases has been reported, and has been shown to be genetically close to the holoprosencephaly locus on chromosome 7q [31-35]. The incomplete form, in which one or two features may be absent, is usually observed, but the very rare complete form may be manifested [31, 34, 36, 37]. The incidence of this triad is unknown, and fewer than 250 cases have been reported [29, 38]. The age at presentation ranges from the neonatal period up into adulthood.

Furthermore, Currarino's triad is frequently associated with other disorders, such as duplication of the urogenital tract, tethered cord, and fistulae such as those between the spinal cord and colon or anterior meningocele, which may lead to meningitis [37-41]. Genitourinary irregularities are the most consistent associated anomalies [19, 34, 36]. Tethered cord has been reported in 18% of cases [39]. The symptomatology of a tethered cord associated with Currarino's triad include abnormal gait, bladder dys-

function, sensory deficit in the lower extremities, and/or pain in the back, legs, or feet.

Constipation is observed in the majority of cases after birth and diagnosed in more than 95% of patients with the syndrome. This incidence of constipation occurs in the presence or absence of a tethered cord. A presacral mass and tethered cord have been suggested as potential causes of constipation in this triad, but resection of the presacral mass has not been reported to provide patients any relief, and constipation is present in all cases without a tethered cord [31, 37-39]. Therefore, the true etiology of constipation in this rare hereditary condition remains unknown. Other clinical manifestations include recurrent urinary tract infections, perianal sepsis, and lower back pain, which can occur at various stages in life [19, 42].

Given the rarity of this syndrome, optimizing the diagnosis is of paramount importance [29]. Infants with intractable constipation should have a rectal biopsy to exclude Hirschsprung's disease. Otherwise, a rectal examination should be performed in which the stenosis may be found distally and a presacral mass palpable. A lumbosacral x-ray and/or computed tomography (CT) should be performed for the detection of the anterior sacral bony defect. Since persistent constipation is a common occurrence, magnetic resonance imaging (MRI) or CT myelography should be conducted to detect the presence of anosacral and spinal cord anomalies. The potential presence of vesicoureteric reflux in this syndrome should be sought with a thorough investigation of the genitourinary system. Vesicoureteric reflux in this triad has a familial occurrence, particularly in affected girls. Urodynamics is recommended to investigate the possibility of a neuropathic bladder. A combined pediatric and neurosurgical assessment should be conducted in all cases along with family screening.

Lateral Meningocele Syndrome

Lateral meningoceles are protrusions of the arachnoid and dura mater through inter- or intravertebral foramina. Multiple lateral meningoceles in the absence of neurofibromatosis and Marfan's syndrome are characteristic of the lateral meningocele syndrome (LMS). LMS was first described by Lehman et al. [43] in 1977 in a 14-year-old girl with lateral meningoceles, distinctive craniofacial features, and other skeletal findings. Nine more cases have been reported since Lehman's original description [4, 44, 45]. An autosomal dominant inheritance pattern has been suggested but the underlying biochemical and molecular defect has yet to be elucidated [3, 4, 45].

A characteristic craniofacial phenotype has been consistently reported. These findings include hypertelorism, downslanting palpebral fissures, ptosis, low-set, posteriorly rotated ears, abnormal palate, micrognathia, and malar hypoplasia [3, 4, 43, 45].

In addition, an underlying connective tissue dysplasia has been suggested through the findings of joint hypermobility, scoliosis, kyphosis, umbilical/inguinal hernias, loose skin, Wormian bones, and pectus deformities [3]. Short stature, cryptorchidism, a short umbilical cord, keloid formation, hypotonia, developmental delay, and conductive hearing loss have also been reported in some patients [3, 4, 43].

Marfan's Syndrome

Marfan's syndrome is an autosomal dominant inherited, systemic disorder of connective tissue that affects many organs. Its prevalence is one in 5,000-10,000 people [46]. Biochemical and molecular studies have shown that affected patients have mutations in the gene for fibrillin, a major component of microfilaments [47]. A combination of major and minor clinical manifestations in different organ systems are utilized as diagnostic criteria. Minor criteria include a high arched palate, scoliosis, joint hypermobility and pectus deformity, while major criteria include a positive family history, ectopia lentis, four of eight skeletal manifestations, aortic dilatation/dissection, and dural ectasia [48, 49].

Dural ectasia has been reported to occur in 63-92% of patients with Marfan's syndrome, predominantly in the lumbosacral spine [50, 51]. It is defined as an enlargement of the neural canal along the spine and can present as thinning of the cortex of the pedicles and lamina of the vertebrae and widening of the neural foramina or as an anterior meningocele. It has been postulated that cerebrospinal fluid pulsations in these patients progressively dilate the dural sac, since the elastin composition of the dura mater is altered [50, 52-54]. Dural sac bulging can lead to vertebral body erosion, or scalloping, and protrusion through the neural foramina [50]. In one prospective study of patients with Marfan's syndrome, lumbosacral spine MRI was performed in 83 patients, of which 12 were younger than 18 years old; dural ectasia was identified in 76 patients (92%) and none in the control group, and eleven of the 12 pediatric patients had dural ectasia [50]. Severe dural ectasia may result in anterior sacral meningoceles in patients with Marfan's syndrome [8, 55-60].

As mentioned previously, anterior meningoceles may be discovered incidentally by imaging for other reasons or with pelvic or rectal examinations, but patients may present with back pain, constipation, and/or urinary dysfunction. This is also the case for Marfan's syndrome, in which the reported prevalence of these meningoceles in documented cases is 28.6% [8, 52, 57, 58, 60-62].

Neurofibromatosis Type 1

NF-1 is an autosomal dominant disorder in which affected individuals display café au lait spots, iris Lisch nodules, freckling in the axilla and groin, and peripheral nerve sheath tumors. In addition, spinal deformity is the most common musculoskeletal complication [63-66]. Although rare in NF-1, lateral and anterior meningoceles can occur at any level of the spine, and it has been postulated that they may occur secondary to trauma, dural ectasia, congenital herniation of the subarachnoid space, elongation of the nerve root sleeve, or cystic degeneration of neurofibroma [67]. Microscopic studies of the wall of meningoceles in NF-1 have been shown to be similar to those of subcutaneous neurofibromas, in which the cystic wall was composed of wavy shaped, mononuclear cells with collagen bundles and subsets of cells were strongly positive for S-100 protein [67, 68]. Thus, it has been proposed that a subset of meningoceles in NF-1 have a tumoral nature as opposed to simple herniation of the meninges [67].

Lateral meningoceles are very rare and associated with NF-1 in up to 85% of cases [69]. They are usually found in the thoracic spine but may also occur in the lumbar region. Bilateral involvement and multiplicity may also be revealed with radiographic studies [19, 20]. Lateral meningoceles are thought to be more frequent in the thoracic region, in which 75% are associated with NF-1, because of poorer development of the paravertebral muscles and a higher pressure differential between the negative thoracic pressure and cerebrospinal fluid (CSF) pressure [70, 71]. Approximately 50% are discovered incidentally on routine chest X-rays [72, 73]. Diffuse back pain may be a clinical manifestation, in addition to dyspnea, cough, and dysphagia as a consequence of pulmonary and mediastinal compression depending upon the size of the thoracic meningocele [11, 15, 72, 73]. Paraparesis can occur from spinal cord involvement. Furthermore, lateral thoracic meningoceles in NF-1 patients have been reported to present as a posterior mediastinal mass associated with kyphoscoliosis. The kyphoscoliosis in NF-1 is notable for the predominance of the kyphotic component [65].

Anterolateral localization of meningoceles is very rare in the cervical spine and usually associat-

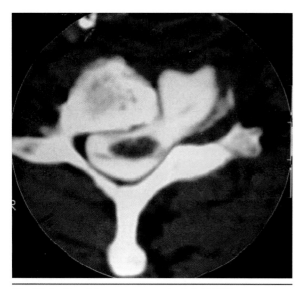

Fig. 35.1. Possible neuroma at the left C6-7 foramen seen on computed tomography myelography. Reproduced from [1]

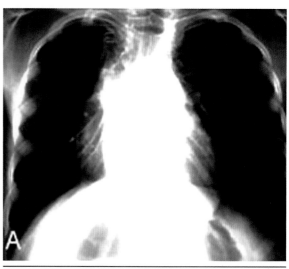

Fig. 35.2. Conventional radiograph of a patient with an anterior thoracic meningocele shows a round homogenous mass in the upper mediastinum. Reproduced from [2], with permission from © American Society of Neuroradiology

Imaging

ed with NF-1 when present [1] (Fig. 35.1). Symptomatology is contingent upon the location, size, and degree of mass effect on nerve roots in the vicinity and possibly the spinal cord itself.

Radiographic studies are pivotal in the diagnostic workup of anterior and lateral spinal meningoceles. Asymptomatic patients harboring these meningoceles usually have incidental findings on imaging that has been obtained for various other clinical reasons. For example, in the case of anterior sacral meningoceles, radiographic studies may be obtained subsequent to the finding of a palpable mass on rectal or pelvic examinations, or a routine plain chest X-ray demonstrating an anterior, anterolateral, or lateral thoracic meningocele.

X-rays, including plain X-rays and myelography, were imaging modalities utilized exclusively in the past for demonstrating associated bony anomalies [74]. Anterior-posterior (AP) and lateral plain X-rays of the cervical, thoracic, and lumbar spine demonstrate widening of intervertebral foramina at the respective levels where anterolateral or lateral meningoceles are present. AP and lateral plain X-rays of the pelvis will demonstrate the presence of a sacral bone defect or absence of a sacral segment(s) in patients with anterior sacral meningoceles. An anterior thoracic meningocele may appear as a round homogenous mass in the mediastinum along with multiple segmental anomalies and widening of the spinal canal (Fig. 35.2). Also, in the past myelography was the most effective technique for confirming the diagnosis of anterior and lateral spinal meningoceles. This radiographic study was useful in the evaluation of morphology and communication with the spinal subarachnoid space.

CT of the spine provides good visualization of the surrounding bony anatomy and its relationship to the lesion. The meningoceles are usually hypodense on CT with Hansfield units similar to that of cerebrospinal fluid. Similar to plain X-rays, CT demonstrates enlargement of intervertebral foramina when lateral meningoceles are present. In the case of anterior spinal meningoceles, this imaging modality reveals, in addition to the hypodense lesion, the sacral bony defect and distortion of surrounding anatomical structures, if present. CT myelography demonstrates a communication between the spinal meningocele and subarachnoid space with filling of the lesion with contrast after it has been injected intrathecally. Myelography is the test of choice to confirm the presence of a spinal meningocele if a contraindication to MRI is present.

MRI is the radiographic study of choice for the diagnosis and operative planning for anterior and lateral spinal meningoceles because it is non-invasive, has multiplanar imaging capability, and has high sensitivity in detecting small associated lesions. Any neurologic signs and symptoms, such as motor weakness, sensory changes, abnormal gait, neck or back pain, bowel/bladder dysfunction, and/or radiculopathy, should be investigated with a spine MRI, with inclusion of the brain in those patients with demonstrable neuroanatomic anomalies. If a mass is palpated with either routine pelvic or rectal examinations, a pelvic and lumbosacral MRI should be performed, if no contraindications are present; otherwise, CT would be the study of choice.

MRI findings vary based upon location and size. T1-weighted images reveal a hypointense lesion(s) while T2-weighted images demonstrate a hyperintense lesion(s). For lateral meningoceles, widening of the intervertebral foramina is demonstrated along with anatomical detail of the relationship of the lesion with the respective exiting nerve root and the spinal cord. In the case of lateral thoracic spinal meningoceles, MRI's provision of sensitive anatomic detail is important in analyzing the relationship to mediastinal structures. If a palpable mass on pelvic and/or rectal examination is confirmed to be an anterior sacral meningocele on MRI, the degree of anatomical distortion, if present, can be assessed, in addition to proximity to vital structures (Figs. 35.3, 35.4).

Furthermore, a lumbosacral spine MRI may reveal a tethered cord in association with an anterior sacral meningocele. Axial T2 imaging is important in the diagnosis of tethered cord, because roots of the cauda equina are normally layered posteriorly in the thecal sac, which can mimic a tethered cord if only sagittal MR imaging is obtained [75].

In patients with neurofibromatosis, detailed radiological studies, such as MRI, are necessary because the spinal meningocele may be associated with a neuroma in the sac [1]. The revelation of a neuroma in the meningocele may change the operative management to address both lesions.

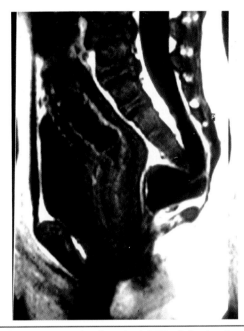

Fig. 35.4. T1-weighted sagittal MRI of the lumbosacral spine demonstrating another anterior sacral meningocele

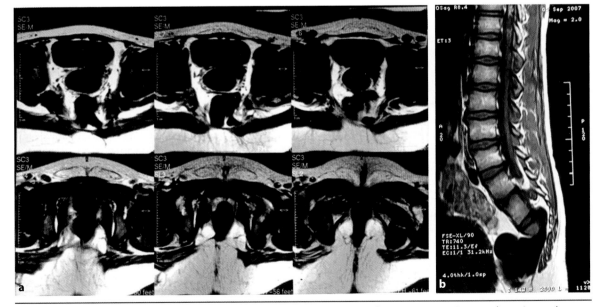

Fig. 35.3 a, b. T1-weighted **a** axial and **b** sagittal MRI of the sacral spine showing an anterior sacral meningocele

Treatment

The prescribed course of treatment for anterior and lateral meningoceles of the spine is contingent upon the clinical scenario and imaging findings for each particular case. Conservative management is usually advised for asymptomatic patients. For patients in which surgery is indicated, the operative approach must be carefully considered and the decision made on the basis of the specific surgical goals for each individual case.

Once radiographic studies have confirmed a cervical anterolateral or lateral meningocele, clinical findings should dictate the next step in the patient's treatment. Symptomatic patients, such as those experiencing any sensory and/or motor abnormalities, should undergo surgical management of the lesion(s). In addition to the presence of a progressive neurologic deficit, rapid increase in the size of the meningocele on serial imaging serves as an indication for surgical resection. A diagnostic puncture of the cyst is not advised, since fatal meningitis may result. For anterolateral cervical meningoceles, an anterior approach should be considered, since the neck of the meningocele may not be able to be repaired by a posterior approach [1].

For isolated lateral meningoceles, the patient should be placed in the prone position with the head held fixed in the Mayfield skull clamp. A preoperative lateral cervical plain x-ray may be taken to minimize the skin incision to the cervical levels of interest. Once the paraspinal muscles have been dissected away from the spine, an intraoperative x-ray should be obtained for confirmation of the appropriate level(s) of interest.

Hemilaminectomy(ies) should be performed to excise the lesion and repair the neck of the meningocele with primary closure of the dura. Fibrin glue should be utilized to reinforce the dural closure, which is the case for subsequent procedures described. In patients with NF-1, a neuroma may be associated with the meningocele and should also be excised. Potential complications include infection, such as that of the wound, meningitis, abscess, CSF leak, and/or nerve root injury leading to weakness and/or sensory disturbance.

Patients with anterior, anterolateral, or lateral thoracic meningoceles have clinical manifestations related to their size and relationship with surrounding structures. Surgical resection is indicated in the presence of progressive neurologic deficit, progressive increase in the size of the meningocele, or respiratory distress [2, 16, 65]. A laminectomy with intradural repair of the meningocele is the most common approach for small and medium-sized lesions. For this posterior approach, the patient is placed in the prone position. A preoperative thoracic lateral plain x-ray is obtained to determine the level of the lesion. After the paraspinal muscles have been dissected away from the spinous processes and lamina, an intraoperative x-ray should be obtained to assess for the correct level(s). Once the appropriate level(s) is confirmed, a laminectomy should be performed with avoidance of injury to the spinal cord. The lesion is identified and excised, and the dura is repaired in a primary fashion. For larger thoracic meningoceles, a transthoracic approach is indicated because it offers a larger operative field while decreasing the chance of injury to the spinal cord [2, 66, 76, 77]. Alternatively, a posterolateral extradural approach can be utilized for moderate to large lateral thoracic meningoceles [73].

The lateral extracavitary approach allows exposure of both the posterior and lateral corridors of the spinal canal. The patient is placed in the prone position, and a preoperative lateral thoracic plain x-ray, or fluoroscopic image, is usually taken for assistance in marking the midline back incision. After the muscle layers are divided, the medial 6-12 cm of one to three ribs are resected laterally with a rib cutter and medially by disarticulation of the costotransverse and costovertebral joints. The parietal pleura is separated from the ribs and spine. The meningocele should be visualized and should be resected at its origin from the thecal sac. A primary dural closure is performed with sutures. Intraoperatively, intrathoracic organ and vascular injury are potential complications. Postoperatively, CSF leak is a major potential complication.

The anterolateral transthoracic approach can be utilized for large anterior and lateral thoracic spinal meningoceles. For meningoceles located in the upper thoracic spine, optimal exposure is achieved by the transpleural transthoracic third rib resection. A thoracic surgeon may be asked to perform this approach for the orthopedic or neurological surgeon. The patient is placed under general anesthesia with standard double lumen endotracheal intubation and then placed in the lateral decubitus position with the appropriate side uppermost. The skin incision is made from the paraspinous area around T1 down the medial border of the scapula to the seventh rib. The third rib is identified after the trapezius and latissimus dorsi are incised and divided. Next, the subscapular space is exposed through retraction of the scapula superiorly. Anterior and posterior subperiosteal dissection of the third rib is conducted, and it is cut using a rib cutter as far anteriorly and posteriorly as feasible. The thoracic cavity is entered after the periosteum, endothoracic fascia, and parietal pleura are incised. The spine and meningocele can be visualized after deflating and retracting the lung. Superior mediastinal structures should be visualized and correctly identified. An incision is made in the parietal pleura overlying the ribs, spinal column, and/or meningocele. The anterior and/or lateral meningocele can then be excised and the dura repaired primarily with sutures. If there is an associated vertebral body anomaly, a vertebrectomy can be performed through this approach, and a distractable cage and plate inserted. Intraoperative electrophysiologic monitoring, through somatosensory (SSEP) and motor evoked potentials (MEP), should be performed if a vertebrectomy is in the operative plan. A chest tube is left in place during closure and can be removed after a satisfactory decrease in drain ouput and no pneumothorax is observed on serial chest x-rays. If a vertebrectomy is necessary, a posterior stabilization procedure is usually required through

pedicle screw and rod fusion. Disadvantages of this procedure include the requirement of mobilization of the scapula and associated muscle dissection, violation of the pleural space and the need for a chest tube, the risk of injury to superior mediastinal structures, such as the sympathetic chain, aorta, esophagus, and trachea, and the inability to perform simultaneous posterior stabilization with this approach. Additional risks include a CSF leak that could potentially lead to a hydrothorax, meningitis, postoperative wound infection, pneumonia, and spinal cord injury during a vertebrectomy. If a CSF leak is observed, the chest tube should be placed on water seal and a lumbar drain inserted.

For large anterior and lateral spinal meningoceles in the mid to lower thoracic spine, the anterolateral open thoracotomy approach can be utilized for resection of the lesion(s) (Figs. 35.5, 35.6). Patient preparation, in-

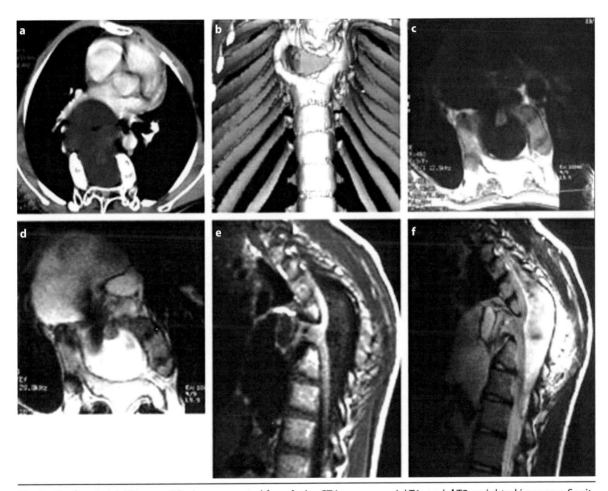

Fig. 35.5 a-f. a Axial CT image, 3D view generated from **b** the CT images , **c** axial T1- and **d** T2-weighted images. **e** Sagittal T1 and **f** T2-weighted images clearly demonstrate multiple segmentation anomalies and a large anterior meningocele herniating through a bone defect at the level of T7-T10 vertebrae. The meningocele is in close proximity to the right main bronchus and the main mediastinal vessels and slightly displaces the heart into the left hemithorax. The spinal cord is displaced toward the neck of the meningocele with a second smaller anterior cyst with fibrous tissue and septa. Reproduced from [2], with permission from © American Society of Neuroradiology

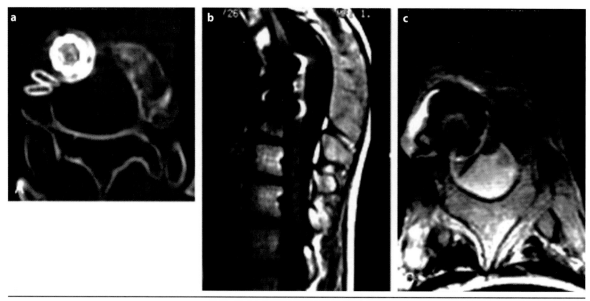

Fig. 35.6 a-c. a In axial CT, **b** sagittal T1-weighted, and **c** axial T2-weighted MR images obtained 2 months after surgery via a right anterolateral thoracotomy, the meningocele cavity is no longer observed and the bone defect is now obstructed by the distraction cage applied. The spinal cord is still displaced anteriorly in the spinal canal. Note the artifacts generated by the surgical implant on MR images. Reproduced from [2], with permission from © American Society of Neuroradiology

tubation, and positioning are similar to that for the transthoracic third rib resection. The correct spinal level of interest and appropriate trajectory is determined by a plain lateral x-ray, or fluoroscopic image, and a curvilinear incision localized over the appropriate level. After the skin incision is made, the muscle layers are cut over the superior aspect of the rib to avoid injury to the neurovascular bundle, and the parietal pleura is divided. Depending upon the exposure needed, a rib may be resected. The ipsilateral lung is collapsed by cessation of ventilation, and the parietal pleura overlying the spinal column and/or meningocele is divided. The meningocele(s) is resected and the dura closed primarily with sutures. A chest tube is placed and managed postoperatively. As mentioned previously, an associated bony anomaly may require a vertebrectomy and subsequent posterior stabilization. Potential complications include injury to the aorta and sympathetic chain, CSF leak, meningitis, postoperative wound infection, persistent pneumothorax, pneumonia, and spinal cord injury if a vertebrectomy is needed.

Additional procedures for anterior and lateral meningoceles of the lower thoracic spine and upper lumbar spine include the transthoracic-transdiaphragmatic approach, which can provide access from the T10 to L3 vertebral bodies, and the transpleural-retroperitoneal approach, which can provide access from the T12 to L2 vertebra. The latter approach is advised when the meningoceles are found at one or two levels, while the former approach should be utilized for the involvement of more than two levels. The crucial aspects of both approaches are retroperitoneal dissection and diaphragmatic dissection. It is important to avoid entrance into the peritoneal cavity, but an opening can be repaired with chromic catgut suture. In the transthoracic-transdiaphragmatic approach, the patient preparation and positioning is similar to that mentioned previously. The skin incision should begin posteriorly near the midline of the back, follow the course of the tenth rib to the costal cartilage, and continue obliquely downward to the abdomen to end at a level between the umbilicus and pubic symphysis. The latissimus dorsi and anterior serratus muscles are incised, subperiosteal dissection and resection of the tenth rib performed, and the pleural cavity is entered. Next, the parietal pleura is reflected at the subcostal diaphragmatic angle with incision of the subjacent insertion fibers of the diaphragm.

After visualization of the peritoneal fat, blunt dissection is utilized to separate the preperitoneal fat, peritoneum, and its contents from the abdominal muscles followed by detachment of the crus from the lumbar vertebrae. The contents of the peritoneum are separated from the psoas and quadratus lumborum muscles after the underlying vertebrae are palpated. The meningocele should be easily visualized and able to be resected. The dura is closed primarily with sutures, the diaphragm reapproximated, and a chest tube left in the chest cavity.

In contrast to the transthoracic-transdiaphragmatic approach, the transpleural-retroperitoneal approach only needs minimal diaphragmatic detachment. An incision in the diaphragm can be made along the ribs and spine parallel to the diaphragmatic insertion. During the retroperitoneal dissection, the psoas muscle is separated from the vertebrae. The meningocele is visualized and extirpated, and the dura is closed. For both approaches, segmental vessels need to be identified, ligated, and divided. Potential complications for both approaches include CSF leak, meningitis, postoperative wound infection, pneumonia, pulmonary injury, respiratory failure requiring re-intubation, segmental vessel bleeding, injury to the inferior vena cava or aorta, injury to the ureter, sympathetic chain injury, genitofemoral nerve injury, nerve root and/or lumbar plexus injury, diaphragmatic hernia, and injury to abdominal contents from entrance into the peritoneal cavity. Morbidity is increased in both approaches, since the thoracic and retroperitoneal regions have to be entered.

Intrathoracic meningoceles in patients with NF-1 may be associated with kyphoscoliosis [65]. In symptomatic patients, laminectomy alone for resection of the meningocele is contraindicated because of the risk for worsening of the kyphosis and potential neurological deterioration. Removal of the posterior tension band leads to unstable postlaminectomy kyphosis. Depending upon where in the thoracic spine the meningocele is located, a transthoracic approach should be used for resection of the lesion and potential vertebrectomy and distractable cage placement for correction of the kyphosis. A posterior pedicle screw fusion with rods is performed for stabilization.

Furthermore, the anterior video-assisted thoracoscopic approach will play a role in the resection of symptomatic lateral and anterior thoracic spinal meningoceles. This procedure is less invasive than an open thoracotomy, with a shorter hospital stay and decreased postoperative pulmonary complications. The patient is placed in the lateral decubitus position with the appropriate side uppermost. A pre-operative lateral thoracic spine image, plain X-ray or fluoroscopic, is obtained for placement of the endoscope portal over the level of the lesion. It is placed between the posterior and midaxillary lines. In addition, a marking on the skin is made in the event an emergent thoracotomy is needed. The endoscope is utilized for visualization within the thoracic cavity to assist in the placement of instrument portals and to avoid injury to the underlying vascular and visceral structures. The parietal pleura is incised and the rib heads of interest removed. The cephalad and caudal pedicles are identified, and bone is removed from the inferior part of the cephalad pedicle. This exposes the spinal canal and dura where the origin of the meningocele is identified. The meningocele can be resected at its origin, and the dura repaired primarily with sutures using endoscopic needle holders and a knot-tying device. Endoscopic clip appliers may be used for dural closure. A chest tube is placed into the thoracic cavity through one of the portal sites. CSF leak is the main potential complication of this procedure, in addition to a persistent air leak.

Small and medium-sized anterior and lateral lumbar spinal meningoceles can be approached and resected through a lumbar laminectomy. Large lesions can be approached through an anterior retroperitoneal procedure. The patient is placed in the lateral decubitus position. Anatomical landmarks can be used to localize the incision depending upon the level of interest, or a plain lateral lumbar x-ray, or fluoroscopic image, can be utilized. An oblique skin incision is made, and the muscle layers divided. The peritoneum is exposed after the transverse fascia is incised, and a plane is formed utilizing blunt dissection. Intra-abdominal contents and retroperitoneal fat are retracted medially to expose the psoas muscle. In the upper lumbar spine, the psoas muscle is dissected off the spine and segmental vessels ligated. The lower lumbar spine requires less psoas muscle dissection, and the common iliac veins, arteries, and branches need to be visualized. The meningocele is identified and resected with primary closure of the dura. Potential complications include CSF leak, meningitis, postoperative wound infection, sympathetic chain injury, ureteral injury, and vascular injury, in which case a general or vascular surgeon should be readily available. The superior hypogastric plexus is at risk of injury in the lower lumbar spine, which can lead to retrograde ejaculation in males.

Various surgical approaches have been applied to anterior sacral meningoceles. A transrectal or transvaginal aspiration of an anterior meningocele is not advised because of the high risk of meningitis, CSF fistula, or death [78]. Preoperative MRI plays a pivotal role in identifying the presence of an associated presacral mass, such as a teratoma or dermoid tumor, and/or abnormalities of the caudal spinal cord, such as tethering of the cord by a thickened filum terminale [79]. This additional radiographic data assists in determining the proper operative technique.

If a tethered cord is present without an associated presacral mass, a sacral laminectomy may be performed to address small and medium anterior sacral meningoceles and any caudal spinal cord anomalies, such as the division of thickened filum terminale (Figs. 35.7, 35.8).

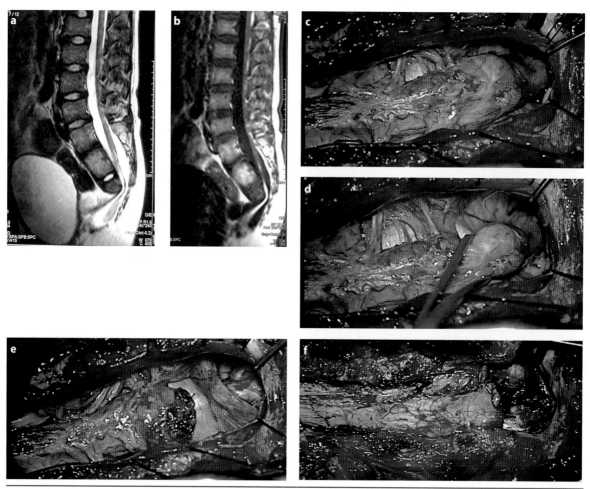

Fig. 35.7 a-f. a Preoperative T2-weighted and **b** T1-weighted MRI of the lumbosacral spine in a patient demonstrating an anterior sacral meningocele with a fatty filum terminale. **c, d** Intra-operative views showing the anterior sacral meningocele prior to resection and **e, f** after surgical extirpation

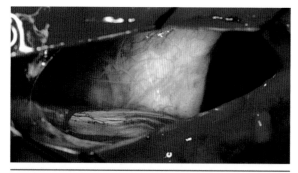

Fig. 35.8. Intra-operative view during resection of an anterior sacral meningocele in a patient

It also allows for preservation of nerve roots. Intra-operative electrophysiologic monitoring should be conducted with SSEPs and MEPs, including the external anal sphincter. The contents of the meningocele and its ostium can be examined with an endoscope for the presence of any neural elements prior to attempting to ligate the ostium. If the anterior meningocele's ostium is less than 10 mm, a simple ligation may be performed. A transdural suture would be the alternative to simple ligation if an abnormal neural structure, confirmed by intra-operative electric stimulation, courses over the ostium. The thecal sac is undermined around the ostium from surrounding tissue followed by approximation ventral to the neural structure [80].

An anterior transabdominal approach may be utilized for large anterior sacral meningoceles associated with a presacral mass. General surgeons and gynecologists usually assist in this procedure. Intra-abdominal and pelvic anatomical structures surrounding the meningocele can be dealt with, particularly if they are adherent. Abnormal neural structures within the thecal sac are not addressed with this approach, and the ostium of the meningocele is not adequately exposed. Thus, caudal spinal cord anomalies demonstrated on preoperative MRI may mean that this approach is not suitable. The risk of meningitis is relatively high with this procedure, and the posterior approach is more frequently utilized, even for large meningoceles, because of its higher cure rate and lower number of complications and mortality [37, 81-85].

The posterior mid-sagittal approach provides excellent exposure to an anterior sacral meningocele [74]. It is normally performed in the pediatric population, and a combined approach with pediatric surgeons is undertaken (Fig. 35.9). This technique is useful in patients with Currarino triad because

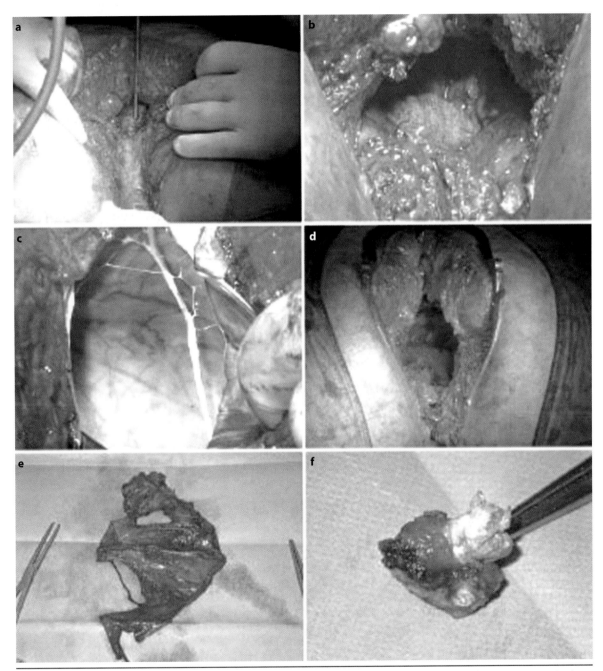

Fig. 35.9 a-f. Intra-operative images of resection of a giant anterior sacral meningocele via the posterior sagittal approach. **a** Coccyx (indicated by the aspirator) reached after splitting of the striated muscle complex; **b** initial view of the meningocele sac in the presacral space after removal of the coccyx and initial dissection from the sacrum; **c** inner appearance of the emptied cyst; **d** large surgical cavity after the excision of the cyst; **e** wall of the meningocele; **f** small associated dermoid tumor. Reproduced from [74]

it allows for the correction of anorectal malformations and extirpation of an associated presacral mass. This technique was first developed in 1982 for the treatment of anorectal anomalies [86, 87]. The perineal region is completely exposed through a median sagittal incision from the sacrum to the anal area. The voluntary striated muscles can be identified and divided without interruption of the fibers with the aid of an electrical stimulator. Sphincter continence can be preserved while reconstruction of the perineal region is performed. A presacral fistula should be excised immediately to prevent the risk of meningitis, and neurosurgical exploration should precede intestinal surgery [29]. The advantage of this approach is that it can be extended to the presacral region and allows easy access to the meningocele without significant risk to neural structures. A disadvantage is the high degree of difficulty in accessing a meningocelic stalk arising high on the sacrum.

Furthermore, an anterior sacral meningocele may be approached by endoscopy if preoperative MRI reveals a stalk 10 mm or less in size, and no neural structural abnormality is present. This form of treatment is less invasive and has an operative mortality close to 0% [12, 88].

In summary, neurosurgical considerations need to be taken into account to formulate a surgical strategy for anterior sacral meningoceles.

Conclusion

Anterior and lateral spinal meningoceles that are found incidentally should be followed expectantly in asymptomatic patients with serial spine MRI scans. If there is progressive enlargement, surgical resection of the meningocele should be strongly considered to preempt the development of clinical sequela. Symptomatic patients should have surgery, in which the technique is determined by the location and size of the meningocele. Although the dura is closed primarily, the additional application of fibrin glue is recommended, given the possibility of a CSF leak.

Postoperative imaging is imperative to determine the degree of cyst reduction. The persistence of cysts early in the postoperative period may occur even in the presence of resolving symptomatology and does not necessarily warrant re-operation. If a persistent cyst is observed on postoperative MRI, then serial imaging over several months is needed to document gradual reduction in the size of the meningocele.

References

1. Gocer A, Tuna M, Gezercan Y et al (1999) Multiple anterolateral cervical meningoceles associated with neurofibromatosis. Neurosurg Rev 22:124-126
2. Oner A, Uzun M, Tokgoz N et al (2004) Isolated true anterior thoracic meningocele. AJNR 25:1828-1830
3. Chen K, Bird L, Barnes P et al (2005) Lateral meningocele syndrome: vertical transmission and expansion of the phenotype. Am J Med Genet 133A:115-121
4. Gripp K, Scott C, Hughes H et al (1997) Lateral meningocele syndrome: Three new patients and review of the literature. Am J Med Genet 70:229-239
5. Kaiser M, De Slegte R, Crezee F et al (1986) Anterior cervical meningocele in neurofibromatosis. AJNR 7:1105
6. Robinson R (1964) Intrathoracic meningocele and neurofibromatosis. Br J Surg 51:432-437
7. So C, Li D (1989) Anterolateral cervical meningocele in association with neurofibromatosis: MR and CT studies. J Comp Assist Tomogr 13:692-695
8. Strand R, Eisenberg H (1971) Anterior sacral meningocele in association with Marfan's syndrome. Radiology 99:653-654
9. Freund B, Timon C (1992) Cervical meningocele presenting as a neck mass in a patient with neurofibromatosis 1. J Laryngol Otol 106:463-464
10. Jaffray D, O'Brien J (1985) A true anterior thoracic meningocele associated with a congenital kyphoscoliosis. J Pediatr Orthop 5:717-719
11. Miles J, Pennybacker J, Sheldon P (1969) Intrathoracic meningocele: Its development and association with neurofibromatosis. J Neurol Neurosurg Psychiat 32:99-110
12. Raftopoulos C, Pierard G, Retif C et al (1992) Endoscopic cure of a giant sacral meningocele associated with Marfan's syndrome: case report. Neurosurgery 30:765-768
13. Voyvodic F, Scroop R, Sanders R (1999) Anterior sacral meningocele as a pelvic complication of Marfan syndrome. Aust NZ J Obstet Gynaecol 39:262-265
14. Ashley W, Wright N (2006) Resection of a giant anterior sacral meningocele via an anterior approach: case report and review of literature. Surgical Neurology 66:89-93
15. Maiuri F, Corriero G, Giampaglia F et al (1986) Lateral thoracic meningocele. Surg Neurol 26:409-412
16. Mizuno J, Nakagawa H, Yamada T et al (2002) Intrathoracic giant meningocele developing hydrothorax: a case report. J Spinal Disord Tech 15:529-532
17. Ilhan H, Tokar B, Atasoy M et al (2000) Diagnostic steps and staged operative approach in Currarino's triad: a case report and review of the literature. Childs Nerv Syst 16:522-524
18. Amornfa J, Taecholarn C, Khaoroptham S (2005) Currarino syndrome: report of two cases and review of the literature. J Med Assoc Thai 88:697-702

19. Gegg C, Vollmer D, Tullous M et al (1999) An unusual case of the complete Currarino triad: Case report, discussion of the literature and the embryogenic implications. Neurosurgery 44:658-662

20. Morimoto K, Kishiguchi T, Ikeda T (2004) Currarino triad as an anterior sacral meningocele. Pediatric Neurosurgery 40:97-98

21. Kontopoulos E, Oyelese Y, Nath C et al (2005) Maternal anterior sacral meningocele in pregnancy. J Matern Fetal Neonatal Med 17:423-425

22. Rigante D, Segni G (2001) Anterior sacral meningocele in a patient with Marfan syndrome. Clin Neuropathol 20:70-72

23. Lynch S, Wang Y, Stracham T et al (2000) Autosomal dominant sacral agenesis: Currarino syndrome. J Med Genet 37:561-566

24. Gardner P, Albright A (2006) "Like mother, like son": hereditary anterior sacral meningocele. Case report and review of the literature. J Neurosurg 104:138-142

25. Brem H, Beaver B, Colombani P et al (1989) Neonatal diagnosis of a presacral mass in the presence of a congenital anal stenosis and partial sacral agenesis. J Pediatr Surg 24:1076-1078

26. Dias M, Azizkhan R (1998) A novel embryogenetic mechanism for Currarino's triad: inadequate dorsoventral separation of the caudal eminence from hindgut endoderm. Pediatr Neurosurgery 28:223-229

27. Dios Seoane J, Amaro S, Fantini M et al (2002) Anterior sacral meningocele with Currarino's syndrome: report of two cases. Neurocirugia (Astur) 13:455-462

28. Gaskill S, Marlin A (1996) The Currarino triad: its importance in pediatric neurosurgery. Pediatr Neurosurgery 25:143-146

29. Samuel M, Hosie G, Holmes K (2000) Currarino triad – Diagnostic dilemma and a combined surgical approach. J Pediatr Surg 35:1790-1794

30. Kennedy R (1926) An unusual rectal polyp; anterior sacral meningocele. Surg Gynecol Obstet 43:803

31. Currarino G, Coln D, Votteler T (1981) Triad of anorectal, sacral and presacral anomalies. AJR 137:395-398

32. Kochling J, Karbasiyan M, Reis A (2001) Spectrum of mutations and genotype-phenotype analysis in Currarino syndrome. Eur J Hum Genet 9:599-605

33. Lynch S, Bond P, Copp A et al (1995) A gene for autosomal dominant sacral agenesis maps to the holoprosencephaly region at 7q36. Nat Genet 11:93-95

34. O'Riordain D, O'Connell P, Kirwan W (1991) Hereditary sacral agenesis with presacral mass and anorectal stenosis: The Currarino triad. Br J Surg 78:536-538

35. Ross A, Ruiz-Perez V, Wang Y et al (1998) A homeobox gene, HLBX9, is the major locus for dominantly inherited sacral agenesis. Nat Genet 20:358-361

36. Kirks D, Merten D, Filston H et al (1984) The Currarino triad: Complex of anorectal malformation, sacral bony abnormality, and presacral mass. Pediatr Radiol 14:220-225

37. Lee S, Chun Y, Jung S et al (1997) Currarino triad: anorectal malformation, sacral bony abnormality, and presacral mass: A review of 11 cases. J Pediatr Surg 32:58-61

38. Kochling J, Pistor G, Marzhauser Brands S et al (1996) The Currarino syndrome: Hereditary transmitted syndrome of anorectal, sacral and presacral anomalies: Case report and review of the literature. J Pediatr Surg 6:114-119

39. Emans P, Aalst J, van Heurn E et al (2006) The Currarino Triad: neurosurgical considerations. Neurosurgery 58:924-929

40. Heij H, Moorman-Voestermans C, Vois A et al (1990) Triad of anorectal stenosis, sacral anomaly and presacral mass: A remedial cause of severe constipation. Br J Surg 77:102-104

41. Yates V, Wilroy R, Whitington G et al (1983) Anterior sacral defects: An autosomal dominantly inherited condition. J Pediatr 102:239-242

42. Kiesemelter W, Nixon N (1967) Imperforate anus: I-Its surgical anatomy. J Pediatr Surg 2:60-84

43. Lehman R, Stears J, Wesenberg R et al (1977) Familial osteosclerosis with abnormalities of the nervous system and meninges. J Pediatr 90:49-54

44. Katz S, Grunebaum M, Strand R (1978) Thoracic and lumbar dural ectasia in a two-year-old boy. Pediatr Radiol 6:238-240

45. Philip N, Andrac L, Moncia A et al (1995) Multiple lateral meningoceles, distinctive facies and skeletal anomalies: a new case of Lehman syndrome. Clin Dysmorphol 4:347-351

46. Pyeritz R (1996) Marfan syndrome and other disorders of fibrillin. In: Emery and Rimoin's principles and practice of medical genetics. D Rimoin, J Connor, R Pyeritz (eds), pp 1027-1065

47. Dietz H, Pyeritz R (1995) Mutations in the human gene for fibrillin-1 (FBN1) in the Marfan syndrome and related disorders. Hum Mol Genet 4:1799-1809

48. Beighton P, De Paepe A, Danks D et al (1986) International Nosology of Heritable Disorders of Connective Tissue, Berlin, 1986. Am J Med Genet 29:581-594

49. De Paepe A, Devereux R, Dietz H et al (1996) Revised diagnostic criteria for the Marfan syndrome. Am J Med Genet 62:417-426

50. Fattori R, Nienaber C, Descovich B et al (1999) Importance of dural ectasia in phenotypic assessment of Marfan's syndrome. Lancet 354:910-913

51. Pyeritz R, Fishman E, Bernhardt B et al (1988) Dural ectasia is a common feature of the Marfan syndrome. Am J Med Genet 43:726-732

52. Raftopoulos C, Delecluse F, Braude P et al (1993) Anterior sacral meningocele and Marfan syndrome: a review. Acta Chir Beig 93:1-7

53. Smith M (1993) Large sacral defect in Marfan syndrome: a case report. J Bone Joint Surg 75:1067-1070

54. Sterm W (1988) Dural ectasia and the Marfan syndrome. J Neurosurg 69:221-227

55. Duncan R, Esses S (1995) Marfan syndrome with back pain secondary to pedicular attenuation. Spine 20:1197-1198

56. Fiandaca M, Ross W, Pearl G et al (1988) Carcinoid tumor in a presacral teratoma associated with an anterior sacral meningocele: case report and review of the literature. Neurosurgery 22:581-589

57. Fishman E, Zinreich S, Kumar A et al (1983) Sacral abnormalities in Marfan syndrome. J Comp Assist Tomogr 7:851-856

58. Nallamshetty L, Ahn N, Ahn U et al (2002) Dural ectasia and back pain: Review of the literature and case report. J Spinal Disorders & Tech 15:326-329

59. Sonier C, Buhe T, Despins P et al (1993) Pseudomeningocele sacre et maladie de Marfan. J Neuroradiol 20:292-296

60. Sonier C, Buhe T, Despins P et al (1993) Sacral pseudomeningocele and Marfan's disease: one case. J Neuroradiol 20:292-296

61. Harkens K, El-Khoury G (1990) Intrasacral meningocele in a patient with Marfan syndrome: case report. Spine 15:610-614

62. Smith H, Davis C (1980) Anterior sacral meningocele: two case reports and discussion of surgical approach. Neurosurgery 7:61-67

63. Allibone D, Illingworth R, Wright T (1960) NF-1 (von Recklinghausen disease) of the vertebral column. Arch Dis Child 35:153-158

64. Calzabara P, Caralion A, Anzola G et al (1988) Segmental neurofibromatosis: a case report and review of the literature. NF-1 J 1:318-322

65. Ebara S, Yuzawa Y, Kinoshita T et al (2003) A neurofibromatosis type 1 patient with severe kyphoscoliosis and intrathoracic meningocele. J Clin Neuroscience 10:268-272

66. Heard G, Holt J, Naylor B (1962) Cervical vertebral deformities in von Recklinghausen disease of the nervous system. A review of necropsy findings. J Bone Joint Surg Br 44:880-885

67. Ogose A, Hirano T, Hasegawa K et al (2002) Tumoral nature of intrathoracic meningocele in neurofibromatosis 1. Neurology 59:1467-1468

68. Nanson E (1957) Thoracic meningocele associated with neurofibromatosis. J Thorac Surg 33:650-662

69. Atlas S (2002) Congenital anomalies of the spine and spinal cord. In: Magnetic resonance imaging of the brain and spine. SW Atlas (ed) Lippincott W&W, Philadelphia, p 1595

70. Atlas S (2002) Central nervous system manifestations of the phakomatoses and other inherited syndromes. In: Magnetic resonance imaging of the brain and spine. SW Atlas (ed) Lippincott W&W, Philadelphia, pp 371-411

71. Reis C, Carneiro E, Fonseca J et al (2005) Epithelioid hemangioendothelioma and multiple thoraco-lumbar lateral meningoceles: two rare pathological entities in a patient with NF-1. Neuroradiology 47:165-169

72. Geerts Y, Marchau M (1992) Intrathoracic meningocele. J Spinal Disord 5:116-121

73. Sonoda Y, Tominaga T, Koshu K et al (1994) Posterolateral extradural approach for lateral thoracic meningocele. Neurol Med Chir (Tokyo) 34:624-627

74. Massimi L, Calisti A, Koutzoglou M et al (2003) Giant anterior sacral meningocele and posterior sagittal approach. Childs Nerv Syst 19:722-728

75. Osborn A (1994) Diagnostic neuroradiology. Mosby, St Louis

76. Erkulurawatra S, Gammal T, Hawkins J et al (1979) Interthoracic meningoceles in NF-1. Arch Neurol 36:557-559

77. Klatte E, Franken E, JA Smith et al (1976) The radiographic spectrum in NF-1. Semin Roentgenol 11:17-33

78. Amacher A, Drake C, McLachlin A (1968) Anterior sacral meningocele. Surg Gynecol Obstet 126:986-994

79. Tani S, Okuda Y, Abe T (2003) Surgical strategy for anterior sacral meningocele. Neurol Med Chir (Tokyo) 43:204-209

80. Dyck P, Wilson C (1980) Anterior sacral meningocele: Case report. J Neurosurg 53:548-552

81. Duthel R, Charret M, Huppert J et al (1988) Anterior sacral meningocele. Report on eleven cases. Neurochirurgie 34:90-96

82. Hino A, Takemoto S, Iwasaki T (1993) Treatment of anterior sacral meningocele - case report. Neurol Med Chir (Tokyo) 33:700-702

83. Simpson B, Glass R, Mann C (1987) Anterior sacral meningocele:magnetic resonance imaging and surgical management. Br J Surg 74:1185

84. Villarejo F, Scavone C, Blasquez M et al (1983) Anterior sacral meningocele: review of the literature. Surg Neurol 19:57-71

85. Wilkins R, Odom G (1978) Anterior and lateral spinal meningoceles. In: Handbook of clinical neurology. P Vinken, G Bruyn (eds) Elsevier North-Holland Biomedical Press, Amsterdam, pp 193-230

86. DeVries P, Pena A (1982) Posterior sagittal anorectoplasty. J Pediatr Surg 17:638-643

87. Pena A (1986) Posterior sagittal approach for the correction of anorectal malformations. Adv Surg 19:69-100

88. Clatterbuck R, Jackman S, Kovoussi L et al (2000) Laparoscopic treatment of an anterior sacral meningocele. J Neurosurg 92:246

CHAPTER 36
Spinal Lipomas

Michel Zerah, Thomas Roujeau, Martin Catala, Alain Pierre-Kahn

Introduction

Congenital lumbosacral lipomas are the most common form of closed neural tube defects. In most cases they are diagnosed prenatally or at birth. They may lead to progressive neurological and urinary deterioration. However, their natural history is poorly understood. Prophylactic surgery has been the gold standard of treatment, but considering the deterioration of prophylactic detethering over time, especially in case of lipoma of the conus, the performance of prophylactic surgery in children has been questioned.

This chapter will discuss the most recent data concerning our knowledge of congenital lipomas of the conus and of the filum. We will try to describe the natural history of the disease compared to the value of early prophylactic surgery by weighing risks of surgery with those of the disease itself, as well as by assessing long-term efficacy of surgery.

Most of the data provided in this chapter come from the authors' experience of 671 consecutive lipomas [1-3] treated between 1984 and 2006 over two periods (1984-1994 retrospectively and 1995-2006 prospectively), regardless of the clinical presentation (Table 36.1).

We will discuss lipomas of the filum (n = 87) and lipomas of the conus (n = 584) separately because they are actually two different lesions.

Table 36.1. Our clinical series

	Filum	Conus	Total
Asymptomatic	60	206	266
	9%*	36%** 31%*	
Symptomatic	27	378*	405
	4%*	64% 56%	
Total	87	584	671
	13%*	100%** 87%*	100%*

* Whole series
** Asymptomatic conus

History of a Controversy

Since the first description by Temoin [4] in 1892, more than 2,500 cases of lipoma have been reported, mainly in the past 50 years. At the end of the nineteenth century, their anatomy was already almost fully described [4-7]. By 1916, their clinical presentation was well known. Risk of progressive neurological deterioration was also widely emphasized and believed to result from compression and/or stretching of the terminal spinal cord and cauda equina [8-10]. In 1918, Brickner [11] operated on the first symptom-free patient. In 1937, Leveuf [12], at the Enfants Malades Hospital in Paris questioned whether early surgery could avoid late deterioration. In 1950, Basset [13] strongly advocated prophylactic surgery. In 1981, Yamada [14] demonstrated that experimental tethering of these structures in cats could lead to neuronal dysfunction at the level of the terminal cord, close to the traction. At present, most of the neurosurgeons [1, 9, 13, 15-123], specifically in North America and Asia are in favor of routine and early removal of these lipomas to decompress and untether the cord. They justify their attitude by the belief that the frequency of spontaneous neurological aggravation becomes more frequent with age, the regression of preoperative deficit is rare and decreases with age, and the surgery is more difficult in children and adults than in the newborn. They also believe that the overall results of this early and prophylactic surgery are good.

This agreement, however, is not as universal as it might appear at first sight, and more and more teams (particularly in Europe) have reconsidered the real benefit of this surgery [45, 46, 112, 123, 124]. The fact that there are only a small number of publications suggesting that surgery should not be performed routinely, or favoring diverse attitudes according to the patient's age does not reflect reality. In fact, more and more surgeons and pediatricians are reluctant to consider routine systematic surgery in asymptomatic patients. Besides the problem of proposing surgery in the absence of deficits, the arguments that they put forward are as follows: The natural risk of the malformation remains unknown, based almost exclusively on symptomatic hospital inpatients. This uncertainty is confirmed by data from the literature, of which there are only two studies, each with a maximum of ten cases, which compare the course of operated and non operated patients, and which draw exactly opposite conclusions. Furthermore, the frequency of healthy asymptomatic carriers of the malformation might not be negligible in old autopsy reports and recent radiological studies. Operative risks and results vary greatly among studies, and postoperative follow-up, when reported, does not exceed an average of 2.5 years. In addition, the pathology reported often covered all the causes of open or occult dysraphism (myelomeningocele, lipoma, diastematomyelia, tethered cord syndrome, neurenteric cyst, etc.), making it difficult to analyze data concerning only lipomas. In addition, the literature never distinguishes between lipomas of the filum and lipomas of the conus, and rarely takes a patient's preoperative clinical status or length of follow-up into account. For all these reasons, the present authors considered it necessary to reappraise the value of routine and preventive surgery.

Embryology [17, 37, 62, 76, 83, 125-148]

Spina bifida with lipoma (SBL) represents a complex morphotype. It associates two single malformative processes: spina bifida and lipoma. The lipoma is made of normal adipocytes, connective tissue and, in 75% of cases, other types of structures coming from the endodermal, mesodermal or ectodermal layers. We want to address two successive questions here in order to establish the origin of such malformations: the embryonic origin of the cells that ultimately differentiate into adipocytes within the lipoma and the basic mechanisms giving rise to such a malformation.

The origin of the adipocytes has been the subject of numerous hypotheses since the nineteenth century (see Catala et al. [134] for a historical review). Most of these hypotheses have been largely anecdotal and are now completely ruled out, particularly the transdifferentiation of adipocytes from meningocytes, endothelial cells or astrocytes. It is now firmly established that lipomas are essentially made up of connective tissues and normal adipocytes. In the body, adipocytes derive from mesoderm in the mediolateral plane. Due to the anatomic relationship between the spinal cord and lipoma, the lipoma can be considered

to be due to an impairment of the normal development of the perineural tube mesoderm; i.e., the mesodermal part that is yielded by dissociation of the somites.

The second question deals with the mechanisms involved in the development of SBL. As the lesion is always located in the dorsal part of the spinal cord, a defect arising during neurulation has been advocated. Lipomas have been interpreted, like dermoid or epidermoid cysts, to result from incarceration of ectodermal tissue into the closing neural groove. Such a hypothesis is unlikely because adipocytes are derived from mesoderm and not from ectoderm. This led Della Rovere [150] to propose an alternative view. He also favored an inclusive mechanism in which the included tissue is mesodermal and not ectodermal. The latter would account for the development of the lipoma. However, as already noted by Stookey [152], it is impossible for the mesodermal anlage to migrate between neurectoderm and surface ectoderm during neurulation. Indeed, at this time, the two epithelia are closely adherent and the interepithelial space is not yet formed. Even if mesodermal anlage were able to migrate between the two epithelia, mesodermal cells, which are not committed to a specific lineage at this stage, would eventually form meninges and cartilage after receiving normal induction from the neural tube. In any case, they would give rise to fatty tissue.

The second hypothesis was put forward by David McLone and Tom Naidich [85]. They proposed that lipoma of the filum arises from a maldevelopment of the so-called tail bud. This structure, which is responsible for secondary neurulation, appears as the posterior neuropore closes, and is considered by these authors to be an undifferentiated mass of multipotent cells. In fact, in the avian embryo it has been demonstrated that the tail bud is made up of different territories with definite developmental potentials, and that the two processes of neurulation proceed concurrently [150]. In conclusion, these two models cannot account for the emergence of SBL and an alternate model is needed. SBL must be considered as a true malformation affecting the dorsal mesoderm, namely the part of the somites that migrates between the neural tube and the surface ectoderm after delamination of these two epithelia.

SBL can be categorized into two groups: those characterized by a normal number of vertebrae and those associated with sacral agenesis. In the first group, which is the most frequent, SBL affects the dorsal moiety of the vertebra, which is the vertebral part produced by the so-called dorsal mesoderm [153]. These cells, which express the *Msx2* gene product [153], differentiate into the dorsal dermis, hypodermis, meninges, and the spinous process of the vertebra. Dorsal mesoderm obeys different molecular regulation from the rest of the somite, making it possible to distinguish two domains in the developing vertebra: dorsal and ventrolateral [154]. The dorsal domain, contrary to the ventral one, is induced by the dorsal neural tube. Its development is inhibited by the ventral neural tube by extranotochord grafting, or by ectopic expression of the HNF3β superfamily [155]. These experiments show that the dorsal part of the vertebra is regulated by different factors from the ventral one.

Catala [151] proposed to interpret SBL without sacral agenesis as a defect of the normal differentiation program of the dorsal mesoderm. The normal structures yielded by this tissue are not formed, explaining spina bifida and the dorsal meningeal defect. Furthermore, the cells forming dorsal mesoderm will receive information that promotes adipocyte differentiation. The source of this information could be the surface ectoderm. According to histologic data gained by pathological examination of lipomas, three subgroups of malformation can be distinguished. First, those in which the lipoma is made up of adipocytes and connective tissue only. In this case, SBL is due to an impairment of the interactions between dorsal mesoderm and neurectoderm. Two basic mechanisms are likely to account for this maldevelopment: either a defect of induction from the neural tube or an impairment of the response from the dorsal mesoderm. In the second group, a dermoid or epidermoid cyst is present within the lipoma. This is due to an impairment of formation of the interepithelial space leading to an adhesion between the surface ectoderm and the neural tube. This promotes development of the cyst. Furthermore, the interactions between dorsal mesoderm and neural tube are defective, leading to formation of the lipoma. The third group is characterized by cells that are not normally derived from the dorsal mesoderm (e.g., renal glomeruli, muscles, cerebellum, endometrium, thyroid). Teratomatous cells could be present within the dorsal mesoderm. Subsequently, this could lead to the formation of the lipoma. Thereafter, these cells could self-differentiate into structures that are not normally found in this region.

In contrast, SBL with sacral agenesis cannot be explained by the sole mechanism of abnormal development of the dorsal mesoderm. This phenotype belongs to the so-called caudal agenesis syndrome. It can be explained by an impairment of the normal movement involved in the formation of the embryonic axial body. It has been recently demonstrated that these movements are continuous during both primary and secondary neurulation. Two different elementary movements are taking place. The first one is a rostrocaudal elongation involving the axial organs (i.e., notochord and neural tube). The second is a movement of lateral divergence. These movements allow the formation of mesodermal derivates. If impaired, they involve both the paraxial mesoderm (somites that yield the vertebrae) and the lateral mesoderm located in the caudal digestive tract. Therefore, the frequent co-occurrence of perineal malformations in this type of SBL can be explained perfectly as in the so-called Currarino Syndrome related to a mutation of the *HLXB9* gene [162].

General Considerations

Sex Ratio

Among the 2,523 cases [2, 3] reported in the literature, there is a significant female predominance (female to male ratio of 1.2:1, p < 0.0001). This contrasts with the equal sex ratio generally found in myelomeningocele (MMC) and the male predominance in isolated osseous spina bifida occulta.

Incidence

The real incidence of sacral lipoma is uncertain. In the literature, the only reported data concerns the incidence of this malformation versus myelomeningocele or other occult dysraphism, which only reflects personal recruitment.

The present authors tried to approach the epidemiology of this malformation in two French regional registers [2, 3] containing data from maternity hospitals. Considering lipomas of the filum and the conus together, and taking into account the universally admitted 10% rate of lipomas covered with normal skin and hence not diagnosed at birth, a minimal incidence of 4-8 per 100,000 was found. This incidence (which means a maximum of 70 new cases per year in France) is clearly under-evaluated, because it does not take into account the unknown incidence of neonates who not only have normal skin on their lower back, but who are also neurologically normal.

Routine autopsy of patients not suspected of spinal disease has provided an incidence of incidentally found lipomas ranging from 0 to 6% with an average of 0.003%. Interestingly, as in our series and in all the clinical studies, lipomas of the conus were ten times more frequent than those of the filum.

Recent magnetic resonance (MR) studies of adults investigated for suspected disk diseases or lumbar stenosis have revealed an incidence for lipomas of 1.5-5%. All of these, however, were of small size and restricted to the filum.

There is therefore a striking discrepancy between the relatively high incidence of lipomas found at autopsy or in radiological studies, and the very low incidence in epidemiologic registers or in our neurosurgical series. This discrepancy could be explained by the existence of a fairly large number of asymptomatic patients.

Familial Data [124, 156-162]

A family study was performed on 71 patients from our retrospective study [2, 3] and has been systematically done in the prospective study in cases of associated malformations (including sacral agenesis). In the retrospective study, in 29 of the 71 cases, lipoma was associated with other anomalies: sacral agenesis in seven, sacral and urogenital abnormalities in ten, and other malformations without sacral agenesis in 12 patients. Plain radiography of the spine was done in all parents. Spina bifida occulta was found in 67% of the relatives. This frequency is higher than that observed in the normal population, estimated to range from 25 to 30%.

In the prospective study, in cases of sacral agenesis in the child, a sacral agenesis in one of the parents was found in 40% of the cases. In the Currarino syndrome, an autosomal dominant mode has been proposed. In our prospective series 47% of the children presented with a familial history of malformation of the lower lumbosacral or perineal region. The most frequent anomalies were sacral agenesia and a mutation of the *HLXB9* gene, found in 50% of the cases [162].

Pathology [5, 6, 29, 76, 134, 140, 163-176]

Lipomas typically consist of normal mature adipocytes separated into clusters by numerous collagen bands. In our series, 77% included, in addition, a wide variety of ectodermal, endodermal or mesodermal tissues (Fig. 36.1). The most common were of mesodermal origin: nerves (63%), striated muscular fibers (37%), Vater Pacini and Krause corpuscles (21%). These formations were always intralipomatous surrounded by dense fibrosis. Tissues of neurectodermal origin were also common, such

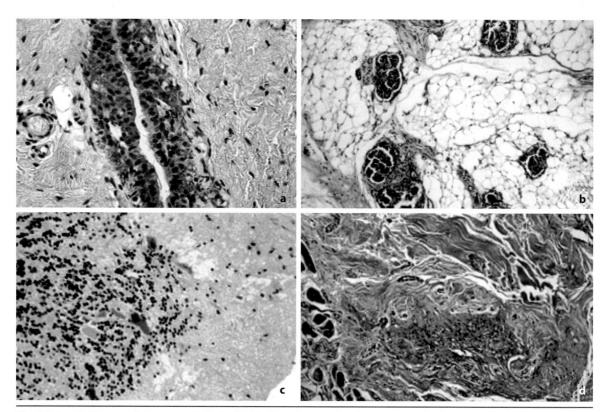

Fig. 36.1 a-d. Lipoma of the conus. Pathological findings in complex forms. **a** Neural tube. **b** Glomerules. **c** Cerebellum. **d** Glia and striated muscle

as glial or neuroglial tissues (18%), arachnoid (7%), ependymal or glioependymal structures (5%). Other tissues were more rare: dermoid or epidermoid cysts (7%), cartilage (6%), smooth muscle fibers (6%), bone (4%), angiomatous formation (4%), lymphatic (3%), cavities lined by respiratory or intestinal epithelia (2%), renal glomerulus (1%), endometrial (1%) and cerebellar tissue (1%). In the literature, similar findings are more rarely reported.

Giudicelli [177] demonstrated that metabolic activities in the lipoma were similar to those observed in the adjacent extraspinal normal adipose tissue. Consequently, if adipocytes from congenital lipomas have no potential evolution of their own, they are capable of growth and regression along the increase or decrease of the rest of the fatty pole, either subcutaneously or intraspinally. In our series, lipomas have been seen to grow subcutaneously in 15% of patients (especially during the first month of life) and intraspinally in 2% of patients. Of these patients, two-thirds were infants, six were obese adolescents, and ten were pregnant women. In three cases the growth of the lipoma provoked a clinical deterioration that disappeared after change of diet. In all these situations, lipomatous growth was easily understandable. When obesity occurs, there is an increase in the fatty pool, including the lipoma. In young infants,

adipocytes increase in size to such a degree that the proportion of fat increases from 14% at birth to 25% at 6 months. At the beginning of gestation, lipogenesis increases as a result of secretion of progesterone and oestradiol, which accelerate the multiplication of preadipocytes and their differentiation into adipocytes. Rarely, growth of complex teratomas may result from other mechanisms such as bleeding of intralipomatous endometrial inclusions, malignant degeneration, or recurrence of a previously incompletely removed dermoid cyst, as seen in two of our patients.

Classification

Among the various anatomic forms of lumbosacral lipoma, lipomas of the filum should be distinguished from lipomas of the conus, the latter being not only much more frequent, but also much more complex to treat than the former.

Lipoma of the Filum

The fatty infiltration of lipoma of the filum (Fig. 36.2) may involve the whole length of the filum or only part of it. Rarely the lipoma, along with the

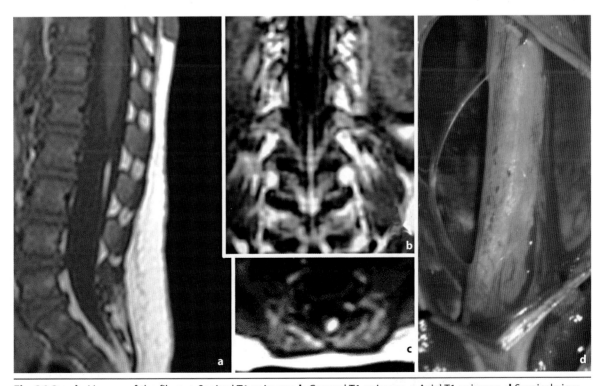

Fig. 36.2 a-d. Lipoma of the filum. **a** Sagittal T1-w image. **b** Coronal T1-w image. **c** Axial T1-w image. **d** Surgical view

filum, has an abnormal course, spreading out of the dura to expand subcutaneously (only three of our 87 cases). Roots of the cauda equina may exceptionally adhere severely to the lipoma, but generally are free and not malformed. In one patient in our series, as in the case of Brophy [178], some of the roots were within the lipoma itself.

Lipoma of the Conus

Different anatomic forms of lipoma of the conus (Fig. 36.3) must be described, but all have in common the description of the insertion of the lipoma on the terminal cord and its relationship with the roots.

Typical Forms

Lipomas of the conus typically spread out of the dura to extend subcutaneously through the defect of a spina bifida. The stalk joining the two parts of the lipoma is frequently severely adherent to the musculoaponeurotic edges of the bony opening. The zone of insertion on the cord is usually wide. It extends typically from L4 to S3 in the majority of our patients. Its median extension is four vertebral levels. The volume of the intraspinal lipoma can be large and may compress the spinal cord. In these cases, the interface is pushed out posteriorly through the dural dehiscence. When small, the interface is usu-

ally within the spinal canal at the level of the dural defect. It is as if the cord was connected to the posterior aspect of the dural sheet and adherences between cord, lipoma, and dura are often severe. This interface is frequently recognizable by its stronger resistance and its whitish color. In our experience the interface is usually flat. In some cases, however, it can be tortuous. Surgery is much more hazardous in these cases.

Chapman [41] classified lipomas into four types according to the interface localization of the cord: dorsal, dorsolateral or lateral, caudal and dorsocaudal. We use a classification in three forms modified from the Chapman classification (Fig. 36.4). In our experience, 35% of the lipomas of the conus were dorsal, 30% caudal and 35% transitional (dorsocaudal or dorsocaudolateral. In the two first forms, in most of the cases the roots had an extralipomatous subdural trajectory. In contrast, in transitional forms, roots were intermingled within the lipoma and were difficult or even impossible to distinguish from fibrotic bands and to separate from the lipoma.

Complex Forms

In our series, complex forms were found in the majority of patients (62.9%).

In lipomyelomeningoceles, a subcutaneous meningocele was associated with an extraspinal extension of the lipoma and the spinal cord. In lipomye-

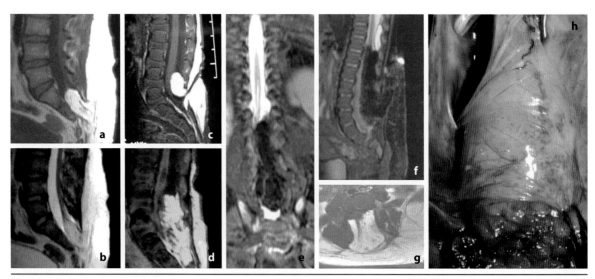

Fig. 36.3 a-h. Lipoma of the conus. **a** Sagittal T1-w image. **b** Sagittal T2-w image. **c** Lipoma associated with a dermal sinus, sagittal T1-w image. **d** Angiolipoma, T1-w image. **e, f** Lipoma of the conus, coronal and sagittal T2 fat saturation T2-w images. **g** Axial T1-w image. **h** Operating view

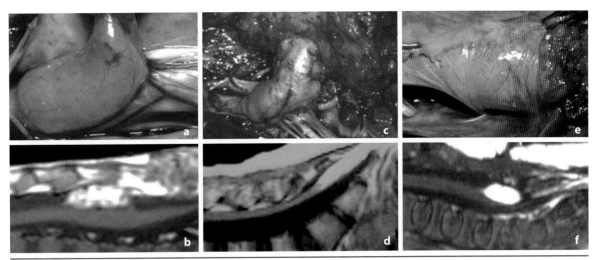

Fig. 36.4 a-f. Modified Chapman Classification. **a, b** Dorsal lipoma. **c, d** Caudal lipoma. **e, f** Transitional lipoma

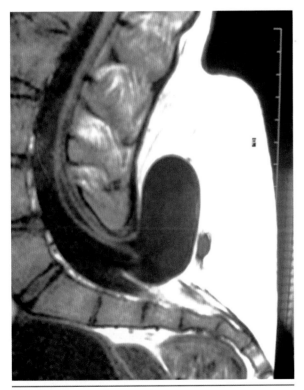

Fig. 36.5 Lipomyelocystocele

loceles, the cord extended extraspinally within the mass of the subcutaneous lipoma.

Lipomyelocystoceles (Fig. 36.5) were much rarer. The terminal cord was the seat of a pseudocystic terminal hydromyelia closed superficially by the dura of the cul-de-sac or the lipoma itself. As already mentioned, the intracystic and subarachnoid cere-brospinal fluid (CSF) never communicated freely. The pseudocyst membranes were described as having an ependymal structure. In our series postnatal MRI failed to diagnose the malformation correctly.

Strictly subdural lipomas were more frequent in the literature (where they accounted for an average of between 7 and 19%) than in our series (6%). Spina bifida in these forms was rare, if not exceptional.

Presacral lipoma was found in 7% of our patients. These were always associated with a sacral agenesis, in 70% of the cases with an anterior meningocele and in 80% with urogenital or digestive tract malformations. In a very few cases the cord may extend in front of the sacrum, but in the large majority of the cases stays within the sacral canal.

Finally, some lipomas are multiple. In our series as in the literature, lumbosacral lipoma can be associated with unique or multiple lipomas of the cord or even of the intracranial space (cerebellopontine angle, tectum or corpus callosum).

Associated Malformations

Associated malformations involve, to varying degrees, the cord and roots, the spine, the skin, the urogenital and digestive apparatus and other viscera.

Cord and Roots Anomalies

The most frequent spinal cord anomaly is a terminal syringomyelia [43, 119, 179-205] (24% in our series compared to the 11-27% reported in the literature). As in the literature, the cavity was almost always localized at the terminal cord and on average extended for two vertebral levels. In 80% of the cases the Vaquero index was under 50%. Dorsal, cervical and bulbar hydromyelia were noted in 3.3%, 0.6% and 0.3% of cases, respectively. Associated diastematomyelia was found in 9% of the cases (in one case, a very complex form with a mosaic spine and a third lower limb).

Roots anomalies [26, 94, 119, 146, 206-219] were found almost exclusively in lipomas of the conus. They were often multiple but unilateral in the same patient. They were considerably more frequent when lipomas were inserted laterally with a rotation of the spinal cord. In 40% of the cases they were short and intralipomatous, in 14% they were agenetic. From a surgical point of view, shortness and intralipomatous trajectory of the roots most frequently prevented the surgeon from freeing the cord on the side of the anomaly correctly.

Three patients in our series had a dorsal arachnoid cyst above the lipoma. In the literature the possibility of enteric cyst, dural arteriovenous malformations, and intramedullary mature teratoma have also been reported.

Spinal Malformations

Spinal malformations are dominated by spina bifida, which was found in 89% of our patients with lipoma of the conus (69% in the literature). It involved L4 in 35% of the cases, L5 in 65% and the whole sacrum in 90% of our patients.

Sacral agenesis [156, 160, 166, 220-243] was more rare (27% of our patients as in the literature), except in patients with urogenital or anorectal malformations in whom it is almost always present (96%).

Scoliosis, when present, was generally related to malformations of the vertebral bodies or shortening of one lower limb.

Other anomalies, such as type I diastematomyelia, hemivertebrae and vertebral fusion, were rare and were found respectively in 8%, 7%, and 6% of our cases.

Brain Malformations

Malformations of the brain are rare in all series (3.6% in ours), in contrast to what is commonly seen with MMC. We observed only five Chiari malformations (0.8%), two hemispheric cysts and one Dandy-Walker malformation (but brain MR was performed in on-

ly 70% of our patients). None of these malformations were symptomatic, except for one Chiari. The malformation was absent at birth and developed with time, so that the patient became symptomatic at the age of 20.

Other Malformations

The incidence of extra-axial malformations ranges from 16% in the literature to 23% in our series. In all series, urogenital and anorectal malformations [47, 63, 82, 105, 132, 134, 141, 158, 166, 206, 231, 235, 244-260] are the most frequent (18%). Cardiac, ear, eye, limb, rib malformations have been found in one or two patients in our series.

Clinical Presentation

Clinical presentation of lumbosacral lipoma is generally associated with cutaneous anomalies and the so-called tethered cord syndrome. The average age at diagnosis was 5 years in our series (3 years in the more recent prospective study). The malformation is usually diagnosed earlier in the presence of cutaneous stigmata (4 months) than in their absence (9 years).

The Cutaneous Syndrome [47, 63, 83, 105, 132, 134, 141, 158, 166, 206, 227, 231, 235, 244-260]

Cutaneous anomalies (Fig. 36.6), when all series are considered together, are present in 90% of cases. These skin anomalies have a considerable diagnostic value. Their absence is often responsible for delayed diagnosis. This explains why, in the literature as well as in our series, adolescents or adults had minor or absent cutaneous stigmata. These anomalies are often on the midline (72%) but when lateral they were predominantly on the left side (75%, p < 0.001). In all series the most common of these anomalies was a subcutaneous lump indicating the subjacent presence of a lipoma or a lipomeningocele. When the subcutaneous lipoma is situated low down, the lump is associated with an intergluteal fold deviation.

The diagnostic value of these lumbosacral cutaneous lesions in asymptomatic children to detect occult spinal dysraphism (OSD) is variable. In a recent study we retrospectively reviewed 54 children referred to the Department of Pediatric Dermatology of our hospital. Occult spinal dysraphysm was detected in three of 36 patients with an isolated con-

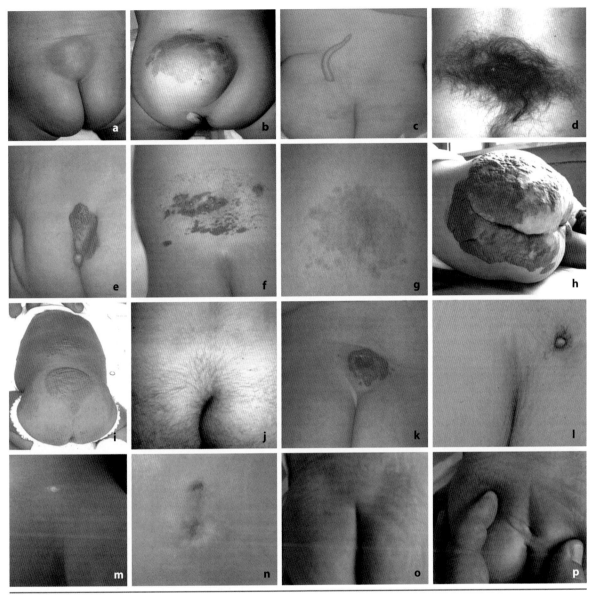

Fig. 36.6 a-p. The cutaneous syndrome. **a** Subcutaneous lipoma. **b** Subcutaneous lipoma associated with an angioma and a dimple. **c** Tail. **d** "Queue de faune". **e-h** Angiomas. **i** Cutaneous hamartoma. **j** Deviation of the gluteal fold. **k** "Meningocele manqué". **l** Lateral dimple. **m** Aplasia cutis. **n** Dermal sinus. **o** Pigmentary naevus. **p** Coccygeal dimple

genital midline lesion and in 11 of 18 patients with combination of two or more different skin lesions. These skin anomalies can be divided into three groups of different risk:
– Group 1 (high risk): two or more lesions (whatever they are), subcutaneous lipoma, tail, dermal sinus, "queue de faune"
– Group 2 (low risk): atypical dimple, aplasia cutis, deviation of the gluteal furrow
– Group 3 (very low risk): hemangioma, port-wine stain, hypertrichosis, fibroma pendulum, pigmentary naevus, coccygeal dimple

The Neurological Syndrome [3, 30, 63, 69, 73, 82, 91, 94, 105, 213, 261-275]

This syndrome is associated in various ways with neurological deficits in the lower limbs, sphincter disturbances and orthopedic deformities.

The extreme difficulty of certifying neurological normality in neonates or infants, as well as neurological deterioration in adolescents must be emphasized. In the very young, sensory impairment, motor deficits when discrete and located in the foot and ankle muscles and voiding difficulties in the absence of clear incontinence or repeated urinary infections may remain clinically undiagnosed. Pain, for example, which is reported in 33% of the adults, was rarely reported in the pediatric population (14 in our series). In young children, neurological deterioration is often difficult to recognize or to confirm. Persistent walking instability, incontinence or development of a clubfoot may indicate a recent aggravation but an undiagnosed deficit may be revealed. Similarly, in older children and in adolescents, the progressive deformation of an already known clubfoot, or the development of trophic ulcerations do not necessarily signify a progressive neurological worsening. All these difficulties explain why all our patients are followed-up by a multidisciplinary team (pediatric neurosurgeon, urologist, orthopedic surgeon, and rehabilitationist) and why electromyography (EMG) and urodynamic studies are performed routinely before and after surgery.

If all the series are included, neurological deficit affects 58% of the patients. In our series, 30% of the lipomas of the filum and 64% of the lipomas of the conus were asymptomatic.

The average age at onset of neurological deficit ranges from 5 to 10 years. In our series, deficits were present at birth in 22% of the cases. In all reports, the numbers of asymptomatic deficits decreases with age. This is generally interpreted as indicating that the older the patient, the worse the neurological condition. This, however, might not be true since healthy carriers never appear in medical statistics, and might signify only those adults, when becoming symptomatic or deteriorating, systematically require care and hospitalization.

Sphincter Disturbances [3, 20, 22, 27, 39, 93, 103, 104, 120, 125, 160, 212, 226, 234, 246, 276-283]

Sphincter disorders are the most common trouble. In our patients, they were particularly frequent in patients with sacral agenesis (69%). Micturition difficulties were more common than any other type of sphincter disorder. Incontinence was rarely passive due to flaccid bladder and sphincter paralysis, but resulted mainly from dysuria, pollakiuria, urgent micturition, and incomplete voiding. Bladder infection or pyelonephritis was also observed frequently, secondary to urinary retention. Urodynamic studies, which must be part of the therapeutic decision-making work-up, frequently revealed both hyperactive bladder and vesicosphincter dyssynergia. Bowel dysfunction is rarely reported in the literature. In our experience severe con-

stipation is not exceptional and sometimes necessitates digital evacuation. Stool leakage was more often due to fecal retention than to sphincter hypotonia, and all patients with such a problem also had urinary disorders (except in Currarino syndrome).

Neuro-Orthopedic Syndrome [36, 79, 88, 116, 124, 160, 284-292]

This syndrome was present in one-third of our patients. As described by Lassman and James [10], it affects the lower limbs and to a lesser degree the spine. Paralysis and sensory deficits usually predominate distally. Thirty percent of our patients had a clubfoot, often with an equinovarus deformity with clawing of the toes, 32% had a muscular atrophy of the leg or foot, and 25% had superficial hypoesthesia. Trophic ulceration secondary to deep anesthesia was much rarer (7%). At examination, 34% of children had a central motor neuron syndrome, but hyperreflexia is often associated with abolished reflexes. Pain, as described by Pang [293] was diffuse to the whole limb, or more often to a distal segment. Occasionally it may occur in a radicular pattern. These troubles are often unilateral, or at least asymmetric. The upper level of the sensory syndrome almost never exceeds L4. In our experience, when patients were asymptomatic, EMGs were normal in only two-thirds of cases. In no case however, was denervation severe. On the other hand, in symptomatic patients, signs of denervation were constant and severe, predominating at the feet and perineum.

Progressive Neurological Deficits

Progressive neurological deterioration has been well documented in patients with lipoma of the filum as well in those with lipoma of the conus. Many authors emphasized that the neurological deterioration could start at any age, including in adults and the elderly. Deterioration usually occurs slowly and insidiously. Rapid evolution and acute onset are rare. They are observed more often in response to sudden effort leading to exaggerated bending of the back, or during pregnancy or the development of obesity. The same findings were observed in our patients: six worsened following sudden and violent effort, two after trauma, five during development of obesity and two during pregnancy.

The real incidence of deterioration is controversial and actually unknown. In the literature, the general impression is that the deterioration is almost unavoidable with age, but "no statistics are available" and data provided are merely subjective. The analysis of our prospective study shows that less than one-third of patients will deteriorate during childhood.

Sexual Dysfunction [16, 53, 59, 96, 164, 212, 294, 295]

Although rarely reported, sexual dysfunction is probably not rare. It was present in 25% of patients in the series of Thomas and Miller [296] and was reported by many adults in our series.

The Caudal Syndrome

Kennedy [297] in 1926, Ashcraft and Holder [298] in 1974 and Currarino [299] in 1981 described a

syndrome associating sacral agenesis, presacral mass (more commonly anterior meningocele, but also teratoma, enteric cyst or lipoma) and perineal malformation (anorectal stenosis in most cases, but also urinary or sexual malformations) (Fig. 36.7). In large series of lipomas, the incidence of caudal syndrome varies from 1.8 to 5.1%. The diagnosis is usually made at birth, due to perineal malformations (anal or rectal imperforation or stenosis, rectoperineal, rectovaginal or rectourethral fistulas, bladder extrophia. However, the diagnosis may be made much later, even during adulthood, after a long period of misdiagnosis, in cases of moderate bowel dysfunction associated with non specific neurological signs.

We recently reviewed 29 patients with Currarino syndrome, including 12 familial cases [162]. All except two patients had a sacral malformation (more often unilateral or asymmetric); 23 had an anorectal anomaly and eight had isolated intestinal pseudo-ob-

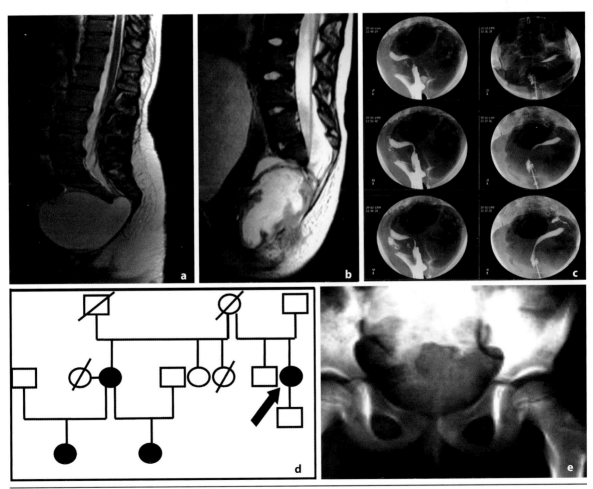

Fig. 36.7 a-e. The caudal syndrome. **a** Presacral meningocele. **b** Secondary presacral abscess. **c** Uterine malformation. **d** Genealogic tree. **e** Sacral agenesis

struction. There were 20 presacral tumors, one of which was malignant. There was a communication between the tumor and the spinal canal in 12 cases and a lipoma in 17 cases (12 filum and five conus). Twenty-five patients underwent surgery with a single stage operation for seven patients on both the intestinal and the presacral malformations and, when required, the spinal malformation. For the other patients, the untethering of the cord was done several months after the perineal surgery. Twelve patients harbored a heterozygous point mutation of the coding sequence of *HLXB9* gene on chromosome 7 (7q36) [162, 300, 301].

Functional Score

To appreciate the functional and social repercussions of these malformations, and to allow rapid comparison between patients and appraise the evolution of the clinical symptoms, we developed a functional scoring system (Table 36.2). This score takes into account four handicaps: motor, sensory, vesical and anal. It is simpler than those previously reported, and differs considerably from some other scores proposed in the neurosurgical literature, which evaluate the neurological level of the deficits but not their functional repercussions. Normality is given a score of 5 for both motor and urinary function and 4 for sensory and anal function. Asymptomatic patients have a score of 18 and a normal life is possible with a score above 15.

Radiology

Ultrasonography and MR have made both antenatal diagnosis and its correct postnatal anatomic analysis possible.

Prenatal Ultrasonography and MRI [3, 128, 135, 141, 158, 161, 196, 244, 301-308]

Prenatal diagnosis is possible from week 17 of gestation on the basis of lumbosacral spina bifida, meningocele, overlying hyperechogenic skin (Fig. 36.8); no hydrocephalus and no cerebral malformation (including Chiari). The meningocele may be echogenic owing to the presence of a low-lying terminal cord. Progressively the meningocele diminishes and the lipoma appears. In no case, in our experience, did prenatal MRI provide more information than echography. In case of antenatal diagnosis of Currarino, a bone computed tomography (CT) scan may be useful to diagnose sacral agenesis.

Plain Radiography

Lack of ossification in neonates and infants makes the interpretation of radiographs difficult, especially with respect to the sacrum, and raises the question of the usefulness of this technique in this age range. Even if they demonstrate the existence of spina bifida poorly, in our opinion they must remain part of the routine work-up when searching for other possible spinal abnormalities such as diastematomyelia, abnormal vertebral segmentation, abnormal spinal curves and sacral agenesis.

Spinal Echography [128, 158, 221, 225, 229, 254, 268, 304-321]

Ultrasonography (US) is the examination of choice in neonates and up to the age of 2 months. Our preference is to recommend US as the first investigation in neonates and infants with lumbosacral stigmata.

Table 36.2. Necker Functional Score

Score	Motor	Sensory	Bladder	Bowel
1	Wheelchair *Major deficit**	Skin ulceration Amputation	Day and night incontinence *Incontinence**	Incontinence
2	Major orthesis Two crutches	Pain	Night incontinence *Retention**	Painful constipation *Digital maneuvers**
3	Distal orthesis	Painless deficit	Intermittent catheterization	Constipation
4	Fatigue on walking	Normal	Dysuria, stress incontinence	Normal
5	Normal		Normal	

* for children under the age of 3

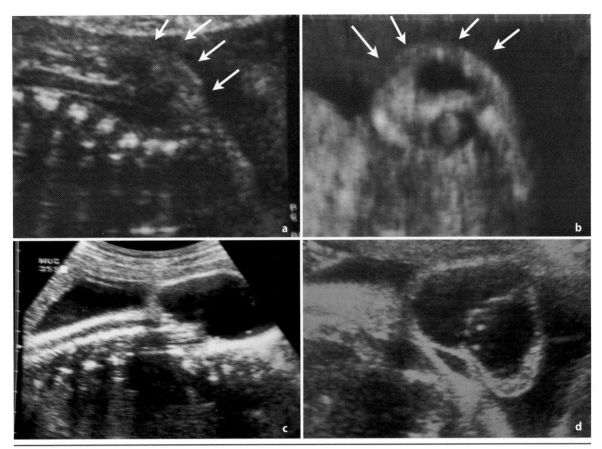

Fig. 36.8 a-d. Antenatal ultrasound. **a, b** Lipoma of the conus (*arrows*). **c, d** Lipomyelocele

In asymptomatic children with grade 2 and 3 skin anomalies, if the US is normal, then MRI can be avoided. In grade 1 or in case of clinical symptoms, the MR can be postponed to the age of 3 months. Echography may show the low cord termination, and the lipoma as an intraspinal hyperechoegenic homogenous and well-demarcated mass or band.

MRI [86, 111, 131, 156, 183, 192, 197, 200, 230, 250, 262, 309, 322-347]

MRI remains the main pretherapeutic investigation. Sagittal and axial views in T1- and T2-weighted images are necessary to analyze relationships between the lipoma and the spinal cord. Special attention must be paid to the insertion of the lipoma on the cord, the rotation of the spinal cord, the relationship of the roots with regard to the lipoma, and to the possible presence of lipomyelocele, lipomyelomeningocele, syringomyelia and other malformations. We do not perform brain MR routinely. On the other hand, special sequence with fat saturation and gadolinium is mandatory when a dermal sinus is suspected. Dynamic MR has been proposed to evaluate the mobility of the spinal cord. In our experience, it has always been useless, both preoperatively and postoperatively.

Surgical Treatment

Principles

Operations must be conducted under optic magnification to untether and decompress the spinal cord, while sparing functional nervous tissue. Ultrasonic aspiration and lasers may be of great help in removing the lipoma and intraoperative monitoring is useful for the large majority of the authors to distinguish functional nerve roots from non-functional ones or from fibrotic bands. To prevent retethering, closure with enlargement of the dural sac is recommended in most cases. Many different types of prosthetic material have been proposed. None has proved superior to autologous material.

Operative Technique

Lipoma of the Filum

In most cases only the lipomatous filum is cut. The approach to the filum is easy. The subcutaneous lipoma is usually absent, the lumbo-sacral aponeurosis intact and the dural sac normal. We routinely make a horizontal incision to put a distance between the scar and the gluteal furrow. An interspinous approach between L5 and S1 is performed to reach the dural sac. A one centimeter incision allows recognition, isolatation and division of the filum.

Lipoma of the Conus

For the last 5 years we have preferred, when possible (less than five levels' exposure), horizontal to vertical or curved incision. When the subcutaneous lipoma is voluminous, the skin incision is split into two at the top of the lump to resect both the excess of skin and fat. The subcutaneous lipoma is usually totally resected. Laminectomy of the lowest normal lamina may be necessary to expose the normal dura and the upper part of the lipoma.

A dural incision is made rostro-caudal to reach the adhesion between the dura and the end of the cord or the upper part of the lipoma. At this level, these adhesions are frequently tight and severe and have to be divided carefully to expose the underlying roots.

Removal of the lipoma is easy in purely dorsal forms. Roots are always extralipomatous and easily recognizable. On the contrary the dissection is difficult in cases of lateral or dorsolateral forms, because roots are often abnormal or absent and the spinal cord is frequently rotated. In addition, dura is often largely missing, replaced by fibromuscular bundles.

In rare cases, dissection may be so difficult that surgery has to be stopped before correct freeing of the cord can be achieved.

Opinions vary from minimal to partial or even total removal of the lipoma. We perform as complete a removal as possible, which we achieved in 66% of the cases of our first series (1984-1994). There is no doubt that "total" removal in an attempt to reach the fibrotic interface is doable, but it carries the intrinsic risk of injuring the posterior columns and provoking a severe and durable postoperative painful syndrome. For that reason, contrary to some authors, we no longer advocate as complete a removal as we did in the past, especially as we have not found any correlation in postoperative results between subtotal and total removal.

Our goal is now to do a subtotal removal decompressing and freeing the cord and allowing a closure of the edge of the placode on itself as in surgery for myelomeningocele. This was achieved in 17% of patients in our retrospective studies and in 80% in the more recent one. This closure is done with non-resorbable sutures (Prolene® 7/0), which make it easy to recognize the midline in case of reoperation. This technique, however, does not seem to prevent patients from late postoperative deterioration.

In patients with severe terminal syrinx, several authors advocated myelotomy and/or drainage. Our experience is different and we had never treated the syringomyelia alone during the first surgery. Cavities were only opened when lipomas were in direct contact with them. Contrary to the results of Iskandar [368], we found no correlation between patients' pre- and postoperative status, and the presence or size of a syringomyelic cavity. Furthermore, many syringes shrink after surgery. These data imply that treating syringomyelia is not necessary in the majority of the cases. Closure with enlargement of the dural sac, as recommended by many, is advised to limit the risk of readhesion and retethering. This procedure may be difficult in case of large intra- and extraspinal lipomas when the dura is largely missing. In such cases, the duroplasty has to be fixed to the paraspinal muscle or to the aponeurosis, making tight and waterproof sutures difficult or even impossible. In these cases, in order to avoid a subcutaneous dead space which can facilitate a postoperative meningocele, leaving a part of the subcutaneous lipoma may be proposed.

Surgical Risks and Complications

Lipoma of the Filum

Surgery for lipoma of the filum is benign in nature. It is a one-hour surgery and children are routinely discharged at day 4 or 5. The incidence of local, general or neurological complication is nil. However, it must be reported that the only death among the 671 patients was for a filum surgery in a young child. A dramatically acute meningitis occurred at day 1 and the child died less than 48 hours after the surgery.

Lipoma of the Conus

The same cannot be said for lipomas of the conus. The operative mortality [48] remains low (0.2% in the literature), but postoperative and permanent morbidity remains a problem.

Local Complications

Local complications were common in our series (15%) as in the literature, where the average incidence was estimated by McLone [78, 85] to be 25%. In all series. these complications are mainly represented by subcutaneous pseudomeningocele, CSF leak and wound reopening and meningitis. Three percent of our patients have had to be reoperated because of these local problems.

Neurological and Urological Complications

Neurological and urological complications are not rare. In our series we considered the following as aggravated by surgery: (1) patients who presented after operation with a new symptom or a symptom that was worse than before operation even when preexisting deficits improved or disappeared following surgery; (2) patients whose functional score was worse after surgery; and (3) infants and young children in whom postoperative EMG or urodynamic studies gave worse results after operation, even in the absence of clinically detectable changes.

Transient Complications

Pain remains the most constant postoperative problem. Only an immediate post-operative aggressive treatment could diminish its intensity. It disappeared usually in 3 or 4 days.

Urinary and motor deficits were observed in 7.5% of the patients. All these troubles regressed completely in a maximum of 6 weeks, while EMG and urodynamic findings always returned to the preoperative status. The incidence of such transient deteriorations has never been reported in the literature but their possibility has been mentioned by many authors.

Permanent Postoperative Deficits

Permanent neurological complications, mainly sphincter-related, occurred in 3.4% of patients in our series. Urinary retention was more frequent than incontinence. It was only severe (score under 13) in six patients. In the literature, the rates of permanent neurological complications vary from 0 to 4%.

Postoperative Outcome of Preoperative Deficits

It is frequently said that preoperative deficits rarely respond to surgery. This is one of the main arguments in favor of prophylactic surgery. In our experience, deficits, regardless of the type, disappeared completely in 41% of symptomatic lipomas of the filum and in 27% of the symptomatic lipomas of the conus, and partly regressed in 12% and 31%, respectively. As already reported, surgery was, however, more frequently efficient with respect to pain than any other deficit.

The only conditions that never improved were clubfoot and scoliosis.

Long-Term Postoperative Outcome in Symptomatic Patients

Up to this point, results of lipoma surgery remain controversial and difficult to analyze. On one hand, the pathology reported often covers all the causes of occult spinal dysraphism or of tethered cord syndrome. On the other hand, follow-up is frequently insufficient to draw conclusions. Very few series have had a follow-up longer than 5 years. In all others, follow-up was either not mentioned or was shorter than 2 years. The results of our retrospective study (1984-1994) with systematic surgery at the moment of diagnosis have been studied separately for lipomas of the filum and lipomas of the conus.

Lipomas of the Filum

Seventeen lipomas of the filum were operated on in symptomatic patients. Results were excellent. At maximum follow-up, no patient had aggravated symptoms. Symptoms disappeared totally in seven patients (41%), improved in two (12%) and stabilized in the remaining eight (47%). These good results remained unchanged in the subgroup followed for more than 5 years.

Lipomas of the Conus

Operations were performed upon a total of 144 symptomatic lipomas of the conus. Results as a whole were satisfactory, but not as good as for lipoma of the filum.

At 1 year follow-up, 26 patients (18%) were cured, 46 (32%) had improved and 59 (41%) had stabilized, but 13 were worse than before the surgery. Of the 13 deteriorations, three were directly secondary to surgery. These relatively good results eroded with time: the percentage of patients who were worse than before operation increased progressively to 20% (n = 29) at maximum follow-up and to 29% (15/51 patients) at follow-up greater than 5 years. In fact, long-term outcome of patients who were symptomatic before operation depended on the immediate postoperative results. The better the immediate results, the better the long-term neurological outcome. Most of those who had clearly improved at one year remained improved. Conversely, most of those who deteriorated with time either were not improved by surgery or only stabilized.

In summary, surgery was nevertheless beneficial as, in the long-term, 70% of patients were improved or stabilized.

Long-Term Postoperative Outcome in Asymptomatic Patients

Lipomas of the Filum

Twenty-one lipomas of the filum were operated upon in the absence of symptoms. As for symptomatic patients, results were excellent. Symptoms were slightly aggravated in only one patient. All others remain symptom free. These good results were maintained with time.

Lipomas of the Conus

Some 101 patients with asymptomatic lipoma of the conus were operated upon. As for symptomatic patients with similar malformations, results were good in the short-term, but eroded with time (Fig. 36.9). At 1 year after surgery, 94% of patients (102/109) were neurologically intact. At maximum follow-up, the proportion was 76% (83/109). At more than 5 years of follow-up, only 53% of the patients (17/32) were still symptom free. This slow decline with time is shown on the actuarial curve (Fig. 36.10). Results at 1 and 5 years following surgery were good or satisfactory. They seem to parallel those in the literature, although strict comparison is difficult because lipomas of the filum and of the conus have never been considered separately. Difference between results in the literature and in our series is found mainly in the very long-term prognosis for patients with asymptomatic lipomas of the conus. It has generally been accepted, mainly since the publication of Bruce [35], that surgery is the major factor determining whether a child will remain symptomatic. These conclusions are in striking contrast with ours,

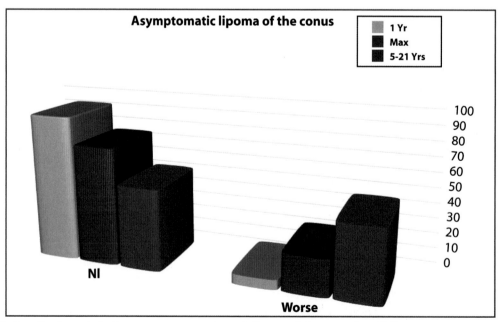

Fig. 36.9. Results of prophylactic surgery on asymptomatic lipoma of the conus (n = 101)

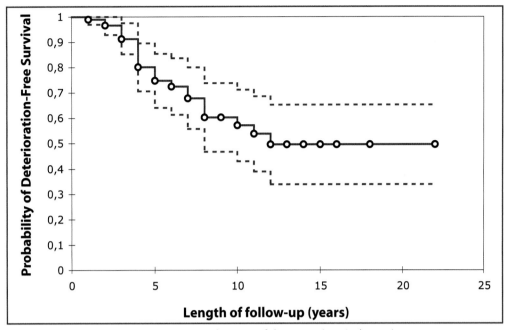

Fig. 36.10. Prophylactic surgery on asymptomatic lipomas of the conus (survival curve)

in which 50% of asymptomatic children developed deficits in the long-term. This divergence could be explained by the fact that our series included more patients than others, follow-up was much longer, and all patients were reviewed systematically by the same multidisciplinary team.

Why did nearly half of asymptomatic patients operated on in our series worsen with time? The answer is unclear. Retethering of the cord may be one reason, but we wonder whether this is the only one or even the major reason. It is striking that postoperative long-term deterioration is a risk only in lipoma of the conus and myelomeningocele but almost never in spinal cord tumor, arteriovenous malformation, or lipoma of the filum. All these operations, nevertheless, led to similar postoperative scarring and adherences. Why then, should the outcome be different? It is possible that the underlying myelodysplasia might play a role, perhaps a major one. Myelodysplasia is indeed absent or minor in case of tumors, arterio-venous malformations (AVM) or even lipoma of the conus, but is probably a constant feature, to varying degrees, in lipoma of the conus. From these observations, we suggest that the risk of late postoperative decompensation may result partly from the degree of underlying myelodysplasia. Postoperative adhesions could be simply an additional contributing factor. In patients with minor myelodysplasia and severe retethering, recurrence of deficits could be improved or even cured by reoperation. In contrast, in patients with se-

vere myelodysplasia, reoperation may have little chance of improving patients or preventing them from developing new postoperative degradation.

Prognostic Factors

A search was undertaken for prognostic factors. Five parameters were studied: type of lipoma (filum versus conus), quality of the surgery (correct or incorrect freeing of the cord), age at surgery, and malformation complex. Two parameters correlated significantly with prognosis: (1) the type of lipoma – when patients who were symptomatic or asymptomatic were grouped together, the rate of deterioration at 5 years or more after surgery was 10% for patients with lipoma of the filum and 36% for those with lipoma of the conus; and (2) the quality of surgery, but only in patients without postoperative deficit ($p < 0.0001$). Contrary to what has been reported in the literature, there was no difference in long-term outcome between patients operated on before or after the age of 1 year. Confirming some previous observations, adults as well as children improved in our series. Finally, the degree of sacral agenesis and perineal and visceral malformations showed no correlation with prognosis. In summary, at present, the long-term prognosis for patients with lipoma of the conus cannot be foreseen before operation.

Reoperation

Most neurosurgeons indicate reoperation in case of postoperative recurrence or deficits [3, 63, 71, 72, 78, 87, 91, 105, 113, 115, 120, 213, 288, 348-353]. In the literature, as in our experience, the rate of reoperation is between 5 and 10%, and the interval between the first and the second surgery is around 6 years. In our hands, as well as in others, this surgery is always difficult because of severe adhesions, and sometimes has to be stopped before complete freeing of the cord. In the literature, postoperative results are often contradictory. In our series, five (31%) of the 16 patients improved, in seven (44%) the deficit stopped evolving, three (19%) continued to deteriorate and one (6%) worsened after surgery. Two patients were operated on twice and one three times because of continuous worsening of the symptoms, finally with no success. Our results were largely the same as those reported by McLone [85] with 33% and 14% improvement for motor and sensory functions, respectively, and by Sakamoto [369] with one improvement and three stabilizations. They were far from being as good as the series of Hoffman [354], Kanev [355], and Herman [288], all of which reported 100% improvement.

In summary, in our experience reoperation, although effective in some cases, often does not lead to improvement. Moreover, reoperation was frequently technically difficult and not without risk, as was found in our study and also in that of Sakamoto, who mentioned three transient aggravations for four reoperations.

Surgical Indications

Surgical indications remain the main subject of controversy, specifically for asymptomatic lipoma of the conus.

Symptomatic Children with Lipoma of the Filum or the Conus

For this group of patients there is a consensus, and we agree fully with all publications that favor early surgery for all these patients.

Symptomatic Adults with Lipoma of the Filum or the Conus [26, 63, 70, 73, 82, 94, 101, 191, 273, 294, 356-366]

For these patients, there is some divergence in the literature. The few who have written on the subject are more reluctant, advocating surgery only when deficits are progressive or show rapid evolution. Our opinion is slightly different. We believe that surgery is mandatory at any age in the presence of deficits, even if these are not progressive. Our results showed that the majority of symptomatic patients, adults as well as children, benefit from surgery. In these patients, surgical risks are clearly counterbalanced by the severity of the condition. In adults, the proposal to wait for progressive symptoms before recommending surgery suggests that, after a certain age, risks of deterioration are small and surgery is ineffective, which is contradicted by our experience and by that of many others.

Asymptomatic Lipomas [1, 36, 45, 84, 112, 124]

For these lesions, opinions are divergent because prophylactic treatments raise major medicoethical problems. This is as true for lipoma as for other pathologies. Examples of prophylactic treatments are exceptional in our medical practice, and prophylactic surgery is justified under only three conditions: (1) very low operative risk, (2) proven protective effect of the treatment; (3) severity of the disorder incompetible with a normal personal and/or social life. To advocate routine surgery in patients with asymptomatic lipoma, we must therefore be able to answer these three questions: Is surgery harmless? Does it prevent patients from further risk of deterioration? Is the prognosis of patients with lipoma poor? Answers to these questions must be considered separately for lipoma of the filum and of the conus.

Asymptomatic Lipoma of the Filum

In asymptomatic lipoma of the filum, the risk of surgery has been shown to be almost nil in all series. Almost all patients remain symptom free, and these good results are stable over time. Does surgery have a truly preventive effect? The data remain insufficient to answer this question because nobody knows the real incidence of the disease and the natural history of these lipoma without surgery. Nevertheless, it may be postulated that surgery is harmless and that the risks of the surgery are less that those of the disease itself. For these reasons, routine surgery is acceptable and advisable and not in contradiction with the ethical rules.

Asymptomatic Lipoma of the Conus

In our retrospective studies, all these lesions were operated on systematically as soon as they were diagnosed, an approach similar to that of many neurosurgeons. However, our results were not as expected, since approximately half the patients developed deficits despite surgery. Considering this, in addition to the risks of postoperative deterioration (almost 4% in lipoma of the conus), routine surgery can no longer be advocated in this group of patients because treatment is not only risky but perhaps not even preventive.

The actuarial curve in our series, showing that approximately 50% of patients had aggravated symptoms with time, cannot be interpreted without knowing the natural history of the disease, and this has been poorly studied. There is a diffuse feeling that aggravations are inevitable but, as already emphasized, the bias of recruitment in all series prevents conclusions from being made, as healthy carriers of the malformation have never been taken into account. The only two series reporting on the spontaneous evolution of asymptomatic lipomas are very small and contradictory. In the series of Bruce [35], seven of eight patients deteriorate, while only one of ten in that of Lagae [367] did so. The number of asymptomatic adults is difficult to know. It could be high if both autopsy and radiological studies are considered. Are the results of surgery any better than the natural history of the disease? The lack of basic information prevents us from answering this question. Until this question is answered, we consider that surgery on patients with asymptomatic lipoma of the conus does not fulfill the ethical rules prevailing in other fields of the medical practice and cannot be advised any longer.

We have therefore modified our approach. Since 1995, we follow a policy of careful surveillance by the same multidisciplinary medical team for these asymptomatic children. At referral they undergo EMG of the lower limbs and perineum, and urodynamic study. Infants are re-examined twice a year until the age of 3 years and once a year later on without limit of age. MRI is repeated at the age of 6 months to ascertain that the lipoma has not grown in the interval and after once a year until the age of 5 years and then every 3 years. Urodynamic studies are also repeated annually until the age of three years. Surgery is decided on in one of the following four circumstances: (1) onset of deficits, foot deformation, amyotrophia, sphincter disturbances, multiple urinary infections with fever, abnormal brisk reflexes, pain; (2) increase of volume of the lipoma; (3) abnormal urodynamic studies; and (4) opposition of the family to follow the surveillance protocol.

This new protocol will be stopped if the incidence of deterioration differs significantly from the results of prophylactic surgery. Comparison of these two groups of patients will hopefully give us the possibility of describing the natural history of the disease scientifically and to define the correct therapeutic approach for patients with asymptomatic lipoma of the conus.

Results at 10 Years of the Prophylactic Study: An Appraisal of the Natural History of Asymptomatic Lipoma of the Conus

Beginning in 1995, all the members of the multidisciplinary team agreed to follow this revised treatment protocol. All asymptomatic children who presented after implementation of the revised protocol were prospectively recorded in a database.

For the current series, there were a total of 106 eligible patients. There were 65 female and 41 male patients. Eighty-nine patients presented at birth and eight prenatally, whereas nine patients presented at ages ranking from 12 months to 19 years. The most common mode of presentation was detection of an obvious lumbosacral mass.

The majority of lipomas were of the transitional type (66%) and all the other data characteristics were identical to those of the previous retrospective study. For 90% of the patients the urodynamic studies were unequivocally normal. For 11 patients (all infants), the results demonstrated sphincter spasticity, which was interpreted as being physiological, rather than pathological.

The children were monitored for a mean of 6.5 years. During that period, 33 children (32%) developed neurological deterioration, a mean of 24 months after presentation (all of them before the age of 10). The deficits developed during a period of months for 30 patients and during a period of weeks for three patients. All of them underwent surgery after they experienced deterioration. Two patients developed acute neurological worsening after surgery. Those 33 children were monitored for an additional mean time of 5 years after the date of the surgery. During that period, 55% of them exhibited improvement and two deteriorated. Overall the mean necker functional score for this group of patients at the last follow-up examination was 16.1. At 10 years of follow-up 90 patients (86%) are strictly normal and only 16 (14%) presented neurological deficit (all except four with a score over 16).

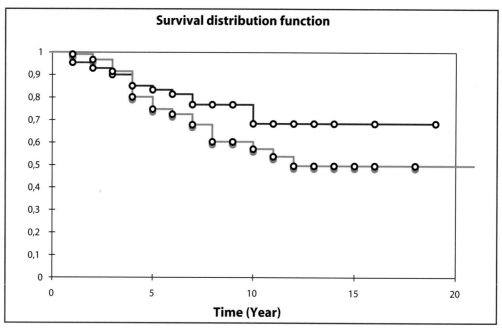

Fig. 36.11. Asymptomatic lipomas of the conus. Comparison between the prophylactic surgery (*old*) and the conservative treatment (*new*)

The survival curves for both surgical retrospective and conservative prospective studies are presented in Figure 36.11. At 10 years, the actuarial risk of deterioration, as determined with the Kaplan-Meier method, was 12% for the conservatively treated patients (33 operated on) and 46% for the surgically treated patients (all operated on).

We think that that this study makes it clear that early surgery for asymptomatic lipoma of the conus is less and less acceptable. On the basis of our nonrandomized study it seems that the pattern of deterioration with or without surgery is at least similar suggesting that aggressive treatment could hardly be reasonable.

In addition to treatment recommendations, the current data force us to reexamine the proposed pathophysiological process of neurological deterioration and the proposed mechanism by which surgery, even theoretically, addresses this pathophysiological process. On the basis of our earlier study, we suggested that tethering might not be the only factor causing neurological worsening. These data seem to reinforce that view: the incidence and timing of patient deterioration are remarkably similar whether or not the patient had undergone early surgery. This certainly suggests that surgery does not ameliorate all of the relevant pathophysiological factors. The potential mechanical benefits of surgery, namely, untethering of the cord and possible relief of mass effect, do seem to be beneficial for at least a subset of patients; in particular, patients whose neurological deficit improves after the mechanical intervention of surgery. Would this group of patients, or perhaps another subset, benefit from early surgery? This question cannot yet be answered, and we currently seem to have no way to prospectively identify such patients.

References

1. Kulkarni AV, Pierre-Kahn A, Zerah M (2004) Conservative management of asymptomatic spinal lipomas of the conus. Neurosurgery 54:868-873; discussion 873-865
2. Pierre-Kahn A, Zerah M, Renier D (1995) Lipomes malformatifs intrarachidiens. Neurochirurgie 41 Suppl 1:1-134
3. Pierre-Kahn A, Zerah M, Renier D et al (1997) Congenital lumbosacral lipomas. Childs Nerv Syst 13:298-334; discussion 335
4. Témoin D (1892) Lipome préméningé simulant un spina bifida. Archives provinciales de chirurgie 1:179
5. Virchow R (1857) Theil in der form des neurons auftretenden fettgeschwülsten. Virchows Archiv für Pathologische Anatomie 11:281-296

6. Gowers W (1876) Myo-lipoma of the spinal cord. Trans Pathol Soc Lond 27:19-22

7. Spiller W (1899) Lipoma of the filum terminale. J Nerv Ment Dis 24:287

8. Spiller W (1916) Congenital and acquired enuresis from spinal lesion : a) myelodysplasia, b) stretching of the cauda equina. Am J Med Sci 151:469-475

9. Jones P, Love J (1956) Tight filum terminale. Arch Surg 73:556-566

10. Lassman LP, James CC (1967) Lumbosacral lipomas: critical survey of 26 cases submitted to laminectomy. J Neurol Neurosurg Psychiatry 30:174-181

11. Brickner W (1918) Spina bifida occulta. Am J Med Sci 315:473-502

12. Leveuf J, Bertrand L, Sternberg H (1937) Spina bifida avec Tumeur: "Etude sur le spina bifida." Masson, Paris, pp 75-88

13. Basset R (1950) The neurologic deficit associated with lipomas of the cauda equina. Ann Surg 131:109-116

14. Yamada S, Zinke DE, Sanders D (1981) Pathophysiology of "tethered cord syndrome". J Neurosurg 54:494-503

15. Al-Mefty O, Kandzari S, Fox JL (1979) Neurogenic bladder and the tethered spinal cord syndrome. J Urol 122:112-115

16. Ammerman BJ, Henry JM, De Girolami U et al (1976) Intradural lipomas of the spinal cord. A clinicopathological correlation. J Neurosurg 44:331-336

17. Anderson FM (1975) Occult spinal dysraphism: a series of 73 cases. Pediatrics 55:826-835

18. Anzai S, Yamaguchi T, Takasaki S et al (1998) Tethered cord associated with intraspinal lipoma and a subcutaneous abscess secondary to a dermal sinus. Int J Dermatol 37:77-78

19. Aoki N (1990) Rapid growth of intraspinal lipoma demonstrated by magnetic resonance imaging. Surg Neurol 34:107-110

20. Arai H, Sato K, Okuda O et al (2001) Surgical experience of 120 patients with lumbosacral lipomas. Acta Neurochir (Wien) 143:857-864

21. Ascher PW, Heppner F (1984) CO2-Laser in neurosurgery. Neurosurg Rev 7:123-133

22. Atala A, Bauer SB, Dyro FM et al (1992) Bladder functional changes resulting from lipomyelomeningocele repair. J Urol 148:592-594

23. Bajpai M (1994) Spina bifida and intraspinal lipomas. Aust N Z J Surg 64:177-179

24. Bajpai M, Kataria R, Gupta DK et al (1997) Occult spinal dysraphism. Indian J Pediatr 64:62-67

25. Bakker-Niezen SH, Walder HA, Merx JL (1984) The tethered spinal cord syndrome. Z Kinderchir 39 Suppl 2:100-103

26. Balagura S (1984) Late neurological dysfunction in adult lumbosacral lipoma with tethered cord. Neurosurgery 15:724-726

27. Bao N, Chen ZH, Gu S et al (2007) Tight filum terminale syndrome in children: analysis based on positioning of the conus and absence or presence of lumbosacral lipoma. Childs Nerv Syst 23:1129-1134

28. Barraquer-Ferre L, Tolosa E, Barraquer-Bordas L et al (1950) Intradural lipoma of the spinal cord. Acta Psychiatr Neurol 25:7-17

29. Barson AJ (1971) Symptomless intradural spinal lipomas in infancy. J Pathol 104:141-144

30. Begeer JH, Wiertsema GP, Breukers SM et al (1989) Tethered cord syndrome: clinical signs and results of operation in 42 patients with spina bifida aperta and occulta. Z Kinderchir 44(Suppl 1):5-7

31. Blount JP, Elton S (2001) Spinal lipomas. Neurosurg Focus 10:e3

32. Bothra ML, Sarin MG, Sharma NK (1976) Intradural lipoma. J Indian Med Assoc 66:128-130

33. Bourque PR, D'Alton JG, Russell NA et al (1986) Congenital lumbosacral lipoma causing primary enuresis in an adult. Cmaj 135:1007-1008

34. Brotchi J, Noterman J, Baleriaux D (1992) Surgery of intramedullary spinal cord tumours. Acta Neurochir (Wien) 116:176-178

35. Bruce DA, Schut L (1979) Spinal lipomas in infancy and childhood. Childs Brain 5:192-203

36. Byrne RW, Hayes EA, George TM et al (1995) Operative resection of 100 spinal lipomas in infants less than 1 year of age. Pediatr Neurosurg 23:182-186; discussion 186-187

37. Caldarelli M, Castagnola D, Ceddia A et al (1992) [Spinal lipomas in childhood]. Minerva Pediatr 44:437-444

38. Caram PC, Carton CA, Scarcella G (1957) Intradural lipomas of the spinal cord; with particular emphasis on the intramedullary lipomas. J Neurosurg 14:28-42

39. Caruso R, Cervoni L, Fiorenza F et al (1996) Occult dysraphism in adulthood. A series of 24 cases. J Neurosurg Sci 40:221-225

40. Chapman P, Stieg PE, Magge S et al (1999) Spinal lipoma controversy. Neurosurgery 44:186-192; discussion 192-183

41. Chapman PH (1982) Congenital intraspinal lipomas: anatomic considerations and surgical treatment. Childs Brain 9:37-47

42. Chapman PH, Davis KR (1993) Surgical treatment of spinal lipomas in childhood. Pediatr Neurosurg 19:267-275; discussion 274-264

43. Chapman PH, Frim DM (1995) Symptomatic syringomyelia following surgery to treat retethering of lipomyelomeningoceles. J Neurosurg 82:752-755

44. Cheng MK (1982) Spinal cord tumors in the People's Republic of China: a statistical review. Neurosurgery 10:22-24

45. Chumas PD (2000) The role of surgery in asymptomatic lumbosacral spinal lipomas. Br J Neurosurg 14:301-304

46. Colak A, Tahta K, Ozcan OE et al (1992) Congenital lumbosacral lipomas presenting as a form of occult spinal dysraphism. A report of 9 surgically treated cases. Zentralbl Neurochir 53:15-19

47. Cornette L, Verpoorten C, Lagae L et al (1998) Closed spinal dysraphism: a review on diagnosis and treatment in infancy. Eur J Paediatr Neurol 2:179-185

48. Cristante L, Herrmann HD (1994) Surgical management of intramedullary spinal cord tumors: functional outcome and sources of morbidity. Neurosurgery 35:69-74; discussion 74-66

49. Crosby RM, Wagner JA, Nichols P, Jr. (1953) Intradural lipoma of the spinal cord. J Neurosurg 10:81-86

50. de Divitiis E, Cerillo A, Carlomagno S (1982) Subpial spinal lipomas. Neurochirurgia (Stuttg) 25:14-18

51. Dinakar I, Seetharam W, Hariprasad P (1978) Tethering of the conus medullaris by lipoma. Neurol India 26:147-149

52. Dincer F, Gokalp HZ, Dincer C et al (1991) Diagnosis and treatment of intraspinal lipomas. Turk J Pediatr 33:221-230

53. Dorward NL, Scatliff JH, Hayward RD (2002) Congenital lumbosacral lipomas: pitfalls in analysing the results of prophylactic surgery. Childs Nerv Syst 18:326-332

54. Dubowitz V, Lorber J, Zachary RB (1965) Lipoma of the cauda equina. Arch Dis Child 40:207-213

55. Emery JL, Lendon RG (1969) Lipomas of the cauda equina and other fatty tumours related to neurospinal dysraphism. Dev Med Child Neurol Suppl 20:62-70

56. Fedun PC (1982) Tethered cord syndrome. J Neurosurg Nurs 14:144-149

57. Feingold M (1984) Picture of the month. Lipomeningocele. Am J Dis Child 138:89-90

58. Foster JJ (1966) Spinal intradural lipomas. A neurosurgical dilemma. Int Surg 46:480-486

59. Giuffre R (1966) Intradural spinal lipomas. Review of the literature (99 cases) and report of an additional case. Acta Neurochir (Wien) 14:69-95

60. Greif L, Stalmasek V (1989) Tethered cord syndrome: a pediatric case study. J Neurosci Nurs 21:86-91

61. Halaby FA, Peterson RB, Leaver RC (1964) Spinal Lipoma. Am J Roentgenol Radium Ther Nucl Med 92:1293-1297

62. Harrison MJ, Mitnick RJ, Rosenblum BR et al (1990) Leptomyelolipoma: analysis of 20 cases. J Neurosurg 73:360-367

63. Huttmann S, Krauss J, Collmann H et al (2001) Surgical management of tethered spinal cord in adults: report of 54 cases. J Neurosurg 95:173-178

64. James HE, Walsh JW (1981) Spinal dysraphism. Curr Probl Pediatr 11:1-25

65. James HE, Williams J, Brock W et al (1984) Radical removal of lipomas of the conus and cauda equina with laser microneurosurgery. Neurosurgery 15:340-343

66. Jindal A, Mahapatra AK, Kamal R (1999) Spinal dysraphism. Indian J Pediatr 66:697-705

67. Johnson DF (1950) Intramedullary lipoma of the spinal cord; review of the literature and report of case. Bull Los Angel Neuro Soc 15:37-42

68. Kang HS, Wang KC, Kim KM et al (2006) Prognostic factors affecting urologic outcome after untethering surgery for lumbosacral lipoma. Childs Nerv Syst 22:1111-1121

69. Kang JK, Lee KS, Jeun SS et al (2003) Role of surgery for maintaining urological function and prevention of retethering in the treatment of lipomeningomyelocele: experience recorded in 75 lipomeningomyelocele patients. Childs Nerv Syst 19:23-29

70. Kaplan JO, Quencer RM (1980) The occult tethered conus syndrome in the adult. Radiology 137:387-391

71. Kasliwal MK, Mahapatra AK (2007) Surgery for spinal cord lipomas. Indian J Pediatr 74:357-362

72. Kirollos RW, Van Hille PT (1996) Evaluation of surgery for the tethered cord syndrome using a new grading system. Br J Neurosurg 10:253-260

73. Klekamp J, Raimondi AJ, Samii M (1994) Occult dysraphism in adulthood: clinical course and management. Childs Nerv Syst 10:312-320

74. Koyanagi I, Iwasaki Y, Hida K et al (1997) Surgical treatment supposed natural history of the tethered cord with occult spinal dysraphism. Childs Nerv Syst 13:268-274

75. Koyanagi I, Iwasaki Y, Hida K et al (2000) Factors in neurological deterioration and role of surgical treatment in lumbosacral spinal lipoma. Childs Nerv Syst 16:143-149

76. Kujas M, Sichez JP, Lalam TF et al (2000) Intradural spinal lipoma of the conus medullaris without spinal dysraphism. Clin Neuropathol 19:30-33

77. Kumar S, Gulati DR, Mann KS (1976) Intradural spinal lipoma. Neurol India 24:188-190

78. La Marca F, Grant JA, Tomita T et al (1997) Spinal lipomas in children: outcome of 270 procedures. Pediatr Neurosurg 26:8-16

79. Lhowe D, Ehrlich MG, Chapman PH et al (1987) Congenital intraspinal lipomas: clinical presentation and response to treatment. J Pediatr Orthop 7:531-537

80. Lunardi P, Missori P, Ferrante L et al (1990) Long-term results of surgical treatment of spinal lipomas. Report of 18 cases. Acta Neurochir (Wien) 104:64-68

81. Maira G, Fernandez E, Pallini R et al (1986) Total excision of spinal lipomas using CO2 laser at low power. Experimental and clinical observations. Neurol Res 8:225-230

82. Maiuri F, Gambardella A, Trinchillo G (1989) Congenital lumbosacral lesions with late onset in adult life. Neurol Res 11:238-244

83. McLone DG (1998) The biological resolution of malformations of the central nervous system. Neurosurgery 43:1375-1380; discussion 1380-1371

84. McLone DG (2000) Congenital malformations of the central nervous system. Clin Neurosurg 47:346-377

85. McLone DG, Naidich TP (1986) Laser resection of fifty spinal lipomas. Neurosurgery 18(5):611-615

86. Merx JL, Bakker-Niezen SH, Thijssen HO et al (1989) The tethered spinal cord syndrome: a correlation of radiological features and peroperative findings in 30 patients. Neuroradiology 31:63-70

87. Mircevski M, Mircevska D, Bojadziev I et al (1983) Surgical treatment of spinal lipomas in infancy and childhood. Childs Brain 10:317-327

88. Morimoto K, Takemoto O, Wakayama A (2005) Spinal lipomas in children-surgical management and long-term follow-up. Pediatr Neurosurg 41:84-87

89. Moufarrij NA, Palmer JM, Hahn JF et al (1989) Correlation between magnetic resonance imaging and surgical findings in the tethered spinal cord. Neurosurgery 25:341-346

90. Murray PJ, O'Gorman AM, Blundell JE (1973) Lumbosacral lipomata producing enuresis. Trans Am Neurol Assoc 98:287-290

91. Ohry A, Azaria M, Zeilig G (1992) Long term follow up of patients with cauda equina syndrome due to intraspinal lipoma. Paraplegia 30:366-369

92. Okai K, Shiraishi S (1969) Spinal cord lipomas. A case report and analysis of 19 cases reported in Japan. Nippon Seikeigeka Gakkai Zasshi 43:395-403

93. Pang D, Casey K (1983) Use of an anal sphincter pressure monitor during operations on the sacral spinal cord and nerve roots. Neurosurgery 13:562-568

94. Pang D, Wilberger JE, Jr. (1982) Tethered cord syndrome in adults. J Neurosurg 57:32-47

95. Pereira W, Araujo RP, Iriya K et al (1964) Spinal intradural lipomas. Considerations on 4 operated cases. Arq Neuropsiquiatr 22:224-230

96. Peter JC (1992) Occult dysraphism of the spine. A retrospective analysis of 88 operative cases, 1979-1989. S Afr Med J 81:351-354

97. Pierre-Kahn A, Lacombe J, Pichon J et al (1986) Intraspinal lipomas with spina bifida. Prognosis and treatment in 73 cases. J Neurosurg 65:756-761

98. Pierre-Kahn A, Renier D, Sainte-Rose C et al (1983) [Lumbosacral lipomas with spina bifida. Anatomo-clinical correlations. Therapeutic results]. Neurochirurgie 29:359-363

99. Rao SB, Dinakar I (1970) Spinal compression. (Analysis of 200 cases). J Assoc Physicians India 18:1009-1013

100. Rogers HM, Long DM, Chou SN et al (1971) Lipomas of the spinal cord and cauda equina. J Neurosurg 34:349-354

101. Salvati M, Orlando Ramundo E, Artico M et al (1990) The tethered cord syndrome in the adult. Report of three cases and review of the literature. Zentralbl Neurochir 51:91-93

102. Satar N, Bauer SB, Scott RM et al (1997) Late effects of early surgery on lipoma and lipomeningocele in children less than 1 year old. J Urol 157:1434-1437

103. Satar N, Bauer SB, Shefner J et al (1995) The effects of delayed diagnosis and treatment in patients with an occult spinal dysraphism. J Urol 154:754-758

104. Sathi S, Madsen JR, Bauer S et al (1993) Effect of surgical repair on the neurologic function in infants with lipomeningocele. Pediatr Neurosurg 19:256-259

105. Sato S, Shirane R, Yoshimoto T (1993) Evaluation of tethered cord syndrome associated with anorectal malformations. Neurosurgery 32:1025-1027; discussion 1027-1028

106. Sattar MT, Bannister CM, Turnbull IW (1996) Occult spinal dysraphism-the common combination of lesions and the clinical manifestations in 50 patients. Eur J Pediatr Surg 6 Suppl 1:10-14

107. Scatliff JH, Kendall BE, Kingsley DP et al (1989) Closed spinal dysraphism: analysis of clinical, radiological, and surgical findings in 104 consecutive patients. AJR Am J Roentgenol 152:1049-1057

108. Schoenmakers MA, Gooskens RH, Gulmans VA et al (2003) Long-term outcome of neurosurgical untethering on neurosegmental motor and ambulation levels. Dev Med Child Neurol 45:551-555

109. Schroeder S, Lackner K, Weiand G (1981) Lumbosacral intradural lipoma. J Comput Assist Tomogr 5:274

110. Schut L, Bruce DA, Sutton LN (1983) The management of the child with a lipomyelomeningocele. Clin Neurosurg 30:464-476

111. Sharma S, Puri S, Das L et al (1988) Intraspinal lumbosacral lipoma: review of literature and report of three cases. Australas Radiol 32:207-213

112. Steinbok P, Garton HJ, Gupta N (2006) Occult tethered cord syndrome: a survey of practice patterns. J Neurosurg 104:309-313

113. Sutton LN (1995) Lipomyelomeningocele. Neurosurg Clin N Am 6:325-338

114. Swanson HS, Barnett JC, Jr. (1962) Intradural lipomas in children. Pediatrics 29:911-926

115. Tobias ME, McGirt MJ, Chaichana KL et al (2008) Surgical management of long intramedullary spinal cord tumors. Childs Nerv Syst 24:219-223

116. Van Calenbergh F, Vanvolsem S, Verpoorten C et al (1999) Results after surgery for lumbosacral lipoma: the significance of early and late worsening. Childs Nerv Syst 15:439-442; discussion 443

117. Villarejo FJ, Blazquez MG, Gutierrez-Diaz JA (1976) Intraspinal lipomas in children. Childs Brain 2:361-370

118. Vinas FJ, Poppen JL (1957) Intradural lipoma of the spinal cord. Surg Clin North Am 37:855-858

119. von Koch CS, Quinones-Hinojosa A, Gulati M et al (2002) Clinical outcome in children undergoing tethered cord release utilizing intraoperative neurophysiological monitoring. Pediatr Neurosurg 37:81-86

120. Xenos C, Sgouros S, Walsh R et al (2000) Spinal lipomas in children. Pediatr Neurosurg 32:295-307

121. Yamada S, Won DJ, Siddiqi J et al (2004) Tethered cord syndrome: overview of diagnosis and treatment. Neurol Res 26:719-721

122. Yashon D, Beatty RA (1966) Tethering of the conus medullaris within the sacrum. J Neurol Neurosurg Psychiatry 29:244-250

123. Zachary RB (1965) Early neurosurgical approaches to spina bifida. Dev Med Child Neurol 7:492-497

124. Cochrane DD, Finley C, Kestle J et al (2000) The patterns of late deterioration in patients with transitional lipomyelomeningocele. Eur J Pediatr Surg 10 Suppl 1:13-17

125. Wu HY, Kogan BA, Baskin LS et al (1998) Long-term benefits of early neurosurgery for lipomyelomeningocele. J Urol 160:511-514

126. Finn MA, Walker ML (2007) Spinal lipomas: clinical spectrum, embryology, and treatment. Neurosurg Focus 23:1-12

127. Donovan DJ, Pedersen RC (2005) Human tail with noncontiguous intraspinal lipoma and spinal cord tethering: case report and embryologic discussion. Pediatr Neurosurg 41:35-40

128. Pierre-Kahn A, Sonigo P (2003) Lumbosacral lipomas: in utero diagnosis and prognosis. Childs Nerv Syst 19:551-554

129. Li YC, Shin SH, Cho BK et al (2001) Pathogenesis of lumbosacral lipoma: a test of the "premature dysjunction" theory. Pediatr Neurosurg 34:124-130

130. Muraszko K, Youkilis A (2000) Intramedullary spinal tumors of disordered embryogenesis. J Neurooncol 47:271-281

131. Tortori-Donati P, Rossi A, Cama A (2000) Spinal dysraphism: a review of neuroradiological features with embryological correlations and proposal for a new classification. Neuroradiology 42:471-491

132. Duru S, Ceylan S, Guvenc BH (1999) Segmental costovertebral malformations: association with neural tube defects. Report of 3 cases and review of the literature. Pediatr Neurosurg 30:272-277

133. Kujas M, Lopes M, Lalam TF et al (1999) Infiltrating extradural spinal angiolipoma. Clin Neuropathol 18:93-98

134. Catala M (1997) Embryogenesis. Why do we need a new explanation for the emergence of spina bifida with lipoma? Childs Nerv Syst 13:336-340

135. Chatelet-Cheront C, Houze de l'Aulnoit D, Ferrant L et al (1997) [Prenatal diagnosis of an intraspinal lipoma. A case report]. J Gynecol Obstet Biol Reprod (Paris) 26:85-89

136. Warf BC, Scott RM, Barnes PD et al (1993) Tethered spinal cord in patients with anorectal and urogenital malformations. Pediatr Neurosurg 19:25-30

137. Hillman J, Bynke O (1992) Description of two informative cases of occult spinal dysraphism with remarks on possible traits in the embryogenesis. Childs Nerv Syst 8:211-214

138. Belzberg AJ, Myles ST, Trevenen CL (1991) The human tail and spinal dysraphism. J Pediatr Surg 26:1243-1245

139. Raghavendra BN, Epstein FJ (1985) Sonography of the spine and spinal cord. Radiol Clin North Am 23:91-105

140. Bale PM (1984) Sacrococcygeal developmental abnormalities and tumors in children. Perspect Pediatr Pathol 8:9-56

141. Lemire RJ (1983) Neural tube defects: clinical correlations. Clin Neurosurg 30:165-177

142. Marques Gubern A, Boix-Ochoa J, Martinez Ibanez V et al (1980) [Lipomeningocele]. Chir Pediatr 21:61-66

143. Suneson A, Kalimo H (1979) Myelocystocele with cerebellar heterotopia. Case report. J Neurosurg 51:392-396

144. Tavafoghi V, Ghandchi A, Hambrick GW, Jr. et al (1978) Cutaneous signs of spinal dysraphism. Report of a patient with a tail-like lipoma and review of 200 cases in the literature. Arch Dermatol 114:573-577

145. Gillespie R, Faithfull DK, Roth A et al (1973) Intraspinal anomalies in congenital scoliosis. Clin Orthop Relat Res:103-109

146. Buchheit WA, Scott M (1971) Surgery of the spinal cord and column. Prog Neurol Psychiatry 26:385-394

147. Dillard BM, Mayer JH, McAlister WH et al (1970) Sacrococcygeal teratoma in children. J Pediatr Surg 5:53-59

148. Matthias FR, Lausberg G (1970) [Clinical features and differential diagnosis of the restricted cranial migration of the spinal cord]. Z Kinderheilkd 108:238-257

149. Till K (1969) Spinal dysraphism. A study of congenital malformations of the lower back. J Bone Joint Surg Br 51:415-422

150. Della Rovere D (1902) Due casi della pia meninge. Studio anatomico e critico. La Clinica Medica Italiana 41:129-143

151. Catala M, Teillet MA, De Robertis EM et al (1996) A spinal cord fate map in the avian embryo: while regressing, Hensen's node lays down the notochord and floor plate thus joining the spinal cord lateral walls. Development 122:2599-2610

152. Stookey B (1927) Intradural spinal lipoma. Arch Neurol Psychiat 18:16-20

153. Takahashi I, Iwasaki Y, Hida K et al (1996) [Clinical study of intraspinal neoplasms in children]. No Shinkei Geka 24:605-611

154. Monsoro-Burq A-H, Montoux M, Teillet M-A, Le Douarin NM (1994) Heterogeneity in the development of the vertebra. Proc Natl Acad Sci USA 91:10435-10439

155. Watanabe Y, Le Douarin NM (1996) A role for BMP-4 in the development of subcutaneous cartilage. Mech Dev 57(1):69-78

156. Kilickesmez O, Gol IH, Uzun M et al (2006) Complete familial Currarino triad in association with Hirschsprung's disease: magnetic resonance imaging features and the spectrum of anorectal malformations. Acta Radiol 47:422-426

157. Bordet R, Ghawche F, Destee A (1991) [Epidural angiolipoma and multiple familial lipomatosis]. Rev Neurol (Paris) 147:740-742

158. Seeds JW, Powers SK (1988) Early prenatal diagnosis of familial lipomyelomeningocele. Obstet Gynecol 72:469-471

159. Farwell J, Flannery JT (1984) Second primaries in children with central nervous system tumors. J Neurooncol 2:371-375

160. Mariani AJ, Stern J, Khan AU et al (1979) Sacral agenesis: an analysis of 11 cases and review of the literature. J Urol 122:684-686

161. Cretolle C, Sarnacki S, Amiel J et al (2007) Currarino syndrome shown by prenatal onset ventriculomegaly and spinal dysraphism. Am J Med Genet A 143:871-874

162. Cretolle C, Zerah M, Jaubert F et al (2006) New clinical and therapeutic perspectives in Currarino syndrome (study of 29 cases). J Pediatr Surg 41:126-131; discussion 126-131

163. Lebkowski WJ, Dudek H, Lebkowska U et al (2000) Neoplasms of the central nervous system of lipoid origin. Pol J Pathol 51:159-163

164. Lellouch-Tubiana A, Zerah M, Catala M et al (1999) Congenital intraspinal lipomas: histological analysis of 234 cases and review of the literature. Pediatr Dev Pathol 2:346-352

165. Ruchoux MM, Kepes JJ, Dhellemmes P et al (1998) Lipomatous differentiation in ependymomas: a report of three cases and comparison with similar changes reported in other central nervous system neoplasms of neuroectodermal origin. Am J Surg Pathol 22:338-346

166. Towfighi J, Housman C (1991) Spinal cord abnormalities in caudal regression syndrome. Acta Neuropathol 81:458-466

167. Chapon F, Hubert P, Mandard JC et al (1991) [Spinal lipoma associated with a neuromuscular hamartoma. Report of one case]. Ann Pathol 11:345-348

168. Theunissen PH, Ariens AT, Pannebakker MA et al (1990) [Late recurrence of a hemangiopericytoma with lipomatous components]. Pathologe 11:346-349

169. Warzok R, Lang G, Schwesinger G (1987) [The relation between melorheostosis and tumors]. Zentralbl Allg Pathol 133:453-458

170. Bardosi A, Schaake T, Friede RL et al (1985) Extradural spinal angiolipoma with secretory activity. An ultrastructural, clinico-pathological study. Virchows Arch A Pathol Anat Histopathol 406:253-259

171. Pasquier B, Vasdev A, Gasnier F et al (1984) [Epidural angiolipoma: a rare and curable cause of spinal cord compression]. Ann Pathol 4:365-369

172. Smith CM, Timperley WR (1984) Multiple intraspinal and intracranial epidermoids and lipomata following gunshot injury. Neuropathol Appl Neurobiol 10:235-239

173. Gerlach H, Janisch W, Schreiber D (1982) [CNS tumors of the perinatal period (author's transl)]. Zentralbl Allg Pathol 126:23-28

174. Johnson DF, Brown DG (1969) Intradural spinal lipoma in an experimental swine. Pathol Vet 6:342-347

175. Brandenburg W (1957) [Lipoblastic meningioma of the spinal cord with the clinical appearance of spastic spinal paralysis.]. Zentralbl Allg Pathol 96:118-123

176. Collins DH, Henderson WR (1949) A case of intradural spinal lipoma. J Pathol Bacteriol 61:227-231

177. Giudicelli Y, Pierre-Kahn A, Bourdeaux AM et al (1986) Are the metabolic characteristics of congenital intraspinal lipoma cells identical to, or different from normal adipocytes? Childs Nerv Syst 2:290-296

178. Brophy JD, Sutton LN, Zimmerman RA et al (1989) Magnetic resonance imaging of lipomyelomeningocele and tethered cord. Neurosurgery 25:336-340

179. Rodriguez-Cano L, Bartralot R, Garcia-Patos V et al (2007) Cervico-thoracic lipoma associated with occult syringohydromyelia. Pediatr Dermatol 24:E76-78

180. Klein O, Thompson D (2007) Spontaneous regression of lipomyelomeningocele associated with terminal syringomyelia in a child. Case report. J Neurosurg 107:244-247

181. Gan YC, Sgouros S, Walsh AR et al (2007) Diastematomyelia in children: treatment outcome and natural history of associated syringomyelia. Childs Nerv Syst 23:515-519

182. Emmez H, Guven C, Kurt G et al (2004) Terminal syringomyelia: is it as innocent as it seems? – Case report. Neurol Med Chir (Tokyo) 44:558-561

183. Scatliff JH, Hayward R, Armao D et al (2005) Pre- and post-operative hydromyelia in spinal dysraphism. Pediatr Radiol 35:282-289

184. Muthukumar N (2004) The "human tail": a rare cause of tethered cord: a case report. Spine 29:E476-478

185. Piatt JH, Jr. (2004) Unexpected findings on brain and spine imaging in children. Pediatr Clin North Am 51:507-527

186. Fujimura M, Kusaka Y, Shirane R (2003) Spinal lipoma associated with terminal syringohydromyelia and a spinal arachnoid cyst in a patient with cloacal exstrophy. Childs Nerv Syst 19:254-257

187. Ng WH, Seow WT (2001) Tethered cord syndrome preceding syrinx formation-serial radiological documentation. Childs Nerv Syst 17:494-496

188. Unsinn KM, Geley T, Freund MC et al (2000) US of the spinal cord in newborns: spectrum of normal findings, variants, congenital anomalies, and acquired diseases. Radiographics 20:923-938

189. Koyanagi I, Iwasaki Y, Hida K et al (1997) Surgical treatment of syringomyelia associated with spinal dysraphism. Childs Nerv Syst 13:194-200

190. Tamaki N, Nagashima T (1995) [Hydrodynamics of syringomyelia]. Rinsho Shinkeigaku 35:1398-1399

191. Fujimura Y, Kimura F, Ishida S et al (1994) [An adult case of tethered cord syndrome with lipoma and thoraco-lumbar syringomyelia presenting slow progressive muscular atrophy in the lower limbs]. Rinsho Shinkeigaku 34:918-921

192. Aguilera Grijalvo C, Bank WO, Baleriaux D et al (1993) Lipomyeloschisis associated with thoracic syringomyelia and Chiari I malformation. Neuroradiology 35:375-377

193. Puca A, Cioni B, Colosimo C et al (1992) Spinal neurenteric cyst in association with syringomyelia: case report. Surg Neurol 37:202-207

194. Aoki N (1991) Syringomyelia secondary to congenital intraspinal lipoma. Surg Neurol 35:360-365

195. Gupta RK, Sharma A, Jena A et al (1990) Magnetic resonance evaluation of spinal dysraphism in children. Childs Nerv Syst 6:161-165

196. Rindahl MA, Colletti PM, Zee CS et al (1989) Magnetic resonance imaging of pediatric spinal dysraphism. Magn Reson Imaging 7:217-224

197. Brunberg JA, Latchaw RE, Kanal E et al (1988) Magnetic resonance imaging of spinal dysraphism. Radiol Clin North Am 26:181-205

198. Szalay EA, Roach JW, Smith H et al (1987) Magnetic resonance imaging of the spinal cord in spinal dysraphisms. J Pediatr Orthop 7:541-545

199. Sutterlin CE, Grogan DP, Ogden JA (1987) Diagnosis of developmental pathology of the neuraxis by

magnetic resonance imaging. J Pediatr Orthop 7:291-297

200. Han JS, Benson JE, Yoon YS (1984) Magnetic resonance imaging in the spinal column and craniovertebral junction. Radiol Clin North Am 22:805-827

201. Ruscalleda J, Rovira A, Guardia E et al (1984) Short review of CT in the study of some intraspinal diseases. Neuroradiology 26:421-427

202. Huk WJ, Gademann G (1984) Magnetic resonance imaging (MRI): method and early clinical experiences in diseases of the central nervous system. Neurosurg Rev 7:259-280

203. Han JS, Kaufman B, El Yousef SJ et al (1983) NMR imaging of the spine. AJR Am J Roentgenol 141:1137-1145

204. Gardner WJ, Bell HS, Poolos PN et al (1977) Terminal ventriculostomy for syringomyelia. J Neurosurg 46:609-617

205. Gold LH, Leach CG, Kieffer SA et al (1970) Large-volume myelography. An aid in the evaluation of curvatures of the spine. Radiology 97:531-536

206. Quinones-Hinojosa A, Gadkary CA, Gulati M et al (2004) Neurophysiological monitoring for safe surgical tethered cord syndrome release in adults. Surg Neurol 62:127-133; discussion 133-125

207. Tsutsumi S, Wachi A, Uto A et al (2000) Infantile arachnoid cyst compressing the sacral nerve root associated with spina bifida and lipoma-case report. Neurol Med Chir (Tokyo) 40:435-438

208. Parlier-Cuau C, Wybier M, Laredo JD (1997) [Secret information provided by lumbosacral myelography]. Ann Radiol (Paris) 40:215-224

209. Meinck HM (1992) Isolated muscle hypertrophy as a sign of radicular or peripheral nerve injury. J Neurol Neurosurg Psychiatry 55:1220-1221

210. Madersbacher H, Ebner A (1992) [Neurogenic disorders of bladder emptying in closed spinal dysraphism]. Urologe A 31:347-353

211. Korsvik HE, Keller MS (1992) Sonography of occult dysraphism in neonates and infants with MR imaging correlation. Radiographics 12:297-306; discussion 307-298

212. Friedli WG, Gratzl O, Radu EW (1992) Lipoma of the cauda equina selectively involving lower sacral roots. Case report. Eur Neurol 32:267-269

213. Barolat G, Schaefer D, Zeme S (1991) Recurrent spinal cord tethering by sacral nerve root following lipomyelomeningocele surgery. Case report. J Neurosurg 75:143-145

214. Roth-Vargas AA, Rossitti SL, Balbo RJ et al (1989) So-called tethered cervical spinal cord. Neurochirurgia (Stuttg) 32:69-71

215. Husson JL, Chales G, Lancien G et al (1987) True intra-articular lipoma of the lumbar spine. Spine 12:820-822

216. D'Haens J, Noterman J, Gerard JM et al (1987) Thoracic spinal epidural cysts. Surg Neurol 27:264-268

217. Stadnik T, De Moor J, Parizel P et al (1986) Diagnostic evaluation of lumbo-sacral lipomas by CT and radiculosaccography. Report of 2 cases and review of the literature. J Belge Radiol 69:87-90

218. Talwalkar VC, Dastur DK (1985) Meningoceles and neurological involvement. Z Kinderchir 40:7-12

219. Marks SM, Miles JB, Shaw MD (1985) Idiopathic spinal extradural lipomas: three cases and review of the literature. Surg Neurol 23:153-156

220. Pilo de la Fuente B, Corral Corral I, Vazquez Miralles JM et al (2007) [Tethered cord syndrome in the adult]. Neurologia 22:201-205

221. Makhoul IR, Soudack M, Kochavi O et al (2007) Anophthalmia-plus syndrome: a clinical report and review of the literature. Am J Med Genet A 143:64-68

222. Nayak PK, Mahapatra AK (2006) Frontal bone agenesis in a patient of spinal dysraphism. Pediatr Neurosurg 42:171-173

223. Pascual-Castroviejo I, Pascual-Pascual SI, Velazquez-Fragua R et al (2005) Oculocerebrocutaneous (Delleman) syndrome: report of two cases. Neuropediatrics 36:50-54

224. Rawashdeh YF, Jorgensen TM, Olsen LH et al (2004) The outcome of detrusor myotomy in children with neurogenic bladder dysfunction. J Urol 171:2654-2656

225. Hughes JA, De Bruyn R, Patel K et al (2003) Evaluation of spinal ultrasound in spinal dysraphism. Clin Radiol 58:227-233

226. Torre M, Planche D, Louis-Borrione C et al (2002) Value of electrophysiological assessment after surgical treatment of spinal dysraphism. J Urol 168:1759-1762; discussion 1763

227. Masjuan Vallejo J, Herrero Valverde AM, Martinez San Millan J et al (2001) [Progressive amyotrophy of a limb as the presenting symptom of anchored spinal cord syndrome with spinal lipoma]. Rev Neurol 32:437-440

228. Jindal A, Mahapatra AK, Kamal R (1999) Spinal dysraphism. Indian J Pediatr 66:697-705

229. Truong BC, Shaw DW, Winters WD (1998) Dilation of the ventriculus terminalis: sonographic findings. J Ultrasound Med 17:713-715

230. Guardiola A, Prates LZ, Ribeiro Mde C et al (1999) [Paraplegia as initial manifestation of tethered spinal cord. Case report]. Arq Neuropsiquiatr 57:101-105

231. Shaul DB, Harrison EA (1997) Classification of anorectal malformations-initial approach, diagnostic tests, and colostomy. Semin Pediatr Surg 6:187-195

232. Muthukumar N (1996) Surgical treatment of non-progressive neurological deficits in children with sacral agenesis. Neurosurgery 38:1133-1137; discussion 1137-1138

233. O'Neill OR, Piatt JH, Jr., Mitchell P et al (1995) Agenesis and dysgenesis of the sacrum: neurosurgical implications. Pediatr Neurosurg 22:20-28

234. Kakizaki H, Nonomura K, Asano Y et al (1994) Pre-existing neurogenic voiding dysfunction in children with imperforate anus: problems in management. J Urol 151:1041-1044

235. Pang D (1993) Sacral agenesis and caudal spinal cord malformations. Neurosurgery 32:755-778; discussion 778-759

236. Bollini G, Cottalorda J, Jouve JL et al (1993) [Closed spinal dysraphism]. Ann Pediatr (Paris) 40:197-210

237. Jamil M, Bannister CM (1992) A report of children with spinal dysraphism managed conservatively. Eur J Pediatr Surg 2 Suppl 1:26-28

238. Rothwell CI, Forbes WS, Gupta SC (1987) Computed tomographic myelography in the investigation of childhood scoliosis and spinal dysraphism. Br J Radiol 60:1197-1204

239. Altman N, Harwood-Nash DC, Fitz CR et al (1985) Evaluation of the infant spine by direct sagittal computed tomography. AJNR Am J Neuroradiol 6:65-69

240. Tihansky DP, Hafeez M (1984) Case report: CT findings in lumbosacral agenesis. J Comput Tomogr 8:325-329

241. Hafeez M, Tihansky DP (1984) Intraspinal tumor with lumbosacral agenesis. AJNR Am J Neuroradiol 5:481-482

242. Naidich TP, McLone DG, Shkolnik A et al (1983) Sonographic evaluation of caudal spine anomalies in children. AJNR Am J Neuroradiol 4:661-664

243. Roller GJ, Pribram HF (1965) Lumbosacral intradural lipoma and sacral agenesis. Radiology 84:507-512

244. James HE, Lubinsky G (2005) Terminal myelocystocele. J Neurosurg 103:443-445

245. Valentini LG, Visintini S, Mendola C et al (2005) The role of intraoperative electromyographic monitoring in lumbosacral lipomas. Neurosurgery 56:315-323; discussion 315-323

246. Mosiello G, Gatti C, De Gennaro M et al (2003) Neurovesical dysfunction in children after treating pelvic neoplasms. BJU Int 92:289-292

247. Tubbs RS, Wellons JC, 3rd, Oakes WJ (2003) Occipital encephalocele, lipomeningomyelocele, and Chiari I malformation: case report and review of the literature. Childs Nerv Syst 19:50-53

248. Barrero-Hernandez FJ, Salazar-Gravan S, Ortega-Molina MJ et al (2002) [Recurrent meningitis as a manifestation of spinal dysraphism in a young adult]. Rev Neurol 35:827-831

249. Ersahin Y, Barcin E, Mutluer S (2001) Is meningocele really an isolated lesion? Childs Nerv Syst 17:487-490

250. Riebel T, Maurer J, Teichgraber UK et al (1999) The spectrum of imaging in Currarino triad. Eur Radiol 9:1348-1353

251. Sakho Y, Badiane SB, Kabre A et al (1998) [Lumbosacral intraspinal lipomas associated or not with a tethered cord syndrome (series of 8 cases)]. Dakar Med 43:13-20

252. Bektas H, Ehrenheim C, Hofmann U et al (1994) [Value of magnetic resonance tomography in diagnosis of tethered cord syndrome in children]. Bildgebung 61:72-80

253. Lewonowski K, King JD, Nelson MD (1992) Routine use of magnetic resonance imaging in idiopathic scoliosis patients less than eleven years of age. Spine 17:S109-116

254. Konner C, Gassner I, Mayr U et al (1990) [Diagnosis of diastematomyelia using ultrasound]. Klin Padiatr 202:124-128

255. Gabay C, van Linthoudt D, Ott H (1989) [Lumbosacral spina bifida associated with an intraspinal lipoma]. Schweiz Med Wochenschr 119:1604-1608

256. Zumkeller M, Seifert V, Stolke D (1989) [Spinal dysraphia and disordered ascension of the spinal cord in adults]. Z Orthop Ihre Grenzgeb 127:336-342

257. Eichler I, Ungersbock K, Waldhauser F et al (1986) [Spinal lipoma with a dural closure defect as a cause of neurogenic bladder and chronic renal failure]. Z Urol Nephrol 79:213-217

258. Isu T, Ito T, Iwasaki Y et al (1979) [Computed tomography in the diagnosis of spinal disease (author's transl)]. No Shinkei Geka 7:1171-1178

259. Selosse P, Granieri U (1968) [Intraspinal lipoma associated with a syndrome of complex craniospinal malformations]. Acta Neurol Psychiatr Belg 68:287-297

260. Cecotto C, De Vito R, Schiavi F et al (1968) [Anterior and posterior myelovertebral malformations]. Minerva Neurochir 12:43-105

261. Rauzzino MJ, Tubbs RS, Alexander E, 3rd et al (2001) Spinal neurenteric cysts and their relation to more common aspects of occult spinal dysraphism. Neurosurg Focus 10:e2

262. Incesu L, Karaismailoglu TN, Selcuk MB (2004) Neurologically normal complete asymmetric lumbar spine duplication. AJNR Am J Neuroradiol 25:895-896

263. Morcuende JA, Dolan LA, Vazquez JD et al (2004) A prognostic model for the presence of neurogenic lesions in atypical idiopathic scoliosis. Spine 29:51-58

264. Pathi R, Kiley M, Sage M (2003) Isolated spinal cord lipoma. J Clin Neurosci 10:692-694

265. Maiuri F, Gangemi M, Cavallo LM et al (2003) Dysembryogenetic spinal tumours in adults without dysraphism. Br J Neurosurg 17:234-238

266. Schizas C, Ballesteros C, Roy P (2003) Cauda equina compression after trauma: an unusual presentation of spinal epidural lipoma. Spine 28:E148-151

267. Botwin KP, Shah CP, Zak PJ (2001) Sciatic neuropathy secondary to infiltrating intermuscular lipoma of the thigh. Am J Phys Med Rehabil 80:754-758

268. Razack N, Jimenez OF, Aldana P et al (1998) Intramedullary holocord lipoma in an athlete: case report. Neurosurgery 42:394-396; discussion 396-397

269. Da Silva LF, Robin S, Guegan-Massardier E et al (1997) Peripheral neurological involvement as the first manifestation of spina bifida occulta. Rev Rhum Engl Ed 64:839-842

270. Kim SK, Chung YS, Wang KC et al (1994) Diastematomyelia-clinical manifestation and treatment outcome. J Korean Med Sci 9:135-144

271. Preul MC, Leblanc R, Tampieri D et al (1993) Spinal angiolipomas. Report of three cases. J Neurosurg 78:280-286

272. Heary RF, Bhandari Y (1991) Intradural cervical lipoma in a neurologically intact patient: case report. Neurosurgery 29:468-472

273. Maiuri F, Corriero G, Gallicchio B et al (1987) Late neurological dysfunction in adult lumbosacral lipoma. J Neurosurg Sci 31:7-11

274. Linder M, Rosenstein J, Sklar FH (1982) Functional improvement after spinal surgery for the dysraphic malformations. Neurosurgery 11:622-624

275. Fearnside MR, Adams CB (1978) Tumours of the cauda equina. J Neurol Neurosurg Psychiatry 41:24-31

276. Subramaniam P, Behari S, Singh S et al (2002) Multiple subpial lipomas with dumb-bell extradural extension through the intervertebral foramen without spinal dysraphism. Surg Neurol 58:338-343; discussion 343

277. Buffa P, Di Rovasenda E, Scarsi PL et al (1997) Vesico sphincteric function in spinal lipomas. Review of 80 cases. Eur J Pediatr Surg 7 Suppl 1:59-60

278. Mimata C, Wada H, Sano Y et al (1992) [Spinal extradural angiolipoma: a case report]. No Shinkei Geka 20:1085-1089

279. Shinomiya K, Fuchioka M, Matsuoka T et al (1991) Intraoperative monitoring for tethered spinal cord syndrome. Spine 16:1290-1294

280. Onishi N, Kiwamoto H, Esa A et al (1989) [Neurogenic bladder dysfunction due to tethered spinal cord syndrome in adults: report of two cases]. Hinyokika Kiyo 35:1229-1234

281. Martino A, Lomiento D (1987) [A case of neurogenic bladder caused by spinal cord traction in childhood. Diagnostic and therapeutic aspects]. Pediatr Med Chir 9:243-246

282. Raco A, Ciappetta P, Mariottini A (1987) Lumbosacral lipoma causing tethering of the conus: case report. Ital J Neurol Sci 8:59-62

283. Rockswold GL, Bradley WE, Timm GW et al (1976) Electrophysiological technique for evaluating lesions of the conus medullaris and cauda equina. J Neurosurg 45:321-326

284. Martinet P, M'Bappe P, Lebreton C et al (1999) Neuropathic arthropathy: a forgotten diagnosis? Two recent cases involving the hip. Rev Rhum Engl Ed 66:284-287

285. Pippi Salle JL, Capolicchio G, Houle AM et al (1998) Magnetic resonance imaging in children with voiding dysfunction: is it indicated? J Urol 160:1080-1083

286. Prandota J, Jarlinska M (1996) [Orthopedic foot abnormalities as a important sign of lumbosacral spinal lipoma in an 11-year-old boy]. Pediatr Pol 71:153-156

287. Lejman T, Harasiewicz M, Sulko J et al (1996) [Orthopedic problems in children after surgical treatment for lipoma of the conus medullaris]. Chir Narzadow Ruchu Ortop Pol 61:39-45

288. Herman JM, McLone DG, Storrs BB et al (1993) Analysis of 153 patients with myelomeningocele or spinal lipoma reoperated upon for a tethered cord. Presentation, management and outcome. Pediatr Neurosurg 19:243-249

289. Tadmor R, Ravid M, Findler G et al (1985) Importance of early radiologic diagnosis of congenital anomalies of the spine. Surg Neurol 23:493-501

290. Garat JM, Aragona F, Martinez E (1985) [Neurogenic bladder caused by spinal cord traction]. J Urol (Paris) 91:145-154

291. Merx JL, Thijssen HO, Bakker-Niezen SH (1983) Tethered conus medullaris in metrizamide myelography. Diagn Imaging 52:179-188

292. Paul DF, Morrey BF, Helms CA (1979) Computerized tomography in orthopedic surgery. Clin Orthop Relat Res 139:142-149

293. Pang D, Wilberger JE Jr (1982) Tethered cord syndrome in adults. J Neurosurg 57:32-47

294. Oi S, Sato O, Matsumoto S (1996) Neurological and medico-social problems of spina bifida patients in adolescence and adulthood. Childs Nerv Syst 12:181-187

295. Di Lorenzo N, Giuffre R, Fortuna A (1982) Primary spinal neoplasms in childhood: analysis of 1234 published cases (including 56 personal cases) by pathology, sex, age and site. Differences from the situation in adults. Neurochirurgia (Stuttg) 25:153-164

296. Thomas JE, Miller RH (1973) Lipomatous tumors of the spinal canal. A study of their clinical range. Mayo Clin Proc 48:393-400

297. Kennedy R (1926) An unusual rectal polyp. Anterior sacral meningocele. Surg Gynecol Obstet 43:803-804

298. Ashkraft K, Holder T (1965) Congenital anal stenosis with presacral teratoma. Ann Surg 162:1091-1095

299. Currarino G, Coln D, Votteler T (1981) Triad of anorectal, sacral, and presacral anomalies. AJR Am J Roentgenol 137:395-398

300. Liang Y, Wang J, Cai W (2007) Clinical features and HLXB9 gene mutation of a sporadic Chinese Currarino's syndrome case. J Pediatr Surg 42:E27-30

301. Nowaczyk MJ, Huggins MJ, Tomkins DJ et al (2000) Holoprosencephaly, sacral anomalies, and situs ambiguus in an infant with partial monosomy 7q/trisomy 2p and SHH and HLXB9 haploinsufficiency. Clin Genet 57:388-393

302. Papadias A, Miller C, Martin WL et al (2008) Comparison of prenatal and postnatal MRI findings in the evaluation of intrauterine CNS anomalies requiring postnatal neurosurgical treatment. Childs Nerv Syst 24:185-192

303. Thorne A, Pierre-Kahn A, Sonigo P (2001) Antenatal diagnosis of spinal lipomas. Childs Nerv Syst 17:697-703

304. Kim SY, McGahan JP, Boggan JE et al (2000) Prenatal diagnosis of lipomyelomeningocele. J Ultrasound Med 19:801-805

305. Sharony R, Aviram R, Tohar M et al (2000) Prenatal sonographic detection of a lipomeningocele as a sacral lesion. J Clin Ultrasound 28:150-152

306. Sattar TS, Bannister CM, Russell SA et al (1998) Prenatal diagnosis of occult spinal dysraphism by ultrasonography and post-natal evaluation by MR scanning. Eur J Pediatr Surg 8 Suppl 1:31-33

307. Chreston J, Sherman SJ (1997) Sonographic detection of lipomyelomeningocele: a retrospective documentation. J Clin Ultrasound 25:50-51

308. Seeds JW, Jones FD (1986) Lipomyelomeningocele: prenatal diagnosis and management. Obstet Gynecol 67:34S-37S

309. Morgan LW, Toal R, Siemering G et al (2007) Imaging diagnosis-infiltrative lipoma causing spinal cord compression in a dog. Vet Radiol Ultrasound 48:35-37

310. Azzoni R, Gerevini S, Cabitza P (2005) Spinal cord sonography in newborns: anatomy and diseases. J Pediatr Orthop B 14:185-188

311. Leung EC, Sgouros S, Williams S et al (2002) Spinal lipoma misinterpreted as a meningomyelocele on antenatal MRI scan in a baby girl. Childs Nerv Syst 18:361-363

312. Lin KL, Wang HS, Chou ML et al (2002) Sonography for detection of spinal dermal sinus tracts. J Ultrasound Med 21:903-907

313. Dick EA, de Bruyn R, Patel K et al (2001) Spinal ultrasound in cloacal exstrophy. Clin Radiol 56:289-294

314. Tsakayannis DE, Shamberger RC (1995) Association of imperforate anus with occult spinal dysraphism. J Pediatr Surg 30:1010-1012

315. Ritchey ML, Sinha A, DiPietro MA et al (1994) Significance of spina bifida occulta in children with diurnal enuresis. J Urol 152:815-818

316. Tenner MS (1994) Case of the day. 1. Diagnosis: tethered spinal cord with hydromyelia terminating at a lipoma. J Ultrasound Med 13:329-330

317. Boop FA, Russell A, Chadduck WM (1992) Diagnosis and management of the tethered cord syndrome. J Ark Med Soc 89:328-331

318. Avni EF, Matos C, Grassart A et al (1991) [Neonatal pilonidal sinuses and screening by medullary ultrasonography: preliminary results]. Pediatrie 46:607-611

319. Zieger M, Dorr U, Schulz RD (1988) Pediatric spinal sonography. Part II: Malformations and mass lesions. Pediatr Radiol 18:105-111

320. Vogl D, Ring-Mrozik E, Baierl P et al (1987) Magnetic resonance imaging in children suffering from spina bifida. Z Kinderchir 42 Suppl 1:60-64

321. Miller JH, Reid BS, Kemberling CR (1982) Utilization of ultrasound in the evaluation of spinal dysraphism in children. Radiology 143:737-740

322. Beall DP, Googe DJ, Emery RL et al (2007) Extramedullary intradural spinal tumors: a pictorial review. Curr Probl Diagn Radiol 36:185-198

323. Erdogan C, Hakyemez B, Arat A et al (2007) Spinal dural arteriovenous fistula in a case with lipomyelodysplasia. Br J Radiol 80:e98-e100

324. Weon YC, Chung JI, Roh HG et al (2005) Combined spinal intramedullary arteriovenous malformation and lipomyelomeningocele. Neuroradiology 47:774-779

325. Choi JY, Goo JM, Chung MJ et al (2000) Angiolipoma of the posterior mediastinum with extension into the spinal canal: a case report. Korean J Radiol 1:212-214

326. Freund M, Thale A, Hutzelmann A (1998) Radiologic and histopathologic findings in a rare case of complex occult spinal dysraphism with association of a lumbar fibrolipoma, neurenteric cyst and tethered cord syndrome. Eur Radiol 8:624-627

327. Matsubayashi R, Uchino A, Kato A et al (1998) Cystic dilatation of ventriculus terminalis in adults: MRI. Neuroradiology 40:45-47

328. Behari S, Banerji D, Gupta RK et al (1997) Problems in differentiating intradural lipoma from dermoid on magnetic resonance imaging. Australas Radiol 41:196-198

329. Schubert F (1996) Intradural lipoma. Australas Radiol 40:61-64

330. Brunelle F, Sebag G, Baraton J et al (1996) Lumbar spinal cord motion measurement with phase-contrast MR imaging in normal children and in children with spinal lipomas. Pediatr Radiol 26:265-270

331. Coulier B, Mailleux P (1994) [Lipoma of the filum terminale: a prospective tomodensitometry study]. J Belge Radiol 77:116-118

332. Kaffenberger DA, Heinz ER, Oakes JW et al (1992) Meningocele manque: radiologic findings with clinical correlation. AJNR Am J Neuroradiol 13:1083-1088

333. Mascalchi M, Arnetoli G, Dal Pozzo G et al (1991) Spinal epidural angiolipoma: MR findings. AJNR Am J Neuroradiol 12:744-745

334. Just M, Schwarz M, Ludwig B et al (1990) Cerebral and spinal MR-findings in patients with postrepair myelomeningocele. Pediatr Radiol 20:262-266

335. Tortori-Donati P, Cama A, Rosa ML et al (1990) Occult spinal dysraphism: neuroradiological study. Neuroradiology 31:512-522

336. Morano JU, Miller JD, Connors JJ (1989) MR imaging of spinal epidural lipoma. AJNR Am J Neuroradiol 10:S102

337. Corr P, Beningfield SJ (1989) Magnetic resonance imaging of an intradural spinal lipoma: a case report. Clin Radiol 40:216-218

338. Taviere V, Brunelle F, Baraton J et al (1989) MRI study of lumbosacral lipoma in children. Pediatr Radiol 19:316-320

339. Fan CJ, Veerapen RJ, Tan CT (1989) Subdural spinal lipoma with posterior fossa extension. Clin Radiol 40:91-94

340. Wright JF, Powell S, Williams MP (1988) Spinal cord compression caused by dual pathology: a close shave with Ockham's razor. Clin Radiol 39:558-559

341. Cecchini A, Locatelli D, Bonfanti N et al (1988) Lipomyelomeningoceles: a neuroradiological approach. J Neuroradiol 15:49-61

342. Altman NR, Altman DH (1987) MR imaging of spinal dysraphism. AJNR Am J Neuroradiol 8:533-538

343. Wippold FJ, Citrin C, Barkovich AJ et al (1987) Evaluation of MR in spinal dysraphism with lipoma: comparison with metrizamide computed tomography. Pediatr Radiol 17:184-188

344. McConnell JR, Holder JC, Mawk JR et al (1986) Spina bifida: the radiology of neural tube defects. Curr Probl Diagn Radiol 15:241-276

345. Gawehn J, Schroth G, Thron A (1986) The value of paraxial slices in MR-imaging of spinal cord disease. Neuroradiology 28:347-350

346. Tadmor R, New PF, Shoukimas G et al (1986) Magnetic resonance imaging of the thoracical spinal cord and spine with surface coils. Acta Radiol Suppl 369:475-480

347. Dooms GC, Hricak H, Sollitto RA et al (1985) Lipomatous tumors and tumors with fatty component: MR imaging potential and comparison of MR and CT results. Radiology 157:479-483

348. Maher CO, Goumnerova L, Madsen JR et al (2007) Outcome following multiple repeated spinal cord untethering operations. J Neurosurg 106:434-438

349. Colak A, Pollack IF, Albright AL (1998) Recurrent tethering: a common long-term problem after lipomyelomeningocele repair. Pediatr Neurosurg 29:184-190

350. Souweidane MM, Drake JM (1998) Retethering of sectioned fibrolipomatous filum terminales: report of two cases. Neurosurgery 42:1390-1393

351. Vernet O, O'Gorman AM, Farmer JP et al (1996) Use of the prone position in the MRI evaluation of spinal cord retethering. Pediatr Neurosurg 25:286-294

352. Goel A, Pandya SK (1993) A shunting procedure for cerebrospinal fluid fistula, employing cannulation of the third and fourth ventricles. Br J Neurosurg 7:299-302

353. O'Neill P, Stack JP (1990) Magnetic resonance imaging in the pre-operative assessment of closed spinal dysraphism in children. Pediatr Neurosurg 16:240-246

354. Hoffman HJ, Taecholarn C, Hendrick EB et al (1985) Management of lipomyelomeningoceles. Experience at the Hospital for Sick Children, Toronto. J Neurosurg 62:1-8

355. Kanev PM, Lemire RJ, Loeser JD et al (1990) Management and long-term follow-up review of children with lipomyelomeningocele, 1952-1987. J Neurosurg 73:48-52

356. Takei K, Suzuki K, Kito H et al (2006) [Two cases of adult tethered cord syndrome with surgical treatment]. Hinyokika Kiyo 52:841-844

357. Harashima S, Taira T, Hori T (2004) [Adult type tethered cord syndrome with chronic attackwise pain in the bilateral feet]. No Shinkei Geka 32:481-485

358. Marushima A, Matsumura A, Fujita K et al (2003) Adult tethered cord syndrome presenting with refractory diarrhoea. J Neurol Neurosurg Psychiatry 74:1596-1597

359. Izumikawa Y (2001) [Lipomeningocele]. Ryoikibetsu Shokogun Shirizu:109

360. Hatayama T, Sakoda K, Tokuda Y et al (1992) [An adult case of intradural lumbo-sacral lipoma]. No Shinkei Geka 20:1075-1078

361. Sperke N, Spring A, Weis G et al (1990) [Tethered cord syndrome in adults as a cause of disorders of bladder function]. Urologe A 29:345-347

362. Yamamura A, Niwa J, Hashi K et al (1989) [Tethered cord syndrome of adult onset: report of a case and a review of the literature]. No Shinkei Geka 17:69-73

363. Lesoin F, Petit H, Destee A et al (1984) Spinal dysraphia and elongated spinal cord in adults. Surg Neurol 21:119-124

364. Boccon-Gibod L, Pierre Kahn A, Hurel JP (1984) [Occult spinal dysraphia with urologic manifestations in adults. 6 cases]. Ann Urol (Paris) 18:17-20

365. Negoro M, Freidberg SR, Yamada H et al (1981) [A case of intradual lumbo-sacral lipona in adult (author's transl)]. No Shinkei Geka 9:410-414

366. Loeser JD, Lewin RJ (1968) Lumbosacral lipoma in the adult: case report. J Neurosurg 29:405-409

367. Lagae L, Verpoorten C, Casaer P et al (1990) Conservative versus neurosurgical treatment of tethered cord patients. Z Kinderchir 45 suppl 1:16-17

368. Iskandar BJ, Oakes WJ, McLaughlin C et al (1994) Terminal syringohydromyelia and occult spinal dysraphism. J Neurosurg 81:513-519

369. Sakamoto H, Hakuba A, Fujitani K, Nishimura S (1991) Surgical treatment of the retethered spinal cord after repair of lipomyelomeningocele. J Neurosurg 74:709-714

CHAPTER 37
Neurenteric Cysts

Ricardo Santos de Oliveira, Giuseppe Cinalli, Christian Sainte-Rose, Helio Rubens Machado, Michel Zerah

Introduction

Neurenteric or enterogenous cysts are uncommon congenital lesions that result from displaced elements of the alimentary canal and are commonly encountered in the posterior mediastinum. These cysts can occur at any level of the neuraxis from the posterior clinoid to the coccyx; they are most commonly found in the lower cervical and upper thoracic regions [1-4]. The lesions are generally located ventral to the spinal cord and at the cervicomedullary junction [1, 5].

The first intraspinal endodermal cyst that was histologically verified was reported by Puusepp [4] and termed "intestinoma" in 1934, but prior to this some authors [6, 7] described a typical case of neurenteric cyst that they designated as a teratomatous cyst of the spinal cord. After the description by Puusepp, the first account of a pediatric cyst of this nature verified histologically was published in 1937 in an autopsy case [8].

The mesodermal disturbance is often reflected by the presence of associated vertebral body anomalies [9, 10]. The cysts consist of mucin-producing, nonciliated epithelium that is simple or pseudostratified and either cuboidal or columnar [11, 12]. The patients may present neurologically with signs of spinal cord compression and meningitis [13], but the clinical symptoms associated with neurenteric cysts depend on the site of the lesion [14, 15].

Classification

There are some discrepancies in the literature regarding the classification of neurenteric cysts in relation to their embryological origin [16]. It is generally accepted that they are lesions of spina bifida occulta typically consisting of an intradural cyst lined by mucin-producing nonciliated epithelium that is simple or pseudostratified (columnar or cuboidal) [17]. The cyst can be ciliated or it can have a mixture of gastrointestinal, pancreatic, and/or squamous epithelium (Fig. 37.1) [1, 12, 18]. Some authors have analyzed scanning electron microscopy images of such cysts and described a possible relation to the respiratory tract [19]. These cysts represent 0.3-0.5% of spinal tumors [20, 21].

In 1929, Feller and Sternberg [22] reviewed a series of infants born with varying degrees of central nervous system (CNS) and intestinal anomalies. They concluded that the neurenteric anomalies appeared after the development of the notochord and the neural tube from a group of cells arising from Hensen's node. They defined a classification for these anomalies. In 1976, neurenteric cysts were reclassified into three types by Wilkins and Odom [12] based on histological features. Type A cysts are lined by a single layer of pseudostratified cuboidal or columnar epithelial cells that mimic gastrointestinal or respiratory epithelium; they appear with or without cilia lying on a basement membrane and are supported by a layer of vascular connective tissue. Type B cysts, constituted by epithelial lining, may be arranged in complex invaginations and have a glandular organization, usually producing mucinous or serous fluid, smooth muscle, striated muscle, fat, cartilage, bone, elastic fibers, lymphoid tissue, nerve fibers, ganglion cells, or Vater–Pacini corpuscles. Type C cysts, the most complex, contain ependymal or glial tissue [23].

Immunohistochemical studies have an important role in the diagnosis of these lesions [24]. Defects in vertebral bodies and intra-abdominal or intrathoracic cysts are frequently encountered in association with these cysts [25]. Neurenteric cysts can be classified based on the relative positions in the spinal cord, vertebral column, and alimentary canal [2]. This classification is applicable to the more severe forms of the anomaly. For anomalies of a lesser degree, the classification of Smith is more practical [26]. This classification comes under the rubric of split noto-

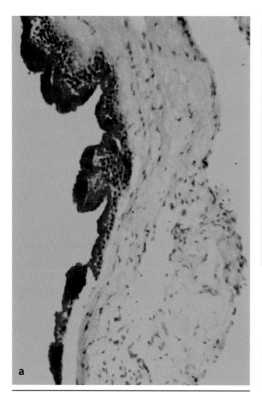

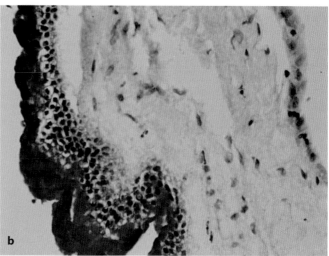

Fig. 37.1 a, b. a Photomicrograph of the cystic lesion (hematoxylin-eosin; original magnification × 200). **b** The wall of the cyst was lined by cuboidal to columnar epithelial cells with intermingled goblet and ciliated cells in the inner layer of the cyst wall

chord syndrome [27, 28, 52] because the concept seems basic to the mechanism underlying the communication between the endoderm and the dorsum of the embryo [29]. The spectrum of anomalies according to Smith's classification includes alimentary diverticula through to prevertebral posterior enteric cysts, to vertebral body malformations with intraspinal cyst, to posterior spina bifida and dermal sinus [27, 30].

Clinical Presentation

In the pediatric age there is a male predominance (60.4%) with a mean age of 6.4 years and a median age of 6 years [21, 31, 49]. Clinically, the more complicated lesions tend to present earlier in life. The mediastinal forms can promote respiratory distress in a newborn [32, 33] or combined neurological symptoms [34-36, 54].

On neurological presentation a patient with these cysts displays no characteristic clinical findings, nor is a particular history associated with this disease. Neurologically, the patients present during the first decade of life with pain and myelopathy [9, 15, 37-39] arising from spinal cord compression [10]. In some cases, neurological signs can be insidious or even absent, despite severe compression of the spinal

cord [40-43]. Meningitis has been the presenting feature in newborns and infants [5, 44] and its symptoms have ranged from low-grade meningeal irritation [45] caused by cystic fluid leakage, to acute pyogenic meningitis [34, 46, 47] with extensive intraspinal and intramedullary abscesses [5]. Meningitis can be found in up to 4.6% of the cases [49]. Ein et al. [48] described a pediatric case of osteomyelitis of the cervical spine that was mistakenly noted to be a neurenteric cyst initially.

Acute neurological deterioration from neurenteric cysts has been described in more than 40% of the cases reported in the literature [24, 45, 50, 53, 56]. This is thought to be due to sudden mechanical compression of a chronically distorted and compressed spinal cord, or an increase in the size of the cyst as the result of an accumulation of intracystic fluid [10, 38, 55]. A history of trauma or repeated infections has been reported [49].

The cranial forms of neurenteric cysts are rarer in the pediatric population [57, 58] and have been described in the posterior fossa [57, 59], at the level of the craniocervical junction [5, 60, 61], within the brainstem [62], and in the cavernous sinus [49].

Neurenteric cysts are most frequently found in the posterior mediastinum [1, 12, 33] and can give rise to neurological defects [18, 63-69]. Superina et al. [69] published a series that included cystic duplications of the esophagus and neurenteric cysts. The series consisted of a total of 15 chest masses and eight lesions of the CNS. They concluded that a spinal component may accompany the mediastinal cyst in as many as 20% of cases and they suggested systematic radiological examination of the spinal canal in cases of chest masses.

In one third of the patients, neurenteric cysts are associated with complex malformations of the CNS and/or gastrointestinal tract and can be detected on prenatal ultrasonographic images [32, 70-75]. Durham et al. [76] have demonstrated that neurenteric cysts can be associated with the Currarino Triad.

Agnoli et al. [1] observed that of 33 intraspinal cysts verified histologically, 18 were located in the cervicothoracic spine (80% were intradural extramedullary and 12% were intramedullary). In a review of the pediatric literature [49], these cysts have been found to be midline benign lesions that can occur at any level of the neuraxis. The most commonly found type and location was intradural in the spinal canal in 122 (94.5%) of 129 instances. The intramedullary form represented 13% of the cases and had a cervical and thoracic predominance [3, 11, 13, 77-85]. A schematic drawing shows the neuraxis distribution of neurenteric cyst (Fig. 37.2).

The cysts have been found predominantly ventral to the spinal cord in the cervical and thoracic spinal subarachnoid space, with a lower incidence at the lumbar and sacral levels [5, 9, 27, 40, 43, 45, 56, 60, 86-91, 93, 103-121] and the craniocervical junction [18, 51, 60, 61, 91, 92]. In one pediatric review, however, the cyst was found dorsal to the spinal cord in 70% of the cases [93]. Other less frequent locations of these cysts include the cerebellopontine angle [62, 94-98], and optic nerve [98]. Multiple intracranial cysts have

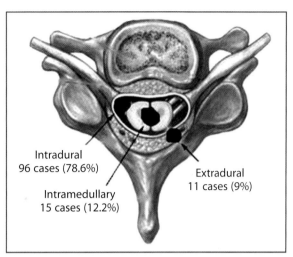

Fig. 37.3. A schematic drawing showing the spinal canal topography of neurenteric cysts in 122 spinal pediatric cases

also been found [99]. A schematic drawing shows the spinal topography of the cyst (Fig. 37.3).

Fusion or malformation of the vertebral bodies at the level of the cyst can occur in up to 50% of patients, and may be associated with intramedullary epidermoid cysts, gastrointestinal tract anomalies (in particular partial duplications of the alimentary tract and fistulas), anal atresia, cardiac anomalies, and renal malformations [100-102].

Radiology

Radiographic diagnosis of neurenteric cysts has included plain spine radiographs, computerized tomography (CT) scans, and magnetic resonance (MR) scans. The frequent bony anomalies mandate a thorough preoperative knowledge of the osseous structures to be encountered during the surgical procedure. Plain x-ray films can disclose a number of deformities of the spine. Ultrasonography could be a useful tool in the diagnosis of spina bifida in neonates [122].

CT scanning and MR imaging may aid in the diagnosis of the neurenteric cyst and associated abnormalities in two respects: the visualization of the cyst itself and the visualization of any associated abnormality [51, 81, 123, 124]. The appearance of the cyst on MR images is that of high protein content without hemorrhage (lower intensity than the spinal cord, higher intensity than cerebrospinal fluid (CSF) on short repetition time spin echo images) [14, 125, 126], resulting more frequently in hypointensity on T1-weighted images and hyperintensity on T2-weighted images (Fig. 37.4) [49].

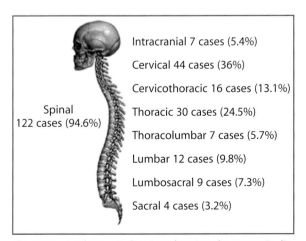

Fig. 37.2. A schematic drawing showing the neuraxis distribution of neurenteric cysts in 129 pediatric cases

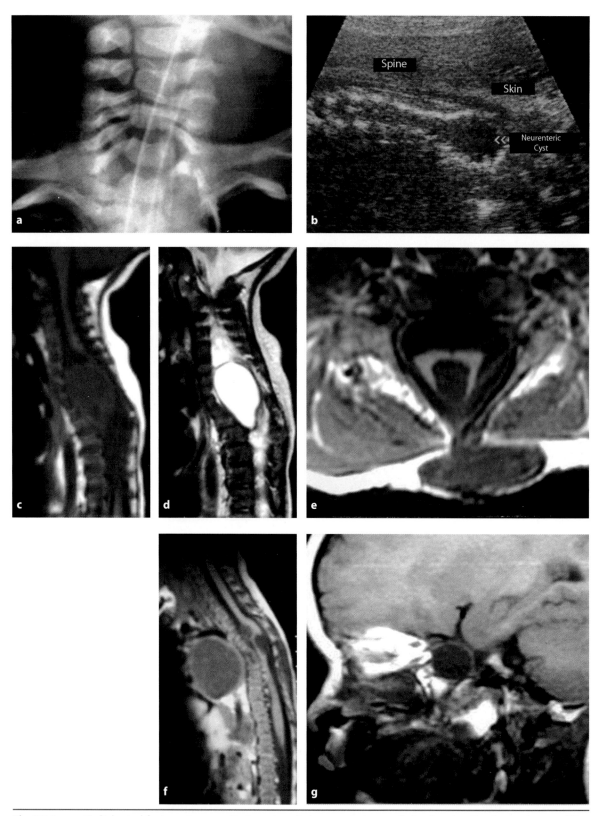

Fig. 37.4 a-g. Radiological features in neurenteric cysts. **a** Antero-posterior cervical spine showing bone abnormalities. **b** Postnatal ultrasonography of the spinal canal showing a dorsal neurenteric cyst. **c** Sagittal T1-weighted and **d** T2-weighted MR scan showing an intradural cyst lying at the level from C5 to T1 and compressing the spinal cord. **e** Axial T1-weighted image of an intradural, dorsal, subcutaneous cyst. **f** Midsagittal T1-weighted image of a mediastinal mass and a prespinal-intramedullary cyst. **g** Sagittal T1-weighted image of an intracavernous cyst

Surgical Treatment

Indications

Complete excision is the aim of surgical intervention. If total removal is achieved, the prognosis is excellent. The surgical management of neurenteric cysts follows the general guidelines for other forms of occult spinal dysraphism. Although the literature purports that the goal of treatment of neurenteric cysts is excision [3, 5, 15, 84, 88, 109], some authors have indicated that its dense adherence to neural structures does not allow for safe total removal [9, 12, 40, 55, 127]. Several authors [38, 50, 83] have described partial excision of intramedullary cysts. Ergun et al. [60] described a partial removal of the anterior lesion in the spinal cord with a T-shaped silastic tube catheter placed to drain the residual cavity to the subarachnoid space. These authors recommended a cystosubarachnoid shunt after partial resection to prevent the possibility of severe neurological deficits due to dense adherence to the neural structures.

Technique and Surgical Approach

The surgical approach to the spinal canal is discussed in the literature, with some authors advocating an anterior approach [9, 31]. These authors reported that total excision of an anterior cyst via a posterior laminectomy is technically difficult without manipulation of the cord, and they recommended an anterior approach to ventral lesions of the spinal canal to avoid the recurrence of the cyst. Menezes and Ryken [5] reported that the posterior approach, due to limited visualization of the cyst walls and the presence of vascular and vertebral bodies, limits the likelihood of complete excision.

The optimal surgical strategy remains controversial. The anterior approach in children is indicated for several reasons: complete resection is easier because the cyst is generally anterior to the spinal cord, and there is less risk of trauma to the spinal cord and of kyphosis. In addition, better management of cases associated with complex vertebral anomalies is possible [55, 66, 128].

On the other hand, a posterior approach has been used as the treatment of choice for some authors [42, 49]. Aggressive removal of the ventrally located cyst may result in spinal cord injury.

We prefer a posterior approach via laminoplasty as a first surgery in all of the spinal cases because this method is technically easier and causes fewer complications for the patient.

After opening the dura mater, the lesion can usually be seen on the side in which the cyst is more visible (although they are usually strictly midline lesions, some asymmetry in the posterior expansion is typically observed), the lesion is gently punctured with a very small needle and the clear fluid content is aspirated slowly to avoid sudden decompression of the spinal cord. After partial aspiration and decompression of the cyst, its wall can be dissected very easily from the spinal roots and from the neural structures of the spinal canal. Often, the spinal cord is so thin that with subtle rotation its anterolateral surface can be easily visualized using adequate inclination of the microscope, allowing gentle dissection of the cyst wall, which is not very adherent in primary cases (i.e., those without previous meningitis). Fig. 37.5 shows a surgical technique in an intramedullary neurenteric cyst.

Except in cases involving previous meningitis (in which adhesions present a problem), the posterior approach can be used in the first instance. There is a consensus in the literature that simple aspiration of the cyst is unacceptable as it generally results in recurrence of the cyst and is unlikely to yield a pathological diagnosis. Incomplete excision may result in excessive scarring and hamper attempts at a repeated excision when the cyst and symptoms recur [5, 25, 116, 127]. On the other hand, Wilkins and Rossitch [127] have indicated that postoperative arachnoiditis is not generally a problem after partial resection. Even if part of the cyst lining remains and the cyst forms again these authors point out that this process may take years to become symptomatic.

Complications

Complications may be observed in up to 23.5% of the cases, namely, diabetes insipidus, CSF leakage and cervical spine deformation despite immobilization, which may require further spine fixation surgery during follow up [49].

One case, misdiagnosed as a retropharyngeal abscess, was surgically addressed five times via the transpharyngeal route. Subsequent referral led to identification of a high-density cystic mass in the clival region. The neurenteric cyst was removed by the transoral route. The patient made an uneventful re-

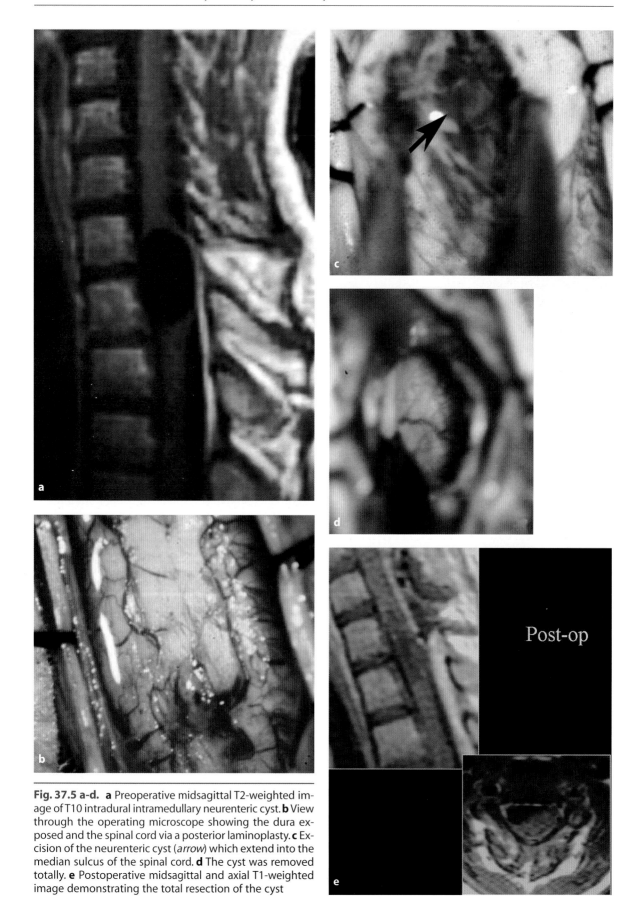

Fig. 37.5 a-d. **a** Preoperative midsagittal T2-weighted image of T10 intradural intramedullary neurenteric cyst. **b** View through the operating microscope showing the dura exposed and the spinal cord via a posterior laminoplasty. **c** Excision of the neurenteric cyst (*arrow*) which extend into the median sulcus of the spinal cord. **d** The cyst was removed totally. **e** Postoperative midsagittal and axial T1-weighted image demonstrating the total resection of the cyst

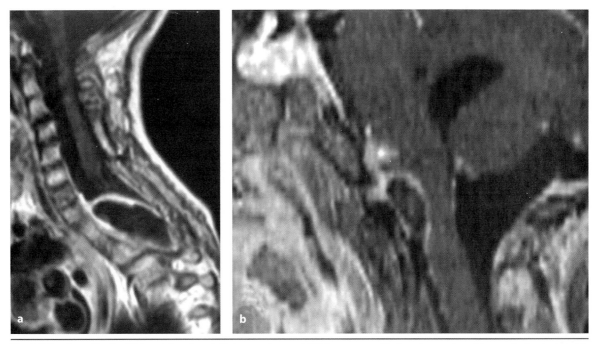

Fig. 37.6 a, b. **a** Sagittal T1-weighted gadolinium-enhanced MR image revealed a recurrent cyst in cervical spine and **b** craniocervical junction with ring enhancement (dense adhesions and scar)

covery and there were no further episodes of meningitis [49]. Similar cases have been described in the literature [5, 47].

Some cases of recurrence have been reported in the literature [6, 8, 19, 31, 57, 63, 79, 83, 93, 110]. Although total removal of the lesion is not always possible, no documented recurrence after such a procedure has been reported in the literature [116]. Chavda et al. [129] reported a recurrence rate of 37% in a series of eight patients (two of whom were pediatric patients) and all recurrences occurred after partial resection of the cyst. The overall recurrence rate in the literature is 11.6%, in all cases due to partial resection of the cyst (Figs. 37.6, 37.7) [49].

Long Term Follow-Up

Early detection and treatment will usually lead to complete neurological recovery [69, 130] but the outcome is not always optimal and authors have reported deaths [35, 63, 66, 102, 103], incomplete recovery with persistence of mild to moderate dysfunction in 18% of the cases and aggravation in 11% of the cases [49]. Recently, Perry and colleagues [132] published reports on widespread craniospinal dissemination associated with the incomplete resection of

neurenteric cysts in the posterior fossa, and, in an adult patient, malignant transformation of a neurenteric cyst that was initially removed in toto into a well-differentiated papillary adenocarcinoma [131, 133].

In conclusion, neurenteric cysts are uncommon congenital anomalies, which may present acutely in the pediatric population. Total removal is usually possible and is associated with a good prognosis.

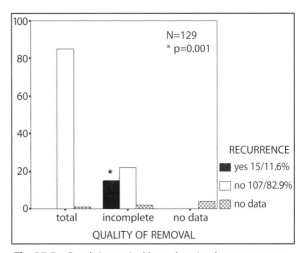

Fig. 37.7. Graph in vertical bars showing how many cases (and percentages) recurred after total removal and the same for incomplete removal. The difference was significant (p=0.001)

References

1. Agnoli AL, Laun A, Schonmayr R (1984) Enterogenous intraspinal cysts. J Neurosurg 61:834-840

2. Batson RA, Scott MR (1986) Neurenteric cysts, teratomatous cysts, teratomas, giant hairy nevi, and their associated anomalies. In: Disorders of the developing nervous system. Diagnosis and treatment, vol 41. Hoffman HJ, Epstein F (eds) Blackwell Scientific Publications, Boston, pp 733-743

3. Odake G, Yamaki T, Naruse S (1976) Neurenteric cyst with meningomyelocele. Case report. J Neurosurg 45:352-356

4. Puusepp M (1934) Variété rare de tératome, sous-dural de la région cervicale (intestinome): Quadriplégie, extirpation, guérison complète. Rev Neurol 2:879-886

5. Menezes AH, Ryken TC (1995) Craniocervical intradural neurenteric cysts. Pediatr Neurosurg 22:88-95

6. Kubie LS, Fulton JFA (1928) A clinical and pathological study of two teratomatous cysts of the spinal cord, containing mucus and ciliated cells. Surg Gynec Obst 48:297-311

7. Bucy PC, Haymond HE (1932) Lumbosacral teratoma associated with spina bifida occulta. Report of a case with review of the literature. Am J Pathol 8:339-345

8. Korff H (1937) Über ein Darmstück in einer Wirbelspalte als Ausdruck einer unvollständigen neurenterischen Verbindung. Arch Path Anat Phys 299:190-202

9. Devkota UP, Lam JM, Ng H et al (1994) An anterior intradural neurenteric cyst of the cervical spine: complete excision through central corpectomy approach-case report. Neurosurgery 35:1150-1154

10. Paleologos TS, Thom M, Thomas DG (2000) Spinal neurenteric cysts without associated malformations. Are they the same as those presenting in spinal dysraphism? Br J Neurosurg 14:185-194

11. Silvernail WI Jr, Brown RB (1972) Intramedullary enterogenous cyst: Case report. J Neurosurg 36:235-238

12. Wilkins RH, Odom GL (1976) Spinal intradural cyst tumors of the spine and spinal cord. In: Vinken PJ, Bruyn GW (eds) Handbook of clinical neurology, vol 20. North-Holland, Amsterdam, pp 55-102

13. Bollini G, Cottalorda J, Jouve JL et al (1993) [Closed spinal dysraphism.] Ann Pediatr (Paris) 40:197-210

14. Geremia GK, Russell EJ, Clasen RA (1988) MR imaging characteristics of a neurenteric cyst. AJNR Am J Neuroradiol 9:978-980

15. Park TS, Kaneu PM, Hanegar MM et al (1996) Occult spinal dysraphism. In: Neurological surgery, vol 2. Youman JR (ed) WB Saunders Co, Philadelphia, pp 873-889

16. Ersahin Y (2002) Thoracolumbar teratoma associated with meningomyelocele: common aetiology or coincidence? Childs Nerv Syst 18:299-301

17. Sarnat HB (1992) Cerebral dysgenesis: Embryology and clinical expression. Oxford University Press, New York

18. Dorsey JF, Tabrisky J (1966) Intraspinal and mediastinal foregut cyst compressing the spinal cord. Report of a case. J Neurosurg 24:562-567

19. Morita Y, Kinoshita K, Wakisaka S et al (1990) Fine surface structure of an intraspinal neurenteric cyst: a scanning and transmission electron microscopy study. Neurosurgery 27:829-833

20. Guilburd JN, Arieh YB, Peyser E (1980) Spinal intradural enterogenous cyst: report of a case. Surg Neurol 14:359-361

21. Sundaram C, Paul TR, Raju BV et al (2001) Cysts of the central nervous system: a clinicopathologic study of 145 cases. Neurol India 49:237-242

22. Feller A, Sternberg H (1929) Zur Kenntnie der Fehlbildungen der Wirbelsaule. I. Die Wirbelkörperspalte und ihre formale Genese. Arch Pathol Anat 272:613-640

23. Gimeno A, Lopez F, Figueira D et al (1972) Neurenteric cyst. Neuroradiology 3:167-172

24. Inoue T, Matsushima T, Fukui M et al (1988) Immunohistochemical study of intracranial cysts. Neurosurgery 23:576-581

25. Lazareff JA, Hoil Parra JA (1995) Intradural neurenteric cyst at the craniovertebral junction. Childs Nerv Syst 11:536-538

26. Smith JR (1960) Accessory enteric formations: a classification and nomenclature. Arch Dis Child 35:87-89

27. Gardner WJ (1973) The dysraphic states: From syringomyelia to anencephaly. Excerpta Medica, Amsterdam, pp 97-111

28. Prop N, Frensdorf EL, van de Stadt FR (1967) A postvertebral entodermal cyst associated with axial deformities: a case showing the "entodermal-ectodermal adhesion syndrome." Pediatrics 39:555-562

29. Nathan MT (1959) Cysts and duplications of neurenteric origin. Pediatrics 23:476-484

30. Langmaid C, Jones R (1963) Enterogeneous cyst of the spinal cord with associated anomalies. J Neurol Neurosurg Psychiatry 26:559 (Abstract)

31. Rauzzino MJ, Tubbs RS, Alexander E III et al (2001) Spinal neurenteric cysts and their relation to more common aspects of occult spinal dysraphism. Neurosurg Focus 10:E2

32. Fernandes ET, Custer MD, Burton EM et al (1991) Neurenteric cyst: surgery and diagnostic imaging. J Pediatr Surg 26:108-110

33. Paterson A, Sweeney LE (1999) Radiological case of the month. Neurenteric cyst. Arch Pediatr Adolesc Med 153:645-646

34. Alrabeeah A, Gillis DA, Giacomantonio M et al (1988) Neurenteric cysts-a spectrum. J Pediatr Surg 23:752-754

35. Chung HD, DeMello DE, D'Souza N et al (1982) Infantile hypoventilation syndrome, neurenteric cyst, and syringobulbia. Neurology 32:441-444

36. Sarkar C, Karaguiosov KL, Simeonov S et al (1996) Spinal enterogeneous cysts: a clinical, morphological

and radiological study of three cases. Ann Saudi Med 16:689-694

37. Fortuna A, Mercuri S (1983) Intradural spinal cysts. Acta Neurochir (Wien) 68:289-314

38. Midha R, Gray B, Becker L et al (1995) Delayed myelopathy after trivial neck injury in a patient with a cervical neurenteric cyst. Can J Neurol Sci 22:168-171

39. Mochida J, Yamada S, Toh E et al (1997) Intradural neurenteric cyst of the cervical spine misdiagnosed as a psychogenic disorder in a 7-year-old-child. Spinal Cord 35:700-703

40. Rebhandl W, Rami B, Barcik U et al (1998) Neurenteric cyst mimicking pleurodynia: an unusual case of thoracic pain in a child. Pediatr Neurol 18:272-274

41. Tubbs RS, Salter EG, Oakes WJ (2006) Neurenteric cyst: case report and a review of the potential dysembryology. Clin Anat 19:669-672

42. Tuzun Y, Izci Y, Sengul G et al (2006) Neurenteric cyst of the upper cervical spine: excision via posterior approach. Pediatr Neurosurg 42:54-56

43. Velasco-Siles JM, Paredes E, Escanero A et al (1986) Spinal cord compression due to cystic duplication of the primitive digestive tract. Childs Nerv Syst 2:157-159

44. Menezes AH Traynelis VC (2006) Spinal neurenteric cyst in the magnetic resonance imaging era. Neurosurgery 58:97-105

45. LeDoux MS, Faye-Petersen OM, Aronin PA et al (1993) Lumbosacral neurenteric cyst in an infant. Case report. J Neurosurg 78:821-825

46. Jackson FE (1961) Neurenteric cysts. Report of a case of neurenteric cyst with associated chronic meningitis and hydrocephalus. J Neurosurg 18:678-682

47. Lieb G, Krauss J, Collmann H et al (1996) Recurrent bacterial meningitis. Eur J Pediatr 155:26-30

48. Ein SH, Shandling B, Humphreys R et al (1988) Osteomyelitis of the cervical spine presenting as a neurenteric cyst. J Pediatr Surg 23:779-781

49. Oliveira RS, Cinalli G, Roujeau T et al (2005) Neurenteric cyst in children: 16 consecutive cases and review of the literature. J Neurosurg 103:512-523

50. Agrawal D, Suri A, Mahapatra AK et al (2002) Intramedullary neurenteric cyst presenting as infantile paraplegia: a case and review. Pediatric Neurosurg 37:93-96

51. Brooks BS, Duvall ER, el Gammal T et al (1993) Neuroimaging features of neurenteric cysts: analysis of nine cases and review of the literature. AJNR Am J Neuroradiol 14:735-746

52. Ebisu T, Odake G, Fujimoto M et al (1990) Neurenteric cyst with meningomyelocele or meningocele. Split notochord syndrome. Childs Nerv Syst 6:465-467

53. Hicdonmez T, Steinbok P (2004) Spontaneous hemorrhage into spinal neurenteric cyst. Childs Nerv Syst 20:438-442

54. Languepin J, Daoud P, Desguerre I (1994) [Cervical intraspinal enterogenous cyst: a rare cause of neonatal syncope.] Arch Pediatr 1:54-56

55. Rizk T, Lahoud GA, Maarrawi J et al (2001) Acute paraplegia revealing an intraspinal neurenteric cyst in a child. Childs Nerv Syst 17:754-757

56. Voth D, Eckert HG, Hohn P (1975) [Intraspinal neurenteric cyst associated with dystopia of lung tissue and myelocele.] J Neurol 208:233-239

57. Husson M, Marchal JC, Hepner H et al (1981) [Kyste intra-cranien d'origine entoblastique. A propos d'une observation.] Ann Med Nancy Est 20:1077-1079

58. van der Wal AC, Troost D (1988) Enterogeneous cyst of the brainstem-a case report. Neuropediatrics 19:216-217

59. Filho FL, Tatagiba M, Carvalho GA et al (2001) Neurenteric cyst of the craniocervical junction. Report of three cases. J Neurosurg 94(1 Suppl):129-132

60. Ergun R, Akdemir G, Gezici AR et al (2000) Craniocervical neurenteric cyst without associated abnormalities. Pediatr Neurosurg 32:95-99

61. Itakura T, Kusumoto S, Uematsu Y et al (1986) Enterogenous cyst of the cervical spinal cord in a child-case report. Neurol Med Chir (Tokyo) 26:49-53

62. Matson DD (ed) (1969) Neurosurgery of infancy and childhood, 2nd edn. Thomas, Springfield, Ill, pp 114-118

63. Kadhim H, Proano PG, Saint Martin C et al (2000) Spinal neurenteric cyst presenting in infancy with chronic fever and acute myelopathy. Neurology 54:2011-2015

64. Laha RK, Huestis WS (1975) Intraspinal enterogenous cyst: delayed appearance following mediastinal cyst resection. Surg Neurol 3:67-70

65. Mam MK, Mathew S, Prabhakar BR et al (1996) Mediastinal enterogenic cyst presenting as paraplegia-a case report. Indian J Med Sci 50:337-339

66. Mooney JF III, Hall JE, Emans JB et al (1994) Spinal deformity associated with neurenteric cysts in children. Spine 19:1445-1450

67. Neuhauser EB, Harris GB, Berrett A (1958) Roentgenographic features of neurenteric cysts. AJR Am J Roentgenol 79:235-240

68. Piramoon AN, Abbassioun K (1974) Mediastinal enterogenic cyst with spinal cord compression. J Pediatr Surg 9:543-545

69. Superina RA, Ein SH, Humphreys RP (1984) Cystic duplications of the esophagus and neurenteric cysts. J Pediatr Surg 19:527-530

70. Bilik R, Ginzberg H, Superina RA (1995) Unconventional treatment of neuroenteric cyst in a newborn. J Pediatr Surg 30:115-117

71. Daher P, Melki I, Diab N et al (1996) Neurenteric cyst: antenatal diagnosis and therapeutic approach. Eur J Pediatr Surg 6:306-309

72. Gilchrist BF, Harrison MW, Campbell JR (1990) Neurenteric cyst: current management. J Pediatr Surg 25:1231-1233

73. Macaulay KE, Winter TC III, Shields LE (1997) Neurenteric cyst shown by prenatal sonography. AJR Am J Roentgenol 169:563-565

74. Rizalar R, Demirbilek S, Bernay F et al (1995) A case of a mediastinal neurenteric cyst demonstrated by prenatal ultrasound. Eur J Pediatr Surg 5:177-179

75. Satyarthee GD, Mahapatra AK (2003) Presacral neurenteric cyst in an infant. Pediatr Neurosurg 39:222-224

76. Durham MM, Chahine AA, Ricketts RR (1998) Presacral neuroenteric fistula presenting with meningitis and vaginal fistula: a case report. J Pediatr Surg 33:1558-1560

77. Carachi R (1982) The split notochord syndrome: a case report on a mixed spinal enterogenous cyst in a child with spina bifida cystica. Z Kinderchir 35:32-34

78. Deshpande DH, Pandya SK, Dastur HM et al (1972) An intraspinal enterogenous cyst. Neurol India 20:217-220

79. Fan YK, Huang JK, Sheu CY et al (2001) MR imaging characteristic of cervical neurenteric cysts: two cases reports. Chin J Radiol 26:39-44

80. Hamamoto O, Guerreiro NE, Nakano H et al (1997) [Intraspinal enterogenous cyst. Case report.] Arq Neuropsiquiatr 55:319-324 (Port)

81. Kantrowitz LR, Pais MJ, Burnett K et al (1986) Intraspinal neurenteric cyst containing gastric mucosa: CT and MRI findings. Pediatr Radiol 16:324-327

82. Knight G, Griffiths T, Williams I (1955) Gastrocystoma of the spinal cord. Br J Surg 42:635-638

83. Mizuno J, Fiandaca MS, Nishio S et al (1988) Recurrent intramedullary enterogeneous cyst of the cervical spinal cord. Childs Nerv Syst 4:47-49

84. Takemi K, Kubo S, Ibayashi N et al (1984) [A case of cervical intramedullary neurenteric cyst.] No Shinkei Geka 12:539-543

85. Yamashita J, Maloney AF, Harris P (1973) Intradural spinal bronchiogenic cyst. Case report. J Neurosurg 39:240-245

86. Hassan AMA, Rahman NA, Awadi YAI et al (1999) Intraspinal neurenteric cyst-report of two cases. Pan Arab J 3:44-48

87. Kim CY, Wang KC, Choe G et al (1999) Neurenteric cyst: its various presentations. Childs Nerv Syst 15:333-341

88. Kumar R, Jain R, Rao KM et al (2001) Intraspinal neurenteric cysts-report of three paediatric cases. Childs Nerv Syst 17:584-588

89. Mendel E, Lese GB, Gonzalez-Gomez I et al (1994) Isolated lumbosacral neurenteric cyst with partial sacral agenesis: case report. Neurosurgery 35:1159-1163

90. Turgutalp H, Ozoran Y, Ozoran AS et al (1991) A case of neurenteric cyst. Turk J Pediatr 33:139-142

91. Kemp SS, Towbin RB (1992) Pediatric case of the day. Neurenteric cyst without associated vertebral anomalies. Radiographics 12:1255-1257

92. Rao MB, Rout D, Misra BK et al (1996) Craniospinal and spinal enterogenous cysts-report of three cases. Clin Neurol Neurosurg 98:32-36

93. Holmes GL, Trader S, Ignatiadis P (1978) Intraspinal enterogenous cysts. A case report and review of pediatric cases in the literature. Am J Dis Child 132:906-908

94. Eynon-Lewis NJ, Kitchen N, Scaravilli F et al (1998) Neurenteric cyst of the cerebellopontine angle: case report. Neurosurgery 42:655-658

95. Shin JH, Byun BJ, Kim DW et al (2002) Neurenteric cyst in the cerebellopontine angle with xanthogranulomatous changes: serial MR findings with pathologic correlation. AJNR Am J Neuroradiol 23:663-665

96. Bejjani GK, Wright DC, Schessel D et al (1998) Endodermal cysts of the posterior fossa. Report of three cases and review of the literature. J Neurosurgery 89:326-335

97. Zalatnai A (1987) Neurenteric cyst of medulla oblongata-a curiosity. Neuropediatrics 18:40-41

98. Scaravilli F, Lidov H, Spalton DJ et al (1992) Neuroenteric cyst of the optic nerve: case report with immunohistochemical study. J Neurol Neurosurg Psychiatry 55:1197-1199

99. Walls TJ, Purohit DP, Aji WS et al (1986) Multiple intracranial enterogenous cysts. J Neurol Neurosurg Psychiatry 49:438-441

100. Arnould G, Lepoire J, Tridon P et al (1965) [Acropathie ulcero-mutilante secondaire et kyste tératomateux du canal sacré.] Rev Neurol 112:373-377

101. Bale PM (1973) A congenital intraspinal gastroenterogenous cyst in diastematomyelia. J Neurol Neurosurg Psychiatry 36:1011-1017

102. Németh K (1965) [Enterogene Zyste des Rückenmarks.] Zentrabl Allg Pathol 108:196-200

103. Brun A, Saldeen T (1968) Intraspinal enterogenous cyst. Acta Pathol Microbiol Scand 73:191-194

104. Evans JA, Lougheed LM (1978) Intradural cysts of the cervical spine: report of three cases. J Bone Joint Surg Am 60:123-125

105. Hoefnagel D, Benirschke K, Duarte J (1962) Teratomatous cysts within the vertebral canal. Observations on the occurrence of sex chromatin. J Neurol Neurosurg Psychiatry 25:159-164

106. Ingraham FD (1938) Intraspinal tumors in infancy and childhood. Am J Surg 39:342-376

107. Kahn AP, Hirsch JF, da Lage C et al (1971) [Intraspinal enteric cysts. 3 cases.] Neurochirurgie 17:33-44

108. Kinoshita K, Tokuda H (1973) Intraspinal enterogenous cyst: a case report and review of the literature. No To Shinkei 25:1857-1859

109. Klump TE (1971) Neurenteric cyst in the cervical spinal canal of a 10-week-old boy. Case report. J Neurosurg 35:472-476

110. Lerma S, Roda JM, Villarejo F et al (1985) Intradural neurenteric cyst: review and discussion. Neurochirurgia (Stuttg) 28:228-231

111. Matsushima T, Fukui M, Egami H (1985) Epithelial cells in a so-called intraspinal neurenteric cyst: a light and electron microscopic study. Surg Neurol 24:656-660

112. Miyagi K, Mukawa J, Mekaru S et al (1988) Enterogenous cyst in the cervical spinal canal. Case report. J Neurosurg 68:292-296

113. Ohwaki K, Shimura T, Murayama K et al (1978) Intraspinal enterogeneous cyst: a case report. Shoni No Noshinkey 3:223-228

114. Okino T, Kito K, Miyazaki T et al (1973) A case of intraspinal neurenteric cyst. No To Shinkei 25:1849-1855

115. Pianetti Filho G, Fonseca LF (1993) [High medular compression caused by neurenteric cyst. Report of a case.] Arq Neuropsiquiatr 51:253-257

116. Prasad VS, Reddy DR, Murty JM (1996) Cervico-thoracic neurenteric cyst: clinicoradiological correlation with embryogenesis. Childs Nerv Syst 12:48-51

117. Rewcastle NB, Francoeur J (1964) Teratomatous cysts of the spinal canal; with "sex chromatin" studies. Arch Neurol 11:91-99

118. Schiffer J, Till K (1982) Spinal dysraphism in the cervical and dorsal regions in childhood. Childs Brain 9:73-84

119. Voth D, Toussaint W, Olbertz S (1963) [Zum formenkreis der neurenterischen kommunikation.] Acta Neurochir (Wien) 9:139-150

120. Woo PY, Sharr MM (1982) Childhood cervical enterogenous cyst presenting with hemiparesis. Postgrad Med J 58:424-426

121. Reddy DR, Subrahmanian MV, Prabhakar V et al (1972) Neurenteric cyst (a case report). Neurol India 20:221-223

122. Appasamy M, Roberts D, Pilling D et al (2006) Antenatal ultrasound and magnetic resonance imaging in localizing the level of lesion in spina bifida and correlation with postnatal outcome. Ultrasound Obstet Gynecol 27(5):530-536

123. Aoki S, Machida T, Sasaki Y et al (1987) Enterogenous cyst of cervical spine: clinical and radiological aspects (including CT and MRI). Neuroradiology 29:291-293

124. O'Neill P, Stack JP (1990) Magnetic resonance imaging in the preoperative assessment of closed spinal dysraphism in children. Pediatr Neurosurg 16:240-246

125. Chaynes P, Thorn-Kany M, Sol JC et al (1998) Imaging in neurenteric cysts of the posterior cranial fossa. Neuroradiology 40:374-376

126. Shakudo M, Inoue Y, Ohata K et al (2001) Neurenteric cyst with alteration of signal intensity on follow-up MR images. AJNR Am J Neuroradiol 22:496-498

127. Wilkins RH, Rossitch E Jr (1995) Intraspinal cysts. In: Pang D (ed) Disorders of the pediatric spine. Raven Press, New York, pp 445-466

128. Arai Y, Yamauchi Y, Tsuji T et al (1992) Spinal neurenteric cyst. Report of two cases and review of forty-one cases reported in Japan. Spine 17:1421-1424

129. Chavda SV, Davies AM, Cassar-Pullicino VN (1985) Enterogenous cysts of the central nervous system: a report of eight cases. Clin Radiol 36:245-251

130. Lee SH, Dante SJ, Simeone FA et al (1999) Thoracic neurenteric cyst in an adult: case report. Neurosurgery 45:1239-1243

131. Ho LC, Olivi A, Cho CH et al (1998) Well-differentiated papillary adenocarcinoma arising in a supratentorial enterogenous cyst: case report. Neurosurgery 43:1474-1477

132. Perry A, Scheithauer BW, Zaias BW et al (1999) Aggressive enterogenous cyst with extensive craniospinal spread: case report. Neurosurgery 44:401-405

133. Sahara Y, Nagasaka T, Takayasu M et al (2001) Recurrence of a neurenteric cyst with malignant transformation in the foramen magnum after total resection. Case report. J Neurosurg 95:341-345

CHAPTER 38
Diastematomyelia

Benedict Rilliet

Introduction – Definitions

The word diastematomyelia (DM) was introduced by Ollivier in his treatise on disease of the spinal cord published in Paris in 1837 [1]. DM takes its origin from the Greek words διαστεμα meaning slit or cleft, and μψελοσ, meaning cord. Ollivier clearly states that this definition applies to a more or less wide division of the spinal cord in two lateral halves. Later Cohen and Sledge [2] emphasised that this term only defines the cleft in the spinal cord and not, as often written, the osseous spur or fibro-cartilaginous tract that separates both hemicords. This common error of interpretation of the original definition has been the source of much confusion. Cases of division of the cauda equina and filum terminale should also be included in the definition of DM [3-5]. Partial DM is characterised by an incomplete sagittal division of the spinal cord whether anteriorly or posteriorly situated [4, 6-8]. The term diplomyelia (DP), invented by von Recklinghausen [9], applies to a completely different malformation where one finds a totally formed spinal cord, situated dorsally or ventrally to the original spinal cord, mostly at the lumbo-sacral level. This malformation occurs in the second phase of the neurulation process, called secondary neurulation. Cases of DP have also been described in mouse mutants [10, 11] and in cat mutants that live in the Isle of Man (Manx cat [12]). Human examples of DP are very rare and only autopsy cases [13-16] fit with the definition of DP. The case reported by Rokos [17] may add to the confusion because this author described an association of a DP and DM in the same patient (namely a slit and an antero-posterior duplication). Hori et al. [16] clearly demonstrated with a schematic classification that case number one from Rokos corresponded to a DM with an antero-posterior rotation of the two hemicords at the middle segment of the malformation, the upper and lower segments to the rotation definitely showing a sagittal division into two

lateral parts. Van Gieson [18] also proposed that the term DP be used to characterise a true duplication of the spinal cord found in double monsters. This definition should also be abandoned and be replaced by dimyelia as proposed by Hori et al. [16]. A recent report of a foetus with trimyelia shows that the complexity of spinal cord malformations is almost infinite [19]. A personal autopsy case of a lumbar trimyelia is shown in Figure 38.1.

The confusion between DM and DP is still present in the recent literature regarding the genetic mutations that can induce congenital spinal cord anomalies. Nait-Oumesmar et al. [20] have produced ectopic spinal cords at the caudal level of mice embryos, which they consider as being similar to those seen in human DM; in fact, what they have pro-

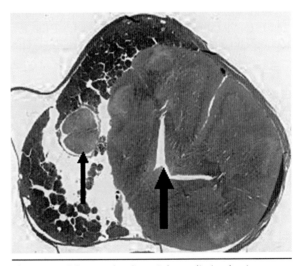

Fig. 38.1. A human lumbar triplomyelia (author's personal observation). On the right side of the image, two complete spinal cords with the recognisable butterfly appearance of the spinal grey matter are facing each other; the cleft (*large black arrow*) is an artefact due to the section of the specimen. A third tiny spinal cord is seen (*small black arrow*) surrounded by nerves of the cauda equina

duced more closely resembles the caudal DP that is due to a faulty involution at secondary neurulation and not a malformation that occurs prior to primary neurulation at the stage of gastrulation.

In the early nineties, Pang [21], dissatisfied with the terms of DM and DP that were often mistaken for each other, decided to create a new classification of the cases of duplication of the spinal cord and coined the term split cord malformation (SCM). This new classification was based on his personal surgical experience in 39 cases and two autopsy cases. He proposed an embryogenetic theory which fitted with all these spinal cord malformations. Apparently, Pang was unaware of the original description of Ollivier of a sagittal cleft in the spinal cord thus creating the concept of a split spinal cord. Nevertheless, credit must be given to Pang to have clearly individualised the two main types of DM (for the sake of reading of this chapter, the term DM will be uniformly used instead of SCM) that we encounter in clinical practice. Type I (Fig. 38.2) is characterised by two hemicords, each one having its own dural envelope, separated by an osteo-cartilaginous septum, whereas in Type II (Fig. 38.3) the two hemicords are contained in a single dural envelope and separated by a fibrous septum. In Type I, the associated bony abnormalities, such as hemi-vertebra, butterfly vertebra and fused vertebrae, are always present, whereas in Type II they are exceptional.

An alternative to these descriptive classifications are those that are based on the supposed pathogenesis of DM and its associated anomalies.

Carcassone et al. [22] grouped all the anomalies that originate due to faulty development of the notochord under the term notochordodysraphia. This

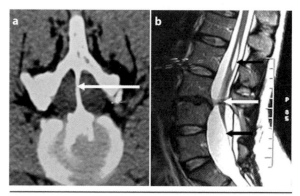

Fig. 38.2 a, b. Type I DM (author's personal observation). **a** Lumbar CT scan without contrast. The bony spur, transfixing the spinal is indicated by a *white arrow*. **b** T2-weighted MRI of the same patient. The large *white arrow* points at the bony spur, the *upper arrow* at the proximal syrinx and the *lower arrow* at the tight filum

notochordodysraphia may show variable pathological expression as listed below:

– Malformations incompatible with life (total encephalomyeloaraphia)
– Enteric fistulae and remnants of these fistulae
– Malformation of the axial skeleton
– Malformation of the neuraxis (including DM) considered as secondary to the aberrant development of the notochord.

The same approach has been proposed by Naidich [23] who individualised three entities under the heading of anomalies of the development of the notochord:

– Split notochord syndrome
– DM
– Segmental spinal dysgenesis.

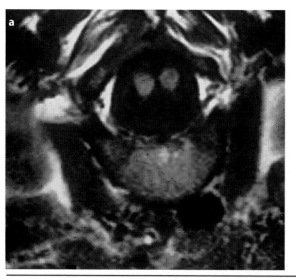

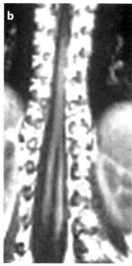

Fig. 38.3 a, b. Type II DM (author's personal observation). **a** T1-weighted axial MRI showing both hemicords without any visible intervening septum in a single dural sac. **b** Long cleft between the two hemi-cords, going down to the conus (same patient)

A Brief History of DM

According to Perret [24], congenital sagittal divisions or duplications of the spinal cord have been known since 1684 with autopsy reports of foetuses and still-born monsters. The oldest specimen of DM, dating back probably more than 18 centuries, has been found in a tomb in the Neguev desert (Israel) [25]. The malformed spine of an approximately 20-year-old person included a bone spur dividing the spinal canal on the sagittal plane associated with a butterfly vertebra and an osseous spina bifida above and below the spur, consistent with what we would now classify after Pang as DM Type I.

After the important monograph of Ollivier [1], several sporadic reports of DM were published at the end of the nineteenth and the beginning of the twentieth century and most of them are included in the work of Herren and Edwards [26] who collected 43 cases, including their own observation. Only one of the cases collected by these two authors had been diagnosed and treated when living by Hamby [27]. Hamby is therefore credited to be the first surgeon to have operated upon a DM. The modern era of DM started with the first surgical series of 11 cases reported in children by Matson in 1950 [28].

Embryology

Firstly it must be emphasised that although several experimental models of DM have been created, an animal counterpart of this rare malformation has yet to be reported.

The embryologists have taught us that the formation of the notochord arises from the invagination of the mesoblast from the primitive node of Hensen between the epiblast and the endoblast. This crucial step of the development of the vertebrate embryo when the bilaminar embryo becomes trilaminar is called gastrulation and occurs before the differentiation of the nervous system (neurulation process) from the ectoderm into surface ectoderm and neuroectoderm. Fibronectin plays an important role at the time of gastrulation. Mutant mice with a knock-out gene responsible for the synthesis of fibronectin have been created [29, 30]. Heterozygotic individuals have a concentration of fibronectin reduced by one half and a normal phenotype, whereas in the homozygotic individual, the mutant allele causes the death of the embryo. Growth seems to be normal until gastrulation but the embryos have a shortened antero-posterior axis. The neural tube is then malformed and severe anomalies concerning all the tissues of mesodermal origin are seen. The notochord and the somites are lacking. According to these authors, the absence of fibronectin results in severe perturbations of migration, adhesion, growth and differentiation of all the tissues of mesodermal origin.

Around the 16th day of life of the human embryo, epiblastic cells that migrate between the epiblastic and the hypoblastic layers will form the notochord. From the blastopore a notochordal canal soon appears. This canal has been described in human and non-human primates but not in amphibians, birds and mammals other than primates. Its exact function is not known [31]. The growth of the notochordal canal is mainly due to the apposition of cells progressing from the level of Hensen's node in a caudal direction as the primitive steak regresses [32]. The ventral part of the notochord then merges into the hypoblastic layer and disappears in such a way that the blastopore comes in direct communication with the yolk sac. The notochord then develops into the notochordal plate by a process called intercalation [33], with the communication between the amniotic sac and the yolk sac called the neurenteric canal or canal of Kovalevski [34]. The neurenteric canal remains open for only 48 hours [33]. At the end of this brief period of time, the notochordal plate wraps itself up again to form a notochord by a phenomenon called excalation [33, 35], which progresses in a caudo-rostral direction, the pharynx being the last part of the endoderm to dissociate from the notochordal plate [31]. The formation of the definitive notochord varies according to authors. Hamilton [36] and later Raybaud [34] state, contrary to McLone [31], that the wrapping up of the notochord occurs in a rostro-caudal direction. The excalation process is a critical step in the development of the spine. The separation between the notochord and the mesoblastic cells from the future gut should be completed so that the mesodermal anlage that will form the vertebral bodies and spine can develop correctly. Incomplete separation of the notochord from the endoderm may give rise to enterogenous cysts that are found anterior to and occasionally interrupting the vertebral body [35]. However, the notochordal canal and intercalation and excalation phenomenon have not been described in the human embryo and non-human primates. This point was also discussed by Klessinger [37], who quoted Steding's personal communication: "The existence of a neurenteric canal is contradictory. However, in recent studies of well-preserved human embryos, no neurenteric canal could be found".

Theories on the Pathogenesis of DM

Disorders of Neurulation

On the basis of observations made in chick embryos, but without clearly providing proof of his hypothesis, Herren [26] postulated that DM resulted from an exaggerated folding of the neural plate. To justify his theory of a primary disorder of the neural tube, Herren stated that the spinal cord formed prior to the spine, a statement which is disputable, if one considers that the chordomesoderm differentiates during gastrulation, that is to say before and during the initiation of neurulation. Another argument given by Herren is that a DM is always associated with an anomaly of the spine, but this does not account for those cases where no septum can be found. Pang [38] rejected Herren's hypothesis stating his own unified theory that is based on the concept of an endomesenchymatous tract and applies to both cases with a bone septum and associated vertebral malformation (DM Type I) and cases where there is only a fibrous tract between the two hemicords and no associated vertebral malformation (DM Type II). The endomesenchymatous tract that determines DM Type II is only constituted by meninx primitiva that does not contains precursors of bone cells. Dryden [39], utilising X-rays as a teratogenic agent, has produced in chick embryos exactly what Herren has postulated, namely a wrapping of the neural folds. However, he was not able to show a separation into two hemicords in any of his chick embryos; both parts of the neural plate remaining joined at the level of the basal plate. Quoting Kapsenberg [40], Rokos [17] also demonstrated that this theory could not explain the disappearance of the tissue of the basal plate at the level of the DM and therefore invented a destructive process that is responsible for the bifurcation of the neural tube or its anlage, this focal destruction representing "one of the earliest and non specific reactions of the embryonic tissue to the teratogenic agents". Gardner [41] hypothesised that the hydromyelic distension of the neural tube and its secondary rupture both on its ventral and dorsal aspect would constitute two neural tubes. Then the fibrous tissue of mesodermal origin that penetrates the space between the two neural tubes would constitute the fibrous or bony spur. This hypothesis has been rejected, particularly by Mann [42], who stated that the production of cerebrospinal fluid (CSF) by the choroid plexus was not yet effective at a time when the neural tube was already closed.

The Neurenteric Canal Theory

Since the beginning of the twentieth century, authors have postulated that the development of an anterior rachischisis can be due to remnants of the neurenteric canal [43, 44]. Bremer [45] presented a theory in 1952 taking into account a dorsal intestinal fistula described by Keen [46]. From the archenteron that gives rise to the gut, a diverticulum develops that, upon expansion, separates the notochord and the neural plate into two parts. If this diverticulum opens at the skin level, it gives rise to the dorsal enteric fistula, that is to say an open form of split notochord syndrome. If the endodermal elements disappear totally, a fibrous or osseous septum between the two hemicords remains. Considering the pathogenesis of DM, Bremer [45] wrote that "this cleft is a magnified neurenteric canal, but since it does not pass through the primitive knot, it is an accessory neurenteric canal; the dorsal intestinal fistula is of this type". Bremer's theory based on the hypothesis of an accessory neurenteric canal can be explained because upon excalation of the notochord, segmental multiple interruption of the ventral part of the notochordal canal may occur.

These variations of morphogenesis of the notochord, all having a transient occurrence, may explain the fact that the neurenteric canal is not always caudally situated in relation to the embryo but can open more rostrally, explaining therefore thoracic, cervical or even occipital clefts. Ancel [47] showed that he could obtain segmental duplication of the chick-embryo if he incubated the eggs not at 37°C but at 40.5°C. In this situation one may ask if this relative hyperthermia has its effect simply on the most important part, in terms of volume, of the egg, namely the vitellus that expands itself because of heat. The vitelline content then herniates between the two parts of the neural plate at the time where the communication between the vitellus and the amnios is open. Cohen and Sledge [2] postulate that the malformations of the spinal cord and the spine that are encountered in DM all originate from the persistence of the neurenteric canal:

- if only the ventral part persists, an intestinal duplication will result;
- if the medial portion persists, an enterogenous (or neurenteric) cyst may persist;
- if only the dorsal portion persists, the result may be a dermal sinus, a dermoid cyst or a teratoma originating from embryonic pluripotential cells.

All combinations of the above can occur. Therefore only one embryological error can explain the association of the DM with cutaneous defects, vertebral malformations, intestinal duplications and mediastinal intra-spinal enterogenous cysts.

Adherence Between Endoderm and Ectoderm

According to Beardmore [48], the initial step of the malformation is an endo-ectodermic adherence occuring at the middle part of the embryo between Hensen's node and the prochordal plate at a presomitic stage. This adherence will partially block the invagination of the chordal cells in the direction of the prochordal plate, causing a slit in the notochord which duplicates around it. At the place where the notochord is duplicated, both paired anlagen of the neural plate fail to fuse on the midline and thus give rise to two hemicords. The growth of the embryo causes this adherence to exert traction on the primitive gut and via this mechanism the formation of an enteric diverticulum with, as a final result, the incorporation of intestinal structures into the spinal cord.

Primitive Steak Abnormally Wide

Dias and Walker [33] have provided an alternative theory for the pathogenesis of DM and other associated complex dysraphic malformations. They postulate that at the time of gastrulation, the primitive streak is, for a reason that is not yet elucidated, abnormally wide. Therefore, the paired anlagen of the notochord together with the neural and somatic material stay separated and develop independently. Pluripotential cells that develop in this enlarged primitive streak may give rise to tissues derived from any of the three embryonic layers. The communication between the amnios and the vitellus that may give rise to the split notochord syndrome does not form by the persistence of a neurenteric canal, but by the disappearance of the cells of the primitive streak.

All the surgical animal models proposed by Dias and Walker [33], Rilliet et al. [49], Klessinger and Christ [37] and Emura et al. [50-52] mimic the features of human DM and are convincing in the sense that they all support that DM is a disorder of gastrulation and not primary neurulation. However, the intrinsic mechanism is still to be elucidated.

Some clues may be derived from the genetic mutations occurring in rare cases of spondylocostal dysplasia (SCD) (Jarcho-Levine syndrome) associated with DM [53-55]. Both conditions are probably due

to a disorder of the chordo-mesoderm. According to Etus et al. [55], autosomal recessive SCD maps to a 7.8-cM interval on chromosome 19q13.1-q13.3 that is homologous with a mouse region containing a gene encoding the Notch ligand delta-like 3 (DLL3). In 2000, Bulman et al. [56] cloned and sequenced human DLL3 to evaluate it as a candidate gene for SCD and identified mutations in three autosomal recessive SCD families. Segmentation of the body, as shown in fish, chick and mouse embryos, relies on a segmentation clock, a molecular oscillator, which depends on Notch signalling for its proper functioning. DLL3 seems to be another gene required for oscillation and the fact that its mutation in humans results in abnormal segmentation of the vertebral column suggests that the segmentation clock also acts during human embryonic development. More recently, Williams [57] has postulated that there could be a genetic link between Sprengel anomaly and DM. This association has been known since the publication of Banizza von Bazan [58]. Williams postulated that the scapula, or more precisely, its medial part, originates from the paraxial mesoderm, as do the ribs, and is not regulated by the homeobox genes that build the upper limb. Moreover, Klippel-Feil anomaly, which represents a disorder of segmentation of the axial skeleton, and the more severe form iniencephaly, are also associated with DM and the Sprengel anomaly. On reviewing the animal models and gene expression studies concerning the limb development and the scapula, however, Williams could not find an example of scapular dysplasia and DM. Nevertheless he concludes that: "The occasional co-occurrence of DM with Sprengel deformity is particularly intriguing, given that Pax1 is involved in the development of the notochord"; and quoting Bentley and Smith [59] that "DM is thought to be due to abnormal development of the notochord". David et al. [60] also hypothesised a role for the Pax1 gene in Klippel-Feil, but showed no evidence for it. Interestingly enough, Banizza von Bazan [61] also reported the association of DM and sacral agenesis or caudal regression syndrome, a condition now classified under the generic name of notochordodysraphy. Hohl's princeps case report [62] of sacral agenesis, published more than 150 years ago, is illustrated by a beautiful sketch, depicting a skeleton with an agenesis of the sacrum and a medial bone spur in a widened lumbar canal.

Although we still have no animal genetic model of DM, we trust the capability of our molecular geneticists to solve this problem in the not too distant future.

Anatomo-Pathology

Level of DM

Analysis of significant series in the literature shows that the lumbar and thoraco-lumbar levels are the most frequently affected segments in this malformation [5, 63-67].

If one considers the largest series reported [67], DM are found at the lumbar or lumbosacral level in 54.33% of cases, at the thoraco-lumbar level in 31.88%, at the thoracic level in 10.23%, at the cervico-thoracic level in 0.78% and at the cervical level in 2.75% of the cases.

Four occipital or basicranial DM are reported in the medical literature: the first description of a very unusual occipital DM, which in fact can be more properly described as a diastematobulbia, was by Malacarne (quoted by Ollivier [1]). "The medulla oblongata was divided by a bone spur at the level of the foramen magnum". To our knowledge, there are only three other reported cases of diastematobulbia. Concurrently, Herman et al. [68] and Pfeiffer et al. [69] reported the same case of a basicranial DM. The female newborn did not survive more than 14 days. The autopsy showed a DM extending from the pons to the thoracic spinal cord and a widened occipital foramen divided in the sagittal plane by a large bone spur that was attached anteriorly to the clivus and posteriorly to the inner occipital prominence. Two recent cases of diastematobulbia have been reported [70, 71].

Multiple DMs, Length of the Cleft, Level of the Conus

Although most of the cases of DM are characterised by a unique cleft, some cases have been described with several clefts [6, 72, 73], each one containing a septum. According to Naidich [72], the occurrence of two spurs in two separated clefts is found in 5-6% of cases. In a series of 41 patients, James and Lassman [6] found 16 patients with a bone spur, three with a fibrous band and 21 where they could not find any septum in the cleft. One case presented three clefts with three of the above described possibilities, namely a bone spur in one cleft, a fibrous septum in another and in the third there was no septum [6]. This coexistence of a DM Type I and DM Type II in the same patient has been very rarely reported [5, 64, 74, 75] and is assigned as composite DM [66, 76, 77].

Keim [74], in a collection of 173 observations

published in the literature before 1973, found 22 cases where the length of the cleft was described. The cleft measured from 1.4 to 6.8 cm (mean size: 4.7 cm). In another 11 cases the length of the cleft was estimated in relation to the vertebral segments, from 2 to 15 (mean: 5.5 vertebral segments). The length of the split segments is longer in patients older than one year of age than it is in younger children [66]. This most likely reflects the dynamic splitting of the cord with increasing age. Hilal [4] emphasised the fact that the clefts and septa that are located at the higher position in the spine are longer than those situated in the more caudal situation.

In the series of Hilal, the conus is situated below the inferior vertebral plate of L2 in 26 of 34 cases and above the same level in only six of 34 cases. In these six cases, the septum is found at the thoracic level in five cases and only one is found at the lumbar level. Conversely, in the 26 children who have a low lying conus, only one septum was found at the thoracic level, all the others had a lumbar septum. The logical deduction of these observations is concordant with the fact that septa, which are situated more superiorly, interfere with the normal ascension of the spinal cord less than those that are located at the lumbar level. Another reason for a low lying conus in DM is the association with a thickened filum that also contributes to spinal cord tethering. Seventy-five percent of the cases reported by Andar et al. had a low lying conus [78].

Bone Spur or Cartilaginous Septum

According to French [79], septa are fibrous in 25% and osseous in 75% of the cases. Several anatomic variations of the bony spur according to their extension and connection in the spinal canal have been described:

– The spur arises from the anterior aspect of the spinal canal where the disk is absent or grossly malformed or from the vertebral body itself; this connection with the vertebra may be narrow or wide, and may have a fibro-cartilaginous part forming a synchondrosis that permits disarticulation of the spur.

– The spur bears no relation with either the anterior or the posterior aspect of the spinal canal and appears to be simply interposed in the slit between the two hemicords with some adherence to the dura.

– The spur is especially wide in the cases of split notochord syndrome, which have a persistent neurenteric fistula, as it is formed by the medial pedicles of the duplicated vertebral bodies.

– The spur takes its origin from the posterior arch of the vertebral body, by duplication of the laminae and fusion of the medial part [80-84] as an attempted spinal segment duplication. A synchondrosis has also been described at the level of the posterior connection with the laminae [2].

– The spur arises from both the anterior and the posterior aspects of several more or less fused or malformed vertebral bodies. The spur may have several nuclei of ossification [85].

According to French [65], the spur or the septum is attached to the anterior and posterior parts of the vertebrae in 68% of cases, only to the posterior parts in 11% and only to the anterior parts in 24%.

In the majority of cases, only one septum lies in the slit, while occasionally there may be two or three and exceptionally four [86]. French considers the distal septum as causing the symptoms. The incidence of ossified spurs varies as to whether the series are reported by orthopaedic surgeons or neurosurgeons. Orthopaedists consider DM to be present, almost exclusively, when a spur is present (DM Type I). In that respect, Keim [74], reviewing 112 patients, observed that most of them had a fibrous septum or an osseous spur and only two had no structure in the cleft. Pang [75], putting forward the neurosurgeon's point of view, says that in DM Type II, according to his classification, at surgery there is always a tract or some fibrous bands that escapes neuroradiological detection, even when a contrasted computed tomography (CT) myelogram is performed.

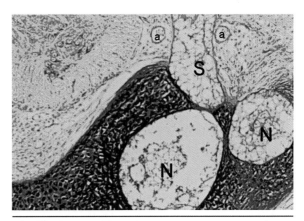

Fig. 38.4. Duplication of the anterior spinal artery in an experimental model of diastematomyelia. Toluidine blue stain. *N*, duplication of the notochord; *S*, grafted notochord; *a*, duplication of the anterior spinal artery. Reproduced from [49]

Asymmetry of the Hemicords and Duplication of the Anterior Spinal Artery

The division of the spinal cord into two asymmetric hemicords may be explained by the fact that the accessory neurenteric canal may be slightly eccentric in the axial plane [38]. At that time the notochord consequently undergoes an asymmetric division, the hemicord developing from the wider neural plate is inevitably thicker than the other one and will push aside the endomesenchymal tract. This could explain the fact that often, in the case of asymmetrical hemicords, the spur has an oblique course on the axial plane. Ersahin et al. [66] found 21 patients out of 74 with one hemicord smaller than the other, with the smaller hemicord almost always associated with an atrophic lower limb on the same side (p = 0.005).

Cohen and Sledge first showed a diagram of a DM where one sees clearly that each hemicord has its own anterior spinal artery [2]. Other examples of

the duplication of the anterior spinal artery have been reported [4, 87] in one case by CTmyelogram [88] and even by spinal angiography [85]. We were also able to demonstrate the same feature in an experimental model of DM (Fig. 38.4) [49].

An embryological explanation has been provided by Naidich [88]. The paired anlagen of the future anterior spinal artery develop at the second to third week of gestation; they eventually migrate to the midline and fuse to give rise to the anterior spinal artery. The presence of an intervening structure (osseous spur or fibrous septum) impedes this fusion and the two duplicated anterior spinal arteries remain, each one supplying its own hemicord.

Scoliosis

Sixty percent of patients with a DM have scoliosis [89, 90]. Conversely, the incidence of intra-spinal malformation in congenital scoliosis varies from 5% [74, 91] to 18% [92]. The association of congenital scoliosis with widening of the spinal canal should urge the clinician to suspect a DM or any dysraphic anomaly. The risk of neurological complications when correcting congenital scoliosis is ten times greater than with idiopathic scoliosis, and orthopaedists [93, 94] have emphasised that every patient with congenital scoliosis must have magnetic resonance imaging (MRI) to rule out these intra-spinal congenital anomalies. Scoliosis is more frequent when the septum is more rostrally situated [4]. Reviewing his series of 34 children with DM, Hilal [4] clearly showed that the incidence and the severity of scoliosis increases with time. This finding suggests that the management of DM in small children may prevent or postpone the appearance of scoliosis. Scoliosis is seldom due to a unique factor. Lapras [95] considered three factors: the first one is attributed to the anomalies of segmentation of vertebrae, like the hemi-vertebrae, the second one is related to the asymmetry of the lower limbs that can induce a secondary scoliosis and the third one, the malformation of the spinal cord by itself with asymmetry of the two hemicords and impaired innervation of the paravertebral muscles by aberrant nerve roots. The association of hemi-vertebrae and DM is considered to be rare [96], representing 5.9% of cases in the Mahapatra and Gupta series [67].

Hydromyelia

Alternatively described as hydromyelia, syringomyelia, syringo-hydromyelia or hydro-syringomyelia, the presence of a syrinx in one of the hemicords or in the adjacent normal spinal cord segment has been reported in autopsy cases [17, 97] and clinical cases, documented by ultrasonography [98], myelography [99], CTmyelogram [100] and above all MRI [23, 98, 101-106]. In large series, the presence of a syrinx may vary from 27.5% [107], 47% [108] to 55% [109] of cases. Repetitive traction and compression by the spur of the spinal cord is postulated as the mechanism of abnormal CSF accumulation in the central canal [109, 110]. In an experimental model of DM, a syrinx of one of the hemicords was found in some embryos (Fig. 38.5) [49]. In this model it is hard to imagine that chronic trauma to one of the hemicords is responsible for the hydromyelia, the more plausible mechanism is malformative and could be related to the dysraphic state, probably a segmental non-regression of the hemi-central neurocele.

Meningomyelocele and DM

Cameron [111], and above all Emery [112, 113], have studied the incidence of DM in cases of open spinal dysraphism. This incidence is particularly high in autopsy series. In the 100 autopsy cases of open myelomeningocoele (MMC) collected by Emery, a duplication of the spinal cord was situated rostral to the open defect in 31% of the cases, at the level of the MMC in 22%, and caudal to the defect in 25%. Mahaprata et al. [67] reported an association with spina bifida aperta in 18.9% of their cases. Kumar et al. [114] found 16 cases, mainly of type I DM

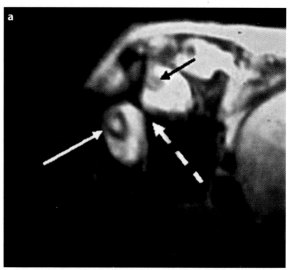

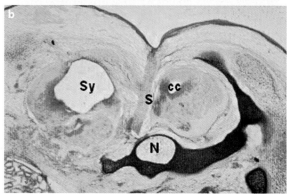

Fig. 38.5 a, b. DM Type I with syrinx in one of the hemicords (author's personal observation). **a** T2-weighted axial MRI of the lumbar spine. *Large white arrow* points at hemicord with syrinx, small black arrows points at the other hemicord with a slightly dilated central canal, notice oblique position of the spur (*large interrupted white arrow*). **b** Experimental DM in a chick embryo with a syrinx in one of the hemicord. Toluidine blue stain. *Sy*, syrinx; *S*, soft eggshell membrane septum; *cc*, central canal of the other hemi-cord; *N*, notochord. Reproduced from [49]

(12/16) out of 106 cases of spinal dysraphism and proposed to add the term "complex spina bifida" to Pang's classification.

Chiari Malformations

In the context of closed spinal dysraphism, DM is very rarely associated with a Chiari I malformation. Some authors state that this association does not exist [4]. In their large series, Mahaprata et al. [67] found 18 of 254 cases of Chiari malformation, five of Chiari I and 13 of Chiari II. If one can easily legitimate the Chiari II malformation in patients who have DM associated with an open defect, it is more difficult to understand why the Chiari I malformation was found associated with DM. Unfortunately, Mahaprata et al. do not specify if the Chiari I malformations were found in association with spina bifida aperta or occulta.

Hemimyelocele

Duckworth [115] described hemimyelocele, a rare type of DM. The spinal cord is separated into two unequal hemicords and one of these hemicords or even both show a defect of closure. The neurological deficit is more pronounced on the side where there has been a defect of neurulation. Duckworth published 16 cases and in ten of them, sphincter control was normal, and all had normal neurological function in one leg. One can deduce that healthy unilateral innervation of the sphincter muscles may be sufficient. All his cases had pronounced scoliosis with hemivertebrae. The embryological explanation of hemimyelocele is difficult to understand, because one has to consider both a defect of gastrulation onto which is superimposed a defect of neurulation on one of the hemi-neural plates, unless credit is given to the hypothesis of Duckworth who speculated that the neuro-ectoderm has a direct influence on the development of the chordo-mesoderm. This assumption is in complete discordance with the usual theory that stipulates that the chordo-mesoderm influences the development of the neural plate and not the contrary. Although this anomaly is very rare, surgeons must be cognisant of its existence and pay particular attention to preserve the healthy hemicord at the time of closure of the side which has remained open. Maguire [116] reported ten cases of hemimyelocele. He also emphasised the fact that all these cases have a scoliosis with a Cobb angle from 20° to 117° due to anomalies of segmentations of the vertebrae. More than half of his patients had malformations of the kidneys. Other cases of hemimyelocele have been reported more recently [38, 117-120]. A unique case of terminal lipomyelocystocele arising from one hemicord was reported by Parmar [121].

Dermal Sinus, Dermoid, Epidermoid and Neurenteric Cysts

If an ecto-endodermic fistula remains (remnant of the accessory neurenteric canal) the surface ectoderm will be in contact with the structures that are interposed between the two hemicords. Pang has demonstrated that the sinus ends in the posterior part of the spur in Type I DM, whereas in Type II DM the occurrence of intradural dermoid cysts must be suspected. The association of a dermal sinus and DM is not frequently observed but complications that may occur following incomplete surgery are well described in one case of Fauré [122]: a 3-year-old girl became tetraplegic immediately after the excision of a cervical dermal sinus: X-rays showed a C2-C3 cervical block and a spina bifida of C1. A second, more extensive operation allowed complete removal of the dermal sinus and showed a DM.

Black [123] reported four cases of congenital intraspinal tumors, one of which was an epidermoid cyst that was found in between a duplicated spinal cord. He quoted a similar case classified as a dermoid cyst published by Harriehausen [124].

Neurenteric cyst (synonyms: gastroenterogenous cyst, foregut cyst, intradural spinal bronchogenic cyst, intraspinal enterogenous cyst) represents a rather rare pathological entity. Until 1989, 26 cases had been reported in the literature [125].The association with a DM is even rarer [126-135]. In a recent review of 16 consecutive cases of neurenteric cysts from Necker Hospital, two cases of associated DM were found [136]. These cases could be an indirect confirmation of the neurenteric canal theory explaining DM.

Lipoma

Cochrane [137] reported the association of a DM and a lipoma in a patient who had a Klippel-Feil anomaly. Another case with the combined defect was also reported by Solanki [138]. A personal example of an association of a DM Type II, a thoracic lipoma and a blind dermal sinus is shown in Fig. 38.6.

Mathieu [127] observed that associated lipomas and lipomeningocele are always situated on the side of the smallest hemicord.

Filum Lipoma or Hypertrophy

The occurrence of a thickened filum or filum lipoma has been reported as a concomitant cause of tethering in most of the series of DM [66, 67, 89, 119, 139-141]. The incidence of a filum terminale that is thicker than 2 mm in cases of DM is, according to Naidich, between 40 to 100% [23]. MRI of the spine should always include all spinal levels to detect this hypertrophied filum. Section of the filum is an inte-

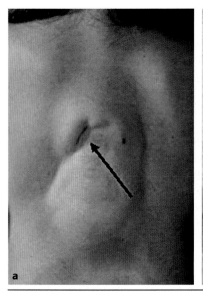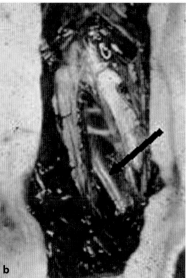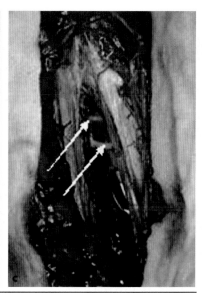

Fig. 38.6 a-c. DM plus lipoma and a blind dermal sinus (author's personal observation). **a** Clinical aspect of the patient with soft subcutaneous lipoma and blind sinus (*black arrow*). **b** Same patient, DM Type II, *black arrow* points at fibrous septum. **c** After the removal of the fibrous septum, demonstration of aberrant medial roots (*white arrows*)

gral part of the treatment [95, 119, 142] and sometimes needs a lower incision over the sacrum, particularly in patients with cervical or dorsal DMs [67].

"Méningomyélocèle Manqué"

Using the French "Méningomyélocèle manqué" (translation = failed meningomyelocele), Lassman and James [143] described an aborted meningomyelocele consisting of a bundle of aberrant roots, fibrous tract and vessels that came out from the posterior part of the spinal cord and were bound to the dura or crossed it to end in the sub-cutaneous tissue. They reported 45 cases of such an anomaly, associated with a DM in 28 cases (ten with a septum and 18 without). Other authors have also mentioned this anomaly [38, 144]. Pang found 24 cases of these fibro-neuro-vascular tracts. He suspected that this malformation is due to the fact that some neural crest cells are driven into the posterior part of the endomesenchymatous tract. The importance of severing these anomalous bands is pointed out by Humphreys et al. [145] and Scatliff et al. [8], especially in patients where no clear septum is found.

Other Associated Anomalies

Ureteral duplication, bifidity of the renal pelvis and anomaly of the origin of the renal artery have been

described by Lassale [85] in cases of DM. Faris [146] reported a case of bifid scrotum and Castillo [147] of uterus didelphis. There could be a remote association between DMs and situs inversus totalis [148].

Association with Other Anomalies of the Development of the Notochord (Notochordodysraphia): Klippel-Feil, Iniencephaly, Spondylocostal Dysplasia (Jarcho-Levine Syndrome), Sprengel Anomaly, Sacral Agenesis (Caudal Regression Syndrome)

The association of a cervical DM with Klippel-Feil malformation (Fig. 38.7) has been reported on several occasions [60, 64, 67, 137, 149-156]. Ulmer et al. [155] systematically reviewed CTs and MRIs of 24 patients presenting with Klippel-Feil syndrome and found signs of dysraphism of the cervical spinal cord or DM in five cases.

Therefore it is obvious that in the presence of clinical signs of Klippel-Feil syndrome (low-lying hair line with limitation of cervical movements, Sprengel deformation, pterygium colli and mirror movements of the upper limbs) the radiological work-up should include MR images of the cervical spine and its contents. Moreover, the split in the cord is not always at the same level as the Klippel-Feil anomaly but sometimes at the lumbar level [74, 155, 157], therefore it is advisable to obtain a MR of the whole spine. Iniencephaly is con-

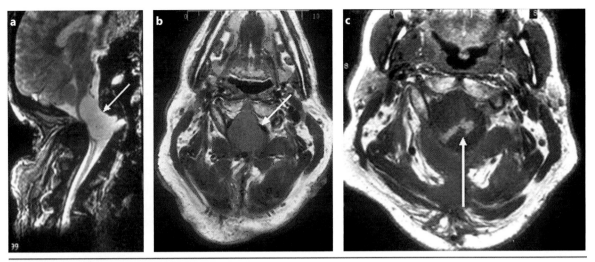

Fig. 38.7 a-c. Patient with Klippel-Feil anomaly, neurenteric cyst and DM (author's personal observation). **a** T2-weighted image: cervical and cranial image. Multiple fused vertebrae, the neurenteric cyst (*white arrow*) causing significant compression of the cervical spinal cord, which is pushed posteriorly. **b** The T1-weighted axial MRI shows that the cyst (*white arrow*) is occupying the major part of the cervical canal. **c** Axial T1 MRI after removal of the cyst shows the posterior partial DM of the cervical spinal cord (*white arrow*)

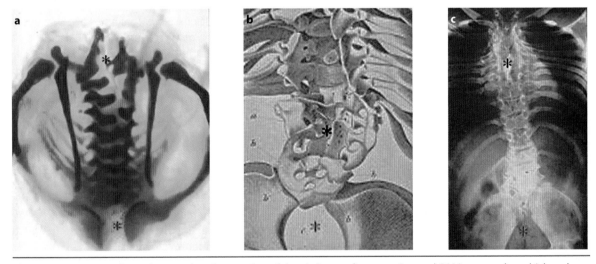

Fig. 38.8 a-c. DM and sacral agenesis. **a** Preparation of the skeleton of an experimental DM in a rumpless chick embryo. Reproduced from [49]. **b** Hohl's princeps observation of a sacral agenesis with a sacral lumbar bone spur. Reproduced from [62]. **c** Plain X-rays of the spine and pelvis showing a sacral agenesis and Type I DM. Reproduced from [61]. *Black asterisk* points at the bony spur, *red asterisk* at the sacral agenesis

sidered as the extreme and non-viable form of the Klippel-Feil syndrome. Following the works of Gardner [158, 159], more recent observations of DM associated with iniencephaly have been reported [160, 161]. Spondylo-costal dysplasia (Jarcho-Levine syndrome) is characterised by an association of multiple vertebral malformations and ribs. This gives rise to a typical clinical picture with a short neck and trunk, and scoliosis with deformation of the thorax. It is inherited in an autosomal recessive fashion [54]. The association with open and occult spina bifida and DM has been found on several occasions [53, 54, 162-164]. Another well accepted feature of notochordodysraphism is the association between sacral agenesis and DM (Fig. 38.8) [22, 61, 62, 165-170].

Ectopic Neural Tissue, Wilms' Tumor, Teratoma

Cells originating from the mesoderm that will transform into anlagen of the excretory system may exceptionally be driven into the cleft and develop as ectopic renal tissue [171-173], or an extra-renal Wilms' tumour [174].The occurrence of teratoma is also well documented [144, 175, 176, 177-187]. Cerebellar heterotopia associated with a split cord and a neurenteric cyst has also been recently described [188]. These associations are certainly not fortuitous: pluripotential cells that give rise to teratomatous tumours may be driven into the neurenteric canal.

Clinical Presentation

Geographical Distribution, Epidemiology, Age at Presentation, Sex Prevalence

DM has been reported in every part of the world, although few reports come from Japan. Kurihara et al. [189] say that DM is rare in their country. This affirmation is also shared in another Japanese report [190]. Fewer than ten papers dealing either with DM or SCM have come from Japan [120, 189-198]. On the other hand, the largest series [66, 67] and recent publications about DM come from India and Turkey. Does this mean anything? As this malformation is rare, definitive conclusions about its geographical distribution cannot be drawn, and speculating upon environmental or ethnic factors as has often been proposed for spina bifida aperta is not possible.

The mean age at presentation was 3.5 years in Matson's series [199], 6.5 years at the Sick Kids Hospital in Toronto [145] and 17 months in the report from Gutkelch [200]. In the series of Ersahin et al. [66], symptomatic patients, either with neurological deficits or orthopaedic deformities present at a significantly older age (43.2 months) than those without deficits (8.2 months). Conversely, the age at presentation is very similar in the Mahapatra and Gupta series [67] when they make a comparison between symptomatic patients with neurological deficits (mean age: 6.66 years) to asymptomatic patients (mean age: 6.7 years). French [65] also studied the age at presentation: he found 57% between birth and 5-years-old, 25% between 6 and 10 years, 12% between 11 and 20 years and only 6% above 21 years of age. Presentation at adult age is therefore rare. Beyerl et al. [201] collected 21 cases published up until 1985. This figure must be compared with all

the 314 collected cases from any age found in the English literature [79]. After the paper of Pang and Wilberger [202], several publications dealing with the adult tethered cord syndrome were published and in each of these reports [83, 203-210], one can find a small proportion of DM as the cause of the tethered cord. DM has even been observed at a geriatric age [211, 212].

The predominance of the feminine gender has been reported in all series. The female/male ratio is between 5/3 [75] and 1.5/1 [67]. There is no explanation in the literature for the predominance of girls. A peculiar susceptibility of the female embryo at a certain stage of development is suspected, although without any proof.

Familial Incidence, Heredity

Most cases of DM are sporadic. A family history has been reported by some authors and Ersahin et al. [213], reporting two sisters with DM of the same family, were able to find three others reports of such an occurrence [41, 214, 215]. The type of genetic transmission is discussed by Ersahin et al., who quote two papers [216, 217] dealing with the sex ratio of affected and transmitting members of multiple case families with neural tube defects; more females are affected and seem to inherit the predisposition to a neural tube defect from their mother. Unfortunately, if one assumes that DM is not due to a neurulation defect, this hypothesis cannot yet be validated.

Among the five cases reported by Kennedy [218], two children suffering from DM had relatives that died from spina bifida aperta. One patient had an especially burdened family history as three of his sisters died with a spina bifida. A patient reported by Kurihara [189] had a sister who had been operated upon for a meningomyelocele.

Carter [219] investigated whether brothers and sisters of children treated for an occult spinal dysraphism (including cases with DM) presented an increased risk of having severe neural tube defects (anencephaly and spina bifida aperta). Of a total of 364 siblings, nine were born with an anencephaly and six with an open spina bifida, thus giving a proportion of 4.12%. This proportion is rather similar to that found in families with previous open neural tube defects. Wynne-Davies [220], analysing a cohort of 337 patients with congenital vertebral anomalies stated that subsequent siblings of patients with multiple vertebral anomalies (without apparent spina bifida), aetiologically related to open tube defects, have a 5-10% risk for any one of these defects. Conversely, solitary hemivertebrae and localised anterior defects of the vertebral bodies (such as one can find in DM Type I) causing kyphoscoliosis are sporadic and carry no risk to subsequent siblings.

It is difficult to form an opinion about a putative genetic transmission of DM. Caspi [221] wrote that familial cases could be attributed to a recessive trait.

Skin Markers

Cutaneous stigmata or markers represent the skin expression of the underlying DM, most often as hypertrichosis (or hairy patch) which resembles a faun's tail (Fig. 38.9), or as a dimple or sinus. A capillary angioma is also seen, especially when the parents shave the hypertrichosis. Most of these cutaneous lesions are often associated and rarely appear as a single entity. Hypertrichosis is the most frequent stigmata [75]. Schropp et al. [222], studying the cutaneous lesions in occult spinal dysraphism, found a strong statistical correlation between the presence of a hairy patch and the underlying DM. These authors also found that of a total of 55 patients where the main diagnosis was DM; only seven did not show any cutaneous stigmata. In Pang's series [75], if one excludes cases of DM associated with meningomyelocele, only two children did not have hypertrichosis. Conversely, the absence of cutaneous stigmata has been reported [223], even in a case with an important malformation [224].

Owing to the cosmetic concerns, if the lesion is small, it can be excised at the time of the treatment of DM. If the area involved is significant as in widespread hypertrichosis, plastic surgery may be scheduled at a second stage [225] or the hairy patch may be treated by electric or laser epilation by a dermatologist [226].

Neurological and Orthopaedic Syndromes, Trophic Changes

Classical descriptions of DM have separated the neurological and the orthopaedic presentations [6, 200] but inevitably there are some patients who have both neurological and orthopaedic symptoms and signs.

The orthopaedic syndrome is characterised by scoliosis and more rarely kyphosis, a congenital elevation of the shoulder blade (Sprengel's deformity), especially when DM is associated with the Klippel-Feil syndrome, hip luxation causing a limp, asymmetry of the length of the inferior limbs and the feet, pes cavus or a pes varus or valgus. According to James and Lassman [227], pes cavus is the most precocious sign, with pes valgus appearing at a later stage. Rachialgia is often a complaint of older patients suffering from DM.

The neurological syndrome is characterised by gait difficulties, frequent asymmetrical weakness and atrophy of the lower limbs, sensory deficits, neurotrophic foot ulcers and sphincter dysfunction. Neurotrophic changes can also occur in the hands as a sign of cervical DM. This has been reported in a patient who presented with self-mutilation of the fingers [228]. Sciatica may be a presenting symptom in older patients as well as, more rarely, neurogenic claudication [229].

Absence of crossed reflexes has been described in 31% of cases of DM associated with spina bifida

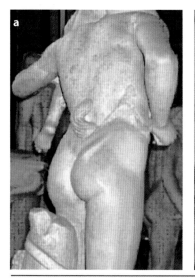
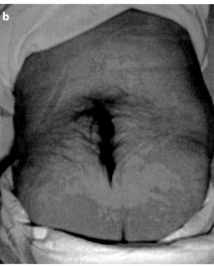

Fig. 38.9 a, b. Hypertrichosis in the lumbar region (faun's tail). **a** Example from the gallery of sculptures, Città del Vaticano. **b** Example in a 3-month-old boy (author's personal observation)

[112, 113]. Birch and McCormick [129] reported a high cervical split cord malformation with a neurenteric cyst associated with congenital mirror movements.

A case where sphincter disturbance was the only presenting symptom was reported [142]. Trophic ulcers in the feet are a relatively rare complication of DM [200, 230, 231]. The most severe form is represented by the acrodystrophic neuropathy [232, 233] with torpid ulcers, distal bone resorption and insensibility to pain.

Presentation at Adult Age

Russel [234] collected 45 cases of DM diagnosed in adulthood having escaped detection at an earlier age due to the clinical signs (cutaneous stigmata, neurological deficit) being very discrete or absent. For some unknown reason, the incidence of cervical DM is increased in adults [153, 201, 235-238]. Cervical DM that are not associated with complex malformations such as Klippel-Feil anomalies typically become symptomatic in the second or third decade of life with neurological signs sometimes revealed by a minor or trivial injury such as a whiplash injury [237]. Brisk aggravation after a trauma with hemiplegia has been reported [235]. The importance of trauma in the revelation of symptoms is emphasised by Garza-Marcado [176] who noticed, in a collection of 12 cases of adult DM, that the symptoms appeared in four of the patients after a blow on the lumbar spine, a long journey in a lorry, a lumbar puncture and a road traffic accident. Conversely, the discovery of a cervical DM in the absence of a traumatic history is rather rare. Ohwada [192] reported an adult case with a cervico-thoracic DM who presented with signs of thoracic myelopathy. In another case of cervical DM, the patient had a bilateral amyotrophy of the upper limbs [191]. Concerning the presentation in adulthood, Maroun [3] proposed that the differential growth of the spine and the spinal cord can explain the occurrence of symptoms during growth, but is insufficient to explain the late presentation. In some cases, albeit fortunately extremely rare, a delay in diagnosis was iatrogenic [239, 240].

Pathophysiology

The three types of factors that have been used to explain the symptoms that occur in DM are discussed below.

1. Mechanical factors:

The most logical explanation is that the osseous or fibro-cartilaginous septum is usually situated in the inferior part of the cleft, anchors the spinal cord and impedes the normal ascension of its distal segments. Therefore a situation of tethered cord is created. The growth of the patient can cause a progressive enlargement of the cleft due to a slow sagittal section of the spinal cord by the bone spur that is fixed in the spinal canal (Fig. 38.10). In small children, plasticity of the nervous system may explain the fact that they can remain asymptomatic or pauci-symptomatic, but after a certain age, particularly in period of rapid growth, the nervous tissue cannot tolerate these constraints and the patient will become symptomatic. The indication to perform prophylactic surgery is mainly based on this hypothesis. Nevertheless, some observations cast doubt on this argument. Guthkelch [200] studied the incidence of deterioration in relation to the level of the DM. He postulated that if the tethering of the spinal cord is greater at the lumbar than the thoracic level, one may deduce that the incidence of neurological deficit would be greater in lumbar than in thoracic DM. In fact, data from his own series did not confirm this difference and analysis of other series, regarding this particular aspect, shows that the mean level of DM is slightly higher in patients who harbour neurological deficits compared to those who are asymptomatic. Another argument forwarded by Guthkelch is that after removal of

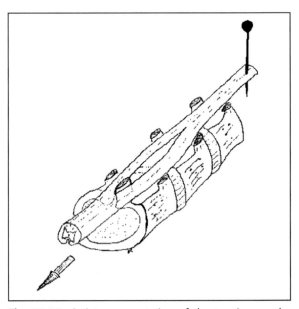

Fig. 38.10. Artist representation of the traction on the spinal cord by a spur situated at the lower end of the cleft

the bone spur and release of the spinal cord, there is no real ascension as one would expect. Moreover, in some cases the septum is situated in the middle portion of the cleft and does not exert any tethering on the spinal cord. Guthkelch also postulated that the progressive increase of physical activity in the lower limbs when the child begins to walk could explain the delay in the presentation of symptoms. Goldberd et al. [241] are also in favour of the mechanical hypothesis. Flexion and extension movements are responsible for local stress on the spinal cord either by traction on neurons and their axons or through involvement of the spinal cord arteries with resultant ischemia of the cord. The aggravating role of spinal canal stenosis and scoliosis on a spinal cord that is not free floating in the CSF spaces due to the constraint imposed by the bone spur is recognised by several authors [139, 202, 242]. Hypertrophy of the laminae associated with the bone spur has also been incriminated [243]. Other mechanical factors such as traction by fibro-glial bands, "méningomyélocèle manqué", associated hypertrophied tight filum or compression due to other associated dysraphic pathologies (dermoid and neurenteric cyst, teratoma) should also be considered.

2. Vascular factors:
   Vandresse [244] thought that compression of the anterior spinal artery or an asymmetrical distribution of the vascular supply to both hemicords could be responsible for ischemic disturbances. The hypothesis of a venous origin of the symptoms has been discussed by Hüsler [245]. Whatever the vascular disturbance, of either arterial or venous origin, the consequences are reduced local flow and eventually the appearance of ischemic lesions. Experiences of Yamada et al. [246] bring a definite credit to this vascular hypothesis. With the help of a spectroscopic technique and applying progressive weights to the cat lumbo-sacral spinal cord, they were able to demonstrate changes in the oxidative metabolism that were reversible when the traction on the spinal cord was released. Non-invasive spectrophotometry performed during surgery before and after cord detethering showed the same results as in experimental conditions.

3. Anatomical factors:
   Pre-operative imagery (CT scan and MRI) and peri-operative findings suggest that hypoplasia of one of the hemicords certainly plays an important role in the pathogenesis, especially for patients with "orthopaedic" presentations [21, 140].

Investigations

Strategy of Imagery

Antenatal Diagnosis

In 2003, Sonigo-Cohen et al. [247] reported three new prenatal cases of DM and reviewed 18 previous cases reported in the literature. Three more reports have been published since then [248-250]. DMs were confirmed either with antenatal or post-natal MRI or post-natal CT scan. Antenatal diagnosis should be capable of separating cases of isolated DM with a favourable prognosis and cases of DM associated with open defects or multiple malformations of less favourable prognosis.

Postnatal Diagnosis

Ultrasonography in newborns is a simple tool to demonstrate a DM and can give an accurate image of the malformation (Fig. 38.11) before an MRI is prescribed. Simple X-rays are not diagnostic in every case and are reserved for the assessment of the spinal curvature especially by the orthopaedic surgeon. MRI allows the shape of the DM to be visualised, as well

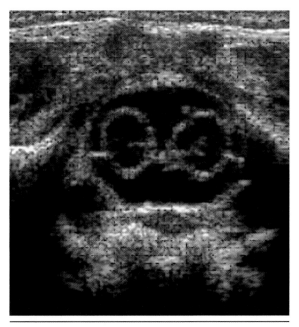

Fig. 38.11. Ultrasonographic axial view of a DM in a 3-month-old baby (author's personal observation, same patient as in Fig. 38.9b)

as the asymmetry of the hemicords, the presence of a syrinx and associated intra-dural malformations such as a tight filum, dermoid and neurenteric cysts, ectopic tissue, teratomas and hydromyelia.

Bone anomalies can also be demonstrated with MRI, but in the presence of a severe scoliosis and vertebral malformations, CT in the axial plane, three dimensional CT and CT with intra-thecal water-soluble iodine contrast may better show the relationship between the spine elements and the malformed spinal cord.

Urodynamic Studies

Few patients with DM present with complaints of urological dysfunction but formal testing of urodynamics can reveal up to 75% of urological abnormalities [251]. Urodynamic studies are mandatory in the follow-up (FU) of patients with tethered cord syndrome; they have been utilised on a routine basis in the author's department for more than ten years [252]. Prospective evaluation of the patients has permitted the establishment of an urodynamic score. This has facilitated the surveillance of these patients either if an operation is pending or in patients that have been already operated upon and present with symptoms of re-tethering.

Surgical Indications

Matson [28] first discussed the indication to operate, saying that the aim of surgery of DM is more prophylactic than curative. The indication to operate is largely accepted for patients presenting a rapid deterioration of neurological, urological or orthopaedic function when they were previously devoid of symptoms. The results of surgery in these patients is particularly rewarding, with a rapid recovery of function to the premorbid state.

Most orthopaedists are clear about the fact that patients presenting with scoliosis and an associated DM Type I should be operated for the intra-spinal anomaly prior to reduction of the scoliosis [92, 243]. Laminectomies to remove a bone spur on a scoliotic spine will aggravate the deformation and thus systematic fixation is recommended. This can be done in the same surgical session after the neurosurgical time [127, 243] or as a separate procedure in some cases, sometimes with a rather long delay between the treatment of DM and the spinal surgery [96]. No patient with such a combined approach suffered from neurological complications [127, 243, 253].

The indication to remove a bony spur or fibrous septum if discovered in a spina bifida aperta patient is obvious [142]; failure to appreciate the spur or the septum in a meningomyelocele closure can lead to delayed complications [118].

In cases of chronic neurological deficit characterised by an orthopaedic syndrome with leg atrophy, foot deformation, absence of reflexes and long-standing sensory deficits, surgery is aimed at preventing further severe deterioration.

Twenty-two patients of Gutkelch [200] with a stable deficit were separated into two groups. Of ten patients who were managed with a conservative wait-and-watch attitude, eight had to be eventually operated upon for aggravation of a pre-existing deficit. In 12 patients with a stable deficit who had the bony spur removed soon after the diagnosis was made, no progression of the deficit had occurred. Therefore surgery is indicated in all patients with a stable deficit, with the expectation of stabilisation of their deficit and not recovery ad integrum of their neurological function.

Patients who present predominantly with deterioration in sphincter functions are also candidates for immediate surgery, especially if the bladder symptoms have appeared recently without evidence of other neurological or orthopaedic deterioration. The systematic utilisation of urodynamic and ano-rectal manometry is proposed by Meyrat et al [252]. In their series of nine cases of tethered cord (two with DM) they claim that the appearance of urodynamic and anorectal manometric signs are the most sensible parameters of deterioration, even in patients that are otherwise asymptomatic, and should urge the surgeon to release the spinal cord.

Very rarely, adult patients with DM complain of sexual disturbances. Chehrazi [254] reported a patient who had sphincter and erectile dysfunction and who was persuaded to have a penile prosthesis implanted. The diagnosis of DM became evident when abnormal hair at the thoraco-lumbar junction was found. The sphincter and sexual disturbances improved after the removal of a fibrous septum. This result is rather exceptional and sphincter disturbances reported in adult tethered cord rarely show such a spectacular improvement [202].

Despite the chronic course of the trophic limb lesions, surgery of DM can lead to healing or regression of the trophic ulcers [6, 67, 230, 233].

Prophylactic surgery must be discussed with the view that surgery should prevent a future deterioration with minimal morbidity or not any morbidity at all.

Mathieu [127] makes a plea for a prophylactic surgery in asymptomatic children because he is convinced that sooner or later they will present with neurological signs. He defends his attitude, emphasising the fact that in some children of his series, surgery was postponed for various reasons and he unfortunately noticed urgency of micturition and even incontinence which according to his own results rarely improved (healed neurogenic bladder in three of 23 cases). It is clear that the results concerning the sphincter dysfunction are proportional to the length of the history of sphincter disturbance. This particular issue is very well analysed in the paper of Proctor and Scott [251] who, in the discussion of their results, insist on the importance of the pre-and postoperative assessment of these patients with urodynamic studies.

Prophylactic treatment of DM is also the recommendation in more recent papers [66, 67, 77, 108, 251]. In contrast and to tone down this uniform way of thinking, Zuccaro [255], in a commentary about another recent series of DM [77], stated that the majority of non-operated asymptomatic patients in her series remained asymptomatic, with a mean FU of seven years.

Most of the cases of cervical DM [153, 201, 235-238] were diagnosed after trauma: it is also justified therefore to propose prophylactic surgery for these patients, and not to wait for a second traumatic event that could further aggravate neurological dysfunction.

Prophylactic surgery is also questioned when the division of the spinal cord is distal to the bone spur or septum and the conus and the filum are separated into two independent hemi-conus and hemi-filia terminalia [77]. According to Harwood-Nash, this situation is found in 10% of cases. If the two hemi-filia are hypertrophic and tether the two hemi-conus, they must be cut [139, 141].

Finally, it is obvious that surgery is indicated in every patient who presents with DM-associated anomalies such as a dermal sinus, a dermoid or neurenteric cyst or a teratoma. These associated pathologies may themselves be the source of important complications if not properly treated.

Technique

For obvious reasons the only position for operation is the prone position. In small children, the vacuum bean bag is modelled to free the abdomen and avoid any compression on the vena cava. Older patients are positioned with a special cushion that also avoids compression of the abdomen. The genu-pectoral position mostly used for disk surgery is not advisable because it can cause unnecessary stretching of the

spinal cord on the bony spur and make the removal of the offending structure more difficult [127]. Neurophysiological monitoring has not been universally utilised and looking back in the literature on DM, the use of intra-operative neurophysiological monitoring depends mainly on the availability of the equipment. A large number of patients with DM have been operated upon without monitoring and it is therefore difficult to estimate if the end results were better in the hands of surgeons who used this equipment. In a recent series of combined DM and hemivertebra reported by a ortho-neuro-surgical team [96] the use of spinal cord monitoring was recommended, albeit only when spinal surgery is performed. Certainly, in Type I DM the surgeon could be more confident if the continuous intra-operative neurophysiological monitoring showed him that the surgical manipulation of the hemicords around the bony spur reduced the amplitude of the evoked potential, thereby urging him to stop dissection until the baseline returned to normal.

A lateral X-ray is recommended when the upper lumbar or dorsal region is being operated upon, as cutaneous lesions may be dissociated several vertebral segments from the bony spur. Laminectomy is centred on the level of the spur, usually corresponding to a hypertrophied or malformed posterior arch of the vertebra. Bone removal begins at the level of the upper and inferior normal lamina where the spinal canal becomes wider. Laminectomy should not be too wide in order to avoid deterioration of the associated spine deformation. When the pre-operative imagery does not show a tight posterior attachment of the bone spur, or in cases of Type II DM, a cautious osteoplastic laminotomy can be done to prevent the deformation of the spine in a growing child. This may be performed with a small reciprocating saw (Fig. 38.12a) or with a high speed drill craniotome (which, for this special use, is more properly called a spinotome). The osteoplastic flap is reflected and the posterior attachment of the bony spur disarticulated (Fig. 38.12b). As soon as the canal is open, the use of magnifying glasses or a microscope is recommended. In type I DM, one may encounter profuse bleeding of the veins that are situated around the dorsal attachment of the spur. This haemorrhage should be managed with bipolar coagulation prior to dural opening and not with patties that may inadvertently compress the underlying hemicords. With the same concern about preservation of neural structures, one should try to remove as much of the bony spur as possible prior to opening the dura (Fig. 38.12c). Morcellation of the spur progresses with fine bone nibblers and a high speed drill, first with cutting burrs, then with diamond burrs. A small artery is sometimes found at the base of the spur [21] and can cause additional difficulties: the bleeding may be significant and haemostasis difficult in the deepest part of the operative field [64, 85]. According to French [65], this problem can be brought under control with application of bone wax or by gentle action of the diamond burr without irrigation.

The dural sleeves of the spur must be removed after opening of the dura down to the anterior part of the dural sac (Fig. 38.12d). This is an important point to mention as there have been several reports of neo-spurs arising from re-ossification from the remaining dural sleeves [28, 64, 256-258]. Section of the arachnoidal adherences and other fibrous bands

is also performed. The filum is cut when there is obvious evidence of a tethering mechanism or in the presence of a low-lying conus, either by the same incision or by a small sacral laminectomy or laminotomy. After the final inspection (Fig. 38.12e), the posterior dura is closed.

Controversy still remains about the management of the associated hydromyelia that can be found in more than 50% of patients in some series [106, 109]. Iskandar et al. [106] promoted the insertion of a syringo-subarachnoid shunt when the syrinx was large enough. Four syringes were shunted at the time when the DM was treated. Three syringes were treated at a second operation. The post-operative MRI showed a significant decrease or even a disappear-

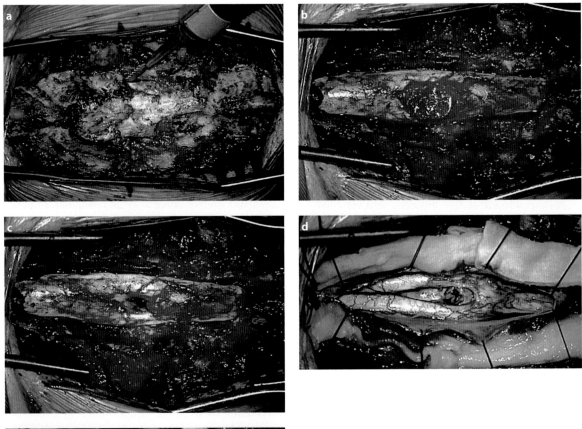

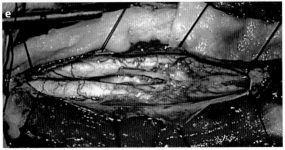

Fig. 38.12 a-e. Osteoplastic laminotomy to cure a Type I DM (Courtesy of Prof. Memet Özek, Istanbul). Rostral side is on the left hand side and caudal side on the right hand side. **a** Cautious laminotomy with a reciprocating mini saw. **b** View after the laminotomy flap has been removed; the posterior attachment of the bony spur has been disarticulated from the lamina. **c** View after extra-dural removal of the bony spur with fine bone nibbler and high speed drill. **d** View after removal of the dural sleeves of the bony spur down to the anterior part of the dural sac to prevent relapse. **e** Final view before closure of the dura

ance of the syrinx but objective clinical improvement was less satisfactory: the neurological and sphincter deficits were better in only one third of the patients. However, the disappearance of back and abdominal pain in these patients justified per se the indication to do these syringostomies. It is difficult to determine, in patients who had in the same sitting detethering of the spinal cord and syringostomy, which of the two procedures was the most efficacious. On the contrary, British neurosurgeons [108, 109], although they also have a high incidence of hydromyelia in their series of DM, state that, even if large, these syringes must be managed in a conservative manner.

Complications

Generally speaking, morbidity and mortality of DM surgery is very low.

Per-operative complications are due to difficulties with haemostasis. Mathieu [127], in the beginning of his experience, reports significant bleeding of the epidural veins in two children less than 2 months of age necessitating cessation of surgery and later re-operation. The message given was that this would not have happened if he had waited longer to do the operation. These two complications occurred prior to the introduction of bipolar coagulation in his department. A more tragic case of uncontrollable bleeding was reported by McCullough [259]. The bleeding appeared at the end of the removal of the superior part of the spur; haemostasis on the vessels that were situated anteriorly to the posterior longitudinal ligament was impossible despite the use of coagulation, bone wax and compression by tamponage. The 4.5-year-old child died on the table, despite multiple transfusions.

The immediate post-operative complications are mainly due to difficulties that are encountered when the bony spur is removed and insufficient water tight-closure of the dura.

One hundred and seventy-eight cases taken from six series of the literature on DM were analysed by McCullough in the eighties [90, 145, 200, 218, 241, 243]. He found an incidence of 2% of permanent neurological deficit, 3% of CSF leak and 1% of meningitis. The incidence of CSF leak in one series rose up to 13% and was particularly elevated in patients who had a duroplasty or an associated lipomeningocele [127]. Children that had already been treated for meningomyelocele and who were re-operated upon for a DM had a higher risk of developing CSF leak because of a previous scar. Two children from Pang's series [75] had such problems later complicated by shunt infection. In a recent series [67] with a huge cohort of patients, the incidence of CSF leak was 9% and wound infection 2%, all these issues were managed conservatively and eventually healed well.

The rate of neurological complication in older series reported by orthopaedists [85, 241] is higher because the majority of the patients they treated had Type I DM. The only case of the series of Pang [75] who had deterioration in the function of one of the lower limbs had a Type I DM with an asymmetric division of the spinal cord and a bone spur that was oblique. The smaller hemicord was inadvertently injured because it was hidden behind the oblique spur. This asymmetrical division of the spinal cord associated with an oblique septum must be recognised prior to surgery. Distorted anatomy can be confusing and Mathieu et al. [127] also reported a case where surgery was particularly laborious due to significant thoraco-lumbar scoliosis. The division of the spinal cord was perpendicular to the surgeon and both dural sleeves were so asymmetric that he had entered the inter-vertebral foramina instead of dissecting around the bony spur.

Mahapatra and Gupta [67] have reconsidered Pang's classification and have proposed a new sub-classification with four types. The classification into four subtypes of Type I DM, based on the location of the bony spur causing the split, is particularly interesting as far as the dissection of the offending structure and the outcome is concerned:
- in Type Ia, the bone spur lays in the centre of the split with an equally duplicated cord above and below the spur;
- in Type Ib, the bone spur is situated at the superior pole with no space above it and a large duplicated cord lower down;
- in Type Ic, the bone spur is situated on the lower pole with a large duplicated cord above;
- in Type Id, a bone spur is straddling the bifurcation of the spinal cord with no space above or below the spur.

Type Id was seen in six of the last 25 patients of their huge series. They noticed that the risk of inflicting a trauma to the hemicords is high in this subtype, four of six patients (67%) had post-operative deterioration.

Urinary retention after surgery is encountered principally in Type I: nine cases in the series of Pang [75] but fortunately permanent in only two cases. Urinary tract infections were seen in 4% in another series [67].

Ersahin et al. [66] report an overall low incidence of complications, and fortunately most of them were transient. The majority of the children in their series remained stable and a clinical improvement was observed in 18/74 patients. Five patients experienced deterioration with time, two had arachnoiditis and three had scoliosis. They lost two patients: one had a meningomyelocele and a DM and was found dead in his bed probably as a result of an apnea, another infant died of ventriculitis.

In the eighties, McCullough reported an operative mortality of 2% [259]. Three authors [74, 243] separately reported cardiac arrest at the time of the laminectomy, with resuscitation successful in only one patient. Mathieu [127] also had to deplore an early death in a child with a DM found during the repair of a meningomyelocele.

Long term mortality is also very low: two out of 40 cases in the series of Gower [64], one due to a urinary infection the other of unknown cause. Two other late deaths, respectively from a pneumonia in Keim's series (1/20 cases) [74] and another due to complication of an associated meningomyelocele in the series of Hood et al. [90] (1/51 cases), were reported.

Results

Analysis of results of surgery for DM unfortunately suffers from a lack of homogeneity of their presentation by the different authors. It is therefore impossible to gather all the information in a table.

The analysis of the series of Gower [64] reports the longest FU (30 patients over 40 years, 21 were operated). Of the condition of these patients, three were considered as better-off (mean FU=4.3 years, extremes 1 month to 11 years), 14 were considered as stable (mean FU=14.6 years, extremes 2 months to 28 years), and four were considered as worse-off (mean FU=17.3 years, extremes 8 to 28 years) after surgery.

The FU duration in the Mahapatra and Gupta series [67] varied from 3 months to 12 years. Of their symptomatic patients, 68 (39%) showed improvement of their motor function, 33 of 57 (60%) improved their sensation, and 20 of 73 (27%) regained continence. Significant healing of trophic ulcers was seen in 13 of 25 (52%) patients. No change in the neurological examination of 160 of 254 (63%) patients was noticed. Fifteen patients (7%) showed neurological worsening immediately after surgery, ten of them having a Type I DM; most of them improved before discharge from the hospital or made a progressive recovery to their preoperative state and only three were left with a permanent deficit. Three patients of this subgroup were lost to FU.

Concerning the result for scoliosis (without associated spine surgery), Gower [64] states that out of seven cases who had a preoperative scoliosis, four did not change in degree of severity, one stopped its progression and two continued to progress. Mathieu's comment about the same issue is the following: "some moderate scoliosis may be stabilised by the surgery on DM, but an improvement cannot occur only with the neurosurgical operation" [127]. Another series including 51 patients who had removal of a bony spur was analysed by Hood et al. [90]. No change in the neurological condition was found in 61% of the patients and 39% showed only a rather modest improvement, e.g., the return of a stretch reflex or a gain of one point on the motor scale. This author concluded that no patient was harmed by the surgery but none of them made a spectacular recovery.

Lapras [95] wrote that patients suffering from an orthopaedic syndrome can be stabilised but not made better. The only exception to this statement is the partial regression of the clubfoot deformity in patients that were operated early in the course of the disease [260].

Conclusion

DM is a fascinating congenital malformation due to faulty development of the notochord. It may be considered as an aborted sagittal duplication of the embryo in the most severe type or as a simple cleft in the spinal cord. DM has not yet revealed the secrets of its origin. The etiology is totally obscure and some simple but important questions remain unsolved; for example, the female predominance. A better knowledge of the intrinsic cell mechanisms, molecular and genetic events that occur during the development of the embryo will sooner or later give the key to the mystery of DM and will allow one to think about preventing this malformation. In this respect, recent progress of antenatal ultrasonography already permit the most severe forms to be detected. Surgical indications are in most cases straightforward, in both symptomatic and asymptomatic patients, to prevent further deterioration. Results of surgery over time have been globally good, with the exception of some rare patients where the bone spur fills all the space between the two hemicords with an extrememly scoliotic distorted anatomy that makes surgery more difficult and the risk of inflicting a permanent neurological deficit greater.

References

1. Ollivier CP (1837) Traité des maladies de la moelle épinière. Paris, Méquignon-Marvis
2. Cohen J, Sledge CB (1960) Diastematomyelia. An embryological interpretation and report of a case. Am J Dis Child 100:257-263
3. Maroun FB, Jacob BC, Haneghan WD (1972) La diastématomyélie, Ses manifestations cliniques et son traitement chirugical. Neurochirurgie 18:285-316
4. Hilal SK, Marton D, Pollack E (1974) Diastematomyelia in children. Radiographic study of 34 cases. Radiology 112:609-621
5. Harwood-Nash DC, McHugh K (1990-1991) Diastematomyelia in 172 children: The impact of modern neuroradiology. Pediatr Neurosurg16:247-251
6. James CCM, Lassman LP (1972) Spinal dysraphism (Spina bifida occulta). London, Butterworth.
7. Leys D, Samain F, Lesoin F et al (1987) Diastématomyélie partielle de l'adulte avec éperon osseux postérieur. Rev Neurol 143:63-67
8. Scatliff JH, Till K, Hoare RD (1975) Incomplete, false and true diastematomyelia. Radiological evaluation by air myelography and tomography. Radiology 116:349-354
9. Von Recklinghausen F (1886) Untersuchungen über die spina bifida. Virchows Arch Path Anat 105:243-330
10. Cogliatti SB (1986) Diplomyelia: Caudal duplication of the neural tube in mice. Teratology 34:343-352
11. Park CHT, Pruitt JH, Bennet D (1989) A mouse model for neural tube defects: The curtailed (Tc) mutation produce spina bifida occulta in Tc/+ animals and spina bifida with meningomyelocele in Tc/t. Teratology 39:303-312
12. James CCM, Lassman LP, Tomlinson BE (1969) Congenital anomalies of the lower spine and spinal cord in Manx cats. J Pathol 97:269-276
13. von Santha K (1930) Ueber das Verhalten des Kleinhirn in einem Falle von endogenen-afamiliärer Idiotie. Zur differential diagnoses der Marieschen und der sonstigne endogenen Kleinhirnerkrankungen, nebst Beitrag zur Lehre der Diplomyelie. Z Neurol Pschiatr 123:717-793
14. Schneiderling W (1938) Unvollkommene dorso-ventrale Verdoppelung des Rückenmarks. Virchows Arch 301:478-489
15. Dominok GW (1962) Zur Frage de Diplomyelie. Deut Zeitsch Nervenheilk 183:340-350
16. Hori A, Fischer G, Dietrich-Schott B, Ikeda K (1982) Dimyelia, diplomyelia and diastematomyelia. Clin Neuropathol 1:23-30
17. Rokos J (1975) Pathogenesis of diastematomyelia and spina bifida. Path 117:155-161
18. Van Gieson I (1892) A study of the artefacts of the nervous system. The topographical alterations of the gray and white matters of the spinal cord caused by autopsy bruises, and a consideration of heterotopia of the spinal cord. New-York Med J 56:337-346; 365-379; 421-437
19. Sandberg G, Wong K, Horkayne-Szakaly I et al (2007) Trimyelia with divergent cord pathways and three foramina magni. Childs Nerv Syst 23:249-253
20. Nait-Oumesmar B, Stecca B, Fatterpekar G et al (2002) Ectopic expression of Gcm1 induces congenital spinal cord abnormalities. Development 129:3957-3964
21. Pang D, Dias MS, Ahab-Barmada M (1992) Split cord malformation: Part I: A unified theory of embryogenesis for double spinal cord malformations. Neurosurgery 31:451-480
22. Carcassonne M, Bergoin M, Choux M et al (1981) Les malformations de la colonne lombo-sacrée et leurs implications viscérales. Les malformations du système nerveux et de ses enveloppes. Chir Pediatr 22:105-108
23. Naidich TP, Gorey M, Raybaud C et al (1989) Malformations congénitales de la moelle. In: C Manelfe (ed) Imagerie du rachis et de la moelle. Vigot, Paris, pp 571-619
24. Perret G (1957) Diagnosis and treatment of diastematomyelia. Surg Gyn Obstet 105:69-83
25. Edelson JG, Nathan H, Arensburg B (1989) Diastematomyelia-the "double barrelled" spine. J Bone Joint Surg 69 (B):188-189
26. Herren RY, Edwards JE (1940) Diplomyelia (duplication of the spinal cord). Arch Pathol 30:1203-1214
27. Hamby WB (1936) Pilonidal cyst, spina bifida occulta and bifid spinal cord. Report of a case with review of the literature. Arch Pathol 21:831-838
28. Matson DD, Woods RP, Campbell JB et al (1950) Diastematomyelia (congenital clefts of the spinal cord): diagnosis and surgical treatment. Pediatrics 6:98-112
29. George EL, Georges-Labouesse EN, Patel-King RS et al (1993) Defects in mesoderm, neural tube and vascular development in mouse embryos lacking fibronectin. Development 119:1079-1091
30. Georges-Labouesse EN, George EL, Rayburn H et al (1996) Mesodermal development in mouse embryos mutant for fibronectin. Dev Dyn 207:145-156
31. McLone D, Dias M (1994) Normal and abnormal early development of the nervous system. In: W Cheek (ed) Pediatric neurosurgery. Surgery of the developing nervous system. WB Saunders Co, Philadelphia, pp 3-39
32. Spratt N (1947) Regression and shortening of the primitive streak in the explanted chick blastoderm. J Exp Zool 104:69
33. Dias MS, Walker ML (1992) The embyogenesis of complex dysraphic malformations: A disorder of gastrulation. Pediatr Neurosurg 18:229-253
34. Raybaud CA, Naidich TP, Mc Lone DG (1989) Développement de la moelle et du rachis. In: C Manelfe (ed) Imagerie du rachis et de la moelle. Vigot, Paris, pp 89-108
35. Fallon M, Gordon ARG, Lendrum AC (1954) Mediastinal cysts of foregut origin associated with vertebral abnormalities. Br J Surg 41:520-533

36. Hamilton WJ, Mossman HW (1976) Human embryology. Macmillan, London and Basingstoke

37. Klessinger S, Christ B (1996) Diastematomyelia and spina bifida can be caused by the intraspinal grafting of somites in early avian embryos. Neurosurgery 39:1215-1223

38. Pang D (1985) Tethered cord syndrome in adults. In: R Holzman, B Stein (eds) The tethered spine. Thieme-Stratton, New-York, pp 99-115

39. Dryden RJ (1980) Spina bifida in chick embryos: ultrastructure of open neural defects in the transitional region between primary and secondary modes of neural tube formation. In: TVN Persaud (ed) Advances in the study of birth defects. Neural and behavioural teratology, vol 4. MTP press limited, Lancaster, pp 75-100

40. Kapsenberg JG, Van Lookeren, Campagne JA (1949) A case of spina bifida combined with diastematomyely, the anomaly of Arnold-Chiari and hydrocephaly. Acta Anat 7:366-388

41. Gardner WJ (1973) The dysraphic states. Excerpta Medica, Amsterdam

42. Mann RA, Persaud TVN (1980) Experimental open defects in the early chick embryo. In: TVN Persaud (ed) Advances in the study of birth defects, vol 4. Neural and behavioural teratology. MTP press limited, Lancaster, pp 63-74

43. Budde M (1911) Die Bedeutung des Canalis Neurentericum für die formale Genese der Rachischisis anterior. Beitr z Path Anat u Z Allg Path 52:91-129

44. Bell HH (1923) Anterior spina bifida and its relation to a persistance of the neurenteric canal. J Nerv Ment Dis 57:445-462

45. Bremer JL (1952) Dorsal intestinal fistula; accessory neurenteric canal; diastematomyelia. Arch Path 54:132-138

46. Keen WW, Coplin WML (1906) Sacrococcygeal tumor. Surg Gynec Obstet 3: 662-671

47. Ancel P (1947) Recherche expérimentale sur le spina bifida. Arch Anat Micr 36:45-68

48. Beardmore HE, Wiglesworth FW (1958) Vertebral anomalies and alimentary duplications. Pediatr Clin North Am 5:457-474

49. Rilliet B, Schowing J, Berney J (1992) Pathogenesis of diastematomyelia: Can a surgical model in the chick embryo give some clues about the human malformation? Childs Nerv Syst 8:310-316

50. Emura T, Asashima M, Hashizume K (2000) An experimental animal model of split cord malformation. Pediatr Neurosurg 33:283-292

51. Emura T, Asashima M, Furue M et al (2002) Experimental split cord malformation. Pediatr Neurosurg 36:229-235

52. Emura T, Hashizume K, Asashima M (2003) Experimental study of the embryogenesis of gastrointestinal duplication and enteric cyst. Pediatr Surg Int 19:147-151

53. Reyes M, Morales A, Harris V et al (1989) Neural defects in Jarcho-Levin syndrome. J Child Neurol 4:51-54

54. Giacoia G, Say B (1991) Spondylocostal dysplasia and neural tube defects. J Med Genet 28:51-53

55. Etus V, Ceylan S (2003) Association of spondylocostal dysostosis and type I split cord malformation. Neurol Sci 24:134-137

56. Bulman M, Kusumi K, Frayling T et al (2000) Mutations in the human Delta homologue, DLL3, cause axial skeletal defects in spondylocostal dysostosis. Nat Genet 24:438-441

57. Williams M (2003) Developmental anomalies of the scapula – The "omo"st forgotten bone. Am J Med Genet 120A:583-587

58. Banizza von Bazan U (1979) The association between congenital elevation of the scapula and diastematomyelia. J Bone Joint Surg 61:59-63

59. Bentley JFR, Smith JR (1960) Developmental posterior enteric remnants and spinal malformations: The split notochord syndrome. Arch Dis Child 35:76-86

60. David KM, Copp AJ, Stevens JM et al (1996) Split cervical spinal cord with Klippel-Feil syndrome: seven cases. Brain 119 (Pt 6):1859-1872

61. Banizza von Bazan U (1978) Kaudales Regressionsyndrome und Diastematomyelie. Was enthält Hohls Erstbeschreibung einer Kreutzbeindysgenesie? Z Orthop 116:65-72

62. Hohl AF (1852) Merkwürdige Verbindung zwischen einem rudimentären Kreuzbein und eigenthümlisch geformten Becken, nebst Spina bifida eigener Art. In: Zur Pathologie des Becken. Engelmann, Leipzig

63. Sheptak PE (1978) Congenital malformation of the spine and spinal cord, vol 32. In: Diastematomyelia – diplomyelia. Elsevier, North-Holland biomedical press, New York

64. Gower DJ, Del Curling O, Kelly DL et al (1988) Diastematomyelia – A 40 year experience. Pediatr Neurosci 14:90-96

65. French BN (1990) Midline fusion defects and defects of formation. In: JR Youmans (ed) Neurological surgery. WB Saunders Co, Philadelphia, pp 1081-1235

66. Ersahin Y, Mutluer S, Kocaman S et al (1998) Split spinal cord malformations in children. J Neurosurg 88:57-65

67. Mahapatra A, Gupta D (2005) Split cord malformations: A clinical study of 254 patients and a proposal for a new clinical-imaging classification. J Neurosurg (6 Suppl Pediatrics) 103:531-536

68. Herman TE, Siegel MJ (1990) Cervical and basicranial diastematomyelia. Am J Roentgenol 154:806-808

69. Pfeifer JD (1991) Basicranial diastematomyelia: a case report. Clin Neuropathol 10:232-236

70. Ciurea AV, Coman T, Tascu A et al (2005) Intradural dermoid tumor of the posterior fossa in a child with diastematobulbia. Surg Neurol 63:571-575

71. Rustamzadeh E, Graupman PC, Lam CH (2006) Basicranial diplomyelia: an extension of the split cord malformation theory. Case report. J Neurosurg 104:362-365

72. Naidich TP, Harwood-Nash DC, Mc Lone DG (1982) Radiology of spinal dysraphism. In: Clinical Neurosurgery. Williams and Wilkins, Baltimore/London, pp 341-365

73. Akay K, Izci Y, Baysefer A et al (2005) Composite type of split cord malformation; two different types at three different levels: case report. J Neurosurg 102 (4 Suppl):436-438

74. Keim HA, Greene AF (1973) Diastematomyelia and scoliosis. J Bone Joint Surg 55(A):1425-1435

75. Pang D (1992) Split cord malformation: Part II: Clinical syndrome. Neurosurgery 31:481-500

76. Vaishya S, Kumarjain P (2001) Split cord malformation: three unusual cases of composite split cord malformation. Childs Nerv Syst 17:528-530

77. Schijman E (2003) Split spinal cord malformations: report of 22 cases and review of the literature. Childs Nerv Syst 19:96-103

78. Andar UB, Harkness WF, Hayward RD (1997) Split cord malformations of the lumbar region. A model for the neurosurgical management of all types of 'occult' spinal dysraphism? Pediatr Neurosurg 26:17-24

79. French BN (1982) The embryology of spinal dysraphism. In: Clinical neurosurgery. Williams and Wilkins, Baltimore/London, pp 295-340

80. Cowie TN (1951) Diastematomyelia with vertebral column defects: Observation on its radiological diagnosis. Br J Radiol 24:156-160

81. Swift DM, Carmel PW (1990) Congenital intradural pathology. Neurosurg Clin N Am 1:551-567

82. Chandra PS, Kamal R, Mahapatra AK (1999) An unusual case of dorsally situated bony spur in a lumbar split cord malformation. Pediatr Neurosurg 31:49-52

83. Akay KM, Ersahin Y, Cakir Y (2000) Tethered cord syndrome in adults. Acta Neurochir (Wien) 142:1111-1115

84. Akay K, Izci Y, Baysefer A (2002) Dorsal bony septum. A split cord malformation variant. Pediatr Neurosurg 36:225-228

85. Lassale B, Rigault P, Pouliquen JC et al (1980) La diastématomyélie (ou syndrome de la double chorde). Etude de 21 cas. Rev Chir Orthoped 66:123-139

86. Konner C, Gassner I, Mayr U et al (1990) Zur diagnose der Diastematomyelie mittels Ultraschall. Klin Padiatr 202:124-128

87. Ross GW, Swanson SA, Perentes E et al (1988) Ectopic midline spinal ganglion in diastematomyelia: A study of its connections. J Neurol Neurosurg Psychiatry 51:1231-1234

88. Naidich TP, Harwood-Nash DC (1983) Diastematomyelia: Hemicords and meningeal sheaths; single and double arachnoïd and dural tubes. AJNR 4:633-636

89. Mathern G, Peacock W (1992) Diastematomyelia, Spinal dysraphism. In: T Park (ed) Contemporary issues in neurological surgery. Blackwell Scientific Publications, Boston, pp 91-103

90. Hood RW, Riseborough EJ, Nehme HM et al (1980) Diastematomyelia and structural spine deformities. J Bone Joint Surg 62(A):520-528

91. Winter RB, Haven JJ, Moe JH et al (1974) Diastematomyelia and congenital spine deformities. J Bone Joint Surg 56(A):27-39

92. McMaster MJ (1984) Occult intraspinal anomalies and congenital scoliosis. J Bone Joint Surg 66(A):588-601

93. Banizza von Bazan UK, Rompe G, Krastel A et al (1976) Diastematomyelie, ihre Bedeutung für die Behandlung von Missbildungsskoliosen. Z Orthoped 114:881-889

94. Bradford DS, Heithoff KB, Cohen M (1991) Intraspinal abnormalities and congenital spine deformities: a radiographic and MRI study. J Pediatr Orthop 11:36-41

95. Lapras C, Bret P, Capdeville J (1978) La diastématomyélie. Réflexion à propos d'une série de 6 observations. Neurochirurgie 24:381-389

96. Leung YL, Buxton N (2005) Combined diastematomyelia and hemivertebra: a review of the management at a single centre. J Bone Joint Surg Br 87:1380-1384

97. Lemire RJ, Loesser JD, Leech RW et al (1975) Normal and abnormal development of the human nervous system. Harper and Row, New York

98. Bruhl K, Schwarz M, Schumacher R et al (1990) Congenital diastematomyelia in the upper thoracic spine. Diagnostic comparison of CT, CT myelography, MRI, and US. Neurosurg Rev 13:77-82

99. Schiffer J, Till K (1982) Spinal dysraphism in the cervical and dorsal regions in childhood. Childs Brain 9:73-84

100. Schlesinger AE, Naidich TP, Quencer RM (1986) Concurrent hydromyelia and diastematomyelia. AJNR 7:473-477

101. Han JS, Benson JE, Kaufman B et al (1985) Demonstration of diastematomyelia and associated abnormalities with MR imaging. AJNR 6:215-219

102. Kuharik MA, Edwards MK, Grossman C (1985-86) Magnetic resonance evaluation of pediatric spinal dysraphism. Pediat Neurosci 12:213-218

103. Chuang HS (1989) Congenital malformations of the spine in children: Neuro-imaging. In: AJ Raimondi, M Choux, C Di Rocco (eds) The pediatric spine II. Springer, New York, pp 251-290

104. Breningstall GN, Marker SM, Tubman DE (1992) Hydrosyringomyelia and diastematomyelia detected by MRI in myelomeningocele. Pediatr Neurol 8:267-271

105. Tripathi RP, Sharma A, Jena A et al (1992) Magnetic resonance imaging in occult spinal dysraphism. Australas-Radiol 36:8-14

106. Iskandar B, Oakes J, McLaughlin C et al (1994) Terminal hydrosyringomyelia and occcult spinal dysraphysm. J Neurosurg 81:513-519

107. Sinha S, Agarwal D, Mahapatra A (2005) Split cord malformation: An experience of 203 cases. Childs Nerv Syst 22:2-7

108. Gan YC, Sgouros S, Walsh AR et al (2007) Diastematomyelia in children: treatment outcome and natural history of associated syringomyelia. Childs Nerv Syst 23:515-519

109. Scatliff JH, Hayward R, Armao D et al (2005) Pre- and post-operative hydromyelia in spinal dysraphism. Pediatr Radiol 35:282-289

110. Castillo M, Quencer R, Green B et al (1987) Syringomyelia as a consequence of compressive extramedullary lesions: postoperative, clinical and ra-

diological manifestations. AJR Am J Roentgenol 8:973-978

111. Cameron AH (1957) Malformations of the neurospinal axis, urogenital tract and foregut in spina bifida attributable to disturbances of the blastopore. J Path Bact 73:213-221

112. Emery JL, Lendon RG (1972) Clinical implications of cord lesions in neurospinal dysraphism. Dev Med Child Neurol 14(suppl 27):45-51

113. Emery JL, Lendon RG (1973) The local cord lesion in neurospinal dysraphysm (myelomeningocele). J Pathol 110:83-96

114. Kumar R, Bansal KK, Chhabra DK (2002) Occurrence of split cord malformation in meningomyelocele: complex spina bifida. Pediatr Neurosurg 36:119-127

115. Duckworth T, Sharrard WJ, Lister J et al (1968) Hemimyelocele. Develop Med Child Neurol 16:69-75

116. Maguire CD, Winter RB, Mayfield JK et al (1982) Hemimyelodysplasia: a report of 10 cases. J Pediatr Orthop 2:9-14

117. Glasier CM, Chadduck WM, Leithiser REJ et al (1990) Screening spinal ultrasound in newborns with neural tube defects. J Ultrasound Med 9:339-343

118. McLone DG, Dias MS (1991-1992) Complications of myelomeningocele closure. Pediatr Neurosurg 17:267-273

119. Ozek MM, Pamir MN, Ozer AF et al (1991) Correlation between computed tomography and magnetic resonance imaging in diastematomyelia. Eur J Radiol 13:209-214

120. Yamanaka T, Hashimoto N, Sasajima H et al (2001) A case of diastematomyelia associated with myeloschisis in a hemicord. Pediatr Neurosurg 35:253-256

121. Parmar H, Patkar D, Shah J et al (2003) Diastematomyelia with terminal lipomyelocystocele arising from one hemicord: case report. Clin Imaging 27:41-43

122. Fauré C, Lepintre J, Michel JR et al (1958) Les fistules dermiques congénitales: à propos de 6 observations. J Radiol Electr 39:481-486

123. Black SPW, German WJ (1950) Four congenital tumours found at operation within the vertebral canal with observation of their incidence. J Neurosurg 7:49-61

124. Harriehausen (1909) Über Dermoïde im Wirbelkanal neben Verdoppelung des Rüchkenmarks. Dtsch Z Nervenheilk 36:268-284

125. Hirsch JF, Hoppe-Hisch E (1989) Neurenteric cysts. In: AJ Raimondi, M Choux, C Di Rocco (eds) The pediatric spine II. Springer, New York, pp 134-143

126. Bale PM (1973) A congenital intraspinal gastro-enterogenous cyst in diastematomyelia. J Neurol Neurosurg Psychiatr 36:1011

127. Mathieu JP, Decarie M, Dube J et al (1982) La diastématomyélie. Etude de 69 cas. Chir Pédiatr 23:29-35

128. Whitney RW, Brenner R, Gulati R (1990) Occult diastematomyelia in adults. Report of two cases. Clin Radiol 41:415-417

129. Birch BD, McCormick PC (1996) High cervical split cord malformation and neurenteric cyst associated with congenital mirror movements: case report. Neurosurgery 38:813-815

130. Prasad V, Reddy D, Murty J (1996) Cervico-thoracic neurenteric cyst: clinicoradiological correlatioon with embryogenesis. Childs Nerv Syst 12:48-51

131. Muthukumar N, Arunthathi J, Sundar V (2000) Split cord malformation and neurenteric cyst--case report and a theory of embryogenesis. Br J Neurosurg 14:488-492

132. Rauzzino M, Tubbs R, Alexander E et al (2001) Spinal neurenteric cysts and their relation to more common aspects of occult spinal dysraphism. Neurosurg Focus 15:10:e2

133. Shenoy S, Raja A (2004) Spinal neurenteric cyst. Report of 4 cases and review of the literature. Pediatr Neurosurg 40:284-292

134. Soni TV, Pandya C, Vaidya JP (2004) Split cord malformation with neurenteric cyst and pregnancy. Surg Neurol 61:556-558

135. Becker G, Battersby R (2005) Spinal neurenteric cyst presenting as recurrent midline sebaceous cyst. Ann R Coll Surg Engl 87:1-4

136. de Oliveira RS, Cinalli G, Roujeau T et al (2005) Neurenteric cysts in children: 16 consecutive cases and review of the literature. J Neurosurg 103:512-523

137. Cochrane D, Haslan R, Myles S (1990-1991) Cervical neuroschisis and meningocoele manqué in type I (no neck) Klippel-Feil syndrome. Pediatr Neurosurg 16:174-178

138. Solanki GA, Evans J, Copp A et al (2003) Multiple coexistent dysraphic pathologies. Childs Nerv Syst 19:376-379

139. Wolf A, Bradford D, Lonstein J et al (1987) The adult diplomyelia syndrome. Spine 12:233-237,

140. Bret P, Patet JD, Lapras C (1989) Diastematomyelia and diplomyelia. In: AJ Raimondi, M Choux, C Di Rocco (eds) The pediatric spine II. Springer, New York, pp 91-112

141. Hoffman HJ (1989) The tethered spinal cord, In: AJ Raimondi, M Choux, C Di Rocco (eds) The pediatric spine II. Springer, New York, pp 177-188

142. Basauri L, Palma A, Zuleta A et al (1979) Diastematomyelia, Report of 18 cases. Acta Neurochir 51:91-96

143. Lassman LP, James CCM (1977) Meningomyelocele manqué. Childs Brain 3:1-11

144. Kaffenberg DA, Heinz ER, Oakes JW et al (1992) Meningocele manque: radiologic findings with clinical correlation. AJNR 13:1083-1088

145. Humphreys RP, Hendrick EB, Hoffmann HJ (1982) Diastematomyelia, vol 30. Williams and Wilkins, Baltimore/London

146. Faris JC, Crowe JE (1975) The split notochord syndrome. J Ped Surg 10:467

147. Castillo M, Hankins L, Kramer L et al (1992) MR imaging of diastematomyelia. Magn Reson Imaging 10:699-703

148. Tubbs RS, Wellons JC, Oakes WJ (2005) Split cord malformation and situs inversus totalis: case report and review of the literature. Childs Nerv Syst 21:161-164

149. Gunderson C, Solitare G (1968) Mirror movements in patients with the Klippel-Feil syndrome. Arch Neurol 18:675-679

150. Levine RS, Geremia GK, McNeill TW (1985) CT demonstration of cervical diastematomyelia. J Comp Ass Tomogr 9:592-594

151. Nagib MG, Maxwell RE, Chou SN (1985) Klippel-Feil syndrome in children: clinical features and management. Childs Nerv Syst 1:255-263

152. Eller TW, Bernstein LP, Rosenberg RS et al (1987) Tethered cervical spinal cord. Case report. J Neurosurg 67:600-602

153. Wolf AL, Tubman DE, Seljeskog EL (1987) Diastematomyelia of the cervical spinal cord with tethering in an adult. Neurosurgery 21:94-98

154. Ritterbusch JF, McGinty LD, Spar J et al (1991) Magnetic resonance imaging for stenosis and subluxation in Klippel-Feil syndrome. Spine 16(Suppl 10):539-551

155. Ulmer J, Elster A, Ginsberg L et al (1993) Klippel-Feil syndrome: CT and MR of aquired and congenital abnormalities of cervical spine and cord. J Comp Assist Tomogr 17:215-224

156. Palmers M, Peene P, Massa G (2003) Cervicothoracic diastematomyelia with Klippel-Feil syndrome. Rofo 175:1579-1581

157. Tubbs R, Wellons JI, Oakes W (2003) Lumbar split cord malformation and Klippel-Feil syndrome. Pediatr Neurosurg 39:305-308

158. Gardner WJ, Collis JS (1961) Klippel-Feil syndrome. Syringomyelia, diastematomyelia, and meningocele – one disease? Arch Surg 83:638-643

159. Gardner WJ (1964) Diastematomyelia and the Klippel-Feil syndrome. Relationship to hydrocephalus, syringomyelia, meningocele, meningomyelocele and iniencephalus. Cleveland Clinic Quarterly 31:19-44

160. Williamson RA, Weiner CP, Yuh WTC et al (1989) Magnetic resonance imaging of anomalous fetuses. Obstet Gynecol 73:952-956

161. Scherrer CC, Hammer F, Schinzel A et al (1992) Brain stem and cervical cord dysraphic lesions in iniencephaly. Pediatr Pathol 12:469-476

162. McLennan JE (1976) Rib anomalies in myelodysplasia. An approach to embryologic inference. Biol Neonate 29:129-141

163. Weaver D, Russel L, Bull M (1981) The axial mesodermal dysplasia spectrum. Pediatrics 67:176

164. Kozlovski K (1984) Spondylo-costal dysplasia. A further report, review of 14 cases. Fortschr Röntgenstr 140:204-209

165. Lichtor A (1947) Sacral agenesis. Report of a case. Arch Surg 54:430-433

166. Lausecker H (1952) Beitrag zu den Missbildungen des Kreuzbeines. Virchows Arch Pathol Anat 322:119-129

167. Williams DI, Nixon HH (1957) Agenesis of the sacrum. Surg Gynecol Obstet 105:84-88

168. Renshaw TS (1978) Sacral agenesis. A classification and review of twenty-three cases. J Bone Joint Surg 60 (A):373-383

169. Jouve JL (1987) Les agénésies sacrées. Mise au point au sujet de 41 cas. Thèse de Doctorat, Marseille

170. Bradford DS, Kahmann R (1991) Lumbosacral kyphosis, tethered cord, and diplomyelia. A unique spinal dysraphic condition. Spine 16:764-768

171. Gaskill SJ, Kagen-Hallet K, Marlin AE (1988) Diastematomyelia associated with ectopic renal tissue. Pediatr Neurosci 14:108-111

172. Ersahin Y (2002) Split cord malformation associated with ectopic renal tissue. Childs Nerv Syst 18:201

173. Sharma MC, Sarat Chandra P, Goel S et al (2005) Primary lumbosacral Wilms tumor associated with diastematomyelia and occult spinal dysraphism. A report of a rare case and a short review of literature. Childs Nerv Syst 21:240-243

174. Fernbach SK, Naidich TP, McLone DG et al (1984) Computed tomography of primary intrathecal Wilms tumor with diastematomyelia. J Comput Assist Tomogr 8:523-528

175. Ugarte N, Gonzalez-Crussi F, Sotelo-Avila C (1980) Diastematomyelia associated with teratomas. J Neurosurg 53:720-725

176. Garza-Mercado R (1983) Diastematomyelia and intramedullary epidermoid spinal cord tumor combined with extradural teratoma in an adult: case report. J Neurosurg 58:954-958

177. Koen J, McLendon R, Geroge T (1998) Intradural spinal teratoma: evidence for a dysembryogenic origin. J Neurosurg 89:844-851

178. Hader WJ, Steinbok P, Poskitt K et al (1999) Intramedullary spinal teratoma and diastematomyelia. Case report and review of the literature. Pediatr Neurosurg 30:140-145

179. Ozer H, Yuceer N (1999) Myelomeningocele, dermal sinus tract, split cord malformation associated with extradural teratoma in a 30-month-old girl. Acta Neurochir (Wien) 141:1123-1124

180. Muthukumar N (2003) Split cord malformation and cystic teratoma masquerading as lipomeningomyelocele. Childs Nerv Syst 19:46-49

181. Jarmundowicz W, Tabakow P, Markowska-Woyciechowska A (2004) Composite split cord malformation coexisting with spinal cord teratoma--case report and review of the literature. Folia Neuropathol 42:55-57

182. Uzum N, Dursun A, Baykaner K et al (2005) Split-cord malformation and tethered cord associated with immature teratoma. Childs Nerv Syst 21:77-80

183. Suri A, Ahmad FU, Mahapatra AK et al (2006) Mediastinal extension of an intradural teratoma in a patient with split cord malformation: case report and review of literature. Childs Nerv Syst 22:444-449

184. Vaishya S, Pandey P (2006) Unusual spinal teratoma with an accessory penis on the back. Childs Nerv Syst 22:440-443

185. Tsitsopoulos P, Rizos C, Isaakidis D et al (2006) Co-existence of spinal intramedullary teratoma and diastematomyelia in an adult. Spinal Cord 44:632-635

186. Elmaci I, Dagcinar A, Ozgen S et al (2001) Diastematomyelia and spinal teratoma in an adult. Neurosurg Focus 10(1):ecp2

187. Guvenc B, Etus V, Muezzinoglu B (2006) Lumbar teratoma presenting intradural and extramedullary extension in a neonate. Spine J 6:90-93

188. Kumar R, Prakash M (2007) Unusual split cord with neurenteric cyst and cerebellar heterotopia over spinal cord. Childs Nerv Syst 23:243-247

189. Kurihara N, Takahashi S, Ogawa A et al (1992) CT and MR findings in diastematomyelia, with embryogenetic considerations. Radiat Med 10:73-77

190. Katoh M, Hida K, Iwasaki Y et al (1998) A split cord malformation. Childs Nerv Syst 14:398-400

191. Okada K, Takeshi F, Yonenbu K et al (1986) Cervical diastematomyelia with a stable neurologic deficit. Report of a case. J Bone and Joint Surg 68A:934-937

192. Ohwada T, Okada K, Hayashi H (1989) Thoracic myelopathy caused by cervicothoracic diastematomyelia. J Bone Joint Surg 71A:296-299

193. Anzai T, Kato I, Shirane R et al (1992) A case of diastematomyelia with meningomyelocele. No Shinkei Geka 20:261-265

194. Sato N, Sato H (2000) [Diastematomyelia]. Ryoikibetsu Shokogun Shirizu 28:387-390

195. Sato K, Yoshida Y, Shirane R et al (2002) A split cord malformation with paresis of the unilateral lower limb: case report. Surg Neurol 58:406-409

196. Moriya J, Kakeda S, Korogi Y et al (2006) An unusual case of split cord malformation. AJNR Am J Neuroradiol 27:1562-1564

197. Hamasaki T, Makino K, Morioka M et al (2006) Histological study of paramedian dorsal root ganglia in an infant with split cord malformation. Case report. J Neurosurg 104:415-418

198. Akiyama K, Nishiyama K, Yoshimura J et al (2007) A case of split cord malformation associated with myeloschisis. Childs Nerv Syst 23:577-580

199. Matson DD (1969) Neurosurgery of infancy and childhood. Charles C Thomas, Springfield, Ill

200. Guthkelch AN (1974) Diastematomyelia with a median septum. Brain 97:729-742

201. Beyerl BD, Ojemann RG, Davis KR et al (1985) Cervical diastematomyela presenting in adulthood. Case report. J Neurosurg 62:449-453

202. Pang D, Wilberger JEJ (1982) Tethered cord syndrome in adults. J Neurosurg 57:32-47

203. Gupta SK, Khosla VK, Sharma BS et al (1999) Tethered cord syndrome in adults. Surg Neurol 52:362-369

204. Yamada S, Lonser RR (2000) Adult tethered cord syndrome. J Spinal Disord 13:319-323

205. Huttmann S, Krauss J, Collmann H et al (2001) Surgical management of tethered spinal cord in adults: report of 54 cases. J Neurosurg 95:173-178

206. Iskandar BJ, Fulmer BB, Hadley MN et al (2001) Congenital tethered spinal cord syndrome in adults. Neurosurg Focus 10:e7

207. van Leeuwen R, Notermans NC, Vandertop WP (2001) Surgery in adults with tethered cord syndrome: outcome study with independent clinical review. J Neurosurg 94:205-209

208. Phi J, Lee D, Jahng T et al (2004) Tethered cord syndrome in adulthood: reconsidering the prognosis. J Korean Neurosurg Soc 36:114-119

209. Quinones-Hinojosa A, Gadkary CA, Gulati M et al (2004) Neurophysiological monitoring for safe surgical tethered cord syndrome release in adults. Surg Neurol 62:127-133

210. Lee GY, Paradiso G, Tator CH et al (2006) Surgical management of tethered cord syndrome in adults: indications, techniques, and long-term outcomes in 60 patients. J Neurosurg Spine 4:123-131

211. Wright B, Gonsalves CG, Marotta JT (1979) Diastematomyelia in a geriatric patient. J Can Assoc Radiol 30:59

212. Pallatroni HF, Ball PA, Duhaime AC (2004) Split cord malformation as a cause of tethered cord syndrome in a 78-year-old female. Pediatr Neurosurg 40:80-83

213. Ersahin Y, Kitis O, Oner K (2002) Split cord malformation in two sisters. Pediatr Neurosurg 37:240-244

214. Kapsalakis Z (1964) Diastematomyelia in 2 sisters. J Neurosurg 21:66-67

215. Balci S, Caglar K, Eryilmaz M (1999) Diastematomyelia in two sisters. Am J Med Genet 86:180-182

216. Chatkupt S, Lucek PR, Koenigsberger MR et al (1992) Parental sex effect in spina bifida: a role for genomic imprinting? Am J Med Genet 44:508-512

217. Mariman EC, Hamel BC (1992) Sex ratios of affected and transmitting members of multiple case families with neural tube defects. J Med Genet 29:695-698

218. Kennedy PR (1979) New data on diastematomyelia. J Neurosurg 51:355-361

219. Carter CO, Evans KA, Till K (1976) Spinal dysraphism: genetic relation to neural tube malformations. J Med Genet 13:343-350

220. Wynne-Davies R (1975) Congenital vertebral anomalies: aetiology and relationship to spina bifida cystica. J Med Genet 12:280-288

221. Caspi B, Gorbacz S, Appelman Z et al (1990) Antenatal diagnosis of diastematomyelia. J Clin Ultrasound 18:721-725

222. Schropp C, Sorensen N, Collmann H et al (2006) Cutaneous lesions in occult spinal dysraphism--correlation with intraspinal findings. Childs Nerv Syst 22:125-131

223. Banizza von Bazan U, Krastel A, Lohkamp F-W (1978) Diastematomyelia – ein harmloser Zufallsbefund oder Ursache später Rückenmarksschäden. Z Orthop 116:72-80

224. Sedzimir CB, Roberts JR, Occleshaw JV (1973) Massive diastematomyelia without cutaneous dysraphism. Arch Dis Child 48:400-402

225. Eid K, Hochberg J, Saunders DE (1979) Skin abnormalities on the back of diastematomyelia. Plast Recontr Surg 63:534-549

226. Wendelin DS, Pope DN, Mallory SB (2003) Hypertrichosis. J Am Acad Dermatol 48:161-179

227. James CCM, Lassman LP (1964) Diastematomyelia: a critical survey of 24 cases submitted to laminectomy. Arch Dis Child 39:125-130

228. Myles LM, Steers AJ, Minns R (2002) Cervical cord tethering due to split cord malformation at the cervico-dorsal junction presenting with self-mutilation of the fingers. Dev Med Child Neurol 44:844-848

229. Kaminker R, Fabry J, Midha R et al (2000) Split cord malformation with diastematomyelia presenting as neurogenic claudication in an adult: a case report. Spine 25:2269-2271

230. Claudy AL, Thivolet J, Meyer F (1976) La diastématomyélie: une cause rare de mal perforant plantaire. Lyon Méd. 6:503-509

231. Tax HR, Person V, Tuccio M (1982) A podiatric presentation of diastematomyelia. J Am Podiatry Assoc 72:337-341

232. Delgado G, Zubieta JL, Martin E et al (1981) Diastematomyelia simulating an acrodystrophic neuropathy: diagnosis by computerised axial tomography. Rev Med Univ Navarra 25:42-43

233. Serratrice G, Gastaux JL, Pouget J (1990) L'acropathie ulcéromutilante de la diastématomyélie. Rev Neurol (Paris) 146:702-704

234. Russell NA, Benoit BG, Joaquim AJ (1990-1991) Diastematomyelia in adults. A review. Pediatr Neurosurg 16:252-257

235. Anand AK, Kuchner EF, James R (1985) Cervical diastematomyelia: uncommon presentation of a rare congenital disorder. Comput Radiol 9:45-49

236. Kuchner EF, Anand AK, Kaufman BM (1985) Cervical diastematomyelia: a case report with operative management. Neurosurgery 16:538-542

237. Rawanduzy A, Murali R (1991) Cervical spine diastematomyelia in adulthood. Neurosurgery 28:459-461

238. Simpson RK, Rose JE (1987) Cervical diastematomyelia; report of a case and review of a rare congenital anomaly. Arch Neurol 44:331-335

239. Freeman LW (1961) Late symptoms from diastematomyelia. J Neurosurg 18:538-541

240. Constantinou E (1963) A case of diastematomyelia. JAMA 185:983-984

241. Goldberg L, Fenelon G, Blake NS et al (1984) Diastematomyelia: A critical review of the natural history and treatment. Spine 9:367-372

242. Maroun FB, Jacob JC, Mangan MA (1982) Adult diastematomyelia: a complex dysraphic state. Surg Neurol 18:289-294

243. Frerebeau P, Dimeglio A, Gras M et al (1983) Diastematomyelia: Report of 21 cases surgically treated by a neurosurgical and orthopedic team. Childs Brain 10:328-339

244. Vandresse JH (1975) Diastematomyelia: report of eight observations. Neuroradiology 10:87-93

245. Hülser PJ, Schroth G, Petersen D (1985) Magnetic resonance and CT imaging of diastematomyelia. Eur. Arch. Psychiatry Neurol Sci 235:107-109

246. Yamada S, Zirke DE, Saunders D (1981) Pathophysiology of the "tethered cord syndrome". J Neurosurg 54:494-503

247. Sonigo-Cohen P, Schmit P, Zerah M et al (2003) Prenatal diagnosis of diastematomyelia. Childs Nerv Sys 19:555-560

248. Cherif A, Oueslati B, Marrakchi Z et al (2003) [Diastematomyelia: antenatal diagnosis with successful outcome, two cases]. J Gynecol Obstet Biol Reprod (Paris) 32:476-480

249. von Koch CS, Glenn O, Goldstein P et al (2005) Fetal magnetic resonance imaging enhance detection of spinal cord anomalies in patients with sonographically detected bony anomalies of the spine. J Ultrasound Med 24:781-789

250. Biri AA, Turp AB, Kurdoglu M et al (2005) Prenatal diagnosis of diastematomyelia in a 15-week-old fetus. Fetal Diagn Ther 20:258-261

251. Proctor MR, Scott RM (2001) Long-term outcome for patients with split cord malformation. Neurosurg Focus 10:e5

252. Meyrat BJ, Tercier S, Lutz N et al (2003) Introduction of a urodynamic score to detect pre- and postoperative neurological deficits in children with a primary tethered cord. Childs Nerv Syst 19:716-721

253. Lapras C, Bret P (1988) Diastématomyélie. Neurochirurgie 34:99-103

254. Chehrazi B, Aldeman S (1985) Adult onset of tethered spinal cord syndrome due to fibrous diastematomyelia: case report. Neurosurgery 16:681-685

255. Zuccaro G (2003) Split spinal cord malformation. Childs Nerv Syst 19:104-105

256. Moes CA, Hendrick EB (1963) Diastematomyelie. J Pediatr 63:238-248

257. Gilmor RL, Batnitzky S (1978) Diastematomyelia – Rare and unusual features. Neuroradiology 16:87-88

258. Pang D, Parrish RG (1983) Regrowth of diastematomyelic bone spur after extradural resection. J Neurosurg 59:887-890

259. McCullough D (1987) Developmental disorders. In: N Horwitz, H Rizzoli (eds) Post-operative complications of extracranial neurological surgery. Williams & Wilkins, Baltimore, pp 138-160

260. Dawson CW, Driesbach JH (1961) Diastematomyelia and acquired clubfoot deformity. JAMA 175:569-572

CHAPTER 39
Spinal Dermal Sinuses

Jonathan Roth, Liana Beni-Adani, Bo Xiao, Liat Ben Sira, Shlomi Constantini

Introduction

Dermal sinuses are congenital malformations, representing a subtype of occult spinal dysraphism (OSD). A short historical review presented by Ackerman et al. [1] in 2002 cited the first description of dermal sinuses by Ogle in 1865. The first description in English literature was by Verebely in 1913. The incidence of dermal sinuses is frequently noted as 1:2,500 live births [2, 3]. However, this number is based on two studies from 1954 and 1975, both of which were done before the MRI era, and before it was recognized that coccygeal pits and dermal sinus are two distinct entities. Thus, the true incidence is not known [1]. Dermal sinuses are thought to develop in response to an abnormal separation of the cutaneous and the neural ectoderm between the third and fifth weeks of gestation [4-6]. When this separation fails, a persistent connection, or tract, occurs between the skin and deeper structures. Depending on the degree of incomplete separation, the deeper end of the tract may reach subcutaneous tissue, fascia, dura, or even intradural neural tissue. Another possible underlying mechanism is a defect in notochordal formation with sagittal splitting of the spinal cord and persistence of a cutaneo-endo-mesenchymal fistula.

There is no clear gender or known genetic predominance among dermal sinus patients. Typically, dermal sinuses are located above the intergluteal line. About 90% are located at the lumbosacral region. However, just under 10% are located at the thoracic level and approximately 1% are located at the cervical level. In rare cases they may occur rostrally up to the nasion [1, 5, 7-9].

Dermal sinuses are associated with other OSD pathologies [7]. 10% of OSDs also have dermal sinuses. Dermal sinuses are seen in 15-40% of split cord malformations [10], and about 40% of patients with dermal sinuses have other occult spinal dysraphism findings. For example, dermal sinuses are associated with tethered cord [7], although they account for less than 1% of patients with tethered cord [11].

Approximately 60-70% of lumbosacral dermal sinuses reach the subarachnoid space, with half attaching to the cauda equina, conus medullaris, or filum terminale. The tract may ascend several spinal levels before penetrating the dura. Thoracocervical dermal sinuses entering the dura may reach the central canal. About 10% of dermal sinuses end in the subcutaneous tissue, 20% between the fascia and the dura, and 10% terminate subdurally. Most dermal sinuses are situated at the midline, although paravertebral locations have been found [12]. A single midline tract is the common form; however, rare cases of two parallel tracts ending at the same or different spinal levels have been described [13, 14].

Histologically, the tract includes both dermal and epidermal elements because the primitive ectoderm has the potential to differentiate to form all skin components [5, 6]. The dermal sinus tract is thus surrounded by stratified squamous epithelium, and it may encompass fat, blood vessels, cartilage, nerve or ganglion cells, and meningeal remnants. Inclusion lesions may arise anywhere along the tract, within focal expansions, in approximately half of all dermal sinuses [7, 15]. These lesions arise from keratin debris from desquamating epithelium and secretions from sebaceous and sweat glands. Dermoid histology is the most common, occurring in about 83% of cases. However, epidermoids are seen in 13%, and teratomas in 4% of cases. Malignant transformations are rare. Above the L1 level, inclusion lesions may be intramedullary. However, below the L1 level they are usually located in the subarachnoid space, adherent to the roots of the cauda equina. When the dermal sinus tract ends at the conus, there seems to be an anatomical continuum between both [13].

Clinical Presentation

As published by French in 1990, up to 79% of patients present before the age of 5 years, 8% between 6-10 years, 9% in second decade, and 4% after the age of 20 [12]. However, with improved diagnostic understanding, we speculate that currently the vast majority are diagnosed before the age of 5 years. Clinical manifestations include neurological, orthopedic, and urological symptoms and signs, and cutaneous findings. Thus, a patient may primarily present to a pediatrician, pediatric neurologist, pediatric orthopedist, or surgeon.

Skin findings are the most common referral reason among young children [7]. Dermal sinuses present as midline dermal dimples, with or without additional dermal stigmata such as hairy tufts, skin hemangiomas or telangiectasias, hypo or hyperpigmentations, asymmetrical gluteal clefts, subcutaneous lipomas, or skin tags (Figs. 39.1, 39.3, 39.4, 39.5, 39.6, 39.7) [16]. The orifice of the dermal sinus may be very small, visible only under close in-spection (Fig. 39.8). Purulent and other debris may drain from the sinus opening (Fig. 39.2). Dermal sinuses may present as incidental findings in a newborn. In an older child, they usually present through secondary complications; infectious, neurological, urological, and orthopedic. Symptoms secondary to tethering of the cord typically appear during growth spurts, mostly during childhood and adolescence. In rare cases, dermal sinuses are diagnosed in the adult population. Interestingly, in the older group the presentation may be back pain [7].

Infectious Complications of Dermal Sinuses

Infections used to be the major referral reason of patients with dermal sinus tracts. In a comprehensive literature review by French in 1990, infections were the referral reason for 61% of patients [12]. However more recently, probably due to increased awareness, patients are usually referred earlier, before infections occur. Dermal sinuses connect the skin surface and deeper layers – subcutaneous fat, epidural

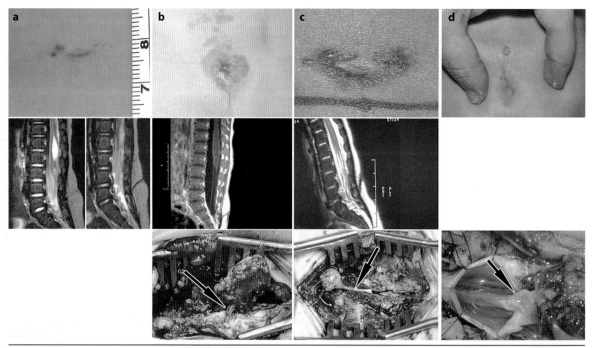

Fig. 39.1 a-d. **a** Midline lumbar dimple and hemangiomas in a five month old child. Incidental finding. MRI – dermal sinus (*lower image*). At surgery – the tract was continuous with the filum and detethering was performed. **b** Midline lumbar dimple and hemangiomas in an eight month old child. Incidental finding. MRI – dermal sinus (*middle image*). At surgery – the tract was continuous with the filum and detethering was performed (*lower image*). **c** Midline lumbar dimple and hemangiomas in a five week old child. The dimple had non infectious secretions. MRI – dermal sinus (*middle image*). At surgery – the tract was continuous with a thickened filum and detethering was performed (*lower image*). **d** Two midline lumbar dimples in a five week old child. The lesion was first diagnosed by a screening US test performed during pregnancy. At surgery – the tract was continuous with a fatty filum and detethering was performed (*lower image*)

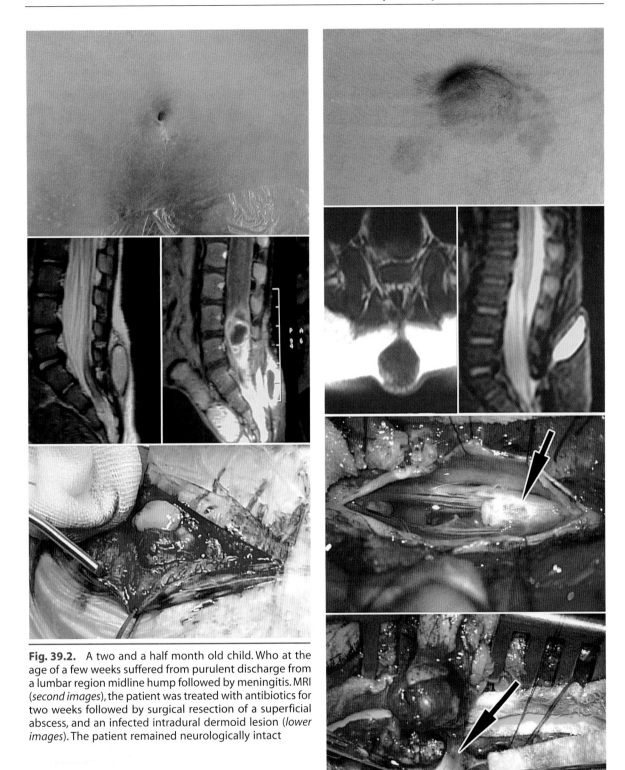

Fig. 39.2. A two and a half month old child. Who at the age of a few weeks suffered from purulent discharge from a lumbar region midline hump followed by meningitis. MRI (*second images*), the patient was treated with antibiotics for two weeks followed by surgical resection of a superficial abscess, and an infected intradural dermoid lesion (*lower images*). The patient remained neurologically intact

space, subarachnoid space, and the spinal cord itself. Secondary infections arising from skin flora may cause meningitis (50%), infected inclusion lesions (30%), spinal abscesses (intramedullary, subdural, or epidural) (20%), or rarely, subcutaneous abscesses (Fig. 39.2). Infections may remain local or spread caudally or rostrally across several spinal segments.

Fig. 39.3. A two month old child. Cutaneous signs – midline lumbar hump and hemangiomas (*upper image*). On MRI – a meningocele adherent to a dermal sinus (*second images*). At surgery – resection of the dermal sinus, untethering of a thickened filum (*arrows*), and resection of the meningocele (*lower images*)

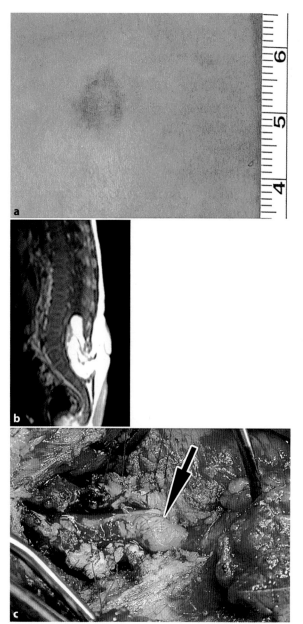

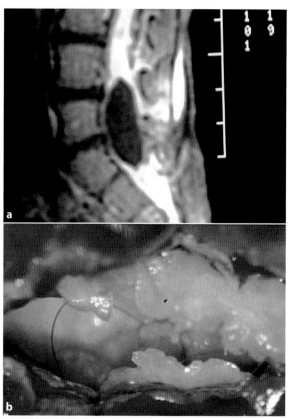

Fig. 39.5 a, b. An eleven month old child. Presented with midline lumbar discoloration, meningitis, and mild paraparesis. On MRI – dermal sinus and an intradural dermoid (**a**). At surgery – resection of an infected dermoid tumor (**b**)

Fig. 39.4 a-c. A three month old child. Local midline lumbar discoloration and subcutaneous irregularity (**a**). On MRI – a subcutaneous lipoma extending intradurally (**b**). At surgery – near total resection of the lipoma (*arrows*) (**c**)

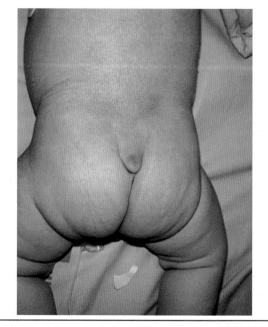

In rare cases, infected lumbosacral dermal sinuses may spread and reach the cervical area [17].

The most common bacterial organisms are *Staphylococcus aureus*, *E. coli*, *Proteus* species, *Klebsiella*, and anaerobic organisms [4, 5]. Multiple organisms are cultured in 20% of cases. When intraspinal infections occur, cultures from cerebrospinal fluid (CSF) obtained via lumbar puncture are more accurate than cultures obtained from superficial discharge from the

Fig. 39.6. A four month old child. Lumbar tail with local discharge. At surgery – resection of the tail and a dermal sinus that reached a fibrotic filum

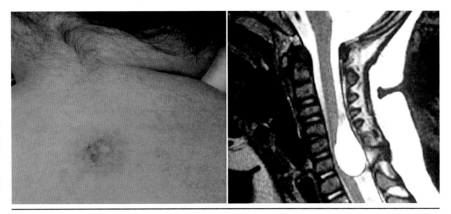

Fig. 39.7. A six month old child. Midline upper thoracic discoloration. On MRI and at surgery – a lower cervical region dermal sinus extending intradurally, and continuous with a local arachnoid cyst

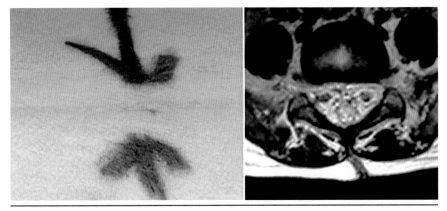

Fig. 39.8. A two year old child. A small midline lumbar dimple with a black hair emerging from it. Recurrent local infections. On MRI and at surgery – superficial dermal sinus extending to the epidural region

sinus orifice. However, due the possibility of an infected intradural inclusion lesion, a lumbar puncture should not be performed until an MRI has been done and the exact anatomy clarified. Inclusion lesions, whether infected or non-infected, may spontaneously rupture, spilling acidic content into the subarachnoid space and causing meningitis (bacterial or chemical) and dense arachnoiditis. Dermal sinuses may also present as recurrent meningitis, in cases where they are small and unnoticed. Other related infections may occur in the urinary tract, secondary to urination disturbances in children with secondary tethered cord.

Neurological Manifestations

Most newborns with dermal sinuses are neurologically intact. However, delayed neurological deterioration may occur secondary to cord compression, arachnoiditis, or tethered cord syndrome (TCS). Neurological deficits are the most common referral reason among older children [7]. Infectious processes may lead to mass effect compressing the cord directly or secondary to infected inclusion lesions, or to local arachnoiditis. Infections may cause local ischemic changes with secondary myelopathy. These effects may lead to rapid neurological deterioration, necessitating urgent treatment. Symptoms due to cord tethering usually emerge during toddler and adolescent growth spurts [7]. Inclusion lesions such as dermoid and epidermoid tumors grow slowly and have relatively few symptoms at the early stages; however, they tend to cause mass effect and compress neural structures – mainly the conus medullaris, and less frequently the cauda equina. In contrast to the rapid neurological deterioration seen secondary to infections, tethered cord and inclusion lesions may cause slower, progressive neurological-urological and orthopedic deterioration, and may present at an older age. Nevertheless, an incidental finding of dermal sinuses in neurologically intact adults is extremely rare.

Neurological manifestations may include distal motor deterioration, usually symmetrical, sensory level, pain, and urinary and bowel incontinence. Note that patchy sensory loss with asymmetrical motor deficits over many years may occur in untreated dermal sinuses. The risk of neurological deterioration exists at all ages, increases with time, and is frequently progressive.

Urological Manifestations

Urinary incontinence and urinary retention may occur at an early or late stage. The mechanism is either detrusor hyperactivity due to upper motor neuron symptoms secondary to cord tethering, or detrusor hypoactivity secondary to root or cauda equina injury. Urinary tract infections may be the presenting symptoms of minor urination disturbances. Hydronephrosis may result from late diagnosis of urinary disturbances.

Orthopedic Manifestations

Scoliosis and asymmetry of legs or feet are the most common orthopedic signs of tethered cord. The signs may be subtle, such as a thinner calf, smaller foot, higher arch, or hammer or claw toes. These signs probably evolve secondary to asymmetric neuromuscular activity.

Differential Diagnosis

Midline skin pits at the sacro-coccygeal region occur in about 2-5% of newborns [18]. These pits, also named coccygeal pits or simple dimples, are located below the cul-de-sac of the subarachnoid space, and do not connect with intraspinal structures. Typically, simple dimples are within 25 mm of the anus, have a diameter of less than 5 mm, and are not associated with other clear skin stigmata [19]. Simple dimples, or the presence of mild skin manifestations such as mild diffuse hypertrichosis or mild bluish discoloration, probably do not necessitate any additional evaluation [18]. Note that coccygeal pits may become infected by fecal material, leading to secondary local infection or pilonidal sinuses. Other occult spina bifida pathologies, which are sometimes associated with dermal sinuses, may sometimes present similar cutaneous stigmata and symptoms of tethered cord even with no dermal sinus involvement. Another presenting symptom with a differential diagnosis is recurrent meningitis. Neuroenteric cysts and CSF fistulas may also cause recurrent meningitis and must be ruled out.

Diagnostic Modalities

Due to the natural history of dermal sinuses and the risk of future infectious and neurological complications, any newborn with a non simple dimple (see *Differential Diagnosis*, above) must be evaluated for occult spina bifida and dermal sinus. This includes a neurological, urological, and in some cases orthopedic evaluation.

Surgical exploration and excision of dermal sinuses must not be attempted before radiological evaluation. Probe insertion and injection of contrast materials may lead to infections or deep tissue injury, are of little diagnostic value, and thus should not be performed [4]. The apparent direction of the dermal sinus may be misleading too; it may initially appear to be directed caudally, but at deeper layers it is usually directed cephalad.

Conventional X-ray studies may demonstrate dysraphic changes such as diastematomyelia and vertebral anomalies that fall into the wider spectrum of occult spina bifida; however, these x-ray studies do not accurately portray the detailed anatomy, which often displays no bony abnormality.

Thin slice computer tomography (CT) including reconstructions may portray the bony components; however, these CTs fail to show the dermal sinus tract and intraspinal components. CT myelography demonstrates the outline of the intradural sinus tract, cord tethering, and grouping of the cauda equina nerve roots secondary to arachnoiditis. However, CT myelography is contraindicated in instances of a superficial infection due to the risk of iatrogenically inducing intraspinal infections and meningitis. In addition, in cases with large inclusion bodies, or when severe arachnoiditis occurs, the contrast material may fail to spread properly. Due to the various functional limitations listed here, as well as the radiation involved in CT scanning, CTs play a very limited role in the evaluation of tethered cord in general and in dermal sinuses in particular.

Ultrasound (US) readily portrays the sinus tract, and in infants below the age of three months the US may show the entire tract length, from the skin to the spinal cord, including the contents of the cauda equina and the exact level of the conus medullaris [20, 21]. In older infants, the content of the neural structure within the spinal canal may not be demonstrated.

Magnetic resonance imaging (MRI) is the radiological study of choice, readily portraying the sinus tract, inclusion lesions, cord tethering, and spinal cord anatomy (Figs. 39.1-39.5, 39.7, 39.8). Typically, dermoid tumors are iso- or hypointense on T1 sequence, enhance with gadolinium, and are hyperintense on T2 [8]. However, dermoid tumors may also be hyperintense on T1 [5]. Note that fatty tissues along the tract or within dermoid tumors are hyperintense on T1. A T2-weighted intramedullary high signal area, rostral to a presumed abscess, may suggest reactive edema or an intramedullary extension of the abscess. Despite the high resolution of MRI images, in some cases the tract may not be clearly illustrated on the MRI if it is small or out of the imaging plane. Barcovich et al. [15] visualized the connection of the dermal sinus tract to the conus in only two of seven cases. In addition, MRI interpretation may be confusing in the presence of infection or arachnoiditis, either of which may masquerade as an intradural lesion with nerve root clumping.

An algorithm for OSD imaging selection that includes a cost-effectiveness analysis, based on evidence-based criteria, has been proposed [16, 22, 23]. For patients with low risk stigmata such as sacro-coccygeal pits (simple dimples), there is probably no need for imaging if the clinical examination is normal. For the intermediate risk group of midline findings such as non-simple dimple, mild skin discolorations, deviated gluteal fold, and light hypertrichosis, an US can serve as a screening tool in children under the age of three months, but an MRI is needed in older children. In children with subcutaneous masses or clinical findings, an MRI is indicated.

Cerebral imaging is not routinely indicated, as hydrocephalus is not associated with dermal sinuses, unless the patient had recurrent meningitis events (bacterial or chemical). However, cervical spinal dermal sinuses may be associated with posterior fossa dermoid and epidermoid tumors, and thus necessitate cerebral imaging [8].

Treatment

Timing and Indications of Surgery

Surgery for dermal sinus may be performed due to an acute neurological deterioration secondary to an infectious event, as a surgical procedure treating symptomatic tethered cord, and as a prophylactic elective procedure in an asymptomatic child.

In the presence of meningitis, antibiotic treatment should be started promptly. The type of antibiotic chosen can occasionally be determined from the flora growth if discharge from the orifice exists. The feasibility of a lumbar tap should be discussed in-

dividually, depending on the intradural anatomy displayed on MRI scans. When dealing with a downward displaced conus medullaris, or in the presence of a large intradural inclusion lesion, empirical broad spectrum antibiotics must be given. The timing of surgery is determined by the neurological status, systemic response to antibiotic treatment, and the specific anatomy. For example, a dermal sinus leading to an infected dermoid may resemble a deep seated abscess in the lack of response to antibiotic treatment alone unless the abscess is drained. In this situation the purpose of the surgical procedure is to open and drain the infected intra and extradural cavities. During these operations the intradural part seems like 'magma', with the nerve roots adherent to dermoid components and pus. True untethering should not be attempted due to an unacceptable risk of neural injury.

A dermal sinus associated with symptomatic tethering should be operated on as soon as possible, since reversal of existing neurological and urological deficits does not always ensue. Untethering should always be scheduled before other planned orthopedic or urological procedures.

Prophylactic surgery in asymptomatic dermal sinus cases is the preferred treatment strategy. The advantages are both technical and clinical, since the surgeon is dealing with non-infected tissue, clearer anatomy, and smaller dermoid lesions. The neurological and urological outcome of surgery is usually favorable. Timely diagnosis and treatment are associated with a favorable outcome and may obviate infectious and neurological complications.

Surgical Technique: Positioning and Monitoring

Place the patient in the prone position, with rolls under upper chest and ramus pubis to relieve abdominal pressure. Patients may be paralyzed for intubation purposes; however, long lasting paralytic agents should not be used when working with electrophysiological monitoring. Prepping and draping should be generous, allowing cephalad elongation of the incision to enable the entire dermal tract to be followed and the normal anatomy to be recognized.

Intraoperative neurophysiological monitoring may be helpful in selected cases. Neurophysiological monitoring includes online somatosensory evoked potentials (SSEPs), motor evoked potentials (MEPs), and specific intraoperative stimulation of roots with concomitant EMG monitoring of the lower extremities (representing L2-S2 roots) and anal sphincter (representing S2-S4 roots). Intraoperative evoked potentials may help to reduce surgical morbidity, especially in cases with distorted anatomy [24-26]. In a straight forward dermal tract continuous with the filum, intraoperative evoked potentials are probably not required.

Resection of the Dermal Sinus Tract and Inclusion Lesions

An elliptical incision encompassing the dermal sinus orifice is made. The incision is elongated cephalad while carefully following the dermal tract as it transverses the fascia. The fascia is dissected rostrally, exposing the laminas and interspinous ligaments. The tract is followed to the spinal canal. A laminectomy is performed following the dermal sinus tract level and exposing the dura at and above the tract point of entry. The dura is opened above the tract entry point and retracted laterally with pull-up sutures. The subarachnoid space is carefully visualized to observe whether the tract terminates at the level of the dura or continues intradurally. Sometimes the intradural tract is a small fibrotic band. Therefore, it may be helpful to use a stimulation probe to differentiate a suspected band from a nerve root of the cauda equine, especially in the presence of previous arachnoiditis and root clumping. Intraoperative ultrasound prior to the dura opening and during surgery may help identify the inclusion lesions. Since these lesions are located along the dermal sinus tract, following the tract should also reveal any inclusion lesions. After dissecting and separating the dermal sinus tract and inclusion lesions from the surrounding nerve roots, they are completely resected (Figs. 39.1, 39.3, 39.5). When the tract terminates in a dermoid tumor at the conus medullaris, it is not uncommon to find an anatomical continuum between the dermoid and the conus [13]. It is therefore critical to define the area of attachment, in order to completely resect the dermoid while preserving neural function. An anatomical landmark of this area may be defined by the lowest rootlets branching off symmetrically from the conus. While it may seem safe to resect the tissue below the rootlets' origin, note that this landmark is somewhat artificial. Another anatomical landmark may be the point of entry of the filum terminale to the conus – the dermoid conglomerate.

In the presence of previous arachnoiditis (infection or aseptic), nerve roots may become firmly attached to the tract and especially to inclusion lesions. It is therefore important to preserve neural function and identify the nerve roots using a stimulation probe and monitoring EMG. If the adhesions are extremely adherent to the inclusion lesion, to the extent that removing the tumor capsule may jeopardize the nerve roots, it is advisable to empty the capsule of its contents and coagulate the capsule remnants. Generally, only about half of dermoid tumors may be completely resected. Similarly, during an acute infectious episode, complete resection of an infected inclusion lesion or an intramedullary abscess may not be feasible without jeopardizing the nerves. In these cases, only a debulking of the abscess and inclusion lesion content is performed, as explained in *Timing and Indications of Surgery* above, followed by antibiotic treatment [13, 27]. Working within these limitations, it is important to try and totally resect the dermoid and tract at the first attempt, as dermoid remnants tend to grow, and postoperative adhesions may preclude total resection at reoperation [4, 5]. In thoracic and cervical dermal sinuses, the tract and inclusion lesions are resected in a similar fashion.

After completion of tract and dermoid removal, the subarachnoid space is irrigated to remove any debris that may cause further arachnoiditis. Dura, fascia, and superficial layers are sutured in a watertight manner. CSF leak prevention is dependent on the fascial closure.

Postoperative Care

Several days of bed rest may be useful to delay challenging the closure with the full height of the CSF column. Steroid treatment is controversial. Prophylactic antibiotics are given by most surgeons.

For simple isolated dermal sinuses, clinical follow up is usually sufficient, and no routine radiological studies are needed.

The most common complications of dermal sinus surgery are incomplete excision, CSF leaks, and postoperative infections; however, their rate is low. Neurological morbidity is low, especially in neurologically intact patients with no previous infectious event, operated prophylactically.

Outcome

Outcome is correlated to the clinical state at the time of surgery. For example, Ackerman and Menezes reported their 30 year experience treating spinal dermal sinuses [1, 7]. Among 11 patients who were preoperatively neurologically intact, no patient developed new neurological deficits following surgery. In addition, 75% of patients with preoperative neurological deficits improved postoperatively. In another series by Elton and Oakes, of 23 operated patients, none suffered from surgery related neurological insults [4]. Ramnarayan et al. [28] recently reported their experience treating delayed diagnosed spinal dermal sinuses. Among nine patients, only one was asymptomatic preoperatively, while the rest had an infectious event (meningitis or an abscess) or neurological deterioration. Five of the nine patients had a good outcome. Note that one of those five cases was operated prophylactically, while the patient was asymptomatic, thus a good outcome occurred in four out of eight symptomatic patients, representing 50% of symptomatic cases. Of the remaining four patients, three had a poor and one had a fair outcome. All nine patients were previously examined by a physician (an average of one year before surgery), and were either misdiagnosed or mistreated.

Summary

Dermal sinuses are a subtype of OSD, presenting as an incidental midline cutaneous dimple above the intergluteal cleft. Infections are the main complication and are associated with rapid and usually irreversible neurological deterioration. Other late complications are tethered cord syndrome and secondary neurological, urological, and orthopedic complications. MRI is the diagnostic tool of choice, demonstrating the dermal sinus tract and related inclusion lesions. Prophylactic resection of dermal sinus tracts and related inclusion lesions is the preferred treatment, and surgical exploration is indicated even in face of a non-diagnostic MRI. Neurological outcome is excellent, especially for prophylactic surgery in neurologically intact patients.

References

1. Ackerman LL, Menezes AH, Follett KA (2002) Cervical and thoracic dermal sinus tracts. A case series and review of the literature. Pediatr Neurosurg 3:137-147
2. Powell KR, Cherry JD, Hougen TJ et al (1975) A prospective search for congenital dermal abnormalities of the craniospinal axis. J Pediatr 5:744-750
3. McIntosh R, Merritt KK, Richards MR et al (1954) The incidence of congenital malformations: a study of 5964 pregnancies. Pediatrics 14:505-522
4. Elton S, Oakes WJ (2001) Dermal sinus tracts of the spine. Neurosurg Focus 1:e4
5. Kanev PM, Park TS (1995) Dermoids and dermal sinus tracts of the spine. Neurosurg Clin N Am 2:359-366
6. French BN (1983) The embryology of spinal dysraphism. Clin Neurosurg 295-340
7. Ackerman LL, Menezes AH (2003) Spinal congenital dermal sinuses: a 30-year experience. Pediatrics 3 Pt 1:641-647
8. Caldarelli M, Massimi L, Kondageski C et al (2004) Intracranial midline dermoid and epidermoid cysts in children. J Neurosurg Pediatrics 100(Suppl 5):473-480
9. Morimoto K, Takemoto O, Nishikawa M et al (2002) Nasal dermal sinus with a dermoid cyst. Pediatr Neurosurg 4:218-219
10. Pang D, Dias MS, Ahab-Barmada M (1992) Split cord malformation: Part I: A unified theory of embryogenesis for double spinal cord malformations. Neurosurgery 3:451-480
11. Swift DM, Carmel PW (1990) Congenital intradural pathology. Neurosurg Clin N Am 3:551-567
12. French BN (1990) Midline fusion defects and defects of formation. In: J Youmans (ed) Neurological surgery. Saunders Company, Philadelphia, pp 1081-1235
13. van Aalst J, Beuls EA, Cornips EM et al (2006) Anatomy and surgery of the infected dermal sinus of the lower spine. Childs Nerv Syst 10:1307-1315
14. Benzil DL, Epstein MH, Knuckey NW (1992) Intramedullary epidermoid associated with an intramedullary spinal abscess secondary to a dermal sinus. Neurosurgery 1:118-121
15. Barkovich AJ, Edwards M, Cogen PH (1991) MR evaluation of spinal dermal sinus tracts in children. AJNR Am J Neuroradiol 1:123-129
16. Guggisberg D, Hadj-Rabia S, Viney C et al (2004) Skin markers of occult spinal dysraphism in children: a review of 54 cases. Arch Dermatol 9:1109-1115
17. Tubbs RS, Frykman PK, Harmon CM et al (2007) An unusual sequelae of an infected persistent dermal sinus tract. Childs Nerv Syst 23:569-571
18. Weprin BE, Oakes WJ (2000) Coccygeal pits. Pediatrics 5:E69
19. Kriss VM, Desai NS (1998) Occult spinal dysraphism in neonates: assessment of high-risk cutaneous stigmata on sonography. AJR Am J Roentgenol 6:1687-1692
20. Cornette L, Verpoorten C, Lagae L et al (1998) Closed spinal dysraphism: a review on diagnosis and treatment in infancy. Eur J Paediatr Neurol 4:179-185
21. Unsinn KM, Geley T, Freund MC et al (2000) US of the spinal cord in newborns: spectrum of normal findings, variants, congenital anomalies, and acquired diseases. Radiographics 4:923-938
22. Medina LS, Crone K, Kuntz KM (2001) Newborns with suspected occult spinal dysraphism: a cost-effectiveness analysis of diagnostic strategies. Pediatrics 6:E101
23. Pacheco-Jacome E, Ballesteros MC, Jayakar P et al (2003) Occult spinal dysraphism: evidence-based diagnosis and treatment. Neuroimaging Clin N Am 2:327-334, xii

24. Kothbauer K, Schmid UD, Seiler RW et al (1994) Intraoperative motor and sensory monitoring of the cauda equina. Neurosurgery 4:702-707; discussion 707
25. Kothbauer KF, Novak K (2004) Intraoperative monitoring for tethered cord surgery: an update. Neurosurg
Focus 2:E8
26. von Koch CS, Quinones-Hinojosa A, Gulati M et al
(2002) Clinical outcome in children undergoing tethered cord release utilizing intraoperative neurophysiological monitoring. Pediatr Neurosurg 2:81-86

27. McComb JG (2005) Excision of a spinal congenital
dermal sinus/dermoid. In: Fessler RG, Sekhar LN (eds)
Atlas of neurosurgical techniques: Spine and peripheral nerves. Thieme, George Verlag, Stuttgart, Germany, pp 715-722
28. Ramnarayan R, Dominic A, Alapatt J et al (2006)
Congenital spinal dermal sinuses: poor awareness
leads to delayed treatment. Childs Nerv Syst 10:1220-
1224

Subject Index